JULIEN'S
PRIMER OF DRUG ACTION

JULIEN'S
PRIMER OF
DRUG ACTION

A Comprehensive Guide to the Actions, Uses, and Side Effects of Psychoactive Drugs

Thirteenth Edition

40th Anniversary Edition

Claire D. Advokat, Ph.D.
Louisiana State University

Joseph E. Comaty, Ph.D., M.P.
Baton Rouge, Louisiana

Robert M. Julien, M.D., Ph.D.
Portland, Oregon

WORTH PUBLISHERS

A Macmillan Higher Education Company

Publisher: Kevin Feyen
Associate Publisher: Jessica Bayne
Senior Acquisitions Editor: Christine Cardone
Marketing Manager: Lindsay Johnson
Interior Designer: Kevin Kall
Cover Designer: Kevin Kall
Director of Development for Print and Digital: Tracey Kuehn
Managing Editor: Lisa Kinne
Associate Media Editor: Anthony Casciano
Editorial Assistant: Catherine Michaelsen
Project Editor: Julio Espin
Illustrations Manager: Matt McAdams
Permissions Manager: Jennifer MacMillan
Production Manager: Barbara Seixas
Composition: TSI Graphics
Printing and Binding: RR Donnelley

Library of Congress Control Number: 2014931532

ISBN-13: 978-1-4641-1171-6
ISBN-10: 1-4641-1171-5

© 2014, 2011, 2008, 2005 by Worth Publishers

Printed in the United States of America

First printing

Worth Publishers
41 Madison Avenue
New York, NY 10010
www.worthpublishers.com

Claire Advokat received her Ph.D. in physiological psychology from Rutgers University, following which she completed an NIH Postdoctoral Fellowship at the College of Physicians and Surgeons of Columbia University in New York City. She then served on the faculty of the Department of Pharmacology at the University of Illinois Health Sciences Center in Chicago. In 1989 she joined the Department of Psychology at Louisiana State University, where she served as the Faculty Senate President (2004–2005), retiring in 2012 as an emerita professor. Her research area is psychopharmacology, specifically drugs used in the treatment of psychiatric and behavioral disorders. She has published over 80 articles, and received funding for her studies from the National Institute of Drug Abuse (NIDA), the Spencer Foundation, the Board of Regents of Louisiana, the State of Louisiana, and the pharmaceutical firm NPS. She received a university teaching award in 2005, served as an ad hoc reviewer for 20 journals, and serves on the editorial board of *The Journal of Attention Disorders*.

Joseph E. Comaty received his M.S. in experimental psychology from Villanova University; his Ph.D. in psychology with a specialization in clinical neuropsychology from the Rosalind Franklin University of Medicine and Science, in Illinois; and his postdoctoral Masters Degree in clinical psychopharmacology from Alliant University/CSPP in California. He is a licensed psychologist under the Louisiana State Board of Examiners of Psychologists (LSBEP) and a licensed medical psychologist under the Louisiana State Board of Medical Examiners. He retired from the Louisiana Department of Health and Hospitals, Office of Behavioral Health in 2013 where he was the Chief Psychologist and Medical Psychologist and Director of the Division of Quality Management. He is an adjunct assistant professor in psychology at Louisiana State University (LSU) in Baton Rouge and serves as emeritus faculty of the Southern Louisiana Internship Consortium (SLIC) in psychology at LSU. He has served as a member and chair of the LSBEP; he is a member and current chair of the RxP Designation Committee of APA, and a site reviewer for APA's Committee on Accreditation. He is a member of the Model Act and Regulation Revision Committee for the Association of State and Provincial Psychology Boards (ASPPB). His research is in the areas of behavior therapy, pharmacology, and clinical psychopharmacology. He is the author of over 50 articles, book chapters, and presentations. He has served on federal grant review committees and has been a reviewer for *Psychiatric Services; The Journal of Gerontology: Psychological Sciences*; and the *Journal of Behavioral Health Services and Research*.

Robert M. Julien, M.D., received his M.S. and Ph.D. in pharmacology from the University of Washington and his medical degree from the University of California at Irvine. His many research articles focus on the psychopharmacology of sedative and anti-epileptic drugs. Formerly an associate professor of pharmacology and anesthesiology at the Oregon Health Sciences University, Dr. Julien has retired from the practice of anesthesiology and is currently a psychopharmacology consultant in Portland, Oregon.

Contents

PREGNANCY AND PSYCHOTROPIC DRUGS

Antidepressants in the Pregnant Female and Neonatal Outcomes / Mood Stabilizers in the Pregnant Female and Neonatal Outcomes / Atypical Antipsychotics in the Pregnant Female and Neonatal Outcomes

PRESCHOOL PSYCHOPHARMACOLOGY

Medications for Treating Attention Deficit/Hyperactivity Disorder (ADHD) in Very Young Children / Medications for Treating Disruptive Behaviors in Very Young Children / Medications for Treating Depression in Very Young Children / Medications for Treating Bipolar Disorder in Very Young Children / Medications for Treating Anxiety Disorders in Very Young Children / Medications for Treating Autism Spectrum Disorders in Very Young Children

CHILD AND ADOLESCENT PSYCHOPHARMACOLOGY

Medications for Treating Autism Spectrum Disorders (ASD) / Medications for Treating Behavioral or Aggressive Disorders / Medications for Treating ADHD; Guidelines for Management of ADHD; Stimulant Treatment for ADHD; Methylphenidate; Amphetamines; Alternative Medications for Treating ADHD; Side Effects of Stimulant Medications / Medications and Medical Issues in Treating Depression Alternative Medications and Treatments; Antidepressants and Suicidal Ideation; Guidelines for Adolescent Depression for Primary Care (GLAD-PC); Calls for Widespread Screening for Youth at Risk / Medications for Treating Anxiety Disorders / Generalized Anxiety Disorder (GAD), Separation Anxiety Disorder (SAD), and Social Phobia (SoP); Obsessive-Compulsive Disorder; Posttraumatic Stress Disorder (PTSD); Panic Disorder / Medications for Treating Bipolar Disorder / Medications for Treating Psychotic Disorders

New in this Thirteenth Edition!

Did You Know? boxes highlight interesting and surprising facts or news related to the chapter content.

Preface

The thirteenth edition of *A Primer of Drug Action* marks nearly 40 years of continuous publication of this now classic textbook. Through these years, *A Primer of Drug Action* has documented the dramatic advances made in the psychopharmacological treatment of mental illness and substance abuse. The initial discoveries that certain chemical compounds could help people who suffer from psychosis, depression, anxiety, mania, and other neurological and psychological conditions, led to the development of medications that greatly improved our treatment of these devastating disorders. There has been a corresponding explosion in our knowledge of the neurological substrates, the receptors and enzymes that are affected by these drugs, and an appreciation that they can be most effective when integrated with appropriate behavioral therapy. Comparable advances have been made in understanding the neurobiological consequences of substance abuse and dependence, which have opened new avenues for pharmacological approaches to addiction.

Each of the prior twelve editions sought to present these developments in a clear, concise, and timely manner. We have strived to maintain this quality in the thirteenth edition, describing the general principles of each class of psychoactive drug, as well as providing specific information about the individual agents. Each chapter includes an overview of the current models of the disorders, background and mechanisms of action of the drugs, and rationales for drug treatment. Chapters on drugs of abuse provide historical context and epidemiological updates, discussions of the classic agents and thorough descriptions of the most recent drugs of concern, as well as the latest developments in regard to pharmacological treatments of these disorders. Addiction is not only a significant behavioral disorder but, in many cases, the same drugs may have addictive properties as well as therapeutic applications.

Features of the Thirteenth Edition

For nearly 40 years of uninterrupted publication, *A Primer of Drug Action* has been the classic psychopharmacology textbook, thanks to the dedication of its founding author, Robert Julien, M.D., Ph.D. For over three decades, Dr. Julien single-handedly accomplished the herculean tasks of revising each edition and maintaining a succinct yet comprehensive and clear review of the most up-to-date advances in psychopharmacology. The book was the premier text for anyone interested in learning about this expanding and important body of science. To acknowledge this accomplishment, we are pleased to announce that the title of this classic text has been modified. Starting from this, the thirteenth edition, the book will be titled, *Julien's Primer of Drug Action*. This change recognizes Dr. Julien's unique achievement in providing a text that has served for decades to make the immense amount of information accessible and timely to all those interested in understanding this important area of study. We are proud to have the privilege of collaborating with Bob in this endeavor, and to be chosen as coauthors of this classic text. We are committed to maintaining its stature as a prominent volume in the field of psychopharmacology.

Dr. Advokat is an emerita professor in the Department of Psychology at Louisiana State University in Baton Rouge. Dr. Comaty recently retired from his position as chief psychologist, HIPAA privacy officer, and director of the Division of Quality Management of the Louisiana State Office of Behavioral Health, Department of Health and Hospitals, in Baton Rouge, Louisiana. He currently serves as a consultant to that office, and also holds an adjunct faculty appointment in the Department of Psychology, Louisiana State University. Dr. Comaty is a clinical and medical psychologist, licensed to prescribe psychotherapeutic drugs in the state of Louisiana. Dr. Julien retired as staff anesthesiologist at St. Vincent Hospital and Medical Center in Portland, Oregon. He is an active consultant and lecturer on pharmacology and anesthesiology.

We three authors worked closely on the last two editions, and we are dedicated to maintaining the high standard in this newest volume, namely, concise description and analysis, clarity of writing, and inclusion of the most current information available. As in earlier editions, each chapter of the thirteenth edition has been revised to reflect the latest developments in the field. A broad overview of these changes since the last edition suggests the following prominent themes.

First, there has been continued expansion in the clinical applications of the major therapeutic drug classes. Distinctions among the accepted indications of major psychotropic drugs have become more diffuse. A parallel reconsideration of the diagnostic categories themselves is evident in the new version of the American Psychiatric Association's *Diagnostic and Statistical Manual*, the *DSM-5*, published in May 2013, and discussed in Chapter 17.

Second, there is a realization that newer medications may not represent better medications. Initial optimism for the most recent (and most expensive) drugs has been tempered by findings that they may not be more effective than the older agents, although they may present a different side effect profile. This understanding has revived interest in the classic agents and in comparisons of therapeutic effectiveness not only among psychiatric medications but also between pharmacological and nonpharmacological treatments.

These developments signal a period of maturation and reassessment in the field of psychopharmacology. Recent challenges (discussed in Chapter 17), have questioned whether the pharmacological revolution in psychiatry has made progress against these disorders. Arguments have been proposed that psychiatric medications have not been successful in mitigating mental illness, and may, in some circumstances, even exacerbate the problems. One practical effect of this pessimistic view is a decrease in current pharmaceutical investment into research and development of new psychotropic medications. Perhaps it is to be expected that the rapid discovery of the first psychiatric drugs would be followed by a more measured analysis of the progress and an appreciation of how much is yet to be accomplished.

Although drug development may be undergoing a hiatus, there has been continuing interest in understanding the genetic basis of the disorders, drug effects, and interactions. This has increased scientific research into the genome and how it is altered by chemical and other environmental stimulation. Increased knowledge of how the environment interacts with our genetic substrate is having a profound effect on all aspects of medicine, and, in our context, especially on theories of addiction and how genetic susceptibility is involved in the etiology of substance abuse. In this edition, we added a new section on epigenetics that includes epigenetic influences in addiction (Chapter 4).

At the same time, there has been a dramatic increase in the variety and extent of drug abuse since the last edition of the *Primer*. Reports of new compounds, often synthetic agents, have appeared worldwide in almost every category of addictive substances, including stimulants (Chapter 7), hallucinogens (Chapter 8), cannabis (Chapter 9), and opiates (Chapter 10), producing novel adverse and sometimes dangerous reactions. For example, in this edition, we explore new research that suggests a link between early-onset cannabis use and psychosis and examine the risks associated with herbal marijuana alternatives (HMAs) (Chapter 9). Meanwhile, the increase in opiate prescription abuse has continued, resulting in an extraordinary effort to develop products that are resistant to misuse and diversion. We discuss the Food and Drug Administration's 2013 *Guidance for Industry: Abuse-Deterrent Opioids—Evaluation and Labeling,* which lists several possible categories of abuse-deterrent formulations (Chapter 10).

As always, we are optimistic that scientific investigation will result in new insights into the etiology of mental illness and addiction and that the future will bring more effective treatments for these devastating disorders. Future editions of this text will parallel the progress.

Finally, we appreciate that keeping current with medical literature is a daunting task and it is unrealistic to expect practitioners to read and analyze the field critically. Therefore, prescribers rely on sources of information that can be presented in compact formats or review articles that provide an informed, comprehensive summary of the important topics. It may be difficult for anyone to know fully whether to trust any article as unbiased. Unfortunately, there is reason to be concerned about this issue.

But, there are some routine things one can do. Look at the disclaimer statement at the bottom of the article; do the authors have any connection to the pharmaceutical company whose products are being tested in the article? Have they received financial support from the company? Are they part of the company's speaker's bureau? When following a particular drug across multiple studies, does the drug perform the same or are the results variable?

In general, drugs that are new to the market have only been examined in small-scale clinical trials using well-defined patient groups treated for short periods of time. Results from these studies may not reflect the broader population of patients to which the drug is going to be prescribed. And, the studies may be too short in duration to allow for the emergence of side effects that will occur under usual clinical prescribing practices when the drug comes to market. Therefore, approaching the use of newly approved drugs with caution is a good idea until there is aftermarket experience with the drug.

Seek out unbiased sources of information. Such resources include publications such as the *Carlat Psychiatry Report,* which does not accept any ads or drug company money;

studies funded by government agencies such as the National Institute of Mental Health (NIMH); reviews of information by the Agency for Healthcare Research and Quality (AHCRQ); and the Cochran Library reviews.

None of the authors of this book have financial ties with the pharmaceutical industry, and we strive to ensure that the information we provide is as objective and unbiased as possible.

Media and Supplements

A free companion Web site for *Julien's Primer of Drug Action,* Thirteenth Edition, is located at www.worthpublishers.com/Julien13e. This free Web site contains resources for both instructors and students and does not require any special access codes or passwords.

Also available is the *Computerized Test Bank* by Mark Hurd, College of Charleston. The *Test Bank* contains approximately 850 items in multiple-choice and true/false formats, as well as separate multiple-choice Web Quiz questions to be made available on the student's book companion site. Each question is keyed to the page in the book on which the answer is located as well as to the Blooms Taxonomy of Learning Levels and the APA Guidelines for the Undergraduate Psychology Major. If you are an instructor and would like to order the *Test Bank,* contact your Worth Publishers sales representative.

Acknowledgments

We thank the following reviewers for their contribution to this edition:

Nicoladie Tam, University of North Texas
Paul J. Wellman, Texas A&M University
Mark W. Hurd, College of Charleston
Vincent Markowski, State University of New York, Geneseo
Trey Asbury, Texas Woman's University
Joshua M. Gulley, University of Illinois, Urbana-Champaign
Rebecca L. Gazda, Newberry College

Claire Advokat, Ph.D.
Baton Rouge, Louisiana
cadvoka@lsu.edu

Joseph Comaty, Ph.D., M.P.
Baton Rouge, Louisiana
drscomatyadvokat@gmail.com

Robert M. Julien, M.D., Ph.D.
Lake Oswego, Oregon
drsjulien@comcast.net

PART 1

Introduction to Psychopharmacology: Biological Basis of Drug Action

Pharmacology is the science of how drugs affect the body. *Psychopharmacology*, a subdivision of pharmacology, is the study of how drugs specifically affect the brain and behavior. To understand the actions, behavioral uses, therapeutic uses, and abuse potentials of psychoactive drugs, we need to know how the body responds when we take them. This understanding involves some knowledge of brain anatomy, the basic principles of drug absorption, distribution, metabolism, and excretion (collectively termed *pharmacokinetics*) as well as the interactions of a drug with its "receptor," or the structure with which the drug interacts to produce its effects (the area of study termed *pharmacodynamics*).

This book specifically concerns drugs that affect the brain and behavior. It is an introduction to psychopharmacology, presenting not only drugs useful in treating psychological disorders but also drugs prone to compulsive use and abuse. The book begins with three chapters devoted to the fundamentals of drug action. For readers without a background in neuroscience, Chapter 1 introduces the structure and function of the nervous system and the neuron, because this is where psychoactive drugs produce their effects. We focus on the connection between two different neurons, the *synapse*, and the chemical substances through which neurons communicate, the *neurotransmitters*. By studying the process of synaptic transmission we begin to understand the mode of action of psychoactive drugs. Furthermore, the phenomenon of synaptic transmission is not static; rather, neurons have the ability to remodel themselves continually, a process called *synaptic plasticity*, which mediates learning and memory as well as such disorders as anxiety, depression, and addiction. A healthy, functioning brain is one that through this process of synaptic plasticity is continually remodeling itself in response to the environment. Healthy neurons continually form new synaptic contacts, maintaining the beautiful architecture that exists through normal interactions with millions of other neurons.

Chapter 2 explores the area of *pharmacokinetics*, the movement of drug molecules into, through, and out of the body. It addresses such questions as: What are the ways by which drugs get into the body, and how does that relate to their actions? Once in the body, how do drugs get to the sites at which they produce their effects? Once a drug exerts its effect, how is that action terminated? Finally, how does the body eventually get rid of the drug?

Chapter 3 explores the area of *pharmacodynamics*. It examines the interaction between drugs and the receptors to which the drugs attach, and through which they produce their effects. Receptors are described both structurally and functionally, and how drugs alter receptor structure and function is discussed. Finally, we summarize the ways in which such actions underlie the therapeutic effects and the side effects of drugs. These three chapters provide the basic foundation for understanding more specific information in subsequent chapters.

Chapter 1

The Neuron, Synaptic Transmission, and Neurotransmitters

All our thoughts, actions, memories, and behaviors result from biochemical interactions that take place in and between *neurons*. Drugs that affect these processes are called *psychoactive drugs*. In essence, psychoactive drugs are chemicals that alter (mimic, potentiate, disrupt, or inhibit) the normal processes associated with neuronal function or communication between neurons. Therefore, to understand the actions of psychoactive drugs, it is necessary to have some idea of how the brain is organized, what a neuron is, and how neurons interact with each other.

Overall Organization of the Brain

The human nervous system consists of two divisions, the central nervous system (CNS) and the peripheral nervous system (PNS). The CNS includes the brain and the spinal cord; the PNS includes the nerves that originate in the spinal cord and that connect the spinal cord to the organs of the body. The drugs discussed in this book exert their primary actions and some of their side effects by acting in the brain. However, many of their side effects are produced by their actions in the PNS, that is, at various organ systems, such as the digestive system and the cardiovascular system, as described in subsequent chapters.

The human brain consists of perhaps 90 billion individual neurons located in the skull and the spinal cord. Figure 1.1A shows the organization of the brain, with the major divisions indicated. There are three primary divisions: the *hindbrain*, the *midbrain*, and the *forebrain*. The hindbrain and the forebrain are further divided, each into two subdivisions, which results in five major sections. Figure 1.1B shows the anatomical arrangement of these structures.

The *spinal cord* is essentially the "information highway of the body," through which messages are sent back and forth between the brain and the rest of the body. This information includes touch, temperature, pain, joint position, and signals telling muscles to move.

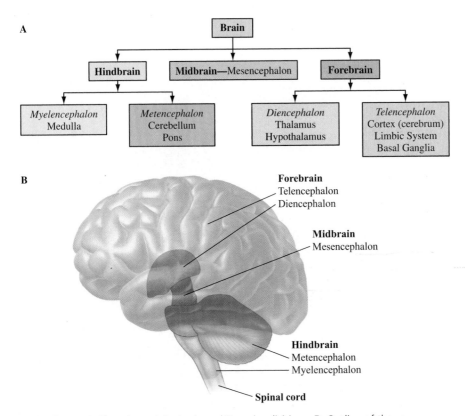

FIGURE 1.1   **A.** Flowchart of the brain and its major divisions. **B.** Outline of the human brain and its primary divisions.

Extending from the bottom of the brain (the medulla), to the sacrum (the bone in the lower part of the spine that forms the back of the pelvis), the spinal cord is made up of neurons and fiber tracts which:

* Carry sensory information from the skin, muscles, joints, and internal body organs to the brain
* Modulate sensory input (including pain impulses)
* Organize and modulate the motor outflow to the muscles (to produce coordinated movement)
* Provide autonomic (involuntary) control of vital body functions

The part of the brain that is attached to the top of the spinal cord is the *brain stem* (Figure 1.2). It is divided into three parts: the *medulla* (its full name is the *medulla oblongata*), the *pons,* and the *midbrain.* All impulses that are conducted in either direction between the spinal cord and the brain pass through the brain stem, which is also important in the regulation of vital body functions, such as respiration, blood pressure, heart rate, gastrointestinal functioning, and the states of sleep and wakefulness. The brain stem is also involved in behavioral alerting, attention, and arousal responses. Depressant

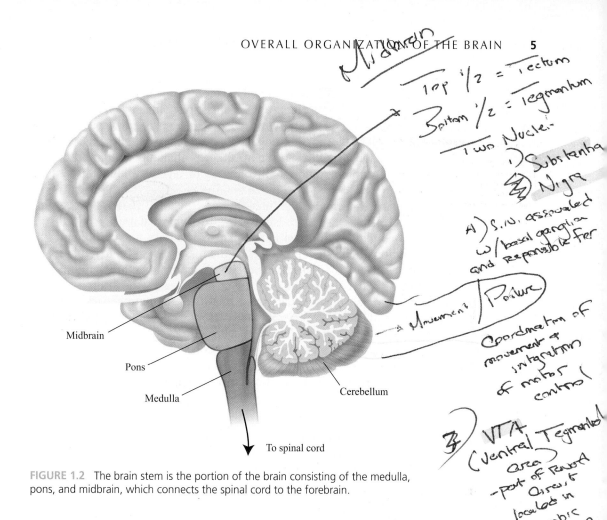

Handwritten annotations:

Midbrain

Top $\frac{1}{2}$ = Tectum

Bottom $\frac{1}{2}$ = Tegmentum

Two Nuclei:
1) Substantia
2) Nigra

A) S.N. associated w/ basal ganglia and responsible for → Movement / Posture

Coordination of movement & integration of motor control

3) VTA (Ventral Tegmental Area) - Part of Reward Circuit, located in limbic system

Both Nuclei Contain Dopamine

FIGURE 1.2   The brain stem is the portion of the brain consisting of the medulla, pons, and midbrain, which connects the spinal cord to the forebrain.

Figure labels: Midbrain, Pons, Medulla, Cerebellum, To spinal cord

drugs, such as the barbiturates (see Chapter 5), depress the brain-stem activating system, which probably underlies much of their hypnotic action.

Behind the brain stem is a large, bulbous structure—the *cerebellum*. A highly convoluted structure, the cerebellum is connected to the brain stem by large nerve tracts. The cerebellum is necessary for the proper integration of movement and posture. The staggering gait that is associated with drunkenness, termed ataxia (loss of coordination and balance), is caused largely by an alcohol-induced depression of cerebellar function.

An important part of the brain stem, even though it is only about 2 centimeters long, is the midbrain, which sits between the forebrain and the hindbrain. The upper half (*tectum*, or "roof") contains pathways that carry sensory information, while the bottom half (*tegmentum*, or "floor") contains two important nuclei, which are connected, respectively, to two other systems, whose primary structures are located in the forebrain. The first of these nuclei, the *substantia nigra*, is associated with the neuroanatomical system called the basal ganglia (discussed below, see Figure 1.4), which is responsible for coordination of movement and integration of motor control. Next to the substantia nigra is a more diffuse group of neurons called the *ventral tegmental area* (*VTA*), which is part of the neuroanatomical system called the *reward circuit*, located in the limbic system (discussed below; see Figure 1.5). As shown in Figure 1.13, on page 21, most of the neurons that make up these two nuclei contain the neurotransmitter dopamine.

The area immediately above the brain stem and covered by the cerebral hemispheres (cerebrum or cortex) is the *diencephalon* (Figure 1.3) consisting primarily of the thalamus and hypothalamus. The *hypothalamus* is a collection of neuronal structures near the junction of the midbrain and the thalamus just above the pituitary gland (whose function it modulates). There are 11 major nuclei that make up the hypothalamus and are responsible for the integration of our entire autonomic (involuntary or vegetative) nervous system. Thus, the hypothalamus controls such vegetative functions as eating and drinking, sleeping, regulation of body temperature, and sexual behavior, in large part by controlling the hormonal output of the pituitary gland. Neurons in the hypothalamus produce substances called *releasing factors,* which travel to the nearby pituitary gland, inducing the secretion of hormones that regulate such processes as the menstrual cycle in females and sperm formation in males. The hypothalamus is a site of action for many psychoactive drugs, either for the primary effect or for the side effects produced by the drug.

The thalamus, located above the hypothalamus, consists of two symmetrical lobes on either side of the midbrain. It is often viewed as a way station, or relay, between multiple subcortical areas and the cerebral cortex. That is because every sensory system (except the olfactory system) passes through a thalamic nucleus, consisting of a group of neurons that receives sensory signals from specific organs (such as the eyes and ears) which sends the information to the appropriate primary cortical area for processing.

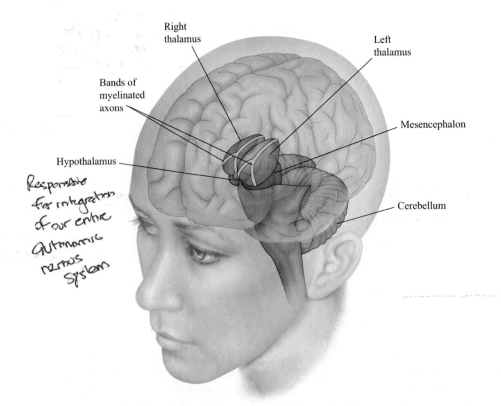

Responsible for integration of our entire autonomic nervous system

FIGURE 1.3   The diencephalon. [After Pinel (2007), p. 53, Figure 2.23.]

The last major division of the brain, the telencephalon, includes two important subdivisions, the *basal ganglia* and the *limbic system*. The major structures of the basal ganglia (Figure 1.4A and B) are the caudate nucleus and putamen (together, often referred to as the striatum) and the globus pallidus, which consists of two parts, the lateral (or external) and the medial (or internal) (see Figure 1.4B). Sometimes all three structures are referred to as the corpus striatum, because of their striated (striped) appearance when the tissue is stained so that it can be studied microscopically. In addition to these primary nuclei the basal ganglia are associated with two additional structures, the subthalamic nucleus and the substantia nigra (see Figure 1.4B; located in the midbrain as noted above).

One major function of the basal ganglia is the integration of movement. Depending on which part of the system is impaired, disorders of the basal ganglia can cause the gradual loss of the ability to initiate movement, such as in Parkinson's disease, or, conversely, an inability to prevent parts of the body from moving unintentionally, as in Huntington's disease.

The second major subdivision of the telencephalon is the *limbic system* (Figure 1.5), the major components of which are the *amygdala* and the *hippocampus*. These structures are involved in memory (hippocampus) and emotion (amygdala). Because the limbic system and the hypothalamus interact to regulate emotion and emotional expression, these structures are the site of action for many psychoactive drugs that alter mood, affect, emotion, or responses to emotional experiences. As discussed in subsequent chapters, this includes drugs used in the treatment of schizophrenia, depression, and Alzheimer's disease. Many side effects of therapeutic drugs also result from actions on the structures in this system. In addition, the limbic system includes the brain structures that make up the *reward circuit* (discussed in Chapter 4). This circuit is believed to be responsible for the feelings of pleasure that we experience in response to activities that we enjoy, such as eating and drinking. Because such activity includes the recreational use of abused drugs, the reward circuit is considered to be the substrate for drug addiction as well as for the more typical sources of pleasurable stimulation.

Almost completely covering the brain stem and the diencephalon is the *cerebrum* (Figure 1.6). In humans the cerebrum is the largest part of the brain. It is separated into two distinct hemispheres, left and right, with numerous fiber tracts connecting the two.

Because skull size is limited and the cerebrum is so large, the outer layer of the cerebrum, the *cerebral cortex*, is deeply convoluted and fissured. Like other parts of the brain, the cerebral cortex is subdivided; it consists of four major lobes, each of which having areas that are responsible for specific functions, such as vision (occipital lobe), hearing (temporal lobe), sensory perception (parietal lobe), and higher-level cognitive functions (frontal lobe).

Did You Know?

Obama's BRAIN Initiative

In April 2013 President Obama announced the BRAIN Initiative to map activity and connections within the brain. Obama's 2014 budget proposal will include $100 million to jumpstart this "big science" initiative, which builds on researchers' interest in understanding the neural circuits that are activated when we perceive, think, and act. The acronym BRAIN stands for Brain Research through Advancing Innovative Neurotechnologies. In his announcement, Obama compared the neuroscience initiative to the Human Genome Project that finished sequencing the entire human genome over a decade ago.

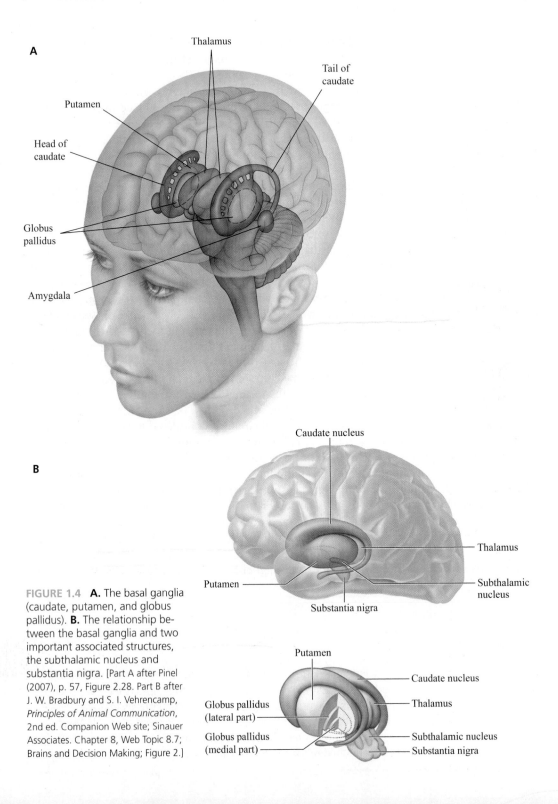

FIGURE 1.4 **A.** The basal ganglia (caudate, putamen, and globus pallidus). **B.** The relationship between the basal ganglia and two important associated structures, the subthalamic nucleus and substantia nigra. [Part A after Pinel (2007), p. 57, Figure 2.28. Part B after J. W. Bradbury and S. I. Vehrencamp, *Principles of Animal Communication*, 2nd ed. Companion Web site; Sinauer Associates. Chapter 8, Web Topic 8.7; Brains and Decision Making; Figure 2.]

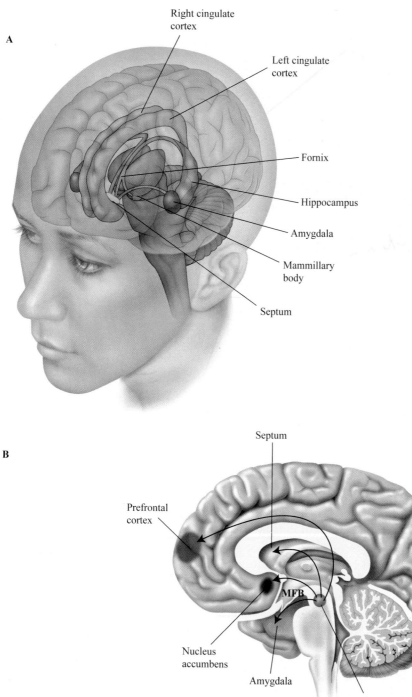

FIGURE 1.5 The limbic system. [After Pinel (2007), p. 57, Figure 2.27.]

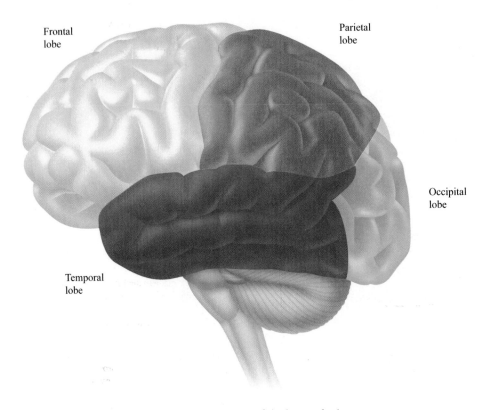

Frontal lobe

Parietal lobe

Occipital lobe

Temporal lobe

FIGURE 1.6 The cerebrum. The four major lobes of the human brain.

Overview of Synaptic Transmission

The central nervous system (CNS) is made up of two types of cells, neurons and a variety of nonneural cells, collectively called *glia*. It had long been thought that glia are more abundant than neurons, and that there were from 10 to 50 times more glia than neurons in the CNS. However, there is recent evidence that the 10:1 glia to neuron ratio is a myth and that the ratio in human and other primate brains is much closer to 1:1. It turns out to be more difficult to determine the ratio of glia to neurons than you might think. For example, some parts of the human brain have a higher ratio than others, and the ratio of other species differs from that of humans. An interesting discussion of this topic can be found at: http://blogs.scientificamerican.com/brainwaves/2012/06/13/know-your-neurons-what-is-the-ratio-of-glia-to-neurons-in-the-brain/.

The neuron is the basic functional unit, while glia primarily provide support and protection. A typical neuron has a *soma* (cell body), which contains the nucleus (within which is the genetic material of the cell) and several other structures or *organelles* that perform vital functions (Figure 1.7A). For example, mitochondria produce energy from nutrients, while Golgi bodies package substances (such as neurotransmitters) into vesicles for storage.

Extending from the soma in one direction are many short fibers, called *dendrites*, which receive input from other neurons through *receptors* located on the dendritic

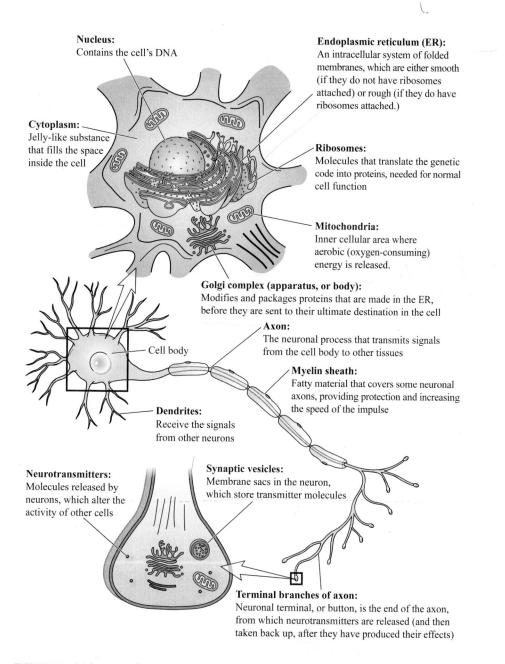

Nucleus:
Contains the cell's DNA

Endoplasmic reticulum (ER):
An intracellular system of folded membranes, which are either smooth (if they do not have ribosomes attached) or rough (if they do have ribosomes attached.)

Cytoplasm:
Jelly-like substance that fills the space inside the cell

Ribosomes:
Molecules that translate the genetic code into proteins, needed for normal cell function

Mitochondria:
Inner cellular area where aerobic (oxygen-consuming) energy is released.

Golgi complex (apparatus, or body):
Modifies and packages proteins that are made in the ER, before they are sent to their ultimate destination in the cell

Axon:
The neuronal process that transmits signals from the cell body to other tissues

Cell body

Myelin sheath:
Fatty material that covers some neuronal axons, providing protection and increasing the speed of the impulse

Dendrites:
Receive the signals from other neurons

Neurotransmitters:
Molecules released by neurons, which alter the activity of other cells

Synaptic vesicles:
Membrane sacs in the neuron, which store transmitter molecules

Terminal branches of axon:
Neuronal terminal, or button, is the end of the axon, from which neurotransmitters are released (and then taken back up, after they have produced their effects)

FIGURE 1.7 Major parts of a neuron. **A.** Internal structures. The genetic material (DNA) is contained in the nucleus, and several specialized organelles are present in the cytoplasm, the material of the cell outside the nucleus. Definitions are included within the figure. The cell is enclosed by a thin wall, or membrane. Mitochondria are present in the cell body, the fibers, and the terminals. The terminals also contain small, round vesicles that contain neurotransmitter chemicals. Synaptic connections from the fibers of other neurons cover the cell body and dendrites. **B.** External structures. [Part A: after Pinel (2007), p. 42, Figure 2.6.] [http://www.brainmaintenanceacademy.com/wpcontent/uploads/2012/06/neuronlarge.png]

membrane (see Figure 1.7B). When a signal arrives from another cell, a message is generated and travels down the dendrite to the soma. Extending in another direction from the soma is a single process called an *axon,* which can vary in length from a few millimeters up to a meter (such as those that run from the motor neurons of the spinal cord out to the muscles that they stimulate). The axon transmits the signal through an electrochemical process (the *action potential)* from the soma to other neurons or to muscles, organs, or glands of the body. Longer axons are usually covered with a *myelin sheath,* produced by specialized types of glia, which increases the speed of the signal.

Information flows from the axon to the next neuron or cell by way of a specialized structure called *a synapse.* A given neuron in the brain may receive thousands of synaptic connections from other neurons. The number of possible different combinations of synaptic connections among the neurons in a single human brain is larger than the total number of atomic particles that make up the known universe. Hence the diversity of the interconnections in a human brain seems almost without limit.

Did You Know?

Growing New Neurons

It may not be as hard as once believed to make new neurons in the brain. Using just two proteins and without any cell divisions, scientists have succeeded in reprogramming brain cells known as pericytes into neurons in both cultured cells from humans and mice. Pericytes help to control the flow of blood in the brain, and they build and maintain the blood-brain barrier. The discovery could have implications for patients with degenerative brain disorders, such as Parkinson's.

It was once thought that the brain has the maximal number of neurons at birth and that once a neuron dies, it is not replaced. This concept has been revised because we now realize that new neurons form every day (a process called *neurogenesis*) (Kempermann et al., 2004; Schaffer and Gage, 2004; Ashraf and Kunes, 2006). Synaptic contacts between neurons are continually being reshaped, with axon terminals and dendrites re-forming new synaptic connections while eliminating old ones. This remodeling probably begins even before birth and continues throughout our lives. The relationship between neuronal "health" and various psychological disorders, such as depression, bipolar disorder, and drug addiction, is discussed in subsequent chapters.

A synapse consists of the presynaptic membrane (typically the axon terminal) of one neuron, the postsynaptic membrane of the receiving neuron (which might be a dendrite, the soma, or the axon terminal of another neuron), and a minute space (the *synaptic cleft*) between them (Figure 1.8). Among the numerous structural elements of the presynaptic side (for our purposes) are the synaptic vesicles, each of which contains several thousand molecules of neurotransmitter chemical that transmits information from one neuron to another. These vesicles serve two functions. They store the transmitter, and protect it from being destroyed by metabolic enzymes, so that it is available for release. When the action potential reaches the axon terminal it triggers a series of biochemical actions, which cause the vesicles to fuse with the presynaptic membrane and release the transmitter, a process

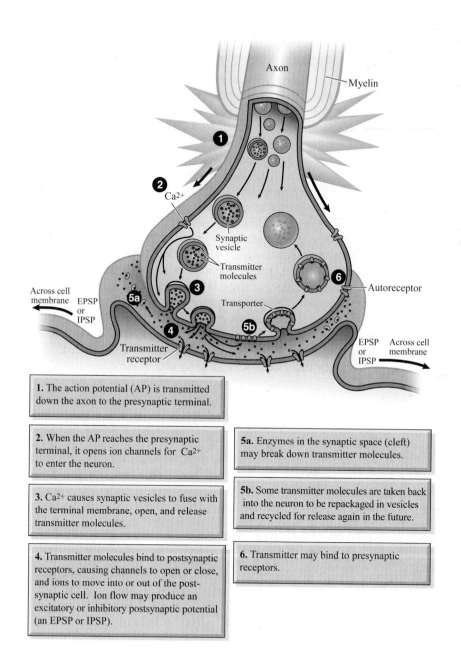

Axon

Myelin

1

2 Ca^{2+}

Synaptic
vesicle

Transmitter
molecules

3

6

Autoreceptor

Across cell
membrane   EPSP
                      or
                      IPSP

5a

Transporter

5b

4

EPSP   Across cell
or   membrane
IPSP

Transmitter
receptor

1. The action potential (AP) is transmitted
down the axon to the presynaptic terminal.

2. When the AP reaches the presynaptic
terminal, it opens ion channels for Ca^{2+}
to enter the neuron.

5a. Enzymes in the synaptic space (cleft)
may break down transmitter molecules.

3. Ca^{2+} causes synaptic vesicles to fuse with
the terminal membrane, open, and release
transmitter molecules.

5b. Some transmitter molecules are taken back
into the neuron to be repackaged in vesicles
and recycled for release again in the future.

4. Transmitter molecules bind to postsynaptic
receptors, causing channels to open or close,
and ions to move into or out of the postsynaptic cell. Ion flow may produce an
excitatory or inhibitory postsynaptic potential
(an EPSP or IPSP).

6. Transmitter may bind to presynaptic
receptors.

FIGURE 1.8 Structure and function of a generic synapse. Neurotransmitter is produced (synthesized) and stored in vesicles within the axon terminal. When an action potential reaches the terminal, it causes channels to open so that calcium can enter and initiate *exocytosis* (release of transmitter molecules) into the synaptic cleft. After release, neurotransmitter molecules bind to and activate receptors on the pre- and postsynaptic membrane. Transmitter effects are terminated either by breakdown of transmitter within the synaptic cleft, or by reuptake back into the axon terminal to be recycled. [Modified after Breedlove et al. (2010), p. 74, Figure 3.12.]

called *exocytosis*. The transmitter molecules diffuse across the synaptic cleft and attach to various types of structures, called receptors, on both the presynaptic terminal and the postsynaptic membrane of the next neuron (see Chapter 3). The neurons do not physically touch each other; synaptic transmission is a chemical rather than an electrical process.

Synaptic transmission is remarkably fast; the entire process may occur over a time span as short as a millisecond for transmitter release (from presynaptic vesicles), diffusion (across the cleft), receptor attachment, and activation. The nature of the response produced by synaptic transmission depends on the characteristics of the receptor that is activated (see Chapter 3). Receptors may respond quickly, within milliseconds, or they may produce responses that last hundreds of milliseconds. The ultimate outcome of receptor activation is a function of the organ or tissue in which it is located. In summary, the arrival of an action potential at the axon terminal induces release of a neurotransmitter into the synaptic cleft, and the transmitter then activates its receptors.

The release of neurotransmitter may be modulated by presynaptic receptors, termed *autoreceptors* (see Figure 1.8). An autoreceptor is a presynaptic site on a neuron that binds the neurotransmitter *released by that neuron*. These receptors regulate the neuron's activity. Autoreceptors serve as negative feedback mechanisms. When stimulated by transmitter or by certain drugs, these receptors *reduce* the synthesis and further release of transmitter. Thus, when large amounts of transmitter are present in the synaptic cleft, excess transmitter acts on the autoreceptors to decrease further production and release. Conversely, if an antagonist blocks an autoreceptor, synthesis and release of transmitter is increased.

Once release has occurred there must be a way to get rid of neurotransmitter; otherwise transmitter would stay in the synaptic cleft and continually bind to and activate receptors. In most cases, transmitter removal occurs through two general types of mechanisms (see Figure 1.8; with some variations as described below for specific transmitters):

1. An enzyme present in the synaptic cleft breaks down any neurotransmitter remaining in the synapse. The metabolites are then taken back up into the presynaptic neuron to be resynthesized and repackaged for release. This is how the effect of the neurotransmitter acetylcholine is terminated. Drugs used in the treatment of Alzheimer's disease act by blocking this process, thereby increasing the amount of acetylcholine in the synapse, which may delay the progression of the dementia (see Chapter 16).

2. The transmitter itself is taken back into the presynaptic neuron and repackaged. The action of the neurotransmitters dopamine, norepinephrine, and serotonin is terminated by this mechanism. Drugs that block this reuptake process represent one class of antidepressant medication. In an alternative version of this process, transmitter is taken up into an adjacent glial cell and metabolized. The metabolites are then recycled back to the neuron where they are resynthesized into neurotransmitter and repackaged for release. The effect of the transmitter glutamate is terminated by this method (Cooper et al., 2003).

Specific Neurotransmitters

Neurons release specific chemical substances from their presynaptic nerve terminals, and it is the interaction between psychoactive drugs and the receptors on which the natural transmitters act that underlies the actions of the drugs. Table 1.1 lists a few of the

TABLE 1.1 Classification of the major neurotransmitter families
with selected neurotransmitters

	Specific neurotransmitters
Family and subfamily	Transmitters
AMINES	
Quaternary amines	Acetylcholine (ACh)
Monoamines	*Catecholamines:* Norepinephrine (NE), epinephrine (adrenaline), dopamine (DA)
	Indoleamines: Serotonin (5-hydroxytryptamine: 5-HT)
AMINO ACIDS	Gamma-aminobutyric acid (GABA), glutamate, glycine
NEUROPEPTIDES	
Opioid peptides	*Enkephalins:* Met-enkephalin, leu-enkephalin
	Endorphins: β-endorphin
	Dynorphins: Dynorphin A
PEPTIDES	Oxytocin, substance P, cholecystokinin (CCK),vasopressin, hypothalamic-releasing hormones
GASES	Nitric oxide, carbon monoxide

From Breedlove et al. (2007), Table 4.1, p. 90.

commonly recognized neurotransmitter families with some of the specific transmitters within each category. The earliest chemicals identified as CNS neurotransmitters were acetylcholine and norepinephrine, largely because of their established roles in the peripheral nervous system. In the 1960s, serotonin, epinephrine, and dopamine were recognized. In the 1970s, gamma aminobutyric acid (GABA), glycine, glutamate, and certain neuropeptides (such as the endorphins) were identified. In the late 1980s, the lipid amide anandamide was identified as the endogenous transmitter for the tetrahydrocannabinol (THC) receptor. For a personal account of this history, see Snyder (2002).

Acetylcholine

Acetylcholine (ACh) was identified as a transmitter chemical first in the peripheral nervous system and later in brain tissue. Deficiencies in acetylcholine-secreting neurons have classically been associated with the dysfunctions seen in Alzheimer's disease. Certainly drugs that either potentiate or inhibit the central action of acetylcholine exert profound effects on memory. For example, scopolamine is a psychedelic drug that blocks central cholinergic receptors and as a result produces amnesia. Conversely, drugs that increase the amount of acetylcholine in the brain appear to improve memory function and are used to delay the progression of Alzheimer's disease.

ACh is synthesized in a one-step reaction from two precursors (choline and acetyl CoA) and then stored within synaptic vesicles for later release (Figure 1.9). Like other neurotransmitters, ACh is released into the synaptic cleft, rapidly diffuses across the cleft, and reversibly binds to postsynaptic receptors. Once ACh has exerted its effect on postsynaptic receptors, its action is terminated by the enzyme *acetylcholinesterase* (AChE), which is located in the postsynaptic side of the synaptic cleft.

The enzymatic reaction that degrades ACh is important not only in the treatment of Alzheimer's disease but also in agriculture and in the military. Drugs that block the action of AChE, referred to as *AChE inhibitors,* include both "reversible" and "irreversible" AChE inhibitors. *Irreversible AChE inhibitors* form a permanent covalent bond with the enzyme and totally inhibit enzyme function. They are usually administered in "toxic" doses, and the result is usually fatal. Some of these toxic drugs (such as *malathion* and *parathion*) have been exploited in gardening and agriculture as insecticides because they kill insects on contact. Other irreversible AChE inhibitors (such as *Sarin* and *Soman*) have been used in the military as lethal nerve gases.

Less toxic and shorter acting are the *reversible AChE inhibitors*. They are used clinically as putative cognitive enhancers, to try to delay memory decline in patients with Alzheimer's disease. Individual agents are discussed in Chapter 16.

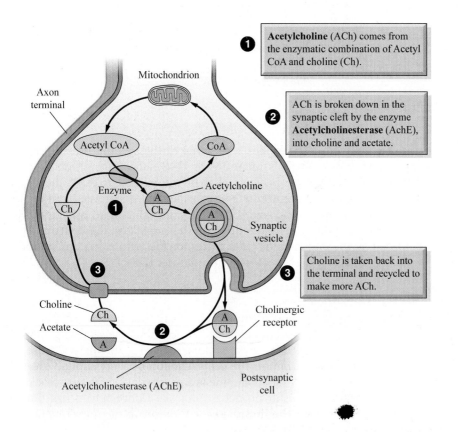

FIGURE 1.9 Schematic of an acetylcholine (ACh) synapse. ACh is made in the axon terminal from acetyl coenzyme A (acetyl CoA) and choline and stored in vesicles for release. After release ACh binds to its receptors and is immediately broken down at the receptors by acetylcholinesterase (AChE) into choline and acetate. [http://faculty. pasadena.edu/dkwon/chap%208_files/images/image61.png]

Cholinergic receptors are subclassified into two categories, nicotinic and muscarinic, named for substances that specifically stimulate each category. Muscarinic receptors are the "slow" type (metabotropic), while nicotinic receptors are the "fast" type (or ionotropic; see Chapter 3). They can be found on both sides of the synaptic cleft (presynaptic and postsynaptic). Muscarinic receptors bind acetylcholine and muscarine, a substance found in certain poisonous mushrooms (it was first isolated in *Amanita muscaria*). Binding studies have identified five subclasses of muscarinic receptors: M_1, M_2, M_3, M_4, and M_5. M_1, M_4, and M_5 are involved in complex CNS responses such as memory, arousal, attention, and analgesia. M_2 are on heart muscle and, when stimulated they slow the heart rate; M_3 are found on a variety of involuntary muscles, such as the bladder and lungs. Nicotinic receptors (nAChR) are subdivided into two types, N_1 (or N_M), found on the voluntary, or skeletal, muscles and N_2 (or N_N), found in the nervous system and in the adrenal glands.

ACh is distributed widely in the brain (Figure 1.10). The cell bodies of cholinergic neurons in the brain lie in two closely related regions. One involves the *septal nuclei* and

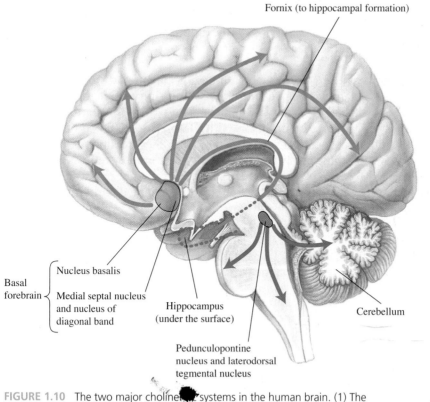

FIGURE 1.10 The two major cholinergic systems in the human brain. (1) The forebrain cholinergic complex composed of neurons in the medial septal nucleus and nucleus basalis which projects to the telencephalon; (2) the pontomesencephalotegmental cholinergic complex, composed of cells in the pedunculopontine and laterodorsal tegmental nuclei which ascend to the thalamus and other diencephalic loci (not shown) and descend to the pons, medulla, cerebellum, and cranial nerve nuclei. [Modified after Breedlove et al. (2007), p. 92, Figure 4.2.]

the *nucleus basalis*. The axons of these neurons project to forebrain regions, particularly the hippocampus and cerebral cortex. The second group of ACh neurons originates in the midbrain region and projects anteriorly (forward) to the thalamus, basal ganglia, and diencephalon (not shown in the figure) and posteriorly (backward) to the medulla, pons, cerebellum, and cranial nerve nuclei. In addition to its generally accepted role in learning and memory, the diffuse distribution of ACh is consistent with suggestions that ACh is involved in circuits that modulate sensory reception; in mechanisms related to behavioral arousal, attention, energy conservation, and mood; and in REM (rapid eye movement, or dreaming) activity during sleep.

Biogenic (Monoaminergic) Neurotransmitters

Catecholamine Transmitters: Dopamine and Norepinephrine

The term *catecholamine* refers to compounds that contain a catechol nucleus (a benzene ring with two attached hydroxyl groups) to which is attached an amine group (Figure 1.11). In the CNS, the term usually refers to the transmitters *dopamine* (DA) and *norepinephrine* (NE). In the peripheral nervous system, *epinephrine* ("adrenaline") is a third catecholamine transmitter. In the brain, a large number of psychoactive drugs (both licit and illicit, therapeutic and abused) exert their effects by altering the synaptic action of NE and DA.

The chemical synthesis of the catecholamines is illustrated in Figure 1.11. Biosynthesis of the catecholamines begins with the amino acid tyrosine (found in foods such as egg whites, cottage cheese, soy products, meat, fish, poultry, mustard greens, and spinach), and involves several steps controlled by specific enzymes. NE is produced from dopamine by an additional step that involves oxidation of the proximal carbon of the ethyl side chain. Following synthesis, these transmitters are stored in vesicles for release into the synaptic space. After release, NE and DA attach to pre- and postsynaptic receptors and initiate responses in the receiving cell or neuron. As noted earlier, inactivation occurs primarily by reuptake of the transmitter from the synaptic cleft into the presynaptic nerve terminal. Within the nerve terminal, catecholamines may be inactivated by enzymes such as *monoamine oxidase* (MAO). The class of antidepressants referred to as MAO inhibitors (MAOIs; see Chapter 12) acts by blocking MAO, thereby increasing the amounts of DA and NE available for synaptic release.

Catecholamine Receptors. Each catecholamine transmitter exerts effects on a number of different receptors. Norepinephrine and epinephrine act on two primary types of receptors (alpha and beta), each of which has at least two subtypes. Dopamine exerts postsynaptic effects on at least six receptors, divided into two families (D_1 type and D_2 type). The D_1 receptor family consists of two subtypes—D_1 and D_5—and the D_2 receptor family consists of four subtypes—D_{2A}, D_{2B}, D_3, and D_4. Postsynaptic dopamine receptors of the D_2 family are responsible for at least part of the antipsychotic activity and side effects of the drugs discussed in Chapter 11. Alterations in dopamine receptor function have been implicated in numerous diseases and behavioral states, including schizophrenia, parkinsonism, affective disorders, sexual activity, addiction, and attention deficit/hyperactivity disorder.

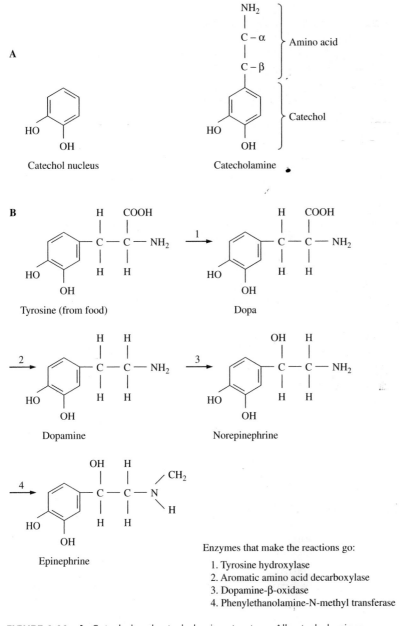

FIGURE 1.11   A. Catechol and catecholamine structure. All catecholamines share the catechol nucleus, a benzene ring with two adjacent hydroxyl (OH) groups. **B.** Structures and synthesis of the catecholamines. Tyrosine, an amino acid found in foods, is converted into dopa, then into dopamine, next into norepinephrine, and finally (in the peripheral nervous system) into epinephrine, depending on which enzymes (1–4) are present in the cell.

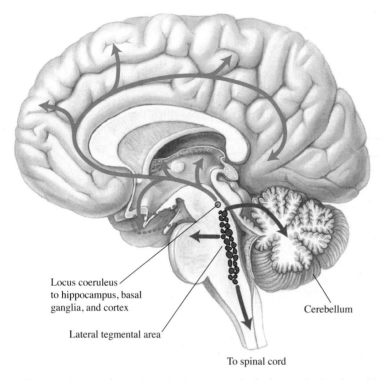

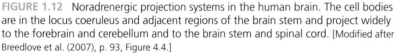

Locus coeruleus
to hippocampus, basal
ganglia, and cortex

Lateral tegmental area

Cerebellum

To spinal cord

FIGURE 1.12 Noradrenergic projection systems in the human brain. The cell bodies are in the locus coeruleus and adjacent regions of the brain stem and project widely to the forebrain and cerebellum and to the brain stem and spinal cord. [Modified after Breedlove et al. (2007), p. 93, Figure 4.4.]

Norepinephrine Pathways. The cell bodies of NE neurons are located in the brain stem, mainly in a structure in the pons called the locus coeruleus (Figure 1.12). From there, axons project widely throughout the brain to nerve terminals in the cerebral cortex, the limbic system, the hypothalamus, and the cerebellum. Axonal projections also travel down the spinal cord, where they exert an analgesic action. The release of NE produces an alerting, focusing, orienting response, positive feelings of reward, and analgesia.

Dopamine Pathways. Dopamine pathways also originate in the brain stem, sending axons both rostral (forward) to the brain and caudal (backward) to the spinal cord (Figure 1.13). Three dopamine circuits are most relevant for our discussions:

1. Neurons in the hypothalamus send short axons to the pituitary gland (not shown in Figure 1.13). These neurons regulate certain hormones. Alterations in hormone function are commonly seen in people with schizophrenia taking various antipsychotics, which block these dopamine receptors (see Chapter 11).

2. Neurons in the substantia nigra (see Figure 1.13) that project to the basal ganglia (see Figure 1.4) play a major role in the regulation of movement. As noted earlier,

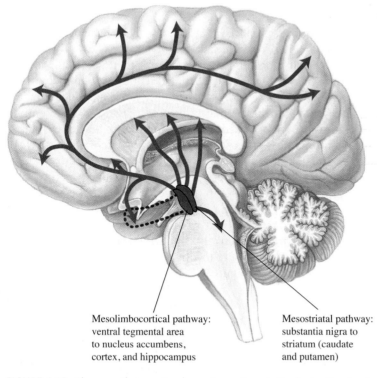

Mesolimbocortical pathway:
ventral tegmental area
to nucleus accumbens,
cortex, and hippocampus

Mesostriatal pathway:
substantia nigra to
striatum (caudate
and putamen)

FIGURE 1.13   There are three major dopamine systems in the brain. One is a local circuit in the hypothalamus (not shown); another, the nigrostriatal pathway, projects from the substantia nigra to the caudate nucleus of the basal ganglia, and is involved in motor functions and Parkinson's disease (see Figure 1.4); the third consists of cell bodies in the brain stem and midbrain (tegmentum) that project widely to the cerebral cortex and forebrain limbic system. [Modified after Breedlove et al. (2007), p. 93, Figure 4.3.]

parkinsonism (see Chapter 16), and parkinsonian side effects produced by antipsychotic drugs (which block these receptors) (see Chapter 11) all involve this pathway.

3. Cell bodies of the VTA (ventral tegmental area) in the midbrain are located next to the substantia nigra (see Figure 1.13). Dopamine neurons of this nucleus extend forward and separate into two pathways. One branch, called the mesocortical, projects to the frontal cortex, and a second branch, called the mesolimbic, projects to the limbic system. These two dopaminergic pathways are extremely important in psychopharmacology. First, alterations in the development of these pathways may be involved in the pathogenesis of schizophrenia and its amelioration by antipsychotic drugs. That is because, as discussed in Chapter 11, drugs used in the treatment of schizophrenia all share the common action of blocking dopamine receptors in this pathway. Second, these dopaminergic pathways also include structures that are activated by drugs (and other stimuli) that produce sensations of pleasure. This group of structures constitutes our "central reward circuit," which is involved in addiction to most drugs of abuse (discussed in Chapter 4).

The Indolamine Transmitter: Serotonin

Serotonin (5-hydroxytryptamine, abbreviated as 5-HT) was first investigated as a CNS neurotransmitter in the 1950s when lysergic acid diethylamide (LSD) was found to resemble serotonin structurally and block the contractile effect of serotonin on the gastrointestinal tract. At that time, it was hypothesized that LSD-induced hallucinations might be caused by alterations in the functioning of serotonin neurons and that serotonin might be involved in abnormal behavioral functioning. Today, drugs that potentiate the synaptic actions of serotonin are widely used as antidepressants and as antianxiety agents (specifically, the serotonergic agents known as *selective serotonin reuptake inhibitors*; SSRIs; see Chapter 12). Serotonin plays a role in depression, anxiety and obsessive-compulsive disorder, panic, phobias, sleep, sex, cardiovascular function, and the regulation of body temperature; use of an SSRI to treat depression can be associated with such side effects as insomnia, anxiety, and loss of libido.

Significant amounts of serotonin are found in the upper brain stem, particularly in the pons and the medulla, in structures collectively called the *raphe nuclei*. Anterior projections from the brain stem terminate diffusely throughout the cerebral cortex, hippocampus, hypothalamus, and limbic system (Figure 1.14). Serotonin projections largely parallel those of DA, although they are not as widespread. Axons of serotonin neurons descending to the spinal cord from cell bodies located in the raphe nuclei may be involved in the modulation of both pain and spinal reflexes.

Serotonin is an indoleamine. Indoleamines all contain indole groups, a benzene ring (six-carbon ring) fused to a pyrrole ring (five-membered ring with four carbons and a nitrogen). Serotonin is synthesized in the brain from the essential amino acid tryptophan (Figure 1.15A). Because the human body cannot make tryptophan we must get it from the foods we eat, such as poultry, bananas, tomatoes, and walnuts. Serotonin is produced by a short metabolic pathway consisting of two enzymes: tryptophan hydroxylase (TPH) and amino acid decarboxylase (DDC).

Several chemically distinct postsynaptic serotonin (5-HT) receptors have been identified. They have been classified in families (designated by a number) and subtypes within a family (designated by a letter). The main families and subtypes of 5-HT receptors are shown in Figure 1.15B. There are 14 different known 5-HT receptors. In 2013, the structures of two of these were uncovered, using X-ray crystallography, by which X-ray beams are fired at crystals of the compound, and the way in which the beams are scattered can allow scientists to determine the structure. The studies found that 5-HT receptors 1B and 2B had similar structures where serotonin binds, but that this space was larger in 1B than in 2B. Although only the width of three helium atoms, this difference was enough to explain why the two receptors bound differently to different drugs. This may be very important for drug safety: because some drugs that stimulate 2B receptors are thought to cause heart problems, it has been nicknamed the "death receptor" (Wang et al., 2013).

Amino Acid Neurotransmitters

There are two amino acid neurotransmitters that are widely distributed in the brain. The first, *glutamic acid* (or *glutamate*), is the major universally excitatory neurotransmitter; the second is *gamma aminobutyric acid* (GABA), which is the major inhibitory

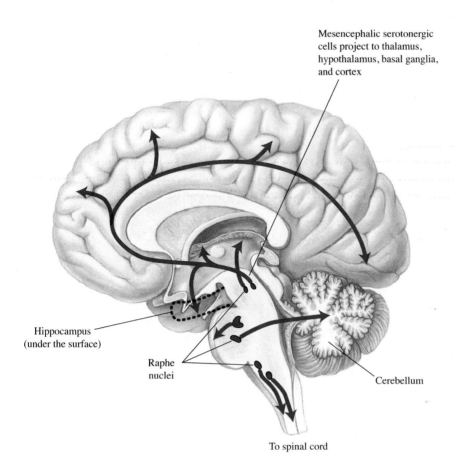

Mesencephalic serotonergic
cells project to thalamus,
hypothalamus, basal ganglia,
and cortex

Hippocampus
(under the surface)

Raphe
nuclei

Cerebellum

To spinal cord

FIGURE 1.14 Serotonin pathways in the human brain. [Modified after Breedlove et al. (2007), p. 94, Figure 4.5.]

neurotransmitter in the brain. Most other amino acids in the brain do not serve as neu-rotransmitters (with the exception of aspartate and glycine) but function as precursor molecules for the biosynthesis of other transmitters (for example, tyrosine for catechol-amines and tryptophan for serotonin).

Both glutamate and GABA function to modulate a number of receptors, maintaining a balance between excitation and inhibition in the brain. The following sections focus on glutamate and GABA because they are involved in the actions of several psychoactive drugs, ranging from the benzodiazepine antianxiety agents (see Chapter 13) to the mood stabilizers (see Chapter 14).

Glutamate. Glutamate is the major excitatory neurotransmitter in the brain, and is also the precursor for the major inhibitory neurotransmitter GABA. GABA is formed from glutamate under control of the enzyme *glutamic acid decarboxylase.*

Glutamate is a nonessential amino acid, meaning that it is easily synthesized in the body and is not required in the diet. It does not readily penetrate the blood-brain barrier,

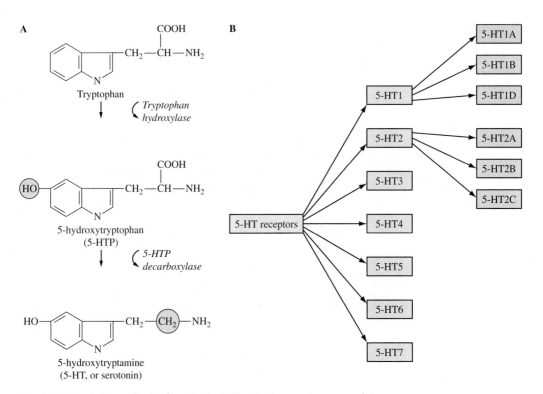

FIGURE 1.15   **A.** Biosynthesis of serotonin. **B.** Serotonin receptor nomenclature.
[http://pharmacologycorner.com/serotonin-5ht-receptors-agonists-antagonist/]

and is produced locally by specialized neuronal mechanisms. It can be synthesized by a number of different chemical reactions, among which is the normal breakdown of glucose. A second reaction, which might be the more important for neuronal glutamate, involves a glutamine cycle in which synaptically inactive glutamine serves as a reservoir of glutamate (Figure 1.16). In this process, after glutamate is released from a neuron and exerts its excitatory effect, it is transported into astrocytes (one type of glial cell) and converted to glutamine. Eventually, the glutamine diffuses out of the astrocytes and enters the presynaptic nerve terminals, where it is converted to glutamate, the active neurotransmitter (Iverson et al., 2009).

Glutamate receptors consist of two families, the *ionotropic* receptors (which respond quickly) that include NMDA and "nonNMDA receptors" (AMPA and kainate receptors), and *metabotropic receptors* (which respond more slowly). Metabotropic glutamate receptors (abbreviated as mGluRs) consist of eight members arranged into three groups (receptor classification is discussed more fully in Chapter 3). In the adult human brain, NMDA and AMPA receptors are colocalized in about 70 percent of their synapses. These receptors mediate rapid excitation of postsynaptic neurons, with especially high concentrations in the cerebral cortex, hippocampus, basal ganglia, septum, and amygdala.

NMDA receptors (Figure 1.17) have some unusual characteristics. First, in addition to glutamate, another amino acid, either glycine or serine, also needs to be present for

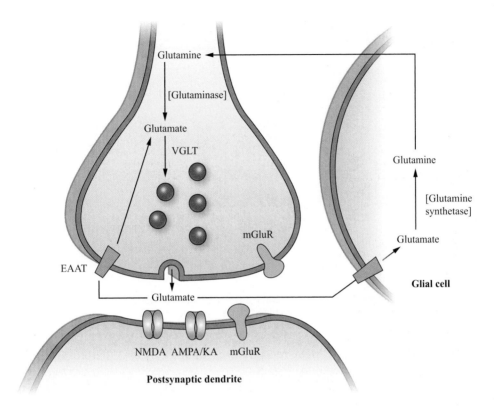

FIGURE 1.16 Schematic of the glutamate synapse. Glutamate (Glu) is released into the synapse and recaptured by excitatory amino acid transporters (EAATs) located on the presynaptic terminal and on adjacent glial cells. Within the glial cells, glutamate is converted to glutamine (Gln) by the enzyme *glutamine synthetase*. Glutamine diffuses back into neuronal terminals to replenish the Glu after conversion by the enzyme *glutaminase* and storage by Vesicular Glutamate Transporters. The "fast" (ionotropic) receptors, NMDA, AMPA, and kainate are shown on the postsynaptic membrane; the "slow" (metabotropic) receptors are shown on both the pre- and postsynaptic membranes. [After Cooper et al. (2003), p. 133.]

the receptor to be activated. Second, in order for NMDA receptors to be activated, they not only need to be stimulated by glutamate, they also need to be sufficiently stimulated electrically. The reason for this is that the NMDA ion channel is normally blocked by magnesium ions (Mg^+). Glutamate alone is not able to activate the receptor because of this block. However, when the neuronal membrane is also electrically stimulated, that is, depolarized (by the activation of AMPA or kainate receptors on the same postsynaptic neuron) the Mg^+ blockade of the ion channel is relieved. Then the NMDA receptor channel opens and permits the entry of both sodium and calcium ions, which further increases neuronal excitation. The NMDA receptor ion channel also has a binding site for phencyclidine (PCP) and ketamine (two "psychedelic" drugs discussed in Chapter 8).

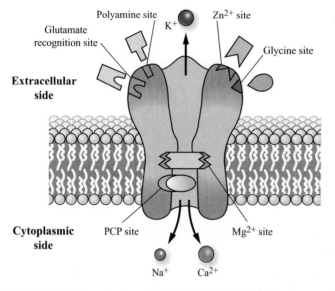

FIGURE 1.17   Schematic drawing of the NMDA (N-Methyl-D-Aspartate) receptor (PCP is discussed in Chapter 8). [http://www.frca.co.uk/article.aspx?articleid=100515]

These two drugs also block the NMDA receptor (see Chapter 3) and therefore prevent glutamate-induced neuronal activation.

NMDA receptors play a critical role in regulating synaptic plasticity. Activation of these receptors is responsible for basal excitatory synaptic transmission and many forms of neurophysiological mechanisms that are thought to underlie learning and memory. Because these receptors are involved in cognitive processes they are potential targets for therapies for Alzheimer's and other dementias. In 2004, the first anti-Alzheimer's drug that acts through a glutamatergic mechanism became available for clinical use (see Chapter 16).

However, although a normal amount of NMDA activity plays an important role in neuronal "health." excessive glutamatergic signaling is also involved in neuronal toxicity, a phenomenon by which nerve cells are damaged. Too much glutamate can lead to neuronal destruction through overactivity of NMDA receptors, which allows high amounts of calcium ions to enter the neuron (see Figure 1.17). Excess calcium activates enzymes, which then cause damage to cell structures and to DNA. For example, ethanol (see Chapter 5) reduces glutamate activity, and alcohol withdrawal markedly increases glutamate release from neurons. Traumatic head injury also results in massive release of glutamate, and attempts to provide "brain protection" after head injury are aimed at preventing glutamatergic overactivity. Anoxia, hypoglycemia, and epilepsy are other glutamate-releasing events that can lead to neuronal damage. Research is also focusing on the possibility of glutamate dysfunction in the pathogenesis of schizophrenia, especially the negative symptoms, and the cognitive dysfunction associated with the disorder (see Chapter 11).

Gamma Aminobutyric Acid. Gamma aminobutyric acid (GABA), the universally inhibitory transmitter, is found in high concentrations in the brain and spinal

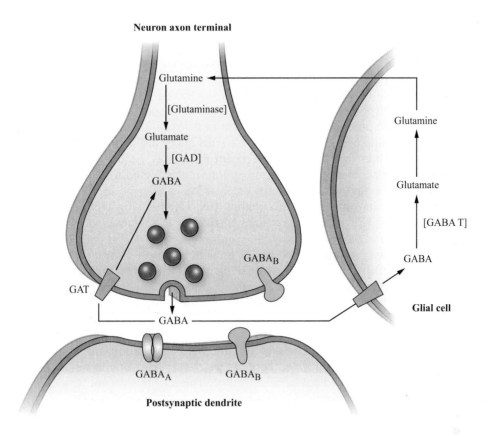

FIGURE 1.18 Schematic of the GABA synapse. GABA$_A$ receptors are fast receptors (ionotropic; Chapter 3) and found on the postsynaptic membrane. GABA$_B$ receptors are metabotropic and found on both pre- and postsynaptic membranes. GAT is the GABA transporter; GAD is glutamic acid decarboxylase, which converts L-glutamic acid to GABA; GABA T is the enzyme that metabolizes GABA.

cord. Two different types of GABA receptors are categorized as GABA$_A$ and GABA$_B$ (Figure 1.18). *GABA$_A$ receptors* are fast receptors. Activation of this receptor by GABA opens an ion channel and leads to an influx of chloride into the cell, hyper-polarizing the cell and reducing its excitability. Barbiturate and benzodiazepine binding to this receptor facilitates the action of GABA (see Chapter 13), which is responsible for the anxiolytic, amnestic, and anesthetic effects of these sedative drugs. GABA$_A$ receptors are found in high density in the cerebral cortex, hippocampus, and cerebellum.

Numerous sub-subtypes of the GABA$_A$ receptor occur, allowing for the development of a variety of agonists and antagonists (see Chapter 13). Such drugs might be novel anti-anxiety agents, anticonvulsants, or cognitive enhancers.

GABA$_B$ receptors are slow-response receptors. Activation of GABA$_B$ receptors in the amygdala is associated with the membrane-stabilizing, antiaggressive properties of valproic acid, a drug widely used to treat bipolar disorder (see Chapter 14).

Peptide Neurotransmitters

Many newly identified neurotransmitters are peptides, which are small proteins (chains of amino acid molecules attached in a specific order). Peptide transmitters can be classified into several groups including the hypothalamic-releasing hormones, the pituitary hormones, and the so-called gut-brain peptides. In this book, one peptide transmitter of interest is the type involved in the actions of the opiates, such as morphine. *Opioid peptides* include the *endorphins* (about 16 to 30 amino acids in length) and the shorter-chain *enkephalins* (5 amino acids in length). These substances are formed from a larger protein produced elsewhere in the body. The endorphins may be involved in a wide variety of emotional states, including pain perception, reward, emotional stability, and energy "highs," and in acupuncture. Opiates such as morphine, codeine, and heroin activate receptors for endorphins and enkephalins (see Chapter 10). Opioid receptors are termed *mu, kappa,* and *delta;* the mu receptor mediates the analgesic and reinforcing properties of morphine and other opiates.

Another peptide transmitter of interest in this book is *substance P,* a *gut-brain peptide* (11 amino acids in length) that plays an important role as a sensory transmitter, especially for pain impulses that enter the spinal cord and brain from a peripheral site of tissue injury. Opioids, serotonin agonists, and norepinephrine agonists exert much of their analgesic effect by acting on substance P nerve terminals to limit the release of this pain-inducing peptide.

From Table 1.1, on page 15, it can be seen that there are some additional transmitter substances that have not been mentioned here, as well as at least one family, the neurotransmitter gases, that have also not been described. These agents do not play a major role in the action of the drugs described in this text.

Until recently, it was believed that only a single neurotransmitter could be produced, stored, and released at each synapse. However, it is now clear that this situation is the exception rather than the rule. "Co-release" of more than one neurotransmitter is now a well-established phenomenon. For example, "GABA and glycine were the first pair of fast-acting neurotransmitters unequivocally proven to be co-released from synapses in the mammalian central nervous system" (Trudeau and Gutiérrez, 2007, p. 139). Most often a peptide is released with one of the "classic" transmitters summarized in this chapter; but a combination of classical transmitters is not uncommon, especially during development of the nervous system or as a postnatal reaction to pathophysiological stimulation (Trudeau and Gutiérrez, 2007).

STUDY QUESTIONS

1. What are the major divisions of the central nervous system?

2. Summarize the major structures of the basal ganglia and the limbic system and their respective functions.

3. Describe the main parts of a neuron, including the components of the synapse.

4. Summarize the processes involved in synaptic transmission. How is synaptic transmitter action terminated? Give examples.

5. What are the six classical neurotransmitters and their major receptor types?

6. Which major brain structures are associated with the neural pathways that release norepinephrine, dopamine, and serotonin?

7. Which diseases and drugs of abuse are associated with each of the major neurotransmitters?

REFERENCES

Ashraf, S. I., and Kunes, S. (2006). "A Trace of Silence: Memory and MicroRNA at the Synapse." *Current Opinions in Neurobiology* 16: 535–539.

Breedlove, M., et al. (2007). *Biological Psychology: An Introduction to Behavioral, Cognitive and Clinical Neuroscience*, 5th ed. Sunderland, MA: Sinauer.

Breedlove, M., et al. (2010). *Biological Psychology, An Introduction to Behavioral, Cognitive and Clinical Neuroscience*, 6th ed. Sunderland, MA: Sinauer.

Cooper, J. R., et al. (2003). *The Biochemical Basis of Neuropharmacology*, 8th ed. New York: Oxford University Press.

Iverson, L. L., et al. (2009). *Introduction to Neuropsychopharmacology*, New York: Oxford University Press.

Kempermann, G., et al. (2004). "Functional Significance of Adult Neurogenesis." *Current Opinions in Neurobiology* 14: 186–191.

Pinel, J. (2007). *Basics of Biopsychology*. New York: Pearson Education.

Schaffer, D. V., and Gage, F. H. (2004). "Neurogenesis and Neuroadaptation." *Neuromolecular Medicine* 5: 1–9.

Snyder, S. H. (2002). "Forty Years of Neurotransmitters: A Personal Account." *Archives of General Psychiatry* 59: 983–994.

Trudeau, L. E., and Gutiérrez, R. (2007) "On Cotransmission & Neurotransmitter Phenotype Plasticity." *Molecular Interventions* 7: 138–146.

Wang, C., et al. (2013). "Structural Basis for Molecular Recognition at Serotonin Receptors." *Science* 340: 610–614.

Chapter 2

Pharmacokinetics: How Drugs Are Handled by the Body

When we have a headache, we take it for granted that after taking some aspirin our headache will probably disappear within 15 to 30 minutes. We also take it for granted that, unless we take more aspirin later, the headache may recur within 3 or 4 hours. This familiar scenario illustrates four basic processes in the branch of pharmacology called *pharmacokinetics*. Using the aspirin example, the four processes are as follows:

1. *Absorption* of the aspirin into the body from the swallowed tablet
2. *Distribution* of the aspirin throughout the body, including into a fetus if a female is pregnant at the time the drug is taken
3. *Metabolism* (detoxification or breakdown) of the drug as the aspirin that has exerted its analgesic effect is broken down into metabolites (by-products or waste products) that no longer exert any effect
4. *Elimination* of the metabolic waste products, usually in the urine

These four processes are sometimes abbreviated as ADME. In concert, they determine the *bioavailability* of a drug, that is, how much of the drug that is administered actually reaches its target.

The goal of this chapter is to introduce these processes of pharmacokinetics, concluding with discussion about how pharmacokinetics can be used to determine the time course of action for drugs. Because many drugs need to be taken chronically, for various periods of time, the chapter also explores the steady-state maintenance of therapeutic blood levels of drugs in the body and the usefulness of therapeutic drug monitoring. Finally, the chapter introduces the concepts of drug *tolerance* and drug *dependence*.

Knowledge of pharmacokinetics and the *dosage* taken allows determination of the concentration of a drug at its *receptors* (sites of action) and the *magnitude* of drug effect on the receptors as a function of time. Thus, pharmacokinetics in its simplest form describes the time course of a particular drug's actions—the time to onset and the duration of effect. Usually, the time course simply reflects the amount of *time* required for the rise and fall of the drug's concentration at the target site. Figure 2.1 illustrates the complexity of drug movement through the body and its equilibrium at its site of action.

The root *kinetics* in the word *pharmacokinetics* implies movement and time. As each of the drugs in this book is discussed, the focus is first on the time course of the drug's movement through the body, particularly its *half-life* and any complications that arise from alterations in its rate of metabolism. Knowledge of movement and time offers significant insight into the action of a drug. At the very least, it helps distinguish a particular drug from other related drugs. For example, the main difference between the two benzodiazepines (see Chapter 13) lorazepam (Ativan) and triazolam (Halcion) is in

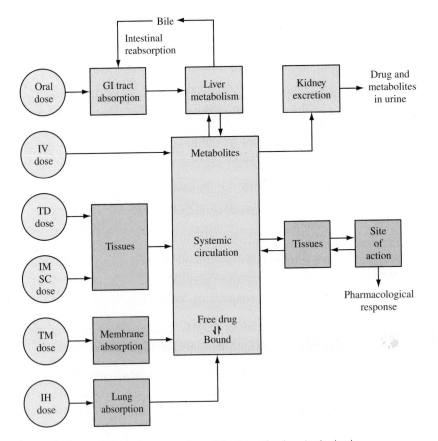

FIGURE 2.1 Schematic representation of the fate of a drug in the body.
IM = intramuscular; IV = intravenous; TM = transmembrane; SC = subcutaneous;
TD = transdermal; IH = inhalational.

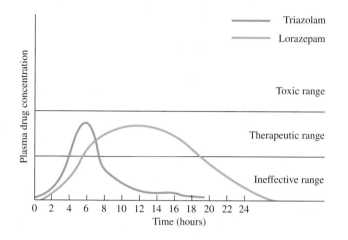

Triazolam
Lorazepam

Toxic range

Therapeutic range

Ineffective range

FIGURE 2.2 Theoretical blood levels of triazolam (a short-acting benzodiazepine) and lorazepam (a longer-acting benzodiazepine) over time following oral administration. Approximations for ineffective, therapeutic, and toxic blood levels are shown.

their pharmacokinetics. Both these drugs depress the functioning of the brain, causing sedative and antianxiety effects. However, lorazepam persists for at least 24 hours in the body, while triazolam persists for only about 6 to 8 hours. If lorazepam is administered at bedtime for treatment of insomnia, daytime sedation the next day can be a problem, because lorazepam persists in the body through the next day. However, for longer, steady action (as might be useful in treating anxiety), lorazepam would be the superior agent to use.[1]

The kinetic differences between lorazepam and triazolam are illustrated in Figure 2.2, which shows three ranges in the blood plasma: an ineffective range (where not enough drug is present to produce either sedative or antianxiety effects), a therapeutic range, and a toxic range (where sedation becomes excessive). Triazolam reaches peak blood level rapidly and is of short duration. Lorazepam, on the other hand, reaches peak blood level later and persists longer in the therapeutic range. In essence, pharmacokinetic differences account for these results and allow two similar drugs to be used to achieve different therapeutic goals.

---

[1] Most drugs used in medicine are known by two or even three names. The most detailed name for a drug is its *structural name*, which accurately describes its chemical structure in words. In this book, the chemical names for drugs are not used. The second name for a drug is its *generic name*, often an abbreviated form derived from the structural name, given to the drug by its discoverer or manufacturer. After a drug's patent protection runs out (usually 17 years after the date of its patent registration by the manufacturer), any other generic drug manufacturer may legitimately sell the drug under this name. The third name is the drug's *trade name*, a unique name given to the drug by its original patent holder. Only that manufacturer can ever sell the drug under that name, even after the patent runs out and others sell the drug under its generic name. For example, many companies sell aspirin, a generic name for acetylsalicylic acid, the structural name. However, only Bayer Pharmaceuticals (the original company that patented acetylsalicylic acid) can call it Bayer Aspirin. In this book, when a drug is introduced, the generic name is given first and is not capitalized. The trade name follows in parentheses, is capitalized, and usually is not given again.

Drug Absorption

The term *drug absorption* refers to processes and mechanisms by which drugs pass from the external world into the bloodstream. For any drug, a route of administration, a dose of the drug, and a dosage form (liquid, tablet, capsule, injection, patch, spray, or gum) must be selected that will both place the drug at its site of action in a pharmacologically effective concentration and maintain the concentration for an adequate period of time. Drugs are most commonly administered in one of six ways, which may be divided into two categories:

1. *Enteral* routes refer to administration involving the gastrointestinal (GI) tract:
    a. Orally (swallowed when taken by mouth)
    b. Rectally (embedded in a suppository, which is placed in the rectum)
2. *Parenteral* routes refer to administration that does not involve the GI tract:
    a. Injected (given in liquid form with a needle and syringe)
    b. Inhaled through the lungs as gases, as vapors, or as particles carried in smoke or in an aerosol
    c. Absorbed through the skin (usually as a drug-containing skin patch)
    d. Absorbed through mucous membranes (from "snorting," or sniffing, the drug, with the drug depositing on the oral or nasal mucosa; termed *insufflation*)

Oral Administration

To be effective when administered orally, a drug must be soluble (able to dissolve) and stable in stomach fluid (not destroyed by gastric acids), enter the intestine, penetrate the lining of the stomach or intestine, and pass into the bloodstream. Because they are already in solution, drugs that are administered in liquid form tend to be absorbed more rapidly than those given in tablet or capsule form. When a drug is taken in solid form, both the rate at which it dissolves and its chemistry limit the rate of absorption. Food in the stomach may slow down absorption, while carbonation may speed up absorption. As an example, absorption of the antipsychotic drug ziprasidone (Geodon) is cut in half if taken without food (Carlat, 2011). In some cases, rather than the active drug itself, the oral formulation contains a precursor (forerunner) of a drug, called a *prodrug*. A prodrug must undergo chemical conversion by metabolic processes before becoming an active pharmacological agent. An example of this type of medication is the drug lisdexamfetamine (Vyvanse), recently approved for the treatment of attention deficit/hyperactivity disorder (ADHD; see Chapter 15).

After a tablet dissolves, the drug molecules contained within it are carried into the upper intestine, where they are absorbed across the intestinal mucosa by a process of *passive diffusion*, passing from an area of high concentration into an area of lower concentration. This process necessitates that the drug molecules, at least to some degree, be soluble in fat (be *lipid soluble*). In reality, even a small amount of lipid solubility allows for absorption after oral administration; the most lipid-soluble drugs are merely absorbed faster than less lipid-soluble drugs. In general, most psychoactive drugs have good solubility in the lipid linings of the stomach and intestine; therefore, about 75 percent (or more) of the amount of an orally administered psychoactive drug is absorbed into the bloodstream within about 1 to 3 hours after its administration.

There are only rare exceptions to this general rule. One involves the antidepressant/antianxiety drug buspirone (BuSpar; see Chapter 13). This drug has limited clinical efficacy, primarily because most of it is rapidly broken down (metabolized) by a drug-metabolizing enzyme located in the walls of the stomach lining. This enzyme (called CYP-3A4, discussed later) reduces the oral absorption of buspirone by over 90 percent. However, should buspirone be taken with grapefruit juice, a component in the juice (furanocoumarin) inhibits the buspirone-metabolizing enzyme, allowing the drug to be more completely absorbed (Figure 2.3) and increasing its therapeutic utility (Lilja et al., 1998; Paine et al., 2006; Rheeders et al., 2006). It has recently been recognized that this interaction affects many more drugs than previously thought. In their review, Bailey et al. (2012) found that more than 85 drugs produce this adverse reaction with grapefruit and 43 have potentially serious consequences. This list, which can be accessed at http://www.cmaj.ca.libezp.lib.lsu.edu/content/early/2012/11/26/cmaj.120951/suppl/DC1 includes drugs from many different categories, not just those that affect the brain. In general, these drugs are usually taken orally, and it may take as little as 200 to 250 milliliters of grapefruit juice to produce an adverse reaction. Such reactions could include loss of drug effect, GI bleeding, urinary retention, dizziness, respiratory depression, and several others.

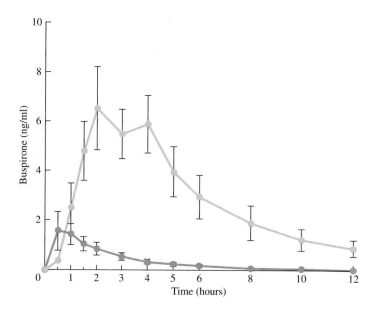

FIGURE 2.3 Plasma concentrations (mean and SEM) of buspirone (in nanograms per milliliter of plasma) in ten healthy volunteers after a single oral dose of 10 mg buspirone, after ingestion of 200 ml (about 7 oz) grapefruit juice (*green circles*) or water (*orange circles*) three times a day for two days, and on the third day with buspirone administration 30 and 90 minutes later. [Data from Lilja et al. (1998).]

> ## Did You Know?
>
> ### Drugs That Interact with Grapefruit on the Rise
>
> The number of drugs that are risky when taken with grapefruit is increasing, as a result of new medications and chemical formulations. Currently, more than 85 drugs may interact with grapefruit. The number that may result in potentially fatal side effects when combined with grapefruit increased from 17 to 43 during the past four years. The list includes some statins that lower cholesterol (such as atorvastatin, lovastatin, and simvastatin), some antibiotics, cancer drugs, and heart medications. Most at risk are older people who use more prescription drugs and eat more grapefruit. The effect can vary. With some drugs, just one serving of grapefruit can make it seem like a person is taking multiple doses of the drug. This interaction can occur even if grapefruit is eaten many hours before taking the medication. For example, simvastatin, when taken with about a 7-ounce glass of grapefruit juice once a day for three days, produced a 330% greater concentration of the drug compared to taking it with water. This can cause life-threatening muscle damage called rhabdomyolysis. It is better to be safe than sorry, therefore patients should double-check with their doctors.

Although oral administration of drugs is common, it does have disadvantages. First, it may occasionally lead to vomiting and stomach distress. Second, although the amount of a drug that is put into a tablet or capsule can be calculated, how much of it will be absorbed into the bloodstream cannot always be accurately predicted because of genetic differences among people (in the amount and in the composition of the enzymes they have that metabolize the drugs) and because of differences in the manufacture of the drugs. Finally, the acid in the stomach destroys some orally administered drugs, such as the local anesthetics and insulin, before they can be absorbed. To be effective, those drugs must be administered by injection.

Rectal Administration

Although the primary route of drug administration is oral, some drugs are administered rectally (usually in suppository form) if the patient is vomiting, unconscious, or is unable to swallow. However, absorption is often irregular, unpredictable, and incomplete, and many drugs irritate the membranes that line the rectum.

Administration by Inhalation

In recreational drug misuse and abuse, inhalation of drugs is a popular method of administration. Examples of drugs taken by this route include nicotine in tobacco cigarettes and tetrahydrocannabinol in marijuana, as well as smoked heroin, crack cocaine, ice methamphetamine, and the various inhalants of abuse, all of which are discussed at length later in the book. The popularity of inhalation as a route of administration follows from two observations:

1. Lung tissues have a large surface area through which large amounts of blood flow, allowing for rapid absorption of drugs from the lungs into the blood (often within seconds).

2. Drugs absorbed into pulmonary (lung) capillaries are carried in the pulmonary veins directly to the left (arterial) side of the heart (Figure 2.4) and from there directly into the aorta and the arteries carrying blood to the brain. As a result, drugs administered by inhalation may have an even faster onset of effect than drugs administered intravenously. If drugs administered in this fashion are behaviorally reinforcing, the rapid onset of effect can be intense and may promote compulsive use.

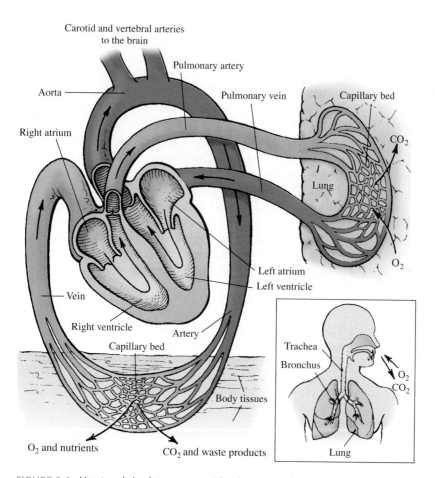

FIGURE 2.4 Heart and circulatory system. Blood returning from the systemic venous circulation to the heart enters the right atrium and flows into the right ventricle. With contraction of the heart, this blood is pumped into the pulmonary arteries leading to the lungs. Once in the pulmonary capillaries, carbon dioxide (CO_2) is lost and replaced by oxygen. The oxygenated blood returns to the heart in the pulmonary veins, which empty into the left atrium. With heart contraction, the oxygenated blood is pumped from the left ventricle into the aorta and is carried to the body tissues and brain, where oxygen and nutrients are exchanged in the systemic capillary beds. Oxygen and nutrients are supplied to the body tissues through the walls of the capillaries; CO_2 and other waste products are returned to the blood. The CO_2 is eliminated through the lungs, and the other waste products are metabolized in the liver and excreted in the urine.

Administration Through Mucous Membranes

Occasionally, drugs are administered through the mucous membranes of the mouth or nose. A few examples:

- Cocaine powder, when sniffed, adheres to the membranes on the inside of the nose and is absorbed directly into the bloodstream (see Chapter 7).
- Nicotine (see Chapter 6) in snuff, nasal spray, or chewing-gum formulations is absorbed through the mucosal membranes directly into the bloodstream.
- For use before and after surgery on children, the opioid narcotic fentanyl (Sublimase; see Chapter 10) became available in 1998 in lollipop form, allowing this pain-relieving drug to be provided without subjecting a child to a painful injection. As the lollipop is sucked, the drug is released and absorbed through the mucous membranes of the mouth. This form of administering fentanyl has also become popular for patients with disabling pain when orally administered pain relievers are insufficient and injection of opioid narcotics is too painful.
- A sublingual (placed under the tongue) combination of buprenorphine (an opioid narcotic) and naloxone (an opioid antagonist) for the office-based treatment of opioid dependency has recently been introduced. The combination product, called Suboxone, is discussed in Chapter 10. The buprenorphine is absorbed through the mucous membranes, but the antagonist, naloxone, is not. When the pill is administered sublingually, the desired narcotic effect is achieved. However, should the pill be crushed, dissolved, and injected, the antagonist naloxone precipitates drug withdrawal. This effect tends to discourage abuse of the buprenorphine and reduce illicit use, providing yet another example of how knowledge of pharmacokinetics can be used to therapeutic benefit in special circumstances.

Administration Through the Skin

Over the past several years, several medications have been incorporated into *transdermal patches* that adhere to the skin. A transdermal patch is a unique bandagelike therapeutic system that provides continuous, controlled release of a drug from a reservoir through a semipermeable membrane. The drug is slowly absorbed into the bloodstream at the area of contact. Following are some examples of drug-containing patches:

- Nicotine (used to deter smoking behaviors)
- Fentanyl (used to treat chronic pain)
- Clonidine (used to treat hypertension)
- Estrogen or other hormones (used to replace reduced hormones in postmenopausal women or for contraception)
- Scopolamine (used to prevent motion sickness)
- Selegiline (Emsam; used to treat depression; see Chapter 12)
- Methylphenidate (Daytrana, a 9-hour patch used to treat attention-deficit/hyperactivity disorder in children; see Chapter 15)

All these transdermal skin patches allow for slow, continuous absorption of the drug over hours or even days, potentially minimizing side effects associated with rapid rises and falls in plasma concentrations of the drug contained in the patch. In all cases, the drug is slowly, predictably, and continuously released from the liquid in the patch and absorbed into the systemic circulation, allowing levels to remain relatively constant over the time of absorption.

Administration by Injection

Administration of drugs by injection can be *intravenous* (directly into a vein), *intramuscular* (directly into a muscle), or *subcutaneous* (just under the skin). Each of these routes of administration has its advantages and disadvantages (Table 2.1), but all share some features. In general, administration by injection produces a more prompt response than does oral administration because absorption is faster. Also, injection permits a more accurate dose because the unpredictable processes of absorption through the stomach and intestine are bypassed.

Administration of drugs by injection, however, has several drawbacks. First, the rapid rate of absorption leaves little time to respond to an unexpected drug reaction or accidental overdose. Second, administration by injection requires the use of sterile techniques. Hepatitis and AIDS are examples of diseases that can be transmitted as a drastic consequence of unsterile injection techniques. Third, once a drug is administered by injection, it cannot be recalled.

Intravenous Administration. In an intravenous injection, a drug is introduced directly into the bloodstream. This technique avoids all the variables related to oral absorption. Intravenous injection can be done slowly, and it can be stopped instantaneously if untoward effects develop. In addition, the dosage can be extremely

TABLE 2.1 Some characteristics of drug administration by injection

Route	Absorption pattern	Special utility	Limitations and precautions
Intravenous	Absorption circumvented Potentially immediate effects	Valuable for emergency use Permits titration of dosage Can administer large volumes and irritating substances when diluted	Increased risk of adverse effects Must inject solutions slowly as a rule Not suitable for oily solutions or insoluble substances
Intramuscular	Prompt action from aqueous solution Slow and sustained action from repository preparations	Suitable for moderate volumes, oily vehicles, and some irritating substances	Precluded during anticoagulant medication May interfere with interpretation of certain diagnostic tests (e.g., creatine phosphokinase)
Subcutaneous	Prompt action from aqueous solution Slow and sustained action from repository preparations	Suitable for some insoluble suspensions and for implantation of solid pellets	Not suitable for large volumes Possible pain or necrosis from irritating substance

precise, and the practitioner can dilute and administer in large volumes drugs that at higher concentrations would be irritants to the muscles or blood vessels.

The intravenous route is the most dangerous of all routes of administration because it has the fastest speed of onset of pharmacological action. Too-rapid injection can be catastrophic, producing life-threatening reactions (such as collapse of respiration or of heart function). Also, allergic reactions, should they occur, may be extremely severe. Finally, drugs that are not completely solubilized before injection cannot usually be given intravenously because of the danger of blood clots or emboli forming. Infection and transmission of infectious diseases are an ever-present danger when sterile techniques are not employed.

Intramuscular Administration. Drugs that are injected into skeletal muscle (usually in the arm, thigh, or buttock) are generally absorbed fairly rapidly. Absorption of a drug from muscle is more rapid than absorption of the same drug from the stomach but slower than intravenous absorption. The absolute rate of absorption of a drug from muscle varies, depending on the rate of blood flow to the muscle, the solubility of the drug, the volume of the injection, and the solution in which the drug is dissolved and injected.

Intramuscular injections are of two types: (1) fairly rapid onset and short duration of action, and (2) slow onset and prolonged action. In the former situation, the drug is dissolved in an aqueous (water) solution. Following injection, the water and dissolved drug are quite rapidly absorbed, with complete absorption occurring over a very few hours. In the latter situation, classically the drug is suspended in an oily solution. The oil and dissolved drug solution is only slowly absorbed, and complete absorption can take days or weeks. Modern manufacturing techniques have allowed the drug to be placed in bioabsorbable polymer microspheres, which release a constant amount of drug each day for a period of a week or more (such as with the antipsychotic Risperdol Consta; see Chapter 11). Similarly, the opioid narcotic antagonist naltrexone suspended in injected microcapsules releases a constant amount of drug into blood over a period of several weeks. This product is marketed under the trade name Vivitrol and is indicated in the treatment of opioid-dependent patients (see Chapter 10).

Subcutaneous Administration. Absorption of drugs that have been injected under the skin (subcutaneously) is rapid. The exact rate depends mainly on how easy it is for the drug to penetrate the blood vessel and the rate of blood flow through the skin. Irritating drugs should not be injected subcutaneously because they may cause severe pain and damage to local tissue. The usual precautions to maintain sterility should be applied.

Drug Distribution

Once absorbed into the bloodstream, a drug is distributed throughout the body by the circulating blood, passing across various barriers to reach its target, that is, its site of action (its receptors) (Figure 2.5). At any given time, only a very small portion of the total amount of a drug that is in the body is actually in contact with its receptors. For example, in the case of a psychoactive drug, most of the drug circulates outside the brain and therefore does not contribute directly to its pharmacological effect. This wide distribution often accounts for many of the side effects of a drug. *Side effects* are results that are different from the primary, or therapeutic, effect for which a drug is taken.

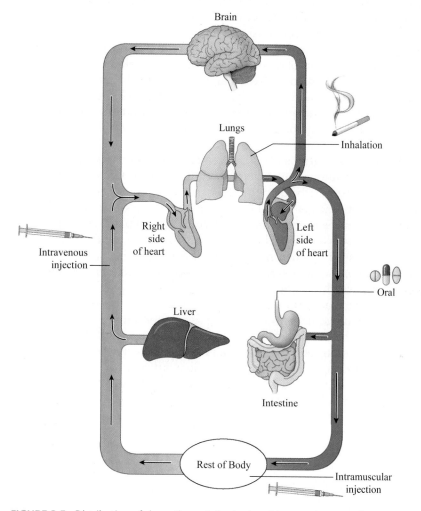

FIGURE 2.5 Distribution of drugs through the body, with several routes of administration indicated. [After Oakley and Ksir, 1996, Figure 6-5, page 122.]

Action of the Bloodstream

Every minute in the average-size adult, the heart pumps a volume of blood that is roughly equal to the total amount of blood in the circulatory system. Thus, the entire blood volume circulates in the body about once every minute. Once absorbed into the bloodstream, a drug is rapidly (usually within the 1-minute circulation time) distributed throughout the circulatory system.

As seen in the schematic diagram of the circulatory system (see Figure 2.4), blood returning to the heart through the veins is first pumped into the pulmonary (lung) circulation system, where carbon dioxide is removed and replaced by oxygen. The oxygenated blood then returns to the heart and is pumped into the great artery (the aorta). From there, blood flows into the smaller arteries and finally into the capillaries, where nutrients (and drugs) are exchanged between the blood and the cells of the body. After blood passes through the capillaries, it is collected by the veins and returned to the heart to circulate again. Psychoactive drugs quite quickly become evenly distributed throughout the bloodstream, diluted not only by blood but also by the total amount of water in the body.

If a drug is taken orally, it passes through the cells lining the GI tract and then through the liver; from there the drug enters the central circulation and is carried to the heart to be distributed throughout the body (see Figure 2.5). Occasionally, drug-metabolizing enzymes in the cells of either the GI tract or the liver can markedly reduce the amount of drug that reaches the bloodstream. This process is called *first-pass metabolism*. One example involves the enzyme that metabolizes alcohol. This enzyme is called *alcohol dehydrogenase*. It is found in the cells lining the GI tract and in cells of the liver. As we will see in Chapter 5, women have less of this enzyme in the GI tract cells than men, and therefore exhibit higher blood alcohol levels for a given amount of alcohol ingested (corrected for body weight) than do men.

When injected (by whatever route), absorbed transdermally, or absorbed from mucous membranes, a drug bypasses intestinal absorption, rapidly enters veins, and is carried in blood to the right side of the heart (with minimal amounts passing initially through the liver). The drug then circulates through the pulmonary vessels, returns to the left side of the heart, and finally travels through the aorta to the brain and the body.

Inhaled drugs are absorbed from the lungs and carried in pulmonary veins directly to the left side of the heart and, from there, rapidly to the brain. The effects of smoked tobacco or smoked marijuana are felt within a breath or two.

Body Membranes That Affect Drug Distribution

Four types of membranes in the body affect drug distribution: (1) cell membranes, (2) walls of the capillary vessels in the circulatory system, (3) the blood-brain barrier, and (4) the placental barrier.

Cell Membranes. The structure and properties of cell membranes determine their permeability to drugs. In Figure 2.6, the two layers of ovals represent the water-soluble head groups of complex lipid molecules called *phospholipids*. The phospholipid heads form a rather continuous layer on both the inside and the outside of the cell membrane. The wavy lines that extend from the heads into the membrane are the lipid chains of the phospholipid molecules. Therefore, for our present purposes, the interior of the cell membrane can be considered to consist of a sea of lipid in which large proteins are suspended.

Cell membranes provide a physical barrier that is permeable to small, lipid-soluble drug molecules but is impermeable to large, lipid-insoluble drug molecules. As a barrier, they are important for the passage of drugs (1) from the stomach and intestine into the bloodstream, (2) from the fluid that closely surrounds tissue cells into the interior

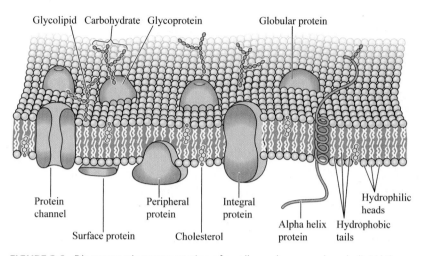

Glycolipid Carbohydrate Glycoprotein   Globular protein

Protein
channel

Surface protein

Peripheral
protein

Cholesterol

Integral
protein

Alpha helix
protein

Hydrophobic
tails

Hydrophilic
heads

FIGURE 2.6 Diagrammatic representation of a cell membrane, a phospholipid bilayer in which cholesterol and protein molecules are embedded. Both globular and helical kinds of protein traverse the bilayer. Cholesterol molecules tend to keep the tails of the phospholipids relatively fixed and orderly in the regions closest to the hydrophilic phospholipid heads; the parts of the tails closer to the core of the membrane move about freely.

of cells, (3) from the interior of cells back into the body water, and (4) from the kidneys back into the bloodstream.

Capillaries. Within a minute or so of entering the bloodstream, a drug is distributed fairly evenly throughout the entire blood volume. From there, drugs leave the bloodstream and are exchanged (in equilibrium) between blood capillaries and body tissues. Figure 2.7 shows a cross-sectional diagram and a schematic of a capillary. Capillaries are tiny, cylindrical blood vessels with walls that are formed by a thin, single layer of cells packed tightly together. Between the cells are small pores (clefts, or fenestra) that allow passage of small molecules between blood and the body tissues. The diameter of these pores is between 90 and 150 angstroms (Å), which is larger than most drug molecules. Thus, most drugs freely leave the blood through these pores in the capillary membranes, moving along their concentration gradient until equilibrium is established between the concentrations of drug in the blood, body tissues, and water.

The transport of drug molecules between plasma and body tissues is independent of lipid solubility because the membrane pores are large enough for even fat-insoluble drug molecules to penetrate. However, the pores in the capillary membrane are not large enough to permit the red blood cells and the plasma proteins to leave the bloodstream. Thus, the only drugs that do not readily penetrate capillary pores are drugs that bind to plasma proteins. The rate at which drug molecules enter specific body tissues depends on two factors: the rate of blood flow through the tissue and the ease with which drug molecules pass through the capillary membranes.

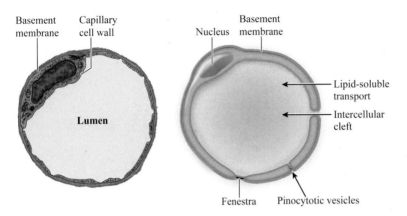

FIGURE 2.7   Cross section of a typical capillary (*left*) and the schematic (*right*), showing the pores (fenestra) and indicating that lipid-soluble substances can pass through the cell wall.

Because blood flow is greatest to the brain and much less to the bones, joints, and fat deposits, drug distribution generally follows a similar pattern. An example might be appropriate. When marijuana is smoked, the active drug, tetrahydrocannabinol (THC; see Chapter 9), achieves plasma concentrations of about 10 to 20 nanograms of drug per milliliter of plasma (ng/ml) soon after initiation of smoking. Within about 30 minutes, it achieves levels of about 50 to 100 ng/ml, which fall off within 1 hour to less than 5 to 10 ng/ml because the drug is rapidly taken up into body fat. From there, it slowly returns to plasma and is metabolized to an inactive metabolite (carboxy-THC) that is excreted in the urine.

Blood-Brain Barrier.   The brain requires a protected environment to function normally, and a specialized structural barrier, called the *blood-brain barrier* (BBB), plays a key role in maintaining this environment (Figure 2.8). In contrast to capillaries in most of the body, the capillary walls in the brain do not have pores. The endothelial cells that make up the capillary walls are tightly joined together and covered on the outside by a fatty barrier called the *glial sheath,* which arises from nearby astrocyte cells.

Thus, to reach the neurons, a drug leaving the capillaries in the brain has to traverse both the wall of the capillary itself (because there are no pores to pass through) and the membranes of the astrocytes. Therefore, the rate of passage of a drug into the brain is generally determined by two factors: (1) the size of the drug molecule, and (2) its lipid (fat) solubility. Large drugs penetrate poorly, while small, fat-soluble drugs penetrate rapidly. Oxygen is small enough and most psychoactive drugs are both small enough and sufficiently lipid soluble to cross the BBB. Drugs that cannot cross the BBB are restricted to structures outside the central nervous system (CNS). Penicillin is an example of such a drug. It does not cross the BBB, and its effectiveness as an antibiotic is restricted to infections located outside the brain.

Unfortunately, some other lipid-soluble drugs, such as steroids and beta blockers, are also unable to pass through capillary walls because they are detected as foreign and

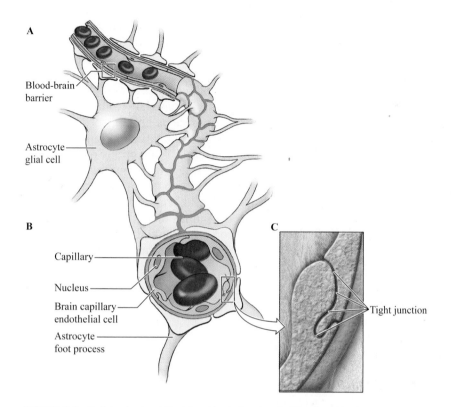

FIGURE 2.8   Cellular basis of the blood-brain barrier. **A.** Blood and brain are separated by capillary cells packed tightly together and by a fatty barrier called the glial sheath, which is made up of extensions (glial feet) from nearby astrocyte cells. A drug diffusing from blood to brain must move through the cells of the capillary wall because there are tight junctions rather than pores between the cells; the drug must then move through the fatty glial sheath. **B.** Cross section of a brain capillary. **C.** Electron micrograph of the section in the box from part B. Arrows point to the tight junctions between the endothelial cells.

expelled by cellular export pumps, transporters (of which at least 15 are known), which protect the brain from toxins. Called P-glycoproteins (Pgps), these are members of a larger group of transporters, called the ATP-binding cassette family or ABCs. It is now known that these transporters are also found in the gut, gonads, and other organs as well as the brain, where they move substances either into or out of the tissue. Some prescription and over-the-counter (OTC) drugs, foods, and substances made by the body may either inhibit or induce these transporters.

Larger molecules, such as glucose, amino acids, and vitamins, reach the brain because they are carried by special transport systems out of the capillaries. Even larger substances like iron and insulin can be transported across the capillary wall by a process called *transcytosis*. In this situation, the substances attach to a receptor that is located in the cell wall membrane. A small segment of this membrane then forms a vesicle, which crosses over to, and fuses with, the membrane on the opposite side of the capillary wall, after which the receptor releases the substance into the brain.

Unfortunately, according to Pardridge (2003) only a few diseases, such as depression and mania, schizophrenia, chronic pain, and epilepsy, consistently respond to molecules that can cross the BBB. In contrast, 98 percent of drugs that would have some effect on the nervous system cannot cross the BBB. Many serious brain disorders do not respond to the conventional lipid-soluble small-molecule model, including Alzheimer's disease, stroke, brain and spinal cord injury, brain cancer, HIV infections of the brain, various ataxia-producing disorders, amyotrophic lateral sclerosis, multiple sclerosis, Huntington's disease, and childhood inborn genetic errors of the brain. Researchers are trying to develop ways in which to "trick" the BBB and "sneak" therapeutic drugs into the brain. Efforts are being made to inhibit specific export pumps or to devise lipid vesicles that could carry drug molecules inside their hollow cores and slide through the capillary walls. Perhaps someday we might be able to overcome the constraints of the BBB and deliver medications for all types of brain disorders.

Did You Know?

Improving Delivery of Medicines to the Brain

New research offers a possible strategy for treating central nervous system diseases, such as brain and spinal cord injury, brain cancer, epilepsy, and neurological complications of HIV.

The experimental method allows small therapeutic agents to cross the blood-brain barrier safely in laboratory rats by turning off P-glycoprotein, one of the main gatekeepers preventing medicinal drugs from reaching their intended targets in the brain.

In a two-stage approach, the researchers first determined that treating rat brain capillaries with the multiple sclerosis drug marketed as Gilenya (fingolimod) stimulated a specific biochemical signaling pathway in the blood-brain barrier that rapidly and reversibly turned off P-glycoprotein. They then pretreated rats with fingolimod, and administered three other drugs that P-glycoprotein usually transports away from the brain. They observed a dramatic decline in P-glycoprotein transport activity, which led to a three- to fivefold increase in brain uptake for each of the three drugs.

Placental Barrier.   Among all the membrane systems of the body, the placental membranes are unique, separating two distinct human beings with differing genetic compositions and differing sensitivities to drugs. The fetus obtains essential nutrients and eliminates metabolic waste products through the placenta without depending on its own organs, many of which are not yet functioning. The dependence of the fetus on the mother places the fetus at the mercy of the placenta when foreign substances (such as drugs or toxins) appear in the mother's blood (Gilstrap and Little, 1998). The placental barrier is discussed further in the discussions of individual drugs.

A schematic representation of the placental network, which transfers substances between the mother and the fetus, is shown in Figure 2.9. In general, the mature placenta consists of a network of vessels and pools of maternal blood into which protrude treelike or fingerlike villi (projections) that contain the blood capillaries of the fetus. Oxygen and nutrients travel from the mother's blood to that of the fetus, while carbon dioxide and other waste products travel from the blood of the fetus to the mother's blood.

The membranes that separate fetal blood from maternal blood in the intervillous space resemble, in their general permeability, the cell membranes that are found elsewhere in the body. In other words, drugs cross the placenta primarily by passive diffusion. Fat-soluble substances (including all psychoactive drugs) diffuse readily, rapidly, and without limitation. The view that the placenta is a barrier to drugs is inaccurate. A more appropriate approximation is that the fetus is to at least some extent exposed to essentially all drugs taken by the mother.

As a general rule, all psychoactive drugs (and all those discussed in this book) will be present in the fetus at a concentration quite similar to that in the mother's bloodstream. However, the presence of the drug in the fetus is not necessarily detrimental to the fetus. Some drugs certainly are detrimental, and their use should be avoided in women who are or might become pregnant. Ethyl alcohol is an obvious example. Many psychoactive medicines have been shown to be relatively safe to fetal growth and development when taken by a pregnant female. The effects of specific psychoactive drugs on the fetus are discussed in Chapter 15.

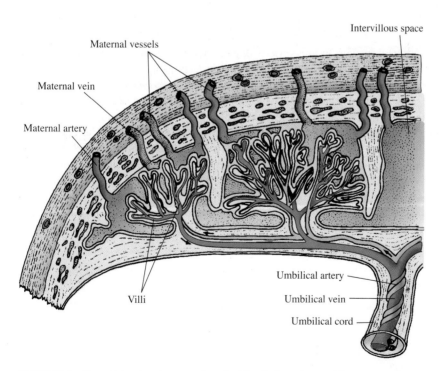

FIGURE 2.9 Placental network separating the blood of mother and fetus. Note the close relationship between fetal and maternal blood in the villus.

Termination of Drug Action

Routes through which drugs can leave the body include (1) the kidneys, (2) the lungs, (3) the bile, and (4) the skin. Excretion through the lungs occurs only with highly volatile or gaseous agents, such as the general anesthetics and, in small amounts, alcohol ("alcohol breath"). Drugs that are passed through the bile and into the intestine are usually reabsorbed into the bloodstream from the intestine. Also, small amounts of a few drugs can pass through the skin and be excreted in sweat (perhaps 10 percent to 15 percent of the total amount of the drugs). However, most drugs leave the body in urine, either as the unchanged molecule or as a broken-down *metabolite* of the original drug. More correctly, *the major route of drug elimination from the body is renal (urinary) excretion of drug metabolites produced by the hepatic (liver) biodegradation of the drug.*[2]

Psychoactive drugs are usually too lipid soluble to be excreted passively with the excretion of urine. They have to be transformed into metabolites that are more water soluble, bulkier, less lipid soluble, and (usually) less biologically active (even inactive) when compared with the parent molecule (the molecule that was originally ingested and absorbed).[3] Thus, for a lipid-soluble drug to be eliminated, it must be metabolically transformed (by enzymes located in the liver) into a form that can be excreted rapidly and reliably.

Role of the Kidneys in Drug Elimination

Physiologically, our kidneys perform two major functions. First, they excrete most of the products of body metabolism; second, they closely regulate the levels of most of the substances found in body fluids. The kidneys are a pair of bean-shaped organs that lie at the rear of the abdominal cavity at the level of the lower ribs. The outer portion of the kidney is made up of more than a million functional units, called *nephrons* (Figure 2.10). Each nephron consists of a knot of capillaries (the *glomerulus*) through which blood flows from the renal artery to the renal vein. The glomerulus is surrounded by the opening of the nephron (*Bowman's capsule*), into which fluid flows as it filters out of the capillaries. Pressure of the blood in the glomerulus causes fluid to leave the capillaries and flow into the Bowman's capsule, from which it flows through the tubules of the nephrons into a duct that collects fluid from several nephrons. The fluid from the collecting ducts is eventually passed through the ureters and into the urinary bladder, which is emptied periodically.

In an adult, about 1 liter (1000 cubic centimeters) of plasma is filtered into the nephrons of the kidneys each minute. Left behind in the bloodstream are blood cells,

---

[2] When evaluating urine for the presence of drugs of abuse, it is the inactive drug metabolites rather than the active drug, which are in the urine. It is often unclear whether there is a correlation between the presence of the metabolite in urine and active drug in plasma *at the time the urine sample was taken.*

[3] Some drugs are exceptions: an administered drug may be metabolized into an "active" metabolite, which is at least as active and possibly more active and may have a longer duration of action than the parent drug. Examples in psychopharmacology include diazepam (Valium; see Chapter 13), which is metabolized to nordiazepam, and fluoxetine (Prozac; see Chapter 12), which is metabolized to norfluoxetine. In both cases, the parent drug has an effect that lasts for two or three days, while the metabolite is active for over a week, until it is eventually biotransformed to an inactive compound that can be excreted.

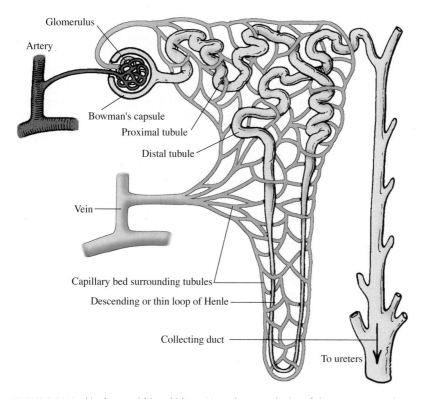

Glomerulus

Artery

Bowman's capsule

Proximal tubule

Distal tubule

Vein

Capillary bed surrounding tubules

Descending or thin loop of Henle

Collecting duct

To ureters

FIGURE 2.10 Nephron within a kidney. Note the complexity of the structure and the intimate relation between the blood supply and the nephron. Each kidney is composed of more than a million nephrons.

plasma proteins, and the remaining plasma. As the filtered fluid (water) flows through the nephrons, most of it is reabsorbed into the plasma. By the time fluid reaches the collecting ducts and bladder, only 0.1 percent remains to be excreted. Because about 1 cubic centimeter per minute of urine is formed, 99.9 percent of filtered fluid is therefore reabsorbed.

Lipid-soluble drugs can easily cross the membranes of renal tubular cells, and they are reabsorbed along with the 99.9 percent of reabsorbed water. Drug reabsorption occurs passively, along a developing concentration gradient—the drug becomes concentrated inside the nephrons (as a result of water reabsorption), and the drugs are themselves reabsorbed with water back into plasma. Thus, the kidneys alone are not capable of eliminating most psychoactive drugs from the body; some other mechanism must overcome this process of passive renal reabsorption of the drug.

Role of the Liver in Drug Metabolism

The reabsorbed drug is eventually picked up by liver cells (*hepatocytes*) and enzymatically biotransformed (by enzymes located in these hepatocytes) into metabolites that are usually less fat soluble, less capable of being reabsorbed, and therefore capable of being excreted in urine. As the drug is carried to the liver (by blood flowing in the hepatic artery and portal vein), a portion is cleared from blood by the hepatocytes and metabolized to by-products that are then returned to the bloodstream (Figure 2.11). The metabolites are then carried in the bloodstream to the kidneys, are filtered into the renal tubules, and are poorly reabsorbed, remaining in the urine for excretion. Mechanisms involved in drug metabolism by hepatocytes are complex, but they have gained increased importance in psychopharmacology, especially because of the increasing number of prescription medications, OTC substances, and supplements being taken by consumers, which can potentially cause many complications from drug-drug interactions.

The *cytochrome P450 enzyme family,* physically located in hepatocytes (with a few located in the cells lining the GI tract), is the major system involved in drug metabolism. This gene family originated more than 3.5 billion years ago and has diversified to accomplish the metabolism (detoxification) of environmental chemicals, food toxins, and drugs. Thus, the cytochrome P450 enzyme system (of which hundreds exist and about 50 of which are functionally active in humans) can detoxify a chemically diverse group of substances. Several P450 enzyme families can be found within any given hepatocyte.

A few of these enzyme families, particularly cytochrome families 1, 2, and 3 (designated *CYP-1, CYP-2,* and *CYP-3*), encode enzymes involved in most drug biotransformations. By definition, because these three families promote the breakdown of numerous drugs and toxins, enzyme specificity is low (the enzymes are nonspecific in action). Thus, the body is enzymatically capable of metabolizing many different drugs. CYP-3A4 (a subfamily of CYP-3) catalyzes about 50 percent of drug biotransformations (Figure 2.12);

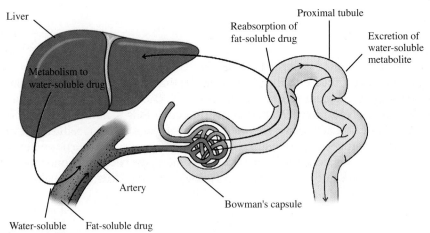

FIGURE 2.11 How the liver and kidneys interact to eliminate drugs from the body. Drugs may be filtered into the kidney, reabsorbed into the bloodstream, and carried to the liver for metabolic transformation to a more water-soluble compound. When the metabolite is filtered into the kidney, it cannot be reabsorbed and is therefore excreted in urine.

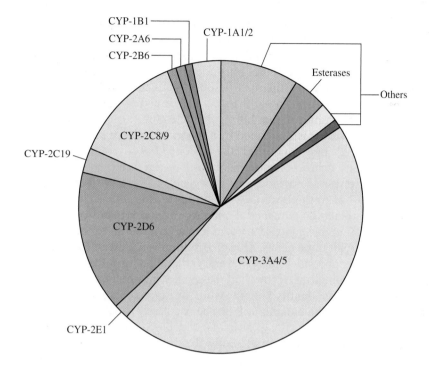

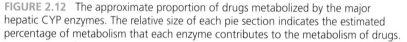

FIGURE 2.12 The approximate proportion of drugs metabolized by the major hepatic CYP enzymes. The relative size of each pie section indicates the estimated percentage of metabolism that each enzyme contributes to the metabolism of drugs.

this variant is found not only in the liver but also in the GI tract, as we saw with the metabolism of buspirone. CYP-2D6 catalyzes about 20 percent of drugs, and CYP-2C variants catalyze an additional 20 percent. Other CYP enzyme variants are responsible for metabolizing the remaining 10 percent of drugs. Even though this may seem like a small proportion, the metabolic effects can be significant, especially considering the various different versions or polymorphisms of the enzymes that can occur genetically. Zanger and Klein (2013), for example, review the pharmacological consequences of the polymorphisms in only one enzyme, CYP-2B6. Stingl and colleagues (2013) update current evidence regarding the effect of different versions of drug-metabolizing enzymes on drug exposure and how testing for these different versions might be clinically useful.

Factors Affecting Drug Biotransformation

Several different factors can alter the rate at which drugs are metabolized, either increasing or decreasing the rate of drug elimination from the body. In general, *genetic, environmental, cultural,* and *physiological factors* are the most relevant.

First, it is now becoming apparent that genetic variations may affect how different people respond to medications. Genetic DNA testing can now identify how a person may metabolize several drugs of different therapeutic classes, including antidepressants, analgesics, and antipsychotics. In general, DNA testing using a simple mouth swab can identify whether a person is a normal metabolizer of a specific drug, a slow metabolizer, or a fast metabolizer. Results provide a scientific basis for understanding why a person might have an unexpectedly toxic reaction after therapeutic doses of a drug or, on the other hand, might fail to respond to what was thought to be a therapeutic dose (Table 2.2). There are currently a number of companies that offer genetic testing.

One example of these developments is illustrated by a report by Villagra and colleagues (2011). These researchers analyzed (they genotyped) the DNA of 1199 psychiatric patients. They found a total of 30 variations, called polymorphisms, among the three genes that code for the enzymes CYP-2C9 (there were 5 variations of this gene), CYP-2C19 (there were 7 variations of this gene) and CYP-2D6 (there were 18 variations of this gene). Their results showed that among the 1199 patients, 7.4 percent did not have variations in any of the three genes; 41 percent had a variation in one gene; 45 percent had a variation in two genes; and 6.6 percent carried a variation in all three genes. This distribution is shown in Figure 2.13. Using this information, the researchers developed several indices, or formulas, to predict how people might metabolize certain drugs if they had these different versions of the genes. By using these methods, they hope to identify patients who, for example, are poor metabolizers, or ultrarapid metabolizers, so the patients will not be needlessly exposed to inappropriate drugs that will produce serious side effects, or inadequate blood levels.

Second, if more than one drug is present in the body, the drugs may interact with one another either in a therapeutically beneficial way or in a way that can adversely affect the patient. Beneficially, two drugs can have additive therapeutic effects; for example, improving antidepressant or antianxiety treatment. In the liver, however, one drug can either increase or reduce the rate of metabolism of a second drug, reducing or increasing the blood level of the second drug. For example, *carbamazepine* (Tegretol; see Chapter 14) is particularly

TABLE 2.2 Significance of genetic testing in the determination of drug dosage for an antidepressant

	Normal metabolizer	Slow metabolizer	Fast metabolizer
Genetic variation	Your genes produce a typical amount of enzyme.	Your genes produce too little enzyme.	Your genes produce too much enzyme.
Effects on you	The antidepressant helps your depression and causes few side effects.	The antidepressant builds up in your body, causing intolerable side effects.	The antidepressant is eliminated too quickly, providing little or no improvement in depression.
Treatment options	Follow the recommended dosage.	Switch antidepressants or reduce your dosage.	Switch antidepressants or increase your dosage.

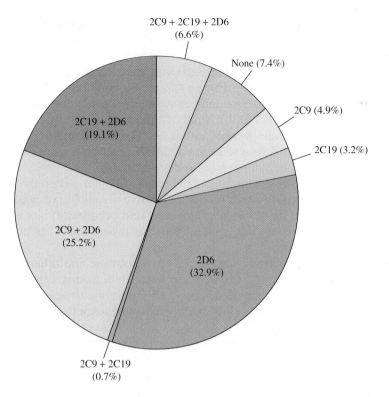

FIGURE 2.13 Combinations of genetic polymorphisms in the *CYP-2C9*, *CYP-2C19* and *CYP-2D6* genes from a population of 1199 psychiatric patients. [Data from Villagra et al., 2011, Figure 1, p. 15.] The graph shows the percent of patients that had a variation in none, one, two or all three genes that code for the three enzymes.

effective in stimulating the production of the drug-metabolizing enzyme CYP-3A3/4 in the liver (a process called *enzyme induction*), inducing an apparent *metabolic tolerance* to other drugs metabolized by CYP-3A3/4. In essence, in the presence of carbamazepine, the rate at which all drugs metabolized by the CYP-3A3/4 enzymes increases. Therefore, metabolic drug *tolerance* develops as the blood level of drug falls more rapidly than would be expected if tolerance had not developed. Thus, increasing doses of a drug must be administered to maintain the same level of drug in the plasma and to produce the same effect as previously administered smaller doses. One consequence of this development of *metabolic tolerance* is that any other drug that is metabolized by the same enzyme will also be broken down more rapidly. In essence, the second drug becomes less effective because it is metabolized more rapidly as a result of the increased amount of metabolic enzyme. As a result, those drugs will also exert less of an effect, a phenomenon termed *cross-tolerance*.

In contrast to carbamazepine (which increases the rate of metabolism of other drugs), some psychoactive drugs *depress* the activity of the CYP enzyme that metabolizes other drugs metabolized by the same enzyme. This process *increases* the blood level of the other drugs and unexpectedly increases their toxicity. For example, antidepressants that are selective serotonin reuptake inhibitors (SSRIs), such as fluoxetine (Prozac; see Chapter 12), inhibit several metabolic enzymes, increasing the toxicity of several other types of antidepressants and certain antipsychotic drugs. This may occur, for example, when an SSRI is given to a person with schizophrenia, to treat obsessive-compulsive symptoms, and who is taking the antipsychotic drug clozapine. By inhibiting the enzymes that metabolize clozapine, the blood level of clozapine may rise, increasing the risk of seizures and other adverse effects (Andrade, 2012b). Similarly, the antibipolar drug *valproic acid* (see Chapter 14) inhibits the metabolism of lamotrigine (Lamictal, another antibipolar drug), increasing the plasma level of lamotrigine and thus potentially increasing its toxicity. Such drug interactions have been known to produce fatalities.

As an interesting aside, the pain-relieving drug codeine (see Chapter 10) needs to be metabolized by CYP-2D6 into morphine, which is codeine's active metabolite responsible for its analgesic effect. Some SSRIs (for example, fluoxetine and paroxetine) block this metabolic conversion of codeine to morphine, and for patients taking SSRIs codeine is ineffective as a pain-relieving agent.

The vast increase in the number of new drugs, both psychotropic and other medications, during the last two decades has increased the number of combinations and the likelihood of drug-drug interactions. Computer programs are now available to help detect and prevent dangerous combinations. Fortunately, not all interactions are common, clinically significant, or dangerous. Demler (2012) summarizes some of the most frequent interactions relating to drug absorption, metabolism, distribution, and elimination, as well as interactions that occur from psychodynamic reactions (see Chapter 3). One interaction that might be worth noting is that between lithium and nonsteroidal anti-inflammatory drugs (NSAIDs). NSAIDS cause a decrease in the renal elimination of lithium and may produce a dangerous increase in lithium blood levels and toxicity. Preskorn and Flockhart (2009) reviewed psychiatric drug interactions and Carlat (2011) provides a very clear overview of pharmacokinetic interactions among commonly prescribed psychiatric drugs.

In addition to prescription drugs, combinations of drugs with herbs and dietary supplements (HDS) can also increase the risk of adverse reactions. It has been estimated that more than 50 percent of patients with chronic disorders use HDS, and that nearly 20 percent of patients take these products together with prescription medications. Tsai et al. (2012) provide an extensive review of such combinations. Most of the documented interactions involved medications that affect the central nervous system and the cardiovascular system. The most frequent adverse interactions involved diseases of the GI tract (16.4 percent), neurological systems (14.5 percent), and the renal/genitourinary system (12.5 percent). They provide an extensive table categorizing these interactions and possible adverse reactions.

Not all psychoactive medications are metabolized by the CYP liver enzymes. Several newer psychotropic medications are not. Moreover, some drugs may have active metabolites that are not further metabolized by this system. Such drugs may be useful in situations in which the normal metabolic enzyme systems are compromised. Examples of this are patients who have liver disease, are rapid metabolizers, or have induced enzymes (such as heavy cigarette smokers). A list of common psychotropic drugs that are not (or are minimally) metabolized by the CYP liver enzymes is shown in Table 2.3 (Andrade, 2012a).

TABLE 2.3 Some neuropsychopharmacologic agents that are not metabolized or are minimally metabolized by CYP enzymes in the liver

Anxiolytics
  Pregabalin
  Lorazepam
Antidepressants
  Milnacipran
  Desvenlafaxine
  Low doses of amisulpride, sulpiride, and levosulpiride
Antipsychotics
  Paliperidone
  High doses of amisulpride, sulpiride, and levosulpiride
Anticonvulsants and mood stabilizers
  Gabapentin
  Levetiracetam
  Lithium
  Lamotrigine
Dementia treatment
  Memantine

From Andrade, C. "Drugs That Escape Hepatic Metabolism." *Journal of Clinical Psychiatry,* Vol. 73, pp. e889-e890, 2012. Copyright © 2012, Physicians Postgraduate Press. Reprinted by permission.

Other Routes of Drug Elimination

Other routes for excreting drugs include the air we exhale, bile, sweat, saliva, and breast milk. Many drugs and drug metabolites may be found in these secretions, but their concentrations are usually low, and these routes are not usually considered primary paths of drug elimination. Perhaps clinically significant, however, is the transfer of psychoactive drugs (such as nicotine) from mothers to their breast-fed babies (see Chapter 15).

Time Course of Drug Distribution and Elimination: Concept of Drug Half-Life

Knowledge about the relationship between the time course of drug action in the body and its pharmacological effects is essential for (1) predicting the optimal dosages and dose intervals needed to reach a therapeutic effect, (2) maintaining a therapeutic drug level for the desired period of time, and (3) determining the time needed to eliminate the drug. The relationship between the pharmacological response to a drug and its concentration in blood is fundamental to pharmacology. With psychoactive drugs, the level of drug in the blood closely approximates the level of drug at the drug's site of action in the brain.

Figure 2.14 illustrates the time-concentration relationship for a drug that is injected intravenously and therefore reaches peak plasma concentration immediately. For our purposes, intravenous injection removes the variability involved with oral absorption and

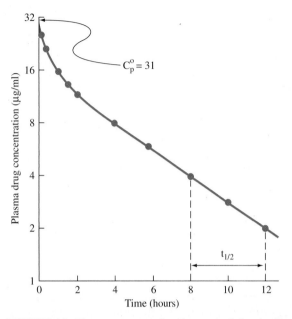

FIGURE 2.14   Plasma concentration time curve following intravenous injection of a drug. In this example, drug concentrations are measured in plasma every 30 minutes for the first 2 hours following drug injection, then every 2 hours until 12 hours after injection. Over the first 2 hours, redistribution occurs as the drug leaves plasma and enters body tissues and equilibrates with those tissues. After redistribution, the fall in plasma level is linear, exhibiting a metabolic half-life of 4 hours, regardless of the plasma concentration of the drug.

slow attainment of peak blood levels. Note that after the immediate peak in the plasma concentration, the concentration appears to fall very rapidly, followed by a slower decline in concentration. The rapid fall reflects the rapid redistribution of the drug out of the bloodstream into body tissues. This process of *redistribution* takes only minutes to spread a drug nearly equally throughout the major tissues of the body. The upper left portion of the curve in Figure 2.14 represents this rapid-distribution phase, which lasts only a few minutes. The shallower part of the curve represents the slower, prolonged decrease in the level of drug in the blood required for the body to detoxify the drug by hepatic metabolism. (The plasma concentration of the drug metabolites is not illustrated.) The calculated elimination half-life is a measure of this process, and it allows the time course of drug action to be determined.

Figure 2.14 shows that the elimination half-life of the drug (the time for the blood level to fall from 4 microg/ml to 2 microg/ml) is about 4 hours. The 4-hour half-life then remains constant over time. In other words, it takes the same amount of time for the blood level to fall from 8 microg/ml to 4 microg/ml as it does to fall from 4 microg/ml to 2 microg/ml or from 2 microg/ml to 1 microg/ml. Thus, although a different absolute amount of drug is metabolized within each half-life, the time interval remains constant.

TABLE 2.4 Half-life calculations

	Amount of drug in the body	
Number of half-lives	Percent eliminated	Percent remaining
0	0	100
1	50	50
2	75	25
3	87.5	12.5
4	93.8	6.2
5	96.9	3.1
6	98.4	1.6

The knowledge of a drug's half-life is important because it tells us how long a drug remains in the body. As shown in Table 2.4, it takes four half-lives for 94 percent of a drug to be eliminated by the body and six half-lives for 98 percent of the drug to be eliminated. At that point, a person is, for most practical purposes, drug free. It is important to remember that even though the blood level of the drug is reduced by 75 percent after two half-lives, the drug persists in the body at low levels for at least six half-lives. The so-called drug hangover is a result.

Throughout this book, drug half-lives are cited to describe the duration of action of psychoactive drugs in the body and allow comparisons between drugs with similar actions but differing half-lives. Most drug half-lives are measured in hours; others are measured in days; and recovery from the drug may take a week or more. For example, the elimination half-life of diazepam (Valium; see Chapter 13) is about 30 hours in a healthy young adult, much longer in the elderly. The half-life of its active metabolite is even longer, on the order of several days to a week. The elderly exhibit even more prolongation of the half-lives of both diazepam and nordiazepam; the duration of action can be four weeks or even longer.

Note that drug half-life is the *time* for the plasma level of drug to fall by 50 percent. Thus, half-life is independent of the absolute level of drug in blood: the level falls by 50 percent every half-life, regardless of how many molecules of drug were actually metabolized during that time. In such cases, called *first-order elimination* (or *kinetics*), the metabolism rate of the drug is a constant fraction of the drug remaining in the body, rather than a constant amount of drug per hour. Therefore, a varying amount of drug is metabolized with each half-life (fewer actual molecules are metabolized per half-life as the plasma level of drug falls).

One of the rare exceptions to this concept is the metabolism of ethyl alcohol by the enzyme alcohol dehydrogenase. In that case, a constant amount of alcohol is metabolized per hour, usually, about 10 cubic centimeters (cc) of absolute alcohol regardless of the absolute amount of alcohol present in blood, and the blood level falls in a straight line. (The metabolism of alcohol is discussed in Chapter 5.) This type of metabolism is called *zero-order elimination* (or *kinetics*).

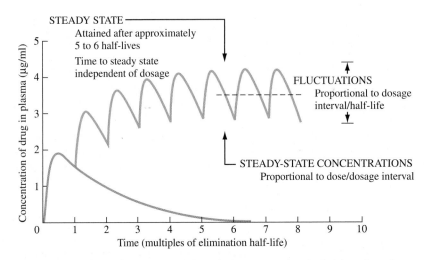

FIGURE 2.15 Plasma drug concentrations during repeated oral administration of a drug at intervals equal to its elimination half-life. The orange curve illustrates elimination if only a single dose is given. Because only 50 percent of each dose is eliminated before the next dose is given, the drug accumulates, reaching steady-state concentration in five to six half-lives. The sinusoidal curve shows the maximal and minimal drug concentrations at the beginning and end of each dosage interval, respectively. The light dashed line illustrates the average concentration achieved at steady state.

Drug Half-Life, Accumulation, and Steady State

The biological half-life of a drug is not only the time required for the drug concentration in blood to fall by one-half; it also determines the length of time necessary to reach a plateau, or *steady-state concentration* (Figure 2.15). If a second full dose of drug is administered before the body has eliminated the first dose, the total amount of drug in the body and the peak level of the drug in the blood will be greater than the total amount and peak level produced by the first dose. For example, if 100 milligrams (mg) of a drug with a 4-hour half-life were administered at 12 noon, 50 mg of drug would remain in the body at 4 P.M. If an additional 100 mg of the drug were then taken at 4 P.M., 75 mg of drug would remain in the body at 8 P.M. (25 mg of the first dose and 50 mg of the second). If this administration schedule were continued, the amount of drug in the body would continue to increase until a plateau (steady-state) concentration was reached.

In general, the time to reach *steady-state concentration* (the level of drug achieved in the blood with repeated, regular-interval dosing) is about six times the drug's elimination half-life and is independent of the actual dosage of the drug. In one half-life, a drug reaches 50 percent of the concentration that will eventually be achieved. After two half-lives, the drug achieves 75 percent concentration; at three half-lives, the drug achieves the initial 50 percent of the third dose, the next 25 percent from the second dose, plus half of the remaining 25 percent from the first dose. At 98.4 percent (the concentration achieved after six half-lives), the drug concentration is essentially at steady state. This is the rationale behind the general rule. The steady-state concentration is achieved when the amount administered per unit time equals the amount eliminated per unit time. The interdependent variables that determine the ultimate concentration (or steady-state blood level of drug) are the dose (which determines the blood level but not the time to steady state), the dose interval, the half-life of the drug, and other more complex factors that can affect drug elimination.

In summary, steady, regular-interval dosing leads to a predictable accumulation, with a steady-state concentration reached after about six half-lives, which is proportional to dose and dosage interval. Clinically, these factors guide drug therapy when blood levels of the drug are monitored and correlated with therapeutic results.

Therapeutic Drug Monitoring

Therapeutic drug monitoring (TDM) can aid a clinician in making critical decisions in therapeutic applications. The basic principle underlying TDM is that a threshold plasma concentration of a drug is needed at the receptor site to initiate and maintain a pharmacological response. Critically important is that plasma concentrations of psychoactive drugs correlate well with tissue or receptor concentrations. Therefore, TDM is an indirect, although usually quite accurate, measurement of drug concentration at the receptor site. To make the correlation between TDM, dosage, and therapeutic response, large-scale clinical trials are performed, and blood samples are drawn at several time periods during both acute (short-term) and chronic (long-term) therapy. Statistical correlation is made between the level of drug in plasma and the degree of therapeutic response. A dosage regimen can then be designed to achieve the appropriate blood level of a drug. A well-defined range of blood levels associated with optimal clinical response is called the *therapeutic window*. The important point is that levels either below *or above* that range are associated with a poor response. Figure 2.16A illustrates the concept of the therapeutic window and Figure 2.16B shows an example of the effective blood level range for the decrease in symptoms of the antipsychotic haloperidol.

The goals of TDM are many. One goal is to assess whether a patient is taking medication as prescribed; if plasma levels of the drug are below the therapeutic level because the patient has not been taking the required medication, therapeutic results will be poor. Another goal is to avoid toxicity; if plasma levels of the drug are above the therapeutic level, the dosage can be lowered, effectiveness maintained, and toxicity minimized. A third goal is to enhance therapeutic response by focusing not on the amount of drug taken but on the measured amount of drug in the plasma. Other goals include possible reductions in the cost of therapy (since a patient's illness is better controlled) and the substantiation of the need for unusually high doses in patients who require higher-than-normal intake of prescribed medication to maintain a therapeutic blood level of a drug.

As a recent example, Sparshatt and coworkers (2010) related the dose, plasma concentrations, receptor binding, and clinical response for the antipsychotic aripiprazole (see Chapter 11).

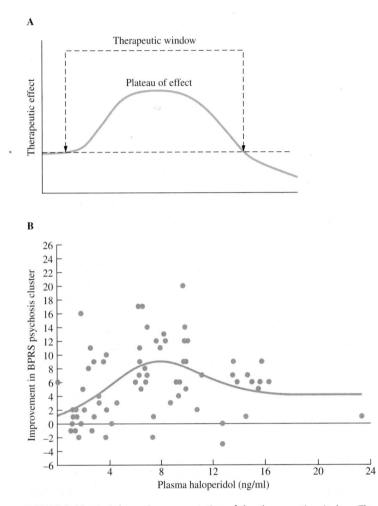

FIGURE 2.16 **A.** Schematic representation of the therapeutic window. The relationship between the therapeutic effect and the drug dose is in the shape of an "inverted U." That is, after the therapeutic effect reaches a plateau, an increase in dose does not produce further improvement, but may actually decrease the drug's effectiveness. **B.** Example of the therapeutic window, showing improvement (of psychotic symptoms) as the plasma level of the antipsychotic drug haloperidol increases, followed by a decrease if the concentration continues to rise. [Data from Van Putten et al., 1991, Figure 1, p. 202.]

Drug Tolerance and Dependence

Drug tolerance is defined as a state of progressively decreasing responsiveness to the same dose of a drug. A person who develops tolerance requires a larger dose of the drug to achieve the effect originally obtained by a smaller dose. At least three mechanisms are involved in the development of drug tolerance—two are pharmacological mechanisms; one is a behavioral mechanism.

In *metabolic tolerance,* the first of the two types of pharmacological tolerance, more enzyme is available to metabolize a drug as a result of *enzyme induction.* This means that more drug must be administered to maintain the same concentration in the body and the same therapeutic response. *Cellular-adaptive,* or *pharmacodynamic, tolerance* is the second type of pharmacological tolerance. Receptors in the brain adapt to the continued presence of the drug, with neurons adapting to excess drug either by reducing the number of receptors available to the drug or by reducing their sensitivity to the drug. Such reduction in numbers or sensitivity is termed *down regulation,* and higher levels of drug are necessary to maintain the same biological effect (see Chapter 3).

Behavioral conditioning processes mediate the third type of drug tolerance. Neither enzyme induction nor receptor down regulation can account for the substantial degree of tolerance that many people acquire to opioids, ethyl alcohol, and other drugs. Instead, such tolerance develops when a drug is consistently administered in the context of predictable predrug cues and not in the context of alternative cues. In such situations, environmental cues routinely paired with drug administration will become conditioned stimuli that elicit a conditioned response that is opposite in direction to or compensation for the direct effects of the drug. Over conditioning trials, the compensatory conditioned response grows in magnitude and counteracts the direct drug effects; that is, tolerance develops.

Physical dependence is an entirely different phenomenon from tolerance, even though the two are often associated temporally. A person who is physically dependent needs the drug to avoid the withdrawal symptoms that occur if the drug is not taken. The state is revealed by withdrawing the drug and noting the occurrence of physical reactions and/or psychological changes (withdrawal symptoms). These changes are referred to as an *abstinence syndrome.* Readministering the drug can relieve the symptoms of withdrawal.

Because physical dependence is often seen after abstinence from drugs of abuse such as alcohol and heroin, the term has been linked with "addiction," implying that withdrawal signs are "bad" and observed only with drugs of abuse. This conclusion is incorrect; withdrawal signs can follow cessation of such therapeutic drugs as the SSRI type of clinical antidepressants (see Chapter 12).[4] In this situation, the phenomenon is more accurately referred to as a discontinuation syndrome. The occurrence of withdrawal signs after drug removal is not necessarily a sign of the drug "addiction" that is usually associated with "bad" drugs such as heroin. Rather, physical dependence is an indication that brain and body functions were altered by the presence of a drug and that a different homeostatic state must be initiated when drug use is discontinued. It takes time (from a few days to about two weeks) for the brain and the body to adapt to the new state of equilibrium without the drug.

---

[4] Discontinuation of SSRI-type antidepressants is followed in many patients by reactions that can be organized into five symptom categories: (1) disequilibrium (dizziness, vertigo, ataxia); (2) GI symptoms (nausea, vomiting); (3) flulike symptoms (fatigue, lethargy, myalgias, chills); (4) sensory disturbances (paresthesias, sensation of electric shocks); and (5) sleep disturbances (insomnia, vivid dreams).

STUDY QUESTIONS

1. What is meant by the term *pharmacokinetics*?

2. Why must a psychoactive drug be altered metabolically in the body before it can be excreted?

3. Discuss the advantages and disadvantages of the various methods of administering drugs.

4. Discuss the blood-brain barrier as a limitation to drug transport.

5. Describe the role of the liver and the hepatic enzyme system in drug metabolism.

6. Define *half-life*. How does *half-life* apply to steady state? If a drug has an elimination half-life of 6 hours, how long does it take for the drug to be essentially eliminated from the body after administration of a single dose?

7. What is meant by the terms *therapeutic drug monitoring* and *therapeutic window*? In what instances might they be useful?

8. What is drug tolerance and why does it occur?

REFERENCES

Andrade, C. (2012a). "Drugs That Escape Hepatic Metabolism." *Journal of Clinical Psychiatry* 73: e889–e890.

Andrade, C. (2012b). "Serotonin Reuptake Inhibitor Treatment of Obsessive-Compulsive Symptoms in Clozapine-Medicated Schizophrenia." *Journal of Clinical Psychiatry* 73: e1362–e1364.

Bailey, D. G., et al. (2012). "Grapefruit-Medication Interactions: Forbidden Fruit or Avoidable Consequences?" *Canadian Medical Association Journal* DOI: 10.1503/cmaj.120951.

Carlat, D. (2011). "Drug Interactions in Psychiatry: A Practical Review." *The Carlat Psychiatry Report* 9: 1–5.

Demler, T. L. (2012). "Psychiatric Drug-Drug Interactions." *US Pharmacist* 37: HS16–HS19.

Gilstrap, L. C., and Little, B. B. (1998). *Drugs and Pregnancy,* 2nd ed. New York: Chapman & Hall.

Lilja, J. J., et al. (1998). "Grapefruit Juice Substantially Increases Plasma Concentrations of Buspirone." *Clinical Pharmacology and Therapeutics* 64: 655–660.

Oakley, R., and Ksir, C. (1996). *Drugs, Society, and Human Behavior,* 7th ed. New York: Mosby.

Paine, M. F., et al. (2006). "A Furanocoumarin-Free Grapefruit Juice Establishes Furanocoumarins as the Mediators of the Grapefruit Juice-Felodipine Interaction." *American Journal of Clinical Nutrition* 84: 1097–1105.

Pardridge, W. M. (2003). "Blood-Brain Barrier Drug Targeting: The Future of Brain Drug Development." *Molecular Interventions* 3: 90–105.

Preskorn, S. H., and Flockhart, D. (2009). "2010 Guide to Psychiatric Drug Interactions." *Primary Psychiatry* 16: 45–74.

Rheeders, M., et al. (2006). "Drug-Drug Interactions After Single Oral Doses of the Furanocoumarin Methoxsalen and Cyclosporine." *Journal of Clinical Pharmacology* 46: 768–775.

Sparshatt, A., et al. (2010) "A Systematic Review of Aripiprazole—Dose, Plasma Concentration, Receptor Occupancy, and Response: Implications for Therapeutic Drug Monitoring." *Journal of Clinical Psychiatry* 71: 1447–1456.

Stingl, J. C., et al. (2013) "Genetic Variability of Drug-Metabolizing Enzymes: The Dual Impact on Psychiatric Therapy and Regulation of Brain Function." *Molecular Psychiatry* 18: 273–287.

Tsai, H.-H., et al. (2012). "Evaluation of Documented Drug Interactions and Contraindications Associated with Herbs and Dietary Supplements." *International Journal of Clinical Practice* 66: 1056–1078.

Van Putten, T., et al. (1991). "Neuroleptic Plasma Levels." *Schizophrenia Bulletin* 17: 197–216.

Villagra, D., et al. (2011). "Novel Drug Metabolism Indices for Pharmacogenetic Functional Status Based on Combinatory Genotyping of CYP2C9, CYP2C19 and CYP2D6 Genes." *Biomarkers in Medicine* 5: 427–438.

Zanger, U. M., and Klein, K. (2013). "Pharmacogenetics of Cytochrome P450 2B6 (CYP2B6): Advances on Polymorphisms, Mechanisms, and Clinical Relevance." *Frontiers in GENETICS* Article 24.

Chapter 3

Pharmacodynamics: How Drugs Act

While the body is trying to rid itself of an ingested psychoactive drug, the drug is exerting effects by attaching to *receptors* in cells in both the brain and the body. As a result of the interactions, the body experiences effects that are characteristic for the drug. *It is a basic principle of pharmacology that the pharmacological, physiological, or behavioral effects induced by a drug follow from their interaction with receptors.*

The study of the interactions, termed *pharmacodynamics,* involves exploring the mechanisms of drug action that occur at the molecular level. While *pharmacokinetics* is the study of what the body does to a drug, *pharmacodynamics* is the study of what the drug does to the body.

To produce an effect, a drug must bind to and interact with specific receptors, which, in the case of psychoactive drugs, are usually located on the surface of neurons in the brain. The occupation of a receptor by a drug (termed *drug-receptor binding*) leads to a change in the functional properties of the neuron, resulting in the drug's characteristic pharmacological response. In most instances, drug-receptor binding is both *ionic* and *reversible* in nature, with positive and negative charges on various portions of the drug molecule and the receptor protein attracting one to the other. The strength of ionic attachment is determined by the fit of the three-dimensional structure of the drug to the three-dimensional site on the receptor,[1] the so-called "lock and key" relationship.

---

[1] Reversible ionic binding is contrasted with the formation of a permanent, irreversible, covalent bond between a drug and a receptor. One of the rare instances in psychopharmacology where an irreversible covalent bond forms is between certain antidepressant drugs and the enzyme monoamine oxidase (see Chapter 12).

Receptors for Drug Action

A *receptor* is a fairly large molecule (usually a protein[2]) at which endogenous transmitters or modulators produce their biological effects. Literally hundreds of different types of receptors are known and the ability to recognize one specific neurotransmitter characterizes each one. Thus, only one neurotransmitter might be specific enough to fit or bind to a specific receptor protein. For example, if only serotonin binds to a specific receptor, that protein is called a serotonin receptor. But although the receptor is specific for serotonin, serotonin, as a neurotransmitter, also binds to other, structurally different *receptor subtypes*.

To date, at least 11 (and perhaps 13 or 14) different serotonin receptor proteins have been identified (see Chapter 1).[3] This diversity makes it possible to develop closely related drugs, each with a slightly different degree of *affinity* (strength of attachment) for the different serotonin receptors. For example, a specific drug might have affinity for a serotonin 1 receptor but not for any other serotonin receptor.

A given drug may even be more specific for a given set of receptors than the endogenous neurotransmitter. Serotonin, for example, must necessarily attach to all its receptors. However, a given drug might attach to only one receptor. For example, buspirone (BuSpar) attaches to 5-HT$_{1A}$ receptors, which results in antianxiety actions. It has no affinity for other serotonin receptors.

It is also a general rule of psychopharmacology that drugs do not create any unique effects; they merely modulate normal neuronal functioning, mimicking or antagonizing the actions of a specific neurotransmitter. Drug binding may mimic or facilitate neurotransmitter action, or drug occupation of a receptor might block access of the neurotransmitter to that receptor and prevent endogenous molecules from attaching, activating, and producing an effect at these sites.

Receptor Structure

What does a receptor look like? Although there are several different configurations of proteins that may serve a receptor function, the following is a brief summary of the major types most relevant to the action of drugs.

Ion Channel Receptors. (Also called *ionotropic receptors.*) This type of membrane-spanning receptor is the kind that forms an *ion channel*. That is, the central portion of the receptor spans the membrane of the neuron and forms a pore, which enlarges when either an endogenous neurotransmitter or exogenous drug attaches to the receptor-binding site. The attachment allows flow of a specific *ion* (such as chloride ions) through the enlarged pore (see Figure 3.1A). (It should be noted that, in some cases, the pore is normally open, and the attachment of a drug or transmitter will close it. Although such situations are beyond the scope of this text, the general phenomenon is the same.)

As shown in Figure 3.1B, the ionotropic receptor is composed of five sections, or subunits, each of which crosses the cell membrane. Each of these sections is labeled, usually

---

[2] A protein is a complex chain of various amino acids, functioning, among other things, as metabolic enzymes and receptors.

[3] Each receptor protein that binds serotonin, for example, has a slightly different amino acid composition; nevertheless, their three-dimensional structures are similar enough that serotonin, for example, still fits a "slot" (like a lock-and-key arrangement) and ionically binds to the protein.

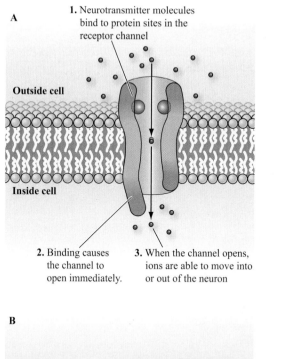

A

1. Neurotransmitter molecules bind to protein sites in the receptor channel

Outside cell

Inside cell

2. Binding causes the channel to open immediately.

3. When the channel opens, ions are able to move into or out of the neuron

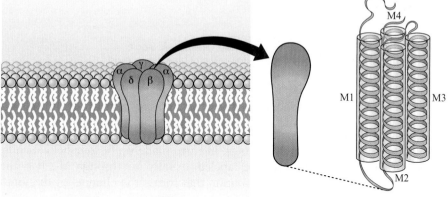

B

M4

M1   M3

M2

FIGURE 3.1   **A.** Schematic of neurotransmitter activation of an ionotropic receptor that contains an ion channel. **B.** Detailed schematic representation of the individual subunits of an ion channel (ionotropic) receptor, showing the helical coils of which they are composed. [Part A after Breedlove et al., 2007, Figure 3.13a, p. 79. Part B after Bear et al., 2007, Figure 6.18a, p. 153.]

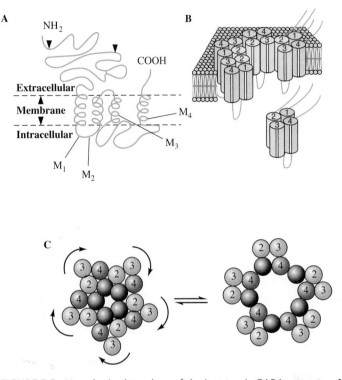

FIGURE 3.2   Hypothesized topology of the ionotropic GABA$_A$ receptor. **A.** Single subunit with its large extracellular terminal part and four transmembrane helical coils. **B.** Arrangement of the transmembrane domains of five subunits to form a central channel. **C.** Transmembrane domain in a transverse section through the membrane when the channel is closed (*left*) and open (*right*).

with a Greek letter. (If they are very similar in composition, two subunits may be given the same Greek letter.) Each of these subunits is, in turn, made up of four helical coils, which also cross the membrane and are also labeled, usually M_1 through M_4. It is the arrangement of these five transmembrane subunits that forms the channel of the ionotropic receptor, as seen in Figure 3.2.

Figures 3.2 and 3.3 illustrate how the neurotransmitter gamma aminobutyric acid (GABA) and various drugs (benzodiazepines, barbiturates) bind to the GABA$_A$ receptor and affect the inward flow of chloride ions. Benzodiazepines (see Chapter 13) serve as allosteric agonists (discussed below) by binding to a site near the GABA-binding site and by facilitating the action of GABA in increasing the flow of chloride ions into the neuron. Because chloride ions are negative, their inward flow hyperpolarizes the neuron and inhibits neuronal function. This action underlies the use of benzodiazepines as sedative, antianxiety, amnestic, and antiepileptic agents.[4]

---

[4] Several other substances, such as barbiturates, also have binding sites on the GABA receptor complex, shown in Figure 3.3. Barbiturates (see Chapter 5) act like benzodiazepines in increasing the effect of GABA on the chloride channel within the GABA receptor. Thus, with a site and mechanism of action similar to that exerted by benzodiazepines, the two classes of drugs might be expected to demonstrate similar clinical and behavioral effects. In general, they do.

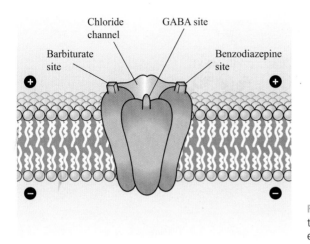

FIGURE 3.3 Schematic of the GABA$_A$ receptor, with its binding sites for GABA, benzodiazepines, and barbiturates.

G-Protein-Coupled Receptors. The second type of membrane-spanning receptor protein is called a *G-protein-coupled receptor.* These receptors are also called *metabotropic* receptors (see Figure 3.4). The activation of these receptors induces the release of an attached intracellular protein (a *G protein*) that, in turn, controls enzymatic functions within the postsynaptic neuron.

G-protein-coupled receptors (sometimes abbreviated as GPCRs) are discussed throughout this book because they mediate the synaptic effects of many neurotransmitters that are involved in the action of psychoactive drugs. The molecular structure of G-protein-coupled receptors consists of a single protein chain of 400 to 500 amino acids arranged as seven transmembrane alpha helices (see Figures 3.4 and 3.5). The endogenous neurotransmitter

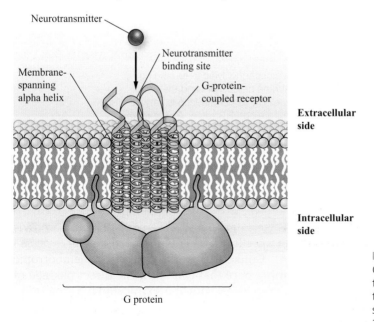

FIGURE 3.4 Schematic of a G-protein-coupled (metabotropic) receptor (GPCR), showing the seven helical, membrane-spanning coils. [After Bear et al., 2007, Figure 6.23, p. 158.]

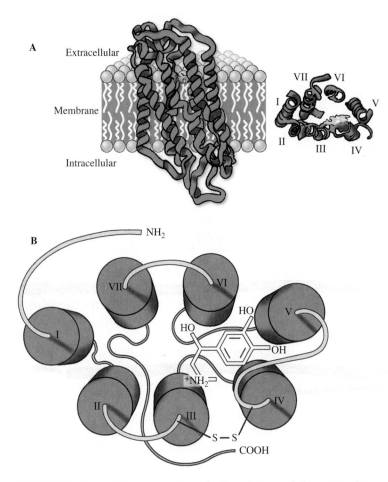

FIGURE 3.5 Schematic representation of a G-protein-coupled transmembrane receptor, with a molecule of neurotransmitter (norepinephrine) lying in its binding site. Note the arrangement of the seven transmembrane helical coils and the site of the transmitter attachment deep within the structure. The ionic interactions between the transmitter and particular amino acid side chains are not illustrated. **A.** The membrane and continuous coils. **B.** The helical coils are represented as cylinders with the molecule of norepinephrine interacting with four of the coils.

(and presumably drugs also) attaches inside the space between these coils (see Figure 3.5) and is held in place by ionic attractions.

G-protein-coupled receptors constitute a large and diverse family of proteins whose primary function is to change extracellular stimuli (transmitters and drugs) into intracellular signals (see Figure 3.6). Unlike ionotropic receptors, metabotropic receptors do not form a membrane-spanning pore that can allow the direct passage of ions. Instead, when a neurotransmitter associates with the extracellular recognition (binding) site the G protein is activated and, either *directly* (see Figure 3.6) or *indirectly*

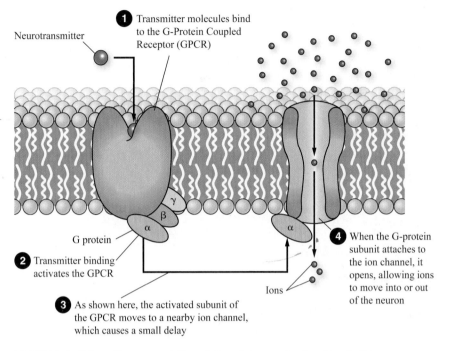

FIGURE 3.6 Schematic representation of G-protein-receptor function. In this situation the ion channel is directly opened by the alpha subunit of the activated G-protein. [After Breedlove et al. (2007), p. 79, Figure 3.13b.]

(see Figure 3.7), through a series of enzymatic reactions, *opens or closes ion channels located at other places on the cell membrane*. Because the effect of metabotropic receptors is not as immediate as that of ionotropic receptors, their action is slower.

The process starts when a hormone, neurotransmitter, or drug attaches to a receptor. This changes the shape of the receptor, which then activates the three-chain G protein on the inside of the cell membrane. One component of the G protein is released and then either *directly* activates an ion channel, or the G protein moves along the membrane until it finds and then *indirectly* activates an enzyme, such as the enzyme adenylyl cyclase. In this example, the activated adenylyl cyclase then produces lots of cyclic AMP, which spreads the signal through the cell. The cyclic AMP is called the *second messenger* (the first being the neurotransmitter). The ultimate cellular response produced by this process may be the opening of ion channels, the alteration of enzyme activities, or changes in gene activation. One major advantage of this approach is that it allows the signal to be amplified; that is, a single molecule of neurotransmitter can stimulate the production of many molecules of a second messenger. By incorporating an enzyme such as adenylyl cyclase into the chain, a weak signal from outside the cell can be translated into a strong signal throughout the inside of the cell. G-protein-coupled receptors are the middlemen, able to effect communication between the neurotransmitter-receptor complex and intracellular enzymes, the *second messengers*, to produce the ultimate biological response.

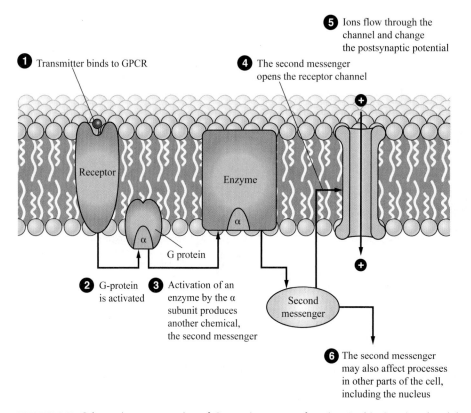

FIGURE 3.7 Schematic representation of G-protein-receptor function. In this situation the alpha subunit of the G-protein activates an enzyme, which then produces a second messenger that opens the channel, or causes other biochemical reactions. [After Carlson, 2010, Figure 2.35b, page 59.]

Furthermore, cyclic AMP is not the only second messenger known to mediate the effects of neurotransmitters. Figure 3.8 summarizes a general model of transmitter-receptor interactions and the resulting cascade of effects produced by second and, in some cases, third messengers (not shown here). Cyclic AMP is shown, associated with its enzyme, adenylyl cyclase; other second messengers are similarly indicated.

Ionotropic and (direct and indirect) metabotropic receptors are not the only receptor types important for understanding drug action. There are additional receptors that mediate the effect of hormones (steroids) and neurotrophic substances (a generic term for any of a family of substances with roles in the maintenance and survival of neurons). Two other types of proteins are also crucial to understanding psychoactive drug mechanisms.

Carrier Proteins. The third type of membrane-spanning protein is a *carrier* (or *transport*) *protein*. This type of receptor transports small organic molecules (such as neuro-transmitters) across cell membranes against concentration gradients. Most important in psychopharmacology are the *presynaptic* carrier proteins that bind dopamine, nor-epinephrine, or serotonin (and other neurotransmitters) in the synaptic cleft and trans-

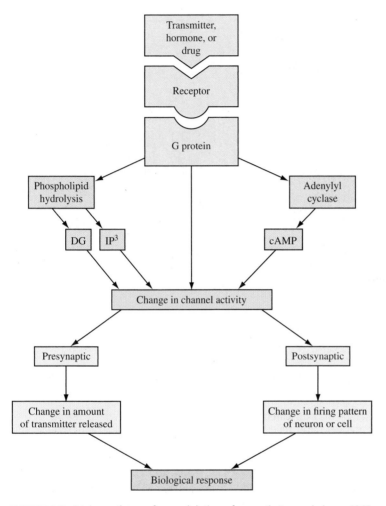

FIGURE 3.8 Major pathways for modulation of synaptic transmission. cAMP = cyclic adenosine monophosphate; IP_3 = inositol triphosphate; DG = diacylglycerol (all three substances are second messengers). [Adapted and modified after Iverson et al., 2009, Figure 4.6, p. 74.]

port them back into the presynaptic nerve terminal, terminating their synaptic action (see Chapter 1). Many drugs discussed in this book, both therapeutic and abused, exert their actions by blocking the carrier protein that is specific for transporting a specific neurotransmitter. Until recently, little was known about these transporters except that they consisted of chains of amino acids (proteins) arranged as 12 helical arrays embedded in the membrane of the presynaptic nerve terminal.

Work by Gouaux and coworkers (Yernool et al., 2004; Gouaux and MacKinnon, 2005; Armstrong et al., 2006) has added considerably to our knowledge of these transporters. To carry molecules of neurotransmitter across presynaptic membranes against a concentration gradient, the transporters are hypothesized to exist in at least three

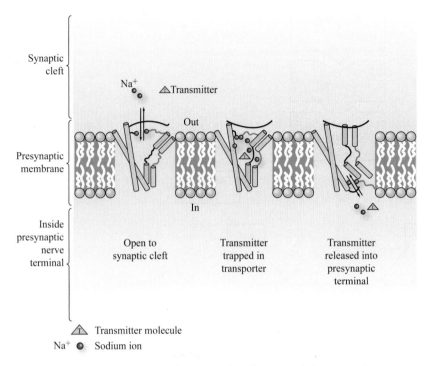

Synaptic cleft

Na$^+$

△Transmitter

Out

Presynaptic membrane

In

Inside presynaptic nerve terminal

Open to
synaptic cleft

Transmitter
trapped in
transporter

Transmitter
released into
presynaptic
terminal

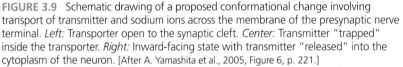

△ Transmitter molecule

Na$^+$ ● Sodium ion

FIGURE 3.9 Schematic drawing of a proposed conformational change involving transport of transmitter and sodium ions across the membrane of the presynaptic nerve terminal. *Left:* Transporter open to the synaptic cleft. *Center:* Transmitter "trapped" inside the transporter. *Right:* Inward-facing state with transmitter "released" into the cytoplasm of the neuron. [After A. Yamashita et al., 2005, Figure 6, p. 221.]

ionic states: open to the synapse, occluded with the transmitter "trapped" inside, and open to the cytoplasm of the presynaptic neuron (see Figure 3.9). The transporter has been conceived as a bowl-shaped structure with a fluid-filled basin (open to the synaptic cleft) extending halfway across the membrane of the presynaptic nerve terminal (see Figure 3.10). At the bottom of the basin are three binding sites for the neurotransmitter, each cradled by two helical "hairpins" reaching from opposite sides of the membrane. In the resting state, the bowl is open to the synaptic cleft. It traps one or more molecules of released transmitter per "cycle," allowing floods of molecules to move from the synaptic cleft into the presynaptic terminal and become available for rerelease. It is proposed that the transport of transmitter is achieved by movements of the hairpins that allow alternating access to either side of the membrane (for example, the outer layer closes, trapping the transmitter, and then the inner layer opens, ejecting the transmitter into the cytoplasm of the presynaptic terminal).

Enzymes. The fourth type of receptor protein for psychoactive drugs is *enzymes*—in particular, enzymes that regulate the synaptic availability of certain neurotransmitters. These enzymes break down neurotransmitters, and their inhibition by drugs increases

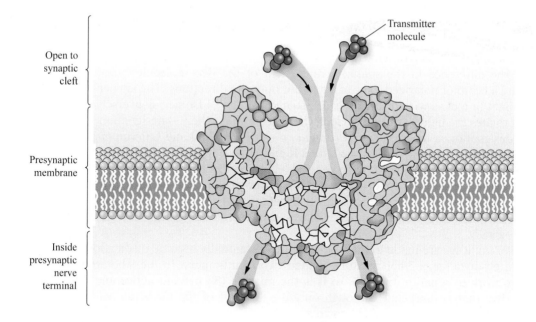

FIGURE 3.10 Schematic drawing of the proposed movement of neurotransmitter molecules through a transporter protein and into the presynaptic nerve terminal. The drawing illustrates the total movement and summarizes the three-step outline in Figure 3.9. The deep aqueous basin reaches halfway across the membrane. [Adapted after Yernool et al., 2004, Figure 2, p. 813.]

transmitter availability. Two examples are *acetylcholine esterase*, the enzyme that breaks down acetylcholine within the synaptic cleft (see Chapter 1), and *monoamine oxidase*, the enzyme that breaks down norepinephrine and dopamine in presynaptic nerve terminals, controlling the amount available for release (see Chapter 1).

Drugs known as *irreversible acetylcholine esterase inhibitors* form covalent bonds with the enzyme, preventing it from functioning, and have been used as insecticides and as lethal "nerve gases." Drugs that *reversibly* inhibit the enzyme *acetylcholine esterase* are used clinically as cognitive enhancers, delaying the progression of Alzheimer's disease (see Chapter 16). Drugs that irreversibly inhibit the enzyme *monoamine oxidase* are called monoamine oxidase inhibitors (MAOIs) and are used primarily as antidepressants (see Chapter 12). [For more advanced discussions of receptor structure and function, see Iverson and coworkers (2009) and Nestler and coworkers (2009).]

Drug-Receptor Specificity

Receptors exhibit high specificity both for one particular neurotransmitter and for certain drug molecules. Modest variations in the chemical structure of a drug may greatly alter the intensity of a receptor's response to it. One important concept in regard to drug specificity is the phenomenon of optical isomers. *Isomers* are molecules formed around a carbon atom that have the same molecular formula but have a different arrangement

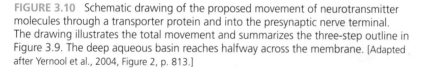

of their atoms in space. Simple substances that show optical isomerism exist as two (or more) isomers known as *enantiomers*. Isomers represent forms of a molecule that are mirror images of each other.

The difference in the spatial arrangement of the two molecules means that they rotate a beam of polarized light in equal but opposite directions. The isomer that rotates the light in a clockwise direction is designated as the (+) isomer; conversely, the isomer that rotates the light in a counterclockwise direction has the (−) designation. Sometimes the designation is made as D (*dextrorotatory*—"to the right") and L (*levorotatory*—"to the left"). Yet another system uses the letters R and S, based on the atomic numbers of molecules, and is not equivalent to the (+) and (−) nomenclatures.

In most cases only one of these optical isomers is biologically active. Therefore, when these molecules interact with a receptor, only one of the isomers would be effective. In other words, optical isomers behave the same way chemically but not biologically.

When drugs are made in the laboratory, and eventually become medications, they are often produced as a 50/50 mixture of their two enantiomers. In the laboratory, it takes more work to separate the two, so it is the mixture (50 percent active and 50 percent inactive) that is marketed, although only the (−) half of the medicine will be biologically active in the body. This is known as a *racemic mixture* or *racemate*. Most medicines are manufactured as racemates. However, sometimes an isomer is also produced. An example is the antidepressant citalopram. This is the racemate version, marketed as the antidepressant Celexa. When the patent on the racemate expired, the active isomer was separated out and is marketed as escitalopram, or Lexapro. As a result, escitalopram doses are approximately half of the clinically comparable citalopram doses (see Chapter 12).[5]

As a consequence of a drug binding to a receptor, cellular function is altered, resulting in changes in physiological or psychological functioning. The total effect of the drug in the body results from drug actions either (1) on one specific type of receptor or (2) at different types of receptors. However, whether the drug is used for therapeutic or recreational purposes, the total action will include additional responses, called *side effects*.

As an example of the side effects produced by the first mechanism, blockade of presynaptic serotonin reuptake, produced by the antidepressant class of selective serotonergic reuptake inhibitors (SSRIs), increases serotonin availability at all postsynaptic serotonin receptors. This single action results not only in relief of depression but also in such side effects as anxiety, insomnia, and sexual dysfunction.

As an example of the side effects produced by the second mechanism, certain other antidepressants (the tricyclic antidepressants) reduce depression by increasing

---

[5] Other drugs discussed in this book that have isomeric formulations include amphetamine and methylphenidate, stimulant drugs used in the treatment of ADHD (see Chapter 15), and modafinil, used in the treatment of narcolepsy (see Chapter 13). Both isomers of amphetamine are active; the D-isomer is familiar as Dexedrine. The L-isomer of methylphenidate is metabolized much faster than the D-isomer, which is marketed separately as Focalin. The racemic mixture of modafinil is marketed as Provigil; the R-isomer is marketed as Nuvigil, which is more soluble in water.

both serotonin and norepinephrine availability. But, in addition, they also produce sedation, dry mouth, and blurred vision because they block cholinergic receptors. The goal is to find an acceptable balance between desirable therapeutic effects and undesirable side effects, and an important reason for understanding receptors is to achieve this outcome.

Acute and Chronic Receptor Effects

When a psychoactive drug binds to a receptor it produces an immediate response. For example, smoking a cigarette containing nicotine, or smoking illicit cocaine or methamphetamine, releases the neurotransmitter dopamine; dopamine activates our reward system, and a stimulant or pleasurable feeling can follow. With respect to medications, ingestion of methylphenidate (Ritalin) can rapidly relieve the symptoms of attention deficit/hyperactivity disorder (ADHD), potent opioid analgesics can rapidly relieve severe pain, and certain sedatives can rapidly induce drowsiness and be used in the treatment of insomnia. Similarly, many of the side effects of drugs (such as dry mouth, unwanted sedation, blurred vision, and so on) follow from acute actions at other receptors, often distinct from those responsible for the desired drug action.

But when the drug is given over a longer period of time, it produces long-term changes in the properties of the receptors. Here, the drug is in contact with its receptors for days to months. As a result, neurons "adapt" to the presence of a drug, resulting in long-term changes in neuronal functioning. There are two types of such adaptations, shown in Figure 3.11. The top panel of the figure shows the normal effect of transmission on receptors. Under normal physiological conditions, neurotransmitter molecules are released intermittently, only when the presynaptic neuron is activated. Therefore, the receptors for that transmitter are only transiently stimulated; the signal is received and then the transmitter molecules are removed.

However, if excessive numbers of transmitter molecules (or molecules of a drug that mimics a transmitter) are available to the receptor over a period of time, changes occur. In the presence of chronic stimulation the number of receptor sites decreases. As indicated in the middle panel, this is called *down regulation* or *desensitization*. This may account for some types of tolerance, for example, when heroin consistently occupies opioid binding sites. Over time, often in a few weeks of continuous exposure, the postsynaptic neuron will no longer respond to average amounts of heroin and increased amounts are required to obtain the opioid effect.

When the reverse occurs, that is, when the number of transmitter molecules available at postsynaptic receptors is decreased, often because they are blocked by an antagonist drug, the opposite result may occur. That is, an *up regulation* or *supersensitivity* may develop, as shown in the bottom panel of Figure 3.11. In this case the number of receptors increases. For example, antipsychotic medications block dopamine receptors, which causes their up regulation. As a result, additional dopamine receptors appear on the postsynaptic membrane. At this point, if the blockade is ended, even average amounts of dopamine can cause overactivity of certain motor responses. This condition may be treated by administration of dopamine agonists (to decrease receptors) or by reestablishing the dopamine blockade.

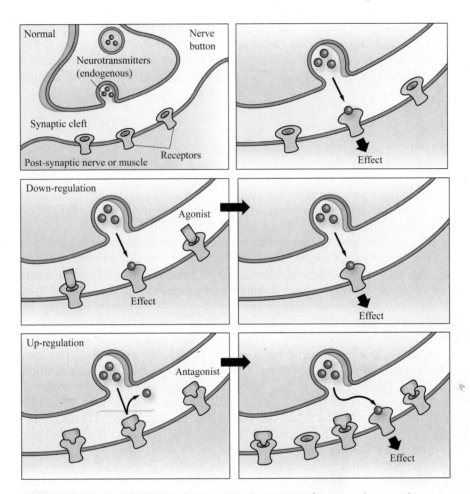

FIGURE 3.11   Schematic diagram depicting the phenomena of receptor downregulation (produced by binding of an agonist drug), and upregulation (produced by binding of an antagonist drug). After http://www.netterimages.com/image/5037.htm

Dose-Response Relationships

One way of quantifying drug-receptor interactions is to use *dose-response curves* (DRCs). A DRC is a function that describes the relationship between the dose of a drug and the magnitude of the drug's effect. A generic graph of a typical DRC is shown in Figure 3.12. Usually (although not always), the horizontal axis indicates the drug dose and the vertical axis shows the magnitude of the response. Figure 3.12 illustrates two different ways of representing response magnitude. In graph A, the dose is plotted against the percentage of people (from a given population) who exhibit a characteristic effect at a given dosage. In graph B, the dose is plotted against the intensity, or magnitude, of the response in a single person.

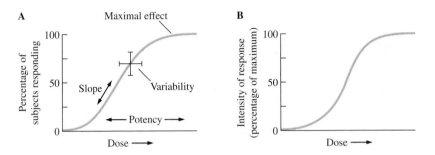

FIGURE 3.12 Two types of dose-response curves. **A.** Curve obtained by plotting the dose of drug against the percentage of subjects showing a given response at any given dose. **B.** Curve obtained by plotting the dose of drug against the intensity of response observed in any single person at a given dose. The intensity of response is plotted as a percentage of the maximum obtainable response.

These curves indicate that a dose exists that is low enough to produce little or no effect; at the opposite extreme, a dose exists beyond which no greater response can be elicited. As indicated in the figure, dose-response curves have several important characteristics:

- *Potency* refers to the amount of drug required to produce a given effect. It is related to the number of molecules of drug required to elicit a biological response at the receptor sites. The location of the dose-response curve along the horizontal axis reflects the potency of the drug. If two drugs produce an equal degree of stimulation, but one exerts this action at half the dose level of the other, the first drug is considered to be *twice* as *potent* as the second drug. This concept is illustrated in Figure 3.13, which shows DRCs for three different stimulant drugs—methamphetamine, d-amphetamine (see Chapter 7), and caffeine (see Chapter 6). The first two are both powerful psychostimulants. Although

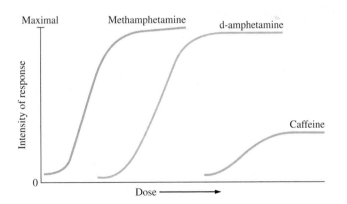

FIGURE 3.13 Theoretical dose-response curves for three psychostimulants illustrates equal efficacy of methamphetamine and dextroamphetamine, increased potency of methamphetamine, and reduced potency and efficacy of caffeine.

their chemical structures are very close, they differ by the simple addition of a methyl (—CH$_3$) group to d-amphetamine, forming methamphetamine. Both drugs attach to the same receptors in the brain, but methamphetamine exerts a much more powerful action on them, at least in milligrams. In pharmacological terms, methamphetamine is more *potent* than d-amphetamine because a lower absolute dose achieves the same level of response as a higher dose of d-amphetamine. However, potency is a relatively unimportant characteristic of a drug, because it makes little difference whether the effective dose of a drug is 1.0 milligram or 100 milligrams as long as the drug is administered in an appropriate dose with no undue toxicity.

- *Variability* refers to individual differences in drug response; some patients respond at very low doses and some require much more drug. As described in Chapter 2, differences in genetic make-up of metabolic enzymes are an important reason for the wide range in response magnitude.

- *Slope* refers to the relationship between the dose of a drug and its effect, as measured within the more or less linear (straight) central portion of the dose-response curve (see Figure 3.12). A flat, or shallow, slope suggests that large increases in dose do not produce big changes in effect. A steep slope on a dose-response curve indicates that there is only a small difference between the dose that produces a barely discernible effect and the dose that causes a maximal effect. This can be good because it may mean that there is little biological variation in the response to the drug. Conversely, it may be a disadvantage if it indicates that even a small increase in dose will produce a toxic reaction.

- *Efficacy* refers to the ability to produce a desired effect. The dose that exerts the maximum effect obtainable has 100 percent efficacy because it is not possible to produce a greater response. The *peak* of the dose-response curve indicates the maximum effect, or efficacy, that can be produced by a drug, regardless of further increases in dose. Not all psychoactive drugs can exert the same level of effect. For example, caffeine, even in massive doses, cannot exert the same intensity of central nervous system (CNS) stimulation as amphetamine (see Figure 3.13). Therefore, caffeine is less efficacious in regard to that reaction. Similarly, aspirin can never achieve the greater analgesic effect of morphine. Thus, the maximum effect is an inherent property of a drug and is one measure of a drug's efficacy. This pharmacological characteristic is essentially what we mean in everyday usage when we ask how *effective* a drug is in regard to its therapeutic benefit. Most psychoactive drugs are not used to the point of their maximum effect because of side effects and toxicities. In other words, sometimes the usefulness of a compound is limited by side effects even though the drug may be inherently capable of producing a greater or more intense response.

These parameters of DRCs allow us to compare the effects of drugs in a variety of different systems, and the effects of different drugs on the same system. They provide a framework for understanding the relationship between drug binding and biological response. Drug-receptor interactions usually produce one of the following outcomes:

- Binding to a receptor site can initiate a cellular response similar or identical to that exerted by the natural, endogenous transmitter; the drug thus mimics the action of the transmitter. This is called an *agonistic action*, and the drug is termed an *agonist*

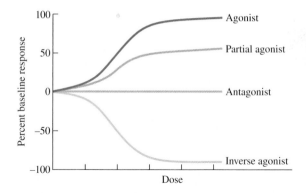

FIGURE 3.14 Dose-response functions produced by different types of drugs. An agonist can produce the maximum possible effect; a partial agonist is not able to elicit the maximum effect at any dose; an antagonist does not produce an overt effect; an inverse agonist produces an effect opposite to that of an agonist.

for that transmitter. If a drug is capable of eliciting the maximum response from a receptor system, then it is referred to as a *full agonist*. A *partial agonist* therefore is an agonist that is unable to induce maximal activation of a receptor population, regardless of the amount of drug applied (see Figure 3.14).

- Binding to a site near the binding site for the endogenous transmitter can indirectly influence transmitter binding. This is termed an *allosteric action*. An allosteric drug may not produce an effect by itself, but, in the presence of the natural transmitter, it may increase (*positive allosteric effect*) or decrease (*inhibitory allosteric effect*) the response of the transmitter. This type of influence may provide a more subtle modulation, something like a "dimmer switch," and might be one way to reduce side effects (Wenner, 2009). Examples of allosteric drugs are the benzodiazepines (such as diazepam), which do not, by themselves, affect the receptor's function, but increase the activity of GABA at the receptor (see Chapter 13).

- Binding to a receptor site may block access of the transmitter to the site. This will prevent the normal effect of the transmitter or will cause transmitter molecules to be displaced from the site and inhibit its normal physiological action. This is called an *antagonistic action*, and the drug is termed an *antagonist* for that neurotransmitter or receptor site (see Figure 3.14).

- Binding to a receptor site normally occupied by the endogenous neurotransmitter may produce the *opposite* pharmacological effect of an agonist. This type of drug is called an *inverse agonist*. The actions of both the agonist and inverse agonist can be reversed by a competitive antagonist (described below). The clinical significance of inverse agonism remains to be explored but inverse agonism has been reported for several systems relevant to this text, including benzodiazepine and cannabinoid receptors.

The hypothetical composite graph of Figure 3.14 indicates the shapes of DRCs for drugs that are full agonists, partial agonists, or inverse agonists. *It also illustrates the point that an antagonist drug by itself produces no response, that is, the effect of the drug on the*

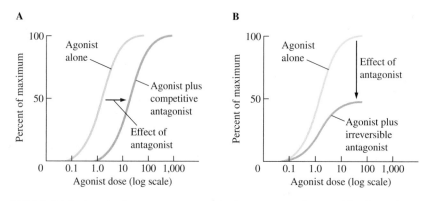

FIGURE 3.15 Agonist dose-response curves in the presence of competitive (Part A) and noncompetitive/irreversible (Part B) antagonists. The effect of a competitive antagonist is to shift the dose-response curve to the right. The noncompetitive/irreversible antagonist shifts the agonist curve down. After http://pharmacologycorner.com/pharmaco dynamics-animation-full-agonists-partial-agonists-inverse-agonists-competitive-antagonists-and-irreversible-antagonists/ Accessed August 4th, 2012.

baseline response level is not different from zero. Therefore, in order to determine if a drug is in fact an antagonist, as opposed to a substance that truly has no effect, it must be given in combination with an agonist. Only in the presence of a measurable response is it possible to determine if a drug has an antagonistic action, by seeing if it *reduces the effect of the agonist.*

There are two primary categories of antagonistic drugs (see Figure 3.15). One type is called a *competitive antagonist.* These are drugs that bind to the receptor in a reversible way. They attach to the receptor yet do not stimulate the effector system for that receptor. In this situation, both the agonist and antagonist bind to the same site on the receptor, hence the term "competitive." The action of a competitive antagonist can be overcome by increasing the dose of the agonist (that is, the block is *surmountable*). In other words, if more molecules of agonist are added then they "compete" with the antagonist for the receptor sites and eventually cause the antagonist to move off the receptor. The effect on the DRC of increasing the dose of agonist to overcome this type of block is to shift it to the right, making the agonist seem less "potent." Therefore, in the presence of a competitive antagonist, the dose-response curve is shifted to higher doses (horizontally to the right on the dose axis) but the same maximal effect is reached (see Figure 3.15A). An example of a competitive antagonist is the drug naloxone, which blocks the opiate receptor responsible for pain relief and for the euphoric effects of opiate drugs. If an overdose of an opiate drug has been taken, such as the analgesic OxyContin, then administration of naloxone will compete with OxyContin for the opiate receptor sites and prevent the overdose from being lethal. To regain the analgesic effect, more of the opiate drug would need to be taken.

In contrast, an *irreversible, or noncompetitive, antagonist* causes a downward shift of the maximum, with no shift of the curve on the dose axis (with some exceptions in more complex situations). (See Figure 3.15B.) As the name implies, the actions of a noncompetitive antagonist cannot be overcome by increasing the dose of agonist. This is because the agonist and antagonist binding sites are different; hence, the agonist will not displace the antagonist molecule. While the actions of an irreversible antagonist are the same as those for a noncompetitive antagonist (and the graphic illustration is the same) the explanation is different; for the irreversible antagonist the binding site may be the same as the agonist, but as it is irreversible (often chemically linked), it cannot be displaced, and therefore cannot be overcome. An example of a noncompetitive antagonist is the recreational drug PCP. PCP attaches to a site on the NMDA receptor for glutamate, but not at the same place as glutamate itself. Nevertheless, PCP prevents glutamate from performing its normal action. (One characteristic of PCP intoxication is memory loss—amnesia—for at least some of the time during which the drug was active. This observation supports the general belief that glutamate is involved in memory functions.) Eventually the antagonist molecules detach from their binding sites and are metabolized. In summary, the important concepts regarding pharmacodynamics are as follows:

- Agonists bind to receptors to produce a functional response.
- Agonists can be full, partial, or inverse.
- Antagonists block or reverse the effects of agonists.
- Antagonists can be competitive or noncompetitive/irreversible.

Variability in Drug Responsiveness— The Therapeutic Index

The dose of a drug that produces a specific response varies considerably among patients. Variability among patients can result from differences in rates of drug absorption and metabolism; previous experience with drug use; various physical, psychological, and emotional states; and so on. Despite the etiology of the variability, any population will have a few subjects who are remarkably sensitive to the effects (and side effects) of a drug and a few who will exhibit remarkable drug tolerance, requiring quite large doses to produce therapeutic results. The variability, however, usually follows a predictable pattern, resembling a Gaussian distribution (also known as a "normal" distribution, sometimes called a "bell-shaped curve"; see Figure 3.16). In a few instances, however, a specific population will show a unique pattern of responsiveness, usually due to genetic alterations in drug metabolism.

From Figure 3.16 it is obvious that, although the average dose required to elicit a given response can be calculated easily, some people respond at very much lower doses than the average and others respond only at very much higher doses. The dose of a drug that produces the desired effect in 50 percent of the subjects is called the ED_{50}, and the lethal dose for 50 percent of the subjects is called the LD_{50}. The LD_{50} is calculated in exactly the same way as the ED_{50}, except that the dose of the drug is plotted against the number of experimental animals that die after being administered various doses of the compound. Both the ED_{50} and the LD_{50} are determined in several species of animals to prevent accidental drug-induced toxicity in humans. The ratio of the LD_{50} to the ED_{50} is

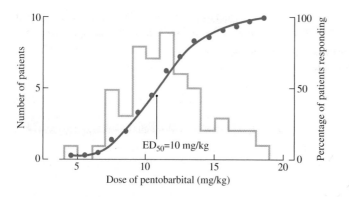

FIGURE 3.16 Example of biological variation. Histogram (*left ordinate*) and cumulative frequency histogram (*right ordinate*) following intravenous administration of pentobarbital, used to cause drowsiness in hospitalized patients. An ED_{50} of about 10 mg/kg body weight is shown. Note, however, that some patients exhibited sedation at about 4 mg/kg, while others required a dose of about 18 mg/kg. The stair-step bars illustrate the data behind the dose-response curve.

used as an index of the relative safety of the drug and is called the *therapeutic index* (TI) or margin of safety. A more precise definition is: the ratio of the highest amount of drug that does not produce toxicity/amount of drug required to produce the desired pharmacological response. Before giving the drug to patients, safety and efficacy data are obtained in nonhuman animals and exposure levels are studied in humans, taking into account species differences. Sometimes humans need more of the drug than expected from animal data and this can reduce the calculated safety margin. As stated by Muller and Milton (2012), in animal studies, the highest level of drug exposure that does not lead to toxicity, called the *no observable adverse effect level* (NOAEL), is usually the value used for the safety endpoint. This is a more conservative value than the lowest level of drug exposure that leads to toxicity, which is known as the *lowest observed adverse effect level* (LOAEL).

To illustrate, two dose-response curves are shown in Figure 3.17. The curve on the left represents the dose of drug necessary to induce sleep in a population of mice, and

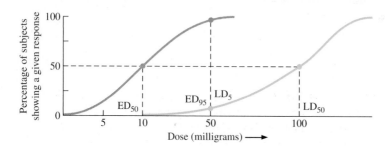

FIGURE 3.17 Illustration of therapeutic index. *Left:* Dose of drug required to induce a given response. *Right:* Lethal dose of the compound. See text for discussion.

the one on the right shows the dose of drug necessary to kill a similar population. In this example, the $LD_{50}:ED_{50}$ ratio is seen to be 100:10, or 10. Although the response in this case is death, a TI can be determined for any drug effect.

The TI of 10 in this example may seem like a rather large margin, but note that at a dose of 50 milligrams, 95 percent of the mice sleep while 5 percent of the mice die. This overlap demonstrates both the difficulty in assessing the relative safety of drugs for use in large populations and the biological variation in individual responses to drugs. With this particular compound, a dose cannot be administered that will guarantee that 100 percent of the mice will sleep and none will die. Thus, a more useful indication of the margin of safety is a ratio of the lethal dose for 1 percent of the population to the effective dose for 99 percent of the population ($LD_1:ED_{99}$). A sedative drug with an $LD_1:ED_{99}$ of 1 would be a safer compound than the drug shown in Figure 3.17. The FDA defines a prescription drug as having a narrow therapeutic index (NTI) if very small changes in dose could cause toxic results in patients. Among these drugs is the class of lithium products (with a therapeutic index of 2 or 3), and some anticonvulsant drugs, used in the treatment of bipolar disorder (see Chapter 14). Usually, although not always, the more selective that a drug is at its site of action, the better its TI.

This is a very simple and basic summary of the TI concept. In actual practice, it is more complicated. After all, even if a new medicine works, it will not be useful if it is not safe, therefore the accuracy of this calculation is very important. The sooner during drug development that a TI can be determined, the sooner any problems can be addressed. It is certainly not desirable to expose human participants to unsafe drugs in the conduct of clinical trials. The expense of developing new medications also argues for early detection of side effects. Unfortunately, rare or idiosyncratic reactions usually will not appear at this stage; they may not be discernible until a large population of patients takes the drug after it is on the market.

Muller and Milton (2012) provide an elegant review of the processes involved in determining and interpreting the therapeutic index in drug development.

Drug Interactions

Combining medications to improve therapeutic outcome, a practice termed *polypharmacy*, is common in psychiatric treatment. As noted by Zigman and Blier (2012), polypharmacy usually occurs because so few patients achieve remission of their illness from current medicines. Unfortunately, prescribing multiple medications may not be desirable because the combinations could be redundant, not useful, or even damaging. Zigmond and Blier (2012) propose several principles to reduce the likelihood of what they call such inappropriate, or "irrational," polypharmacy:

- *Pharmacodynamic redundancy*, in which two drugs have the same or overlapping mechanism of action. For example, alcohol taken after ingesting a benzodiazepine tranquilizer or smoking marijuana increases sedation and loss of coordination. This action may have little consequence if the doses of each drug are low, but higher doses of either or both drugs can be dangerous both to the user and to others. Even though a person may normally be able to ingest a limited amount of alcohol and still drive a car without significant loss of control or coordination, the concurrent use of tranquilizers or marijuana may profoundly impair driving performance, endangering the driver, passengers, other motorists, and pedestrians.

- *Pharmacodynamic interactions* may occur when the effect of two medications oppose each other. This may happen when antipsychotics, which block dopamine type 2 receptors (among other actions; see Chapter 11), are combined with ADHD stimulant medications, which increase dopamine levels (see Chapter 15).

- *Pharmacokinetic interactions*. Chapter 2 explained how certain drugs might either increase or decrease the rate of hepatic metabolism of other drugs and how this interaction can affect the plasma levels of other drugs metabolized by the same enzymes. For example, carbamazepine increases the rate of metabolism of certain other medicines, reducing the blood concentration and effectiveness of the second drug. Conversely, valproic acid can inhibit the metabolism of other drugs, such as lamotrigine, increasing its blood concentrations and potentially increasing its toxicity or side effects.

- *Inadequate dosing* may be a cause of irrational polypharmacy. Sometimes doses are too low because of side effects, or concern about possible side effects. Sometimes the medication is given at a dose that is sufficient for one action, but not high enough for a second pharmacological action to be effective. For example, the dose at which the antidepressant venlafaxine blocks the reuptake of dopamine is lower than the dose at which it blocks the reuptake of norepinephrine.

- *Clinical evaluation and oversight* should be ongoing. Drugs started during exacerbation of an illness might need to be reassessed after the patient has restabilized. The natural history of a disorder might produce spontaneous remission, allowing dose reduction or elimination. The appearance of new symptoms might be a result of long-term drug exposure (tolerance, or development of a side effect), which would be better treated by reassessment of the medication instead of adding a new agent.

Consideration of these possibilities can reduce unnecessary exposure to combinations that may be more harmful than helpful.

One of the most common types of adverse drug reaction is the phenomenon known as the *serotonin syndrome*. This is a rare, but potentially serious untoward response caused by excess serotonergic action at 5-HT2A and 5-HT1A receptors in the central and peripheral nervous systems. Symptoms may develop relatively quickly, within hours of exposure. The syndrome may include altered mental states, such as delirium, clonus, tremor, hyperthermia, tachycardia, and akathisia among other reactions. As noted in Chapter 12, many antidepressant drugs are often involved in this adverse reaction because they inhibit serotonin reuptake. However, other drug classes that may promote this syndrome include drugs that increase 5-HT release, such as stimulants (see Chapter 7) and hallucinogens (see Chapter 8), drugs that are direct agonists, particularly the triptan category of migraine medications (sumatriptan, rizatriptan, naratriptan, and others), and drugs that decrease 5-HT metabolism, such as the MAOI category of antidepressants. It is not known why some people can tolerate the combination of serotonergic drugs while others do not. Patients are reminded to communicate with their prescribers and practitioners are advised to be aware of which drugs are associated with the syndrome, which drugs their patients are taking that might cause the condition, and to check the available resources, which are now accessible electronically, to be familiar with the risky combinations (Bishop and Bishop, 2011). An illustrative case study was presented in the *New York Times Magazine* (Sanders, 2013).

Drug Toxicity

All drugs can produce harmful effects as well as beneficial ones. Unwanted effects can either be related to the principal and predictable pharmacological actions of a drug (for example, the sedation caused by drinking alcohol or the dry mouth experienced while taking certain antidepressants) or unrelated to the expected actions of a drug (for example, a severe allergic reaction). It is important to categorize harmful effects of drugs in terms of their severity and to distinguish between effects that cause temporary inconvenience or discomfort and effects that can lead to organ damage, permanent disability, or even death.

Most drugs exert effects on several body functions. To achieve the desired therapeutic effect or effects, some side effects often must be tolerated. Toleration is possible if the side effects are minor, but if they are more serious, they may be a limiting factor in the use of the drug. The distinction between therapeutic effects and side effects is relative and depends on the purpose for which the drug is administered: one person's side effect may be another person's therapeutic effect. For example, in one patient receiving morphine for its pain-relieving properties, the intestinal constipation that morphine induces may be an undesirable side effect that must be tolerated. For a second patient, however, morphine may be used to treat severe diarrhea, in which case the constipation induced is the desired therapeutic effect and relief of pain is a side effect. In addition to side effects that are merely irritating, some drugs may cause reactions that are very serious, including serious allergies, blood disorders, liver or kidney toxicity, or abnormalities in fetal development. Damage to the liver and kidneys results from the role of these organs in concentrating, metabolizing, and excreting toxic drugs. Examples of drug-induced liver damage include damage caused by alcohol and certain inhalants of abuse (see Chapter 5).

Allergies to drugs may take many forms, from mild skin rashes to fatal shock. Allergies differ from normal side effects, which can often be eliminated or at least made tolerable by a simple reduction in dosage. However, a reduction in the dose of a drug may have no effect on a drug allergy because exposure to any amount of the drug can be hazardous and possibly catastrophic for the patient.

Placebo Effects: Powerful or Problematic?

Placebos have a long history in medicine. Translated from the Latin, the word means "I will please," and, in fact, the first modern definition, appearing in 1811, described placebos as "any medicine adopted more to please than to benefit the patient" (Scheindlin, 2009, p. 108). Since then, the extent to which, or even whether, placebos are beneficial for patients has been the subject of much research and controversy.

Among the first to study the placebo response scientifically were Louis Lasagna and colleagues, who attempted to determine experimentally whether certain subgroups of patients were more likely to be placebo responders and, if so, whether they could be differentiated from nonresponders (Lasagna et al., 1954). Using a measure of post-operative pain, the researchers recorded the consistency of the placebo response and conducted thorough psychological evaluations of the patients. They concluded that their subjects could be divided into three groups: those who sometimes responded to placebo treatment (55 percent), those who always responded (16 percent), and those who never responded (29 percent). A colleague of Lasagna's, Henry Beecher, after further analyz-ing the data from 15 studies, reported that placebo reactions generally occurred in 30 to 40 percent of all patients (Beecher, 1955). Although placebo responders occurred in both sexes and across all ages, there was no clearly defined set of traits that differentiated them from nonresponders.

Support for the classic Beecher-Lasagna studies was provided by Ernst and Resch (1995), who analyzed the results of studies in which placebo effects were compared with that of "no treatment." They appreciated the fact that, even without placebo treatment, patients may improve for many reasons, such as spontaneous recovery, waxing and wan-ing of symptoms, decrease in anxiety, or other, nondrug interventions, such as rest, exer-cise, diet, hot baths, and meditation or other relaxation techniques. Of the six papers that included sufficient information, all of which used a pain rating as the clinical measure, Ernst and Resch (1995) found that four reported a substantial placebo response, one showed a borderline effect, and only one showed no effect.

In fact, even when patients are *told* that they are receiving a placebo, it may still work. In one study, patients with *irritable bowel syndrome* were either given no treatment or placebo pills, honestly labeled as "sugar pills." By the end of the three-week trial almost twice as many patients given the placebo reported sufficient symptom relief (59 percent) compared to the control (35 percent) (Kaptchuk et al., 2010).

One reason placebos worked even in this situation might be that, as a result of previous associations between a medicine and symptom relief, a patient develops a conditioned response. That is, because taking a pill produced relief in the past, the behavior of pill taking acquired the power to elicit at least some amount of relief all by itself. In fact, conditioned responses to pain relief are not unique to humans but have even been seen in a study with rats. Nolan and colleagues (2012) trained rats to lick a metal tube for a highly desirable solution of milk. However, the rats got an uncomfort-able facial heat stimulus when they licked the spout. When the rats got an injection of morphine on each of two days, they licked more, presumably because of the analgesic effect of the opiate. On the third day, a placebo was substituted for the morphine. About 30 to 40 percent of the rats that had previously received morphine acted as though they had again received the drug, and licked more than they had before experiencing the analgesic.

Interestingly, positive treatment effects may not be the only type of response affected by placebo. In one study, placebo therapy improved sleep difficulty, relative to a no-treatment group. But participants also reported experiencing placebo-induced side effects they had been warned about (Colagiuri et al., 2012).

Brain imaging studies, usually of placebo-induced analgesia, have shown that the re-duced pain ratings are associated with a reduction in the activity of those brain areas that normally process pain signals. In fact, there is evidence that the change in the subjective pain state during placebo analgesia is correlated with changes in classical pain pathways, and is produced by active inhibition of spinal cord pain pathways by higher centers in the brain (Meissner and coworkers, 2011).

On the other hand, the validity of the placebo response has also been questioned. In their analysis of 32 clinical trials, Hrobjartsson and Gotzsche (2001) argued that there was little support for placebo treatment, except for a small beneficial effect in pain conditions. They concluded that only in the clinical trial setting was placebo treatment justified.

The *double-blind, randomized, placebo-controlled clinical trial* is currently the gold standard for studying the effectiveness and safety of drugs in humans. First reported in 1937 (Scheindlin, 2009) and accepted as the standard by the 1950s, controlled trials were intended to remove the bias, expectations, and even fraud associated with clinical studies in which uncontrolled variables led to much subjective and presumably biased outcomes (Lakoff, 2002).

But even in double-blind, randomized, controlled trials, placebo effects may be substantial. As summarized by Walsh and coworkers (2002) in an analysis of clinical trials of drugs used to treat depression, about 28 percent of patients treated with placebo respond positively and significantly. This compares with 50 percent of patients who responded similarly when treated with active medication, illustrating that placebo effects contributed significantly (perhaps half or more) to the clinical response.

A possible biological cause for the large placebo effect often seen in antidepressant drug studies was reported by Leuchter and colleagues (2009) who found evidence for a genetic basis for the placebo response in people suffering from major depressive disorder. In fact, Kaptchuk and colleagues found the same type of genetic link in their study of the placebo response in irritable bowel syndrome (IBS) (Hall et al., 2012). That is, people in their study were more likely to show a placebo response of IBS symptom relief if they had a certain genetic make-up.

The large placebo response in clinical trials of antidepressants also illustrates the usefulness of including a "no treatment" condition in addition to comparisons between placebo and active comparators. If there is little or no separation between the placebo and the experimental treatment, then it is not clear whether the placebo response was especially powerful, or the experimental treatment was ineffective, or both (Finniss and coworkers, 2010).

Nevertheless, there are situations in which placebo treatment is not required by the FDA to be included, even in clinical trials. Antipsychotic drugs may be approved on the basis of a comparison between the new agent and an antipsychotic that is already approved. Orphan drugs (drugs that treat rare diseases—that is, diseases that occur in fewer than 200,000 people in the United States) may be approved on the basis of comparisons with historical controls, derived from what is known about the course of the disorder in the absence of treatment. Moreover, if other effective treatments are available, placebo treatment may be unethical.

Enck and colleagues (2013) argue that it may be time to use the placebo phenomenon to benefit medicinal drug use. They suggest that placebos should be minimized in clinical trials, but maximized once the drug is approved and being used. Moreover, by considering the genetic make-up and predisposition of each person, it might be possible to use placebos to maximize the total therapeutic outcome.

Did You Know?

Nocebo Effects

Although placebo effects have received a great deal of attention, the opposite phenomenon, the nocebo, has not been studied as much. For example, nocebo responses can occur as a result of unintended negative suggestion by doctors or nurses when they inform a patient about the possible complications of a proposed treatment. In addition, some of the undesired effects of drugs may be due to nocebo effects.

This may cause an ethical dilemma for doctors in clinical practice, between their obligation to reveal the possible side effects of a treatment, and their duty to minimize the risk of a medical intervention and thus to avoid triggering nocebo effects. One possible solution might be to emphasize the tolerability of the treatment. Another option, if the patient allows, would be to refrain from discussing undesired effects during the patient briefing.

STUDY QUESTIONS

1. Distinguish between the terms *pharmacodynamics* and *pharmacokinetics*.

2. What is a drug receptor? What are the major types and how do they differ?

3. Discuss the receptor phenomena of *up regulation* and *down regulation*.

4. What are the major components of a dose-response function and what do they represent?

5. Define the terms *full, partial,* and *inverse agonist; allosteric drug;* and *antagonist.*

6. What is the difference between a *competitive* and *noncompetitive/irreversible* antagonist?

7. Which factors influence drug safety and toxicity and how is drug safety measured?

8. What is "irrational polypharmacy" and how can it be avoided?

9. Define the placebo response and discuss the history and the major factors that influence it.

REFERENCES

Armstrong, N., et al. (2006). "Measurement of Conformational Changes Accompanying Desensitization in an Ionotropic Glutamate Receptor." *Cell* 127: 85–97.

Bear, M., et al. (2007). *Neuroscience: Exploring the Brain*, 3rd ed. New York: Lippincott, Williams and Wilkins.

Beecher, H. K. (1955). "The Powerful Placebo." *Journal of the American Medical Association* 159: 1602–1606.

Bishop, J. R., and Bishop, D. L. (2011). "How to Prevent Serotonin Syndrome from Drug-Drug Interactions." *Current Psychiatry* 10: 81–83.

Breedlove, M., et al. (2007). *Biological Psychology: An Introduction to Behavioral, Cognitive and Clinical Neuroscience*, 5th ed. Sunderland, MA: Sinauer.

Carlson, N. R. (2010). *Physiology of Behavior*, 10th ed. New York: Allyn & Bacon.

Colagiuri, B., et al. (2012). "Warning About Side Effects Can Increase Their Occurrence: An Experimental Model Using Placebo Treatment for Sleep Difficulty." *Journal of Psychopharmacology* 26: 1540–1547.

Enck, P., et al. (2013). "The Placebo Response in Medicine: Minimize, Maximize or Personalize?" *Nature Reviews Drug Discovery* 12: 191–204.

Ernst, E., and Resch, K. L. (1995). "Concept of True and Perceived Placebo Effects." *British Medical Journal* 311: 551–553.

Finniss, D. G., et al. (2010). "Biological, Clinical and Ethical Advances of Placebo Effects." *Lancet* 375: 686–695.

Gouaux, E., and MacKinnon, R. (2005). "Principles of Selective Ion Transport in Channels and Pumps." *Science* 310: 1461–1465.

Hall, K. T., et al. (2012). "Catechol-O-Methyltransferase val158met Polymorphism Predicts Placebo Effect in Irritable Bowel Syndrome." *PLoS ONE* 7: e48135.

Hrobjartsson, A., and Gotzsche, P. C. (2001). "Is the Placebo Powerless? An Analysis of Clinical Trials Comparing Placebo with No Treatment." *New England Journal of Medicine* 344: 1594–1602.

Iverson, L. L., Iverson, S. D., Bloom, F. E., and Roth, R. H. (2009). *Introduction to Neuropsychopharmacology.* New York: Oxford University Press.

Kaptchuk, T. J., et al. (2010). "Placebos Without Deception: A Randomized Controlled Trial In Irritable Bowel Syndrome." *PLoS One* 5: e15591.

Lakoff, A. (2002). "The Mousetrap: Managing the Placebo Effect in Antidepressant Trials." *Molecular Interventions* 2: 72–76.

Lasagna, L., et al. (1954). "A Study of the Placebo Response." *American Journal of Medicine* 16: 770–779.

Leuchter, A. F., et al. (2009). "Monoamine Oxidase A and Catechol-O-Methyltransferase Functional Polymorphisms and the Placebo Response in Major Depressive Disorder." *Journal of Clinical Psychopharmacology* 29: 372–377.

Meissner, K., et al. (2011). "The Placebo Effect: Advances from Different Methodological Approaches." *The Journal of Neuroscience* 31:16117–16124.

Muller, P. Y., and Milton, M. N. (2012). "The Determination and Interpretation of the Therapeutic Index in Drug Development." *Nature Reviews Drug Discovery* 11: 751–761.

Nestler, E. J., et al. (2009). *Molecular Pharmacology. A Foundation for Clinical Neuroscience*, 2nd ed. New York: McGraw-Hill Medical.

Nolan, T. A., et al. (2012). "Placebo-Induced Analgesia in an Operant Pain Model in Rats." *Pain* 153: 2009–2016.

Sanders, L. (2013, February 17). "Sudden-Onset Madness." *New York Times Magazine* pp. 14, 16.

Scheindlin, S. (2009). "The Problematic Placebo." *Molecular Interventions* 9: 108–113.

Walsh, B. T., et al. (2002). "Placebo Response in Studies of Major Depression: Variable, Substantial, and Growing." *Journal of the American Medical Association* 287: 1840–1847.

Wenner, M. (2009). "A New Kind of Drug Target." *Scientific American* August: 70–76.

Yamashita, A., et al. (2005). "Crystal Structure of a Bacterial Homologue of Na+/Cl-Dependent Neurotransmitter Transporters." *Nature* 437: 215–223.

Yernool, D., et al. (2004). "Structure of a Glutamate Transporter Homologue from *Pyrococcus horikoshii*." *Nature* 431: 811–818.

Zigman, D., and Blier, P. (2012). "A Framework to Avoid Irrational Polypharmacy in Psychiatry." *Journal of Psychopharmacology* 26: 1507–1511.

PART 2

Pharmacology of Drugs of Abuse

This section is composed of seven chapters that cover the pharmacology of drugs subject to compulsive use, abuse, and dependency. Some have no recognized medical use (for example, LSD and alcohol), while others have well-recognized therapeutic uses (for example, methylphenidate and amphetamines for the treatment of attention deficit/hyperactivity disorder).

The section begins with an overview of the neurobiology of addiction, in Chapter 4, which describes current thinking about the neuroanatomical and neurotransmitter basis of substance abuse. Chapter 5 discusses ethyl alcohol, a sedative-hypnotic quite similar in its pharmacology to the sedatives discussed later in Chapter 13. Alcohol differs, however, in that it has few indications and is most often used as a recreational intoxicant.

The psychostimulants are discussed in two chapters. Chapter 6 details the pharmacology of caffeine and nicotine, the most widely used recreational drugs. Neither drug has much therapeutic value, but both are used because of their psychostimulant properties. The toxicities associated with tobacco use, and the treatments for nicotine dependence are included in this chapter. Chapter 7 describes the psychostimulants cocaine, amphetamine, methamphetamine, and several related agents. These drugs present significant abuse issues as well as continuing uses in medicine.

Chapter 8 presents the pharmacology of drugs characterized by their ability to produce altered states of consciousness, the so-called psychedelic drugs, including those found in nature as well as those produced synthetically.

Chapter 9 presents the pharmacology of tetrahydrocannabinol and other compounds found in the marijuana plant. Current research is uncovering medical uses of psychedelic cannabinoids (for example, THC), nonpsychedelic marijuana alkaloids (for example, cannabidiol), and cannabinoid antagonists (for example, rimonabant). Medical and abuse issues related to these products are discussed.

Finally, Chapter 10 addresses the opiate analgesics. Although these drugs provide significant therapeutic benefit for alleviation of pain, they also have substantial abuse liability. During the last few years the dramatic increase in abuse of opiate medications has become a major public health problem, creating serious concerns about how to deal with an epidemic of illicit prescription opiates. Fortunately, there are indications that the epidemic has peaked and the extent of the abuse is decreasing.

Chapter 4

Epidemiology and Neurobiology of Addiction

Drug abuse has been a societal problem for thousands of years, ever since grain was fermented (ethyl alcohol) and natural substances that produced euphoria (cocaine), pain relief (morphine), or altered states of consciousness for divination (psilocybin, mescaline) were found. As history suggests, as long as these drugs persist in society, they will be associated with compulsive use, dependency, and addiction. This chapter reviews the current trends in regard to drug abuse in the United States, introduces the relevant concepts and neurobiological mechanisms believed to be responsible for addiction, and summarizes current approaches to treatment of dependency and abuse. The individual drugs discussed in their respective chapters are brought together in this overview of principles that apply to all drugs of abuse. Table 4.1 summarizes the current schedules of categories for controlled substances included in this section.

Extent of the Drug Problem

Drug abuse and addiction are a major burden to society. The estimated cost of drug use to society in the United States in lost productivity, health care expense, and crime-related and other costs, exceeds half a trillion dollars annually. Staggering as these figures are, however, they do not fully describe the breadth of deleterious public health—and safety—implications, which include family disintegration, loss of employment, failure in school, domestic violence, child abuse, and other crimes.

To address the nation's drug abuse and addiction problems, in 2010 President Obama inaugurated the National Drug Control Strategies describing the recommendations and proposals of the current administration for reducing the toll of addiction in the United States. This document was based on the premise, supported by scientific evidence, that

---

TABLE 4.1 Definition of controlled substance schedules

Drugs and other substances that are considered controlled substances under the Controlled Substances Act (CSA) are divided into five schedules. An updated and complete list of the schedules is published annually in Title 21 Code of Federal Regulations (C.F.R.) §§ 1308.11 through 1308.15. Substances are placed in their respective schedules based on whether they have a currently accepted medical use in treatment in the United States, their relative abuse potential, and likelihood of causing dependence when abused.

Schedule I

Substances in this schedule have:

- No currently accepted medical use in the United States
- A lack of accepted safety for use under medical supervision, and
- A high potential for abuse.

Examples include: heroin, lysergic acid diethylamide (LSD), marijuana (cannabis), peyote, and 3,4-methylenedioxymethamphetamine ("Ecstasy").

Schedule II

Substances have a high potential for abuse, which may lead to severe psychological or physical dependence.

Examples of opiates include: methadone (Dolophine®), oxycodone (OxyContin®, Percocet®), fentanyl (Sublimaze®, Duragesic®), morphine, opium, and codeine.

Examples of stimulants include: amphetamine (Dexedrine®, Adderall®), methamphetamine (Desoxyn®), and methylphenidate (Ritalin®).

Schedule III

Substances have less potential for abuse than substances in Schedules I or II and abuse may lead to moderate or low physical dependence or high psychological dependence.

Examples include: combination products containing less than 15 milligrams of hydrocodone per dosage unit (Vicodin®), products containing not more than 90 milligrams of codeine per dosage unit (Tylenol with Codeine®), buprenorphine (Suboxone®), ketamine, and anabolic steroids such as Depo®-Testosterone.

Schedule IV

Substances have a low potential for abuse relative to substances in Schedule III.

Examples include: alprazolam (Xanax®), clonazepam (Klonopin®), diazepam (Valium®), lorazepam (Ativan®), midazolam (Versed®), and triazolam (Halcion®).

Schedule V

Substances have a low potential for abuse relative to substances listed in Schedule IV and consist primarily of preparations containing limited quantities of certain opiates.

Examples include: cough preparations containing not more than 200 milligrams of codeine per 100 milliliters or per 100 grams (Robitussin AC®, Phenergan with Codeine®), and ezogabine.

drug addiction is not a moral failing but rather a disease of the brain that can be prevented and treated. The aim of the 2010 and 2011 National Drug Control Strategies was to establish and promote a balance of evidence-based public health and safety initiatives focusing on key areas such as substance abuse prevention, treatment, and recovery. The 2012 National Drug Control Strategy, released in April 2012, continued the efforts of the previous two strategies and serves as the blueprint for reducing drug use and its consequences in the United States.

Since 2009, the federal government has spent more than $31 billion on drug control, including $10.1 billion in fiscal year 2012 for substance abuse prevention and treatment programs. According to Assistant Secretary of the Department of Health and Hospitals, Howard Koh, MD, MPH, the second term of President Obama will focus on public health, particularly obesity and smoking cessation. The Healthy People 2020 initiative, which monitors national health trends and sets public health goals, aims to reduce adult smoking rates from the current level of about 19 percent, to 12 percent.

A major source of information on substance use, abuse, and dependence among Americans aged 12 and older is the annual National Survey on Drug Use and Health (NSDUH) conducted by the Substance Abuse and Mental Health Services Administration. Survey respondents report whether they have used specific substances ever in their lives (lifetime), over the past year, and over the past month. It is generally believed that past year and past month are the better indicators of actual use; past month use is also referred to as "current use." Approximately 67,500 people responded to the survey in 2011.

The results show that in 2011 an estimated 22.5 million Americans aged 12 or older—or 8.7 percent of the population—had used an illicit drug or abused a psychotherapeutic medication (such as a pain reliever, stimulant, or tranquilizer) in the past month. This is up slightly from 8.3 percent in 2002. The increase mostly reflects a recent rise in the use of marijuana, the most commonly used illicit drug (from 14.4 past month users in 2007 to 18.1 million past month users in 2011).

The results show that most people use drugs for the first time when they are teenagers (51 percent of new users were under 18 years of age), and more than half begin with marijuana. Next most common are prescription pain relievers, followed by inhalants (whose use is most common among younger teens).

Drug use is highest among people in their late teens and twenties. However, as shown in Figure 4.1, drug use is increasing among people in their fifties. This is, at least in part, due to the aging of the baby boomers, whose rates of illicit drug use have historically been higher than those of previous cohorts.

The Monitoring the Future study is the nation's largest survey of drug use among young people. The most recent results confirm the NSDUH data showing prescription drugs are the second most abused category of drugs after marijuana. Overall, the use of most illicit drugs, including tobacco, alcohol, and ecstasy either declined or remained steady from 2011 to 2012. However, 5-year trends are showing significant increases in current marijuana use. This increase is thought to be partly due to the perception that the substance is not harmful. This year's survey also captured the use of synthetic marijuana (known as K2 or "Spice"; see Chapter 9), for the first time among eighth and

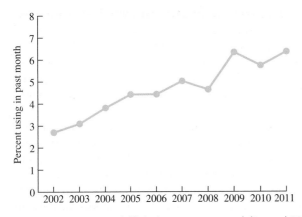

FIGURE 4.1   Past month illicit drug use among adults aged 50 to 59: 2002–2011.

tenth graders. Past year use was reported by 4.4 percent of eighth graders and by 8.8 percent of tenth graders. About 1 in 9, or 11.3 percent of high school seniors reported use of synthetic marijuana—unchanged from 2011. Also new in the survey this year was the past year use of bath salts (see Chapter 8) reported by 0.8 percent of eighth graders, 0.6 percent of tenth graders, and 1.3 percent of twelfth graders. Although this year's survey showed a long-term drop in past year nonmedical use of the opiate drug Vicodin (see Chapter 10) among students in all grades, its use remains high (for example, at 7.5 percent among high school seniors).

The abuse of prescription stimulants is also a cause for concern. In the past several years the percent of twelfth graders reporting the nonmedical use of Adderall has increased from 5.4 percent in 2009 to 7.6 percent in 2012. As in nearly all cases, attitudes toward substance abuse are often seen as harbingers of change in reported use. In 2012 nearly 6 percent fewer high school seniors reported that trying Adderall occasionally was harmful—an indication that use may continue to rise.

The survey further shows that most teens (like adults) obtain prescription drugs, such as amphetamines, tranquilizers, or narcotics other than heroin, free from friends and family; roughly 68 percent of twelfth graders, for example, report getting prescription pain relievers this way.

Nosology and Psychopathology of Substance Abuse

Published in 2000 in its revised fourth edition, the *Diagnostic and Statistical Manual of Mental Disorders* (DSM-IV-TR) (American Psychiatric Association, 2000) presented commonly accepted criteria for what constitutes substance dependence and substance abuse. The two substance use disorders involve maladaptive patterns of substance use, leading to clinically significant impairments or distress. The revision of this manual in May 2013 (DSM-5; see Chapter 17), combines substance abuse and substance dependence into one overarching category, "Substance Use Disorder" (SUD). It was felt that this change allowed experts to diagnose people with an alcohol and/or drug problem more easily by looking at a continuum of severity. This may also lead to earlier diagnoses, which could allow appropriate interventions to be applied more easily. The criteria have not only been combined, but also strengthened. Previously, only one symptom was required, whereas the new DSM-5's mild substance use disorder requires two to three symptoms. In addition, a new diagnosis, "Internet Use Gaming Disorder," is included in Section 3, a category of disorders that are not yet agreed on, but need further research.

Approximately one-third of people addicted to an illicit drug or alcohol have a diagnosed *comorbid* psychiatric disorder, a situation covered by the term *dual diagnosis*. Among people with a lifetime diagnosis of schizophrenia, 47 percent have met criteria for substance abuse or dependence; those with an anxiety disorder, 23.7 percent; those with obsessive-compulsive disorder, 32.8 percent; those with bipolar disorder, 50 percent; and those with depression, 32 percent—with distribution equal for males and females. Current evidence indicates that managing mood symptoms with pharmacotherapy can help those with a substance abuse problem, although results are not always consistent (Pettinati et al., 2013).

Neurobiology of Addiction

Introduction

Recognition of the existence of a neural system responsible for the biological basis of "pleasure" originated with the discovery in the 1950s (by the scientists Olds and Milner, 1954) that rats would work (often very hard) to get electrically stimulated in certain brain sites. Gradually, the anatomical pathways and the neurochemical substances that comprised this system were determined and mapped. This circuit is believed to be the neurobiological basis for the experience of pleasure, satisfaction, or reward. Although presumably this system mediates the pleasures experienced from natural stimuli, such as food and sex, drugs that can stimulate these brain areas activate this system more intensely and directly. According to this interpretation, despite their specific pharmacological effects, all drugs of abuse act through this "reward" system, and such activation promotes repeated use. Unfortunately, in vulnerable people, repeated use can lead to addiction—a loss of control over drug use. Withdrawal of the drug will produce unpleasant emotional reactions regardless of the specific substance. Even after all traces of the specific abused drug are gone from the body (through the process of detoxification), the addicted individual experiences urges to use the drug again and is at risk of relapsing. The development of such cravings indicates that something in the brain has changed as a result of long-term drug use; some process of neuroadaptation has occurred. It is these neurobiological changes that are responsible for craving and relapse, even after long periods of abstinence. Appreciation of this phenomenon, which occurs with all abused drugs, has led to increased research into the mechanisms responsible for craving and relapse; the recognition that such processes are similar to other types of learned reactions; and the realization that these mechanisms may also be relevant to other types of nondrug addictions, such as gambling, and other compulsive behaviors. Efforts are currently ongoing to develop new treatments for these maladaptive learned responses.

Common Effects of Abused Drugs on Brain Reward Circuits

The core of the reward circuit is one of the brain pathways for dopamine, called the *mesolimbic dopamine pathway* (Figure 4.2). As shown in the figure, this pathway begins with a group of dopamine neurons in the ventral tegmental area (VTA), a structure that is located in the midbrain (see Chapter 1). The axons of these dopamine neurons extend to several other brain structures, where they release dopamine when the VTA is activated. The most relevant structures, in this context, are the nucleus accumbens (NAc), the amygdala, the hippocampus, and the prefrontal cortex. The dopamine pathway from the VTA to the NAc is critical to addiction: if these brain regions are lesioned, animals will no longer become addicted (Nestler and Malenka, 2004). This pathway is integrated with the other structures. The amygdala is involved in mediating the emotional characteristics of drug use, the hippocampus is crucial to recording memories of such experiences, and the frontal regions of the cortex synthesize and coordinate information and are involved in planning and the inhibitory control of behavior.

In addition to dopamine neurons, there are also other neurons within the VTA that interact with the dopamine neurons. Some release the neurotransmitter GABA. The release of GABA inhibits dopamine neurons and normally suppresses dopamine release.

During the last few decades a converging body of evidence has indicated that, regardless of their specific effects, most abused drugs share a common action with respect to

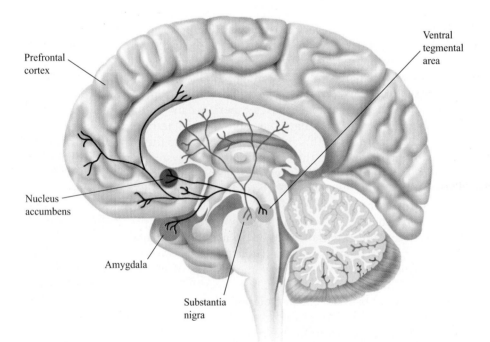

FIGURE 4.2 The reward circuit. The major structures involved in the subjective sensation of pleasure and reward. The pathway starts with dopamine-releasing neurons in the ventral tegmental area (VTA). Axons from the VTA neurons release dopamine onto the amygdala, nucleus accumbens, and prefrontal cortex.

this mesolimbic dopamine pathway. That is, most abused drugs increase the amount of dopamine that is released from the VTA onto the NAc, amygdala, hippocampus, and frontal lobe. However, they do not all increase dopamine activity in the same way. In some cases the dopamine increase is direct; in others, dopamine is increased indirectly. Some drugs may increase dopamine by more than one mechanism, and some may produce other, nondopaminergic responses as well (Pierce and Kumaresan, 2006).

For example, cocaine (and other stimulants; see Chapter 7) increases the amount of dopamine on NAc neurons by blocking dopamine reuptake into VTA neurons after the transmitter has been released. Nicotine (see Chapter 6) may stimulate the dopamine neurons directly and cause them to release dopamine. Heroin and other opioids (see Chapter 10) act on receptors located on GABA neurons and inhibit GABA release. When GABA release is reduced, there is less inhibition of dopamine neurons, and dopamine release increases. Opioids can also act directly on the NAc to produce a positive "reward" signal. Drugs that are CNS depressants, such as benzodiazepines (see Chapter 13), and alcohol (see Chapter 5) may also increase dopamine by inhibiting GABA release as well as by other actions (Nestler and Malenka, 2004). In fact, benzodiazepines were recently shown to activate a specific subtype of $GABA_A$ receptor, a subtype that contains the α1 subunit. These specific subtypes are found on the same neurons as the receptors for opiates. In other words, both benzodiazepines and opiates increase dopamine release by inhibiting GABA neurons (and disinhibiting the VTA dopamine neurons) (Riegel and Kalivas, 2010).

How do we know that the effect of drugs on dopaminergic activity is related to their pleasurable subjective effects? Compelling and extensive evidence from studies done for over 30 years in nonhuman animals supports this relationship. However, in 1997 a particularly relevant observation was made in cocaine addicts, which showed that dopamine was also related to the sensation of pleasure in humans. In this study, methylphenidate (Ritalin; see Chapter 15) was given to cocaine addicts while they underwent a brain scan. Methylphenidate, like cocaine, blocked the dopamine transporter and increased the amount of dopamine in the synapse. The addicts rated the "high" they experienced after receiving methylphenidate, while the brain scans showed the percent of transporters blocked by each dose. There was an excellent correlation—the greater the subjective rating of the "high," the greater the proportion of transporters blocked, which meant the greater the increase in the amount of dopamine in the brain (Volkow et al., 1997).

As noted above, the VTA-NAc pathway and the other limbic regions are also presumed to be responsible, at least in part, not only for the positive effect of drugs but also for the pleasurable effects of natural rewards, such as food, sex, and other enjoyable activities. Consequently, these same regions have also been implicated in the so-called natural addictions (that is, compulsive behaviors in regard to natural rewards), such as pathological overeating, pathological gambling, and sexual addictions (Nestler, 2005).

Research indicates that long-term, chronic exposure to any of several drugs of abuse will impair this dopamine pathway such that eventually the system becomes less responsive to normal, naturally rewarding stimulation. In other words, excessive drug use alters the response to naturally rewarding stimuli such that they are not as enjoyable as they once were. Essentially, tolerance develops within the pathway (Nestler, 2005), and naturally rewarding stimuli do not increase dopaminergic activity as much as they used to. These changes may contribute to the unpleasant emotional state that develops between drug exposures or when drugs are withdrawn.

Did You Know?

Talking About Yourself Online Is as Rewarding to the Brain as Sex or Eating

According to a new study reported in the *Proceedings of the National Academy of Sciences* (Tamir and Mitchell, 2012), boasting about your activities sparks the "primary reward" center of your brain. Diana Tamir, a Harvard researcher, wondered what would happen to brain activity when people answered questions about their favorite subject: themselves.

Tamir asked really mundane questions, such as "Do you prefer coffee over tea?" or "Do you like to snowboard?" And when people were answering those questions, Harvard researchers saw activity in the part of the brain associated with reward. That area lit up when they answered those questions. It is the same thing you would see when someone is laughing or getting good food or money.

The Harvard researchers then offered money to their test subjects. They would offer them four cents to answer questions about someone else and only two cents if they continued to talk about themselves. You guessed it; the test subjects consistently opted for the two pennies.

In brief, drugs, like other rewarding experiences, cause release of dopamine from VTA neurons to NAc neurons. When released, dopamine causes animals to feel good, prompting them to repeat the pleasurable action, leading to compulsive use and addiction.

But this raises another question. Many people use legal drugs, such as alcohol. Yet why do only some drug users become addicted? Is there something different about their brains? Some evidence suggests that this might be the case. In one study, normal male subjects were given methylphenidate and asked if they found the experience pleasant, unpleasant, or neutral. At the same time, they underwent a brain scan that measured their dopamine receptors. It turned out that the subjects who reported that they found methylphenidate to be pleasant had *lower* D_2 receptor levels than those who reported that the drug injection was unpleasant. In fact, the subjects who enjoyed the drug experience had receptor levels similar to those previously reported in cocaine abusers, even though these subjects were not abusing drugs (Volkow et al., 2004).

Does this result mean that, if a person has a low density of receptors he or she is biologically vulnerable to drug abuse? In other words, do people at risk for acquiring addictions have a weaker response to "pleasure" than people who are not as vulnerable, perhaps because of a dopamine receptor deficiency? The implication is that such individuals may have a biological deficit and may require a more powerful stimulus (a drug) to experience a normal pleasurable sensation, while, for others the same drug experience may actually be too strong to be enjoyable. This interpretation is consistent with studies in which methylphenidate (or, in different experiments, amphetamine) was given to different groups of nonaddicts, and either detoxified or nondetoxified addicts. In these cases, the addicts reported a less intense "high" and showed less dopamine (DA) increase in their brains, suggesting that the addict's brain is less responsive to the drug (Volkow et al., 2011).

From Abuse to Addiction

Regardless of the mechanism responsible, however, repeated drug use may develop into chronic drug use that can become compulsive and result in addiction. Because the frontal lobe is one of the areas of the brain that is part of the reward circuit, it is also profoundly altered by chronic drug abuse. One common change that occurs after long-term drug use is cortical "hypofrontality." This means that the normal baseline activity of several regions of the frontal cortex is reduced. Brain scans have shown that addicts not only have fewer dopamine receptors in the NAc than normal, they also have a lower metabolic rate in the frontal lobe. This has been interpreted to mean that their frontal lobe responses to normal, nondrug stimuli are "sluggish." However, even though this brain area is "sluggish" when activated by natural rewards, the frontal lobes become more activated than normal when drug abusers are exposed to stimuli that cause craving, such as drugs or drug cues. For example, when methylphenidate was injected into addicts and nonaddicted subjects, metabolism increased in the frontal areas of the addicts' brains but decreased in the brains of nonaddicted subjects.

Did You Know?

Decreased Dopamine in Addicted Brains

Brain images showing decreased dopamine (D2) receptors in the brain of a person addicted to cocaine versus a nondrug user. The dopamine system is important for conditioning and motivation, and alterations such as this are likely responsible, in part, for the diminished sensitivity to natural rewards that develops with addiction. (NIH Publication Number 10-4166. Revised September 2010).

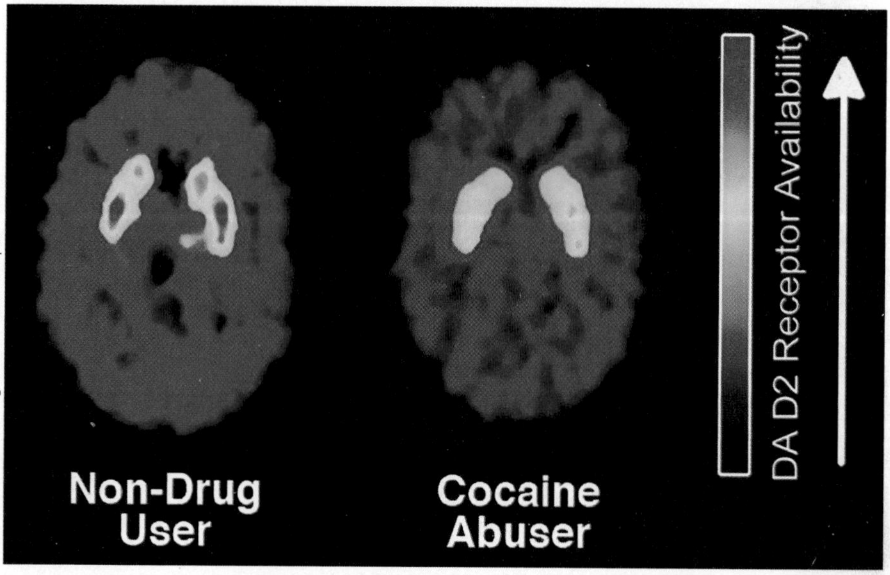

National Institute on Drug Abuse Research Report Series

Non-Drug User

Cocaine Abuser

DA D2 Receptor Availability

Even after three or four months of abstinence, the prefrontal cortex may not recover. Recently Durazzo and coworkers (2011) have found support for this in alcohol addicts. These investigators used magnetic resonance imaging (MRI) of the brain to examine the reward system in addicts one week after abstinence and again 12 months later. They found that the cortex of the brain was thinner in all of the addicts compared with control subjects, but, in addition, those with less volume and surface area were more likely to relapse after one year.

In summary, as a result of chronic drug use natural rewards become *less* pleasurable, and release less dopamine but, in response to drugs and especially to cues that are associated with drugs, there is a *greater response* in dopaminergic transmission than normal (Volkow et al., 2004, 2011; Nestler, 2005). The frontal cortex becomes inherently less active and less responsive to normal rewards, but it is *overactive* in response to drugs or the stimuli that predict drugs.

Of course, for drug use to continue, the user has to remember the positive feelings produced by the drugs and the environmental situation in which it occurred. Even after the drug is no longer present in the body, this memory provides the motivation for compulsive use, and is believed to be responsible for relapse.

This memory is mediated by the other structures associated with the reward circuit, the amygdala and hippocampus (Figure 4.3). In fact, over time, stimuli that "predict" drugs or were associated with the environment in which drugs were used produce a greater response in the reward pathway than the rewarding stimuli themselves. It is proposed that such conditioned, or learned, responses elicit powerful *craving* sensations in the frontal cortex. The frontal lobes are said to become *sensitized* to drug-related stimuli. For example, addicted people frequently relapse after returning to an environment in which they have previously taken drugs, even after they have gone through detoxification and recently spent time in a rehabilitation program.

Furthermore, the brain structures involved in addiction are hypersensitive not only to activation by drugs of abuse and drug-associated stimuli but also to environmental *stressors*. In fact, studies in humans and animal models indicate that stress is significantly

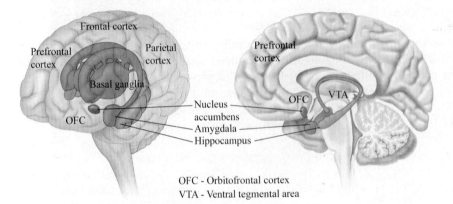

OFC - Orbitofrontal cortex
VTA - Ventral tegmental area

FIGURE 4.3 Major brain structures involved in addiction. The ventral tegmental area (VTA) and nucleus accumbens are key components of the reward system. These, together with the amygdala, hippocampus, and prefrontal cortex (PFC), coordinate drives, emotions, and memories. [Modified after Fowler et al., 2007, Figure 1, p. 5.]

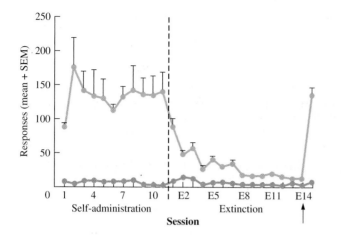

FIGURE 4.4 Variables that promote relapse. This figure illustrates the development, extinction, and relapse phases of addiction in an animal model. Some animals were trained for 12 days to self-administer cocaine in response to a lever press (blue circles). Control animals (orange circles) received no cocaine in response to a lever press. At the vertical dashed line, all animals underwent extinction training (lever presses no longer produced the drug) for 14 days. At the end of this phase (arrow at session E14), all animals were presented with either (1) a cue that accompanied the previous cocaine administration in the training stage; (2) a mild stressor, such as a brief electrical stimulus; or (3) a small amount of intravenous cocaine. All three stimuli overcame extinction in animals that had received cocaine before the extinction period (blue circle at day E14). Cue, stress, or cocaine resulted in resumption of lever pressing in an attempt to obtain cocaine ("reinstatement" of drug seeking). In control animals (orange circle at days E14 and E15), presentation of a cue at day E14 did not result in drug-seeking behavior. [Modified data from Kalivas et al., 2006, Figure 1, p. 340.]

involved in the vulnerability to develop addiction and in relapse in addicted persons (Haass-Koffler and Bartlett, 2012). In humans, stress may eventually result in a mood disorder, such as depression, especially during periods of drug withdrawal, leading to the development of a co-occurring situation (Yadid et al., 2012). An example of the importance of stress and learned reactions in triggering relapse is shown in Figure 4.4, a composite summary of the results of numerous animal experiments. It shows three phases of drug abuse. In the first phase, rats responded on one lever for cocaine infusions but did not respond on a second lever that produced only a saline injection (self-administration). In the second phase, when responding no longer produced cocaine (extinction), the rats eventually stopped pressing the lever. Finally, in the third phase, separate groups of animals were exposed to either (1) direct injection of cocaine, (2) an environmental stimulus previously associated with the drug, or (3) a stressful stimulus (for example, electric shock). Each of these three treatments reinstated responding on the lever that had previously been associated with cocaine injections. (Although not shown, cocaine responding also increased even more after a period of abstinence, that is, after drug injections were stopped but without the extinction responses.) This summary figure shows that even when drug abuse is extinguished, relapse can be readily elicited by three major conditions:

- Reexperience with the drug
- Conditioned drug cues
- Stress (including withdrawal-induced reactions)

Glutamatergic Substrates of Addiction

Regardless of whether they are triggered by drugs, by conditioning, or by stress, these heightened craving sensations are transmitted from the frontal cortex through downstream nerve pathways that feed back onto the reward pathway. In this case, however, the nerve fibers that connect the frontal lobe structures with the downstream reward circuit are not primarily dopaminergic. Rather, they release the transmitter *glutamate* onto the NAc and VTA (Figure 4.5). Evidence from animal experiments and from human brain scans shows that chronic exposure to any of several drugs of abuse causes complex changes in these frontal cortical regions and their glutamatergic outputs. For example, studies with rats showed that the glutamate synapse between the frontal lobes and the NAc *actually became stronger* (responded more intensely) when tested 24 hours after a single exposure to cocaine. To be specific, the increased strength was measured as an increase in the response of AMPA receptors relative to that of NMDA receptors. Most important, the increased reaction was not restricted to cocaine, but was also produced

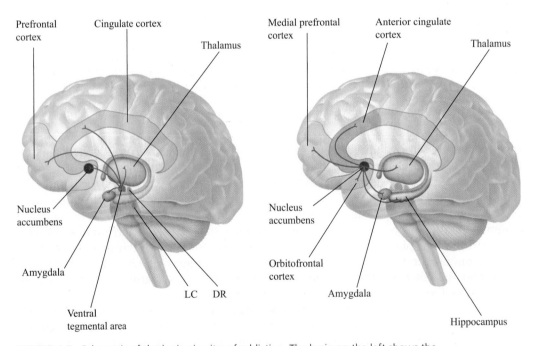

FIGURE 4.5 Schematic of the brain circuitry of addiction. The brain on the left shows the dopamine fibers that originate from the ventral tegmental area (VTA) and which release dopamine in the nucleus accumbens (NAc) and other structures in the limbic system. Other brain structures that influence these sites are also indicated: the noradrenergic nucleus of the locus coeruleus (LC) and the serotonergic dorsal raphe nucleus (DR). The right side indicates the excitatory glutamatergic structures that interact with the VTA and mediate the development of drug addiction: the medial prefrontal cortex (mPFC), the orbitofrontal cortex (OFC), the anterior cingulate cortex (ACC), the thalamus (Thal), hippocampus, and amygdala. [After Robison and Nestler, 2011, Figure 1, p. 624.]

by other abused drugs including amphetamine, morphine, alcohol, nicotine, and benzodiazepines, while drugs that were not abused did not produce this increase in synaptic strength (Madsen et al., 2012).

Other postsynaptic glutamate receptors, notably the mGluR5 subtype, are also altered in addiction. It has been shown that mice lacking this receptor were less prone to relapse after becoming addicted to cocaine (Novak et al., 2010). This was interpreted to mean that without the mGluR5 receptor, mice could not "learn" the association between drug administration and reward that occurred in normal mice (Duncan and Lawrence, 2012).

Glial cells associated with the synapse also play an important role in maintaining the normal concentration of glutamate. [There is increasing recognition that glia may be involved in the effect of a variety of addictive drugs (Cooper et al., 2012).] In particular, there are some structures located on glial cells that modulate the amount of glutamate in the vicinity of the synapse. One of these is a transporter, called GLT-1, which carries glutamate into the glial cell so that it can eventually be returned to the presynaptic neuron. Another structure on the glial cell is a protein, called xCT. This protein pushes glutamate out of the glial cell in exchange for an amino acid, cysteine, and is therefore called the *cystine-glutamate exchanger*. These two proteins, the glial-glutamate transporter-1 (GLT-1) and the cystine-glutamate exchanger (xCT) maintain a balance between glutamate inside and out of the synapse. Chronic drug exposure can decrease the levels of these two proteins. As a result, the amount of glutamate in the synapse resulting from addiction unbalances the normal regulatory processes that control glutamate release.

In summary, the *hypersensitivity of the frontal cortex to drugs or drug cues (learning), which develops in addiction, is the basis of the phenomenon of craving. Craving is biologically mediated as increased glutamatergic reactivity within the reward circuit.* These changes are believed to be responsible for the profound impulsivity (acting on sudden urges to take a drug) and compulsivity (being driven by irresistible inner forces to take a drug) that define addiction.

The increased activation of these pathways also causes some biochemical changes within the VTA-NAc and other brain reward regions. One of the most dramatic examples is that chronic exposure to all drugs of abuse, including cocaine, amphetamine, opiates, alcohol, nicotine, cannabinoids, and phencyclidine, increases the amount of a protein, called ΔFosB, which builds up in the NAc. In fact, chronic exposure to natural rewards, such as high ingestion of sweets, will also increase ΔFosB.

Another substance in the brain that is increased by chronic drug use is brain-derived neurotrophic factor (BDNF). Recently, blood levels of BDNF were found to be significantly increased in opiate-dependent patients, and this increase was significantly associated with craving for heroin (Heberlein et al., 2011).

To summarize: according to current views, several types of functional changes are involved in the development of addiction. These include alterations in dopaminergic reward systems (VTA), which signal the significance or desirability of a stimulus (its "saliency"), the motivational circuits (the NAc, amygdala), which provide incentive for obtaining the reward, the conditioning/learning pathways (hippocampus), which strengthen the behaviors that obtain the reward, and the inhibitory processes (frontal lobe), which normally exert control over inappropriate or destructive behavior. In addition to these processes, there are influences of stress, including the physiological consequences of withdrawal and the emotional mood states of anxiety and depression, which can also reduce the inhibitory control, exerted by the frontal lobes on the reward pathways.

As a result of chronic abuse, this model proposes that drugs acquire increased motivational value, indicated by the development of conditioned reactions (cravings), while the motivational value of normal reinforcers becomes weaker. The ability to inhibit craving is impaired and drug taking becomes compulsive. Although the initial effect of the drug is to activate dopamine release, it is the descending pathways from the frontal lobes, amygdala, and hippocampus, back to the NAc in the striatum (corticostriatal pathway), connections that involve glutamate, which is responsible for the drug-related learned associations. This model therefore predicts that addiction involves some alteration of glutamatergic function in corticostriatal pathways, and that correction of this impairment should promote abstinence (Kalivas, 2009; Mameli and Lüscher, 2011). Cai and colleagues (2013) provide an experimental example that supports this model. In their study, rats were trained to associate a morphine injection with a specific environmental location. When the researchers increased the amount of AMPA receptors in the amygdala of the rats, the animals learned this relationship more quickly; when the receptors were reduced, learning was impaired.

Treatment approaches derived from this model, discussed below, could address any or all of these processes. For example, therapy might decrease the rewarding effect of drugs, or increase the reward intensity of natural stimuli. Other approaches might be to interfere with learned associations between drugs and the environment, to enhance motivation for nondrug-related activities, or to increase inhibitory control. In this regard, evidence has been reported that cortical stimulation reduces responding for drugs in rats that compulsively self-administered cocaine (Chen et al., 2013), and that stimulating specific dopamine receptors in the nucleus accumbens of mice reduced cocaine seeking (Bock et al., 2013).

Introduction to Epigenetics

Drug craving and the risk of relapse can persist throughout an addict's life, even after decades of abstinence. Such persistence means that drugs produce long-lasting changes in the brain that maintain addiction. It is currently believed that the mechanisms for those changes involve the interaction of the environment with our genetic code. Family, twin, and adoption studies suggest that the heritability of addiction is moderate to high, ranging from 0.30 to 0.70. Accordingly, current research into addiction, and other psychiatric disorders, has greatly expanded to include the study of the relationship between environment and genetics. Ultimately, the goal is to develop new therapeutic approaches that will prevent these behavioral problems. This section provides an overview of this new approach with regard to addiction.

Inside the nucleus of each cell in our bodies is our DNA, our genetic code. That DNA represents the blueprints, or instructions, that makes us who we are. But, if each cell in our body has the same DNA, how does a cell that is supposed to become a skin cell actually turn into a skin cell, instead of some other type of cell, like a neuron? In other words, during gestation, when the embryo develops into a fetus and eventually a complete human being, what is responsible for the process that makes sure a liver cell does not turn into a blood cell? That question has led to the realization that the DNA sequence is only one part of the story, and that the answer involves the phenomenon of *epigenetics*, which literally means "over or above genetics." Although there is still debate about the specific meaning of this term, most sources agree that at its simplest, epigenetics is the study of changes in gene activity that do not involve changes in the genetic code itself (DNA or genome), but that still get passed down to at least one successive generation.

One way to conceive of this concept is to think of the DNA code as a musical score, which cannot be heard without an orchestra (the cells of the body) or a conductor that controls the performance. Epigenetics represents the "conductor." Another common analogy is that the DNA (the genome) is the "hardware" while the epigenome is the "software" of our genetic makeup. But, regardless of the way it is expressed, it has become clear that epigenetics may help us to understand the answer to some scientific questions that are not explained by the genome alone. For example, if identical twins have the same DNA, how come only one might develop schizophrenia or bipolar disorder (or any other disorder, such as cancer)? Although monozygotic twins have the same genes, we have come to realize that some genes might be active (or inactive) in one twin but not the other. In other words, they are *genetically* identical but not *epigenetically* the same.

Structure of the Genome

To begin to understand how this might work, it is helpful to know something about the structure of the genome. If all of the DNA in our cells were stretched out, it would be over 6 feet in length. But, the nucleus of the cell is only 1/10,000th of an inch across. Obviously, our DNA has to be packaged very tightly to fit into such a small space. Furthermore, in spite of this cramped environment, there has to be some way for all the functions to be performed for normal development—some genes need to be activated and copied and others turned off at appropriate times. Scientists have been studying how genes are compacted for over a century and our current understanding of how this is accomplished is shown in Figure 4.6.

As indicated in the figure, the strands of our DNA are wound around "spools" of protein, called *histones,* of which there are different versions. These proteins are positively charged, which helps to attract the negatively charged DNA. There is also a thin "tail" that extends from each histone. Together, the combination of histones and DNA is called *chromatin.* The basic repeating structural (and functional) unit of chromatin is the *nucleosome,* which consists of a group of eight histones plus about 166 base pairs of DNA. (In Figure 4.6, we can see only one side of the nucleosomes, which shows four of the eight histones.)

The fact that each chromosome contains an average of over 100 million base pairs of DNA means that every chromosome contains hundreds of thousands of nucleosomes (and the DNA that runs between them). In other words, the *chromosome* is made up of *chromatin,* which is a long chain of *nucleosomes,* composed of *histones,* which looks like a string of beads under an electron microscope. Many higher-order levels of chromatin

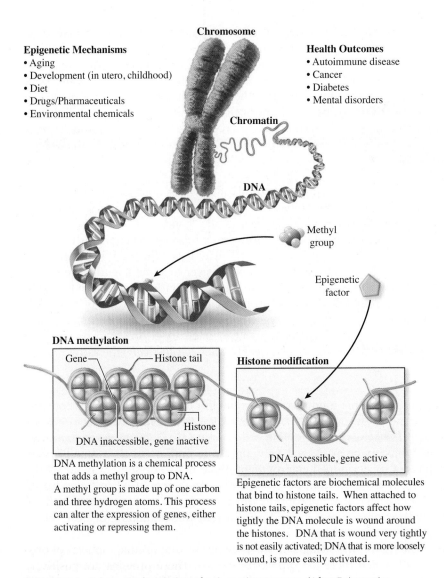

Epigenetic Mechanisms
• Aging
• Development (in utero, childhood)
• Diet
• Drugs/Pharmaceuticals
• Environmental chemicals

Chromosome

Health Outcomes
• Autoimmune disease
• Cancer
• Diabetes
• Mental disorders

Chromatin

DNA

Methyl group

Epigenetic factor

DNA methylation

Gene — Histone tail

Histone

DNA inaccessible, gene inactive

DNA methylation is a chemical process that adds a methyl group to DNA. A methyl group is made up of one carbon and three hydrogen atoms. This process can alter the expression of genes, either activating or repressing them.

Histone modification

DNA accessible, gene active

Epigenetic factors are biochemical molecules that bind to histone tails. When attached to histone tails, epigenetic factors affect how tightly the DNA molecule is wound around the histones. DNA that is wound very tightly is not easily activated; DNA that is more loosely wound, is more easily activated.

FIGURE 4.6   Schematic description of epigenetic processes. (After Epigenetics - Wikipedia, the free encyclopedia)

folding are required for the incredible compaction necessary for the DNA to fit into the nucleus.

As indicated in the figure, under normal conditions, when histones are tightly compacted, genes on the DNA are "hidden" within the nucleosome and not exposed, which means that they cannot be activated and turned on. To turn genes on ("read" them or express them) and off ("not read" them or silence them), the structure of chromatin has to be altered. This is the job of epigenetic processes. Currently, there are several different types of epigenetic processes, which include the biochemical mechanisms of *methylation, acetylation, phosphorylation, ubiquitylation,* and *sumolyation,* and more will likely be discovered. However, for this introduction, only the first two will be described to provide an overview of the importance of these phenomena.

Epigenetic Function

The best-known epigenetic process so far is DNA methylation. As seen in the figure, certain sites on the DNA strands (associated with certain cytosine bases on the DNA) are "tagged" with a *methyl* group, a fundamental unit of organic chemistry. A methyl group consists of one carbon atom attached to three hydrogen atoms ($-CH_3$). Histones may also be methylated. Methyl groups, and other epigenetic factors associated with histones, are located on the small extensions of the histone tails. When DNA or histones are methylated, this compacts the chromatin, which makes DNA inaccessible and means that the gene(s) in this region is (are) silenced (not expressed). (In some situations, histone methylation may activate a gene, depending on location.) Methyl groups are attached to the DNA by enzymes, often near the beginning of a gene—the same place where proteins attach to activate the gene. If the protein cannot attach due to a blocking methyl group, then the gene usually remains off.

Histones are methylated by enzymes called histone methyltransferases, and enzymes called histone demethylases reverse this. Methylation of DNA is regulated by DNA methyltransferase (DNMT) enzymes and demethylation of DNA by DNA demethylase enzymes. There are many forms of methyltransferase enzymes.

Another epigenetic process is histone acetylation. This biochemical reaction removes positive charges, thereby reducing the affinity between histones and DNA. This makes it easier to access genes, therefore, in most cases, histone acetylation enhances gene activation while histone deacetylation represses gene activation. Histone acetylation is catalyzed by histone acetyltransferases (HATs) and histone deacetylation is catalyzed by histone deacetylases (designated as HDs or HDACs). Furthermore, the two processes of methylation and acetylation may affect each other. That is, methylation of DNA can eventually lead to deacetylation of histones, by activating HDACs. (These are not the only known interactions. There are substances that can expose DNA by sliding or even detaching histones.)

In summary, methylation and deacetylation compress chromatin and silence genes. On the other hand, demethylation and acetylation do the opposite; they decompress chromatin and thus activate genes. Effects on chromatin will determine how accessible the chromosomes are to the molecules, such as RNA, that perform all the necessary functions of copying, synthesizing, and repairing our genetic machinery.

Epigenetic Effects

It is epigenetic "marks" such as these that tell your genes to switch "on" or "off," and this is how environmental factors such as diet, stress, and toxins can have an effect on genes that may be passed on to other generations. For example, the body cannot make methyl groups, but gets them from dietary sources. Methyl groups are important in the synthesis of nucleic acid bases, which are not only important for DNA and RNA, but also for a critical cofactor required by the enzymes that make the neurotransmitters dopamine (DA), norepinephrine (NE), and serotonin (5-HT). Methyl groups are also involved in the synthesis of melatonin and epinephrine, and in the inactivation of DA and NE, the latter by the methyltransferase enzyme known as catechol-o-methyl transferase (COMT). Thus, *methylomics* is critically involved in genetics, epigenetics, and neurotransmitters, and, as such, may be relevant to psychiatric disorders.

While the psychiatric implications of epigenetics have yet to be determined, scientists have discovered that some diseases such as Prader–Willi syndrome, Angelman syndrome, and Rett syndrome have epigenetic etiologies. The most extensive amount of research has been in the area of cancer. Because some cancers are caused by deactivation of tumor-suppressing genes, researchers have worked to develop medications that reactivate them. The drug azacitidine, for instance, treats leukemia in this manner. Unfortunately, it also produces serious side effects of nausea, anemia, vomiting, and fever, which might be expected for substances that have such a nonspecific action. Nevertheless, research continues on epigenetic mechanisms in immune disorders, aging-related changes, including Alzheimer's disease, and the possibility of abnormal methylation in schizophrenia. One of the most active areas of epigenetic research in psychiatry is that of addiction. More generally, the possibilities are being explored that unfavorable epigenetic mechanisms may be triggered when someone becomes addicted to drugs or acquires other forms of "abnormal learning," such as developing an anxiety disorder or a chronic pain condition (for more detailed discussions of epigenetics, see Maze et al., 2013, and Moore et al., 2013).

Epigenetic Influences in Addiction

Detailed descriptions of epigenetic processes in regard to drug addiction have been published (Robison and Nestler, 2011; Wong et al., 2011), in which dozens of drug-induced epigenetic changes have been identified. Multiple drugs of abuse produce changes in histone acetylation in the brain, including cocaine, alcohol, and cannabis (THC), although such effects may be different depending on the brain site. The diversity of actions makes it difficult to interpret the possible behavioral relevance of the drug-induced changes. However, a couple of examples may offer some insight into current approaches. Damez-Werno and colleagues (2012), from Dr. Nestler's research group, provide an example of an epigenetic influence. As previously discovered (by their laboratory), and noted above, chronic cocaine use increases the amount of ΔFosB in the NAc. These investigators found that prior exposure to cocaine, followed by extended withdrawal from the drug, produced a greater increase of ΔFosB when rats were reexposed, relative to nonpretreated rats. The increased sensitivity after reexposure was associated with changes in the chromatin in the part of the gene responsible for making ΔFosB. In other words, initial use of cocaine changed the activity of the gene that produced ΔFosB, by making it more responsive when the animal was reexposed to the drug. Similar kinds of changes occurred in regard to natural rewards, such as sexual behavior—at least in male rats (Pitchers et al., 2013)! Another, particularly intriguing, study investigated epigenetic modulation of the unpleasant memory produced by morphine withdrawal in rats. In this study, the association between morphine and a specific environment was extinguished by exposing the animals to the environment without the drug (a process called *conditioned morphine withdrawal*).

The scientists found that this training increased BDNF in the brain and that this increase could be modulated by drugs that affected HDACs and by drugs (such as D-cycloserine) that affected the NMDA receptor (Wang et al., 2012).

Pharmacotherapy of Substance Use Disorders

In spite of their intellectual sophistication and creativity, these new theoretical ways of thinking about addiction have not yet produced novel treatments for this disorder. Current approaches still consist mostly of traditional, relatively specific therapies, focusing on medications that directly affect the biological actions of the primary drug of abuse (Pierce et al., 2012). This section includes an overview of classic approaches to drug treatment of addiction, which will be discussed further in the relevant chapters of this book, and then describes some recent efforts that fall outside of these categories.

Agonist Substitution Treatment

Prescribing a substitute drug for the abused agent is one of the most well-established pharmacological interventions for addiction. This approach has been most commonly used to treat opioid and nicotine addiction. The method originated with early studies of the opiate methadone, which was found to reduce heroin use, crime, and the spread of HIV infections as well as helping to get addicts involved in their treatment (see Lingford-Hughes et al., 2004; Nutt and Lingford-Hughes, 2008). Methadone can substitute for heroin because it is a (relatively) full opioid agonist, but it has a slower onset of effect. Although the oral route produces less of a "rush" than does heroin, its long half-life allows once-daily dosing, which reduces both cravings for and the effect of (and the need to obtain) heroin. Nevertheless, because methadone is still a very addictive drug, which can be fatal in overdose and diverted into street use, it is usually given in supervised situations. This practice is expensive; often addicts are allowed to take doses home over the weekend, which leads to diversion and accidental overdoses, often in children.

Agonist substitution has also long been used effectively for treating nicotine addiction. A variety of formulations have been developed, including nicotine lozenges, gum, and patches (see Chapter 6). A "substitution" approach may also be effective for treating stimulant addiction (Herin et al., 2010). The drug modafinil, currently approved for treating narcolepsy, is a mild stimulant and enhances glutamate neurotransmission. Although there is some evidence that modafinil might blunt some of the psychological and physiological effects of stimulants, clinical results have been inconsistent (see Chapter 7). A parallel approach may be seen with disulfiram (Antabuse), which is a traditional agent for treating alcoholism. Disulfiram blocks an enzyme that is involved in alcohol metabolism. If alcohol is taken with disulfiram, the substance acetaldehyde is not metabolized; it builds up and produces an unpleasant reaction that presumably prevents subsequent alcohol use. However, it has been shown that disulfiram can also block dopamine β-hydroxylase in the brain, thereby increasing dopamine and depleting noradrenaline. Both changes may be beneficial in stimulant dependence (Gaval-Cruz and Weinshenker, 2009). In fact disulfiram has shown promise in treating cocaine addiction and it is hypothesized that this may be due to its effects on the dopaminergic system, although clear evidence of this is needed (Preti, 2007). One disadvantage is that disulfiram also blocks the metabolism of cocaine as well as dopamine, which apparently increases the aversive anxiogenic effects of cocaine.

Partial Agonist Substitution Treatment

Instead of substituting one full agonist for another, an alternative approach is to use a partial agonist such as buprenorphine for opiate addiction (discussed in Chapter 10). Like methadone, such treatment reduces intravenous injecting, because the addict is exposed to sufficient drug to overcome the need for additional opiate use. Buprenorphine produces less severe withdrawal than methadone, but that may be due to its long half-life, which may "protect" an addict from heroin use for two to three days. There is still the risk of potentially fatal respiratory depression (overdose death) if buprenorphine is combined with other sedative hypnotics. This risk can be reduced if an opiate antagonist is added to buprenorphine, which has been done.

Partial agonists have also been successfully developed for nicotine addiction, for which varenicline (an $\alpha_4 \beta_2$ partial nicotinic agonist) was approved (see Chapter 6). The concept is the same as with buprenorphine for opioid dependence in that the agent provides sufficient stimulation to reduce smoking but does not support self-administration. Interestingly, there is emerging evidence that varenicline may also reduce alcohol consumption (Steensland et al., 2007).

As discussed by Nutt and Lingford-Hughes (2008), dopamine partial agonists would presumably be an interesting target for stimulant addiction. Such drugs should provide enough dopamine activation to reduce the effects of withdrawal yet block the consequences of illicit stimulant use. The antipsychotic aripiprazole is such a drug, and it was reportedly effective in preventing relapse in an animal model of cocaine administration (Feltenstein et al., 2007), but was not found effective, in one study, for stimulant abuse in addicts (Tiihonen et al., 2007).

Antagonists as Treatments for Addiction

Another standard approach to treating addiction is to administer an antagonist of the abused drug. By directly blocking the reinforcing effect, an antagonist would eventually reduce the compulsive behavior. The opiate antagonists naloxone, naltrexone, and nalmefene have long been available for such treatment. However, a major difficulty with these agents is compliance—because they offer no positive reinforcement, it is hard to maintain adherence. If the addict continues to take an antagonist, it will be very effective in reducing abuse. But if the patient stops the antagonist and then relapses to heroin, there is a possibility that the opiate will be even more dangerous than it was before the antagonist treatment: the tolerance that developed during prior opiate use (before the antagonist treatment) will have worn off, and renewed opiate use may produce serious problems, such as respiratory depression. Nutt and Lingford-Hughes (2008) discuss the advantages of a long-acting naltrexone implant, although they acknowledge that even this formulation would not eliminate the problems produced by rapid termination of antagonist exposure.

Nevertheless, opiate-specific antagonists, such as naloxone and naltrexone, can be effective for treating heroin abuse. The use of opiate antagonists to also treat different classes of drugs of abuse (e.g., alcohol, stimulants) is perhaps not obvious but has theoretical and practical support. Tiihonen and coworkers (2012) report the results of a 10-week clinical trial assessing the effects of the opiate antagonist naltrexone (in a sustained-release, implantable form) on individuals with dual dependence on heroin and amphetamine. The naltrexone-treated group had significantly more heroin-free urine samples at the 10-week assessment, and the difference in amphetamine-free samples approached significance. Fifty-two percent of the urine samples were heroin free versus 20 percent in the placebo-treated group, and 40 percent of the samples were amphetamine free versus 24 percent in the placebo-treated group. Interestingly, patients in the naltrexone-treated group who continued to use amphetamine reported a significantly reduced amphetamine effect, indicating that naltrexone suppressed the euphoric effect more than placebo.

Antagonists of other abused drugs are available, notably the benzodiazepine antagonist flumazenil (Anexate, Romazicon). As yet this approach has not been used for treating benzodiazepine abuse.

As Nutt and Lingford-Hughes (2008) note, a similar case could be made in regard to cannabis dependence. A number of potent and selective antagonists have been made for the CB_1 receptor. One of them, rimonabant (Acomplia), was approved for weight loss, but it was subsequently pulled off the market because of reports of depression and suicidality (see Chapter 9). Other cannabinoid antagonists and inverse agonists are currently under development, and may eventually be tested as medications for treating cannabis addiction.

Targeting Nondopaminergic Neurotransmitter Systems

GABAergic System. As noted above, the dopaminergic cell bodies in the ventral tegmental area are under GABAergic control, and the GABA-B receptor is involved in this interaction (Cousins et al., 2002). GABA-B agonists, such as baclofen, can reduce the reinforcing effects of several different classes of abused drugs (for example heroin, psychostimulants, alcohol) in animal models under a variety of conditions. Studies in humans have also shown baclofen to be promising in treating cocaine addiction and alcoholism (Nutt and Lingford-Hughes, 2008) although current outcomes do not recommend its use as a first-line treatment for alcoholism (Muzyk et al., 2012).

Other GABAergic medications being tested as possible agents for preventing cocaine relapse are anticonvulsants. One such drug is gamma-vinyl-GABA (Vigabatrin), an anticonvulsant that blocks the enzyme that breaks down GABA. This drug had shown some benefit in small trials and was subsequently found to be effective in a randomized, placebo-controlled clinical trial (Brodie et al., 2009). Because it appears to cause visual field defects, it has not been approved for use in the United States.

Treatment Approaches Derived from the Glutamatergic Model of Addiction. The proposed glial dysfunction involving the xCT exchange process and GLT-1, led to the consideration of the drug N-acetylcysteine for addiction. This drug is currently prescribed for pulmonary disease as well as acetaminophen overdose; it was found to *increase the brain's production of xCT*. In a similar manner, the drug ceftriaxone is an antibiotic that appears *to increase levels of GLT-1*. Laboratory experiments with these drugs indicated that they could reduce the likelihood of relapse to cocaine (Abulseoud et al., 2012).

Because acetylcysteine is already available for human use, several small clinical trials have been conducted in people who are nicotine addicts, marijuana users, cocaine addicts, and pathological gamblers (Dean et al., 2011). The drug is well-tolerated, but although many of the participants reported that they had less craving or desire to use their respective drug or engage in gambling, objective results from these studies were not impressive (Olive et al., 2012). Recent data from animal studies may provide an explanation. The latest experiments reveal what happens when N-acetylcysteine raises extracellular glutamate in the critically important nucleus accumbens region of the reward system. As predicted, at lower doses of the medication the released glutamate stimulates presynaptic glutamate autoreceptors (mGluR2/3) on neurons. The presynaptic stimulation dampens neuronal activity in the nucleus accumbens and, in rats, reduces the tendency to respond to cocaine-associated cues. However, at higher doses, more glutamate is released and an additional, postsynaptic, glutamate receptor (mGluR5) is also stimulated. The postsynaptic stimulation has opposite effects: it intensifies neuronal activity and partly offsets the positive effect. The researchers proposed that a medication (or combination of medications) that both increases nonsynaptic extracellular glutamate to stimulate mGluR2/3, and inhibit mGluR5 receptors, might reduce the risk of relapse more effectively than N-acetylcysteine alone (Kupchik et al., 2012).

Affecting the glial control of glutamate by ceftriaxone has also been reported to prevent relapse in laboratory animals. However, this drug has to be given by intramuscular injection, which limits its practical benefit.

Another medication in this class is the drug modafinil (Provigil), used to treat narcolepsy. Although its mechanism of action is not known for certain, it seems predominantly to be a reuptake blocker of dopamine and norepinephrine, and it also increases glutamate levels. In animals it reduced drug responses for cocaine and amphetamine and it blocked a measure of relapse in morphine-treated animals (Mahler et al., 2012). Clinically, however, the effects of modafinil on cocaine use have been inconsistent. [One explanation of why such a drug that increases glutamate might be antiaddictive is that it might "normalize" glutamate function in addicts during withdrawal (Olive et al., 2012).]

Acamprosate (used clinically to maintain alcohol abstinence; see Chapter 5) has also been found, in animal models, to reduce glutamate overactivity or release in the nucleus accumbens and hippocampus during early ethanol withdrawal and to prevent associated toxicities (Mason and Heyser, 2010). Although electrophysiological studies of its mechanism of action have been inconsistent, it is considered to be an NMDA modulator. However, a large multicenter study did not find that acamprosate was any more effective than placebo in treating alcohol addicts (Olive et al., 2012).

Several antiepileptic drugs also reduce glutamatergic actions and may have some benefit against addiction. Topiramate has been tested in studies of cocaine abstinence and found to be modestly effective. This drug not only facilitates GABA function, it reduces transmitter release, including glutamate, and blocks AMPA receptors. It can cause sedation and memory problems and should not be used in persons with a history of kidney stones (Lingford-Hughes et al., 2004; Sofuoglu and Kosten, 2006; Johnson et al., 2007). Several reports during the last decade found topiramate useful in reducing subjective effects, craving, and heavy consumption in alcohol addicts. There are also some positive results in regard to behavioral addictions such as gambling, overeating, and sex. Topiramate's benefit for addiction may be related to its ability to reduce impulsivity and promote behavioral inhibition (Olive et al., 2012).

Gabapentin and lamotrigine are two other anticonvulsants that inhibit the release of various transmitters, including glutamate. Both drugs can relieve some somatic symptoms of alcohol withdrawal. The results of studies assessing their ability to treat addiction are inconsistent (gabapentin) and very limited (lamotrigine). Lamotrigine can also produce an uncommon but serious skin rash (Olive et al., 2012). Memantine is a noncompetitive antagonist at NMDA receptors, and is used primarily to treat cognitive decline in Alzheimer's disease. Current evidence is inconsistent in regard to alcohol addiction (Olive et al., 2012).

Other approaches involving glutamate include agonists that act directly on the presynaptic glutamate receptor, the mGluR2/3 subtype. By stimulating this autoreceptor, glutamate agonists decrease glutamate release, which might prevent relapse. Interestingly, these receptors are also found on dopamine terminals, where they reduce dopamine release. This could mean that they might also reduce the probability of even initiating drug use. In animals, these agents reduced the self-administration of cocaine, alcohol, and nicotine (Kalivas and Volkow, 2011). Several reviews of animal experiments have recently been published, supporting the involvement of metabotropic glutamate receptors in addiction (Brown et al., 2012; Cleva and Olive, 2012; Duncan and Lawrence, 2012; Li et al., 2013).

In addition to the metabotropic types of glutamate receptor, studies are also examining the effects of ionotropic glutamate receptors, the AMPA and NMDA subtypes. Excessive AMPA activity may contribute to relapse. The drug tezampanel is an AMPA/kainate receptor antagonist that is being tested for relief of acute migraine, and it reduced cocaine self-administration in animal experiments. Two other drugs, talampanel (an AMPA/kainate antagonist) and perampanel (a noncompetitive AMPA antagonist) are being evaluated in some neurological disorders, and might be usefully tested for addiction. In October 2012, perampanel was approved for use in patients aged 12 years and older with partial-onset seizures.

A group of substances called ampakines modulate the AMPA receptor; they maintain its sensitivity in the presence of stimulation, preventing desensitization. These compounds might counteract some of the toxic effects of drug exposure; for example, they might prevent the possible development of Parkinson's disease in people who abuse methamphetamine.

NMDA receptors might affect addiction because of a general enhancement of learning and memory (Sofuoglu et al., 2013). This would include extinction, in which an animal learns that a behavior, or context, is no longer associated with a drug. For this reason the NMDA coagonist drug, D-cycloserine (DCS), has been tested in various studies, in human and nonhuman experiments, in extinction procedures, in an effort to help addicts "unlearn" the association between the drug and the environment of illicit use (Hammond et al., 2013). For example, in cigarette smokers, DCS facilitated extinction compared to the placebo treatment. In another study, the drug showed a slight effect in reducing cravings in cocaine addicts. However, so far, the clinical application of DCS has not been as effective as suggested by the preclinical animal models (Myers and Carlezon, 2012; Olive et al., 2012).

A specific subtype of NMDA receptor, containing the NR2B subunit, has been most implicated in the association between drugs and drug cues. The drug ifenprodil blocks this receptor subtype, and has been reported to reduce relapse in animal models of drug abuse (Kalivas and Volkow, 2011).

Opioid System. μ opioid receptors are also located on GABA neurons in the VTA, and they play a key role in modulating ventral tegmental area dopaminergic activity. A link between alcohol use and endogenous opioid activity was suggested by animal models, in which the opioid antagonist naltrexone reduced alcohol self-administration by blocking this μ opioid receptor. Naltrexone has now been shown in several clinical trials in alcoholism to reduce the risk of a full-blown relapse (Pettinati et al., 2006). It does not work for everyone and may be most effective for people who are more severely alcohol dependent. Jayaram-Lindström and coworkers (2008) and now Tiihonen and colleagues (2012) have shown that naltrexone may also promote abstinence from amphetamine. Evidence has been reviewed showing that other drugs of abuse, such as nicotine, other stimulants, and cannabis may also interact with the endogenous opioid system. The μ opiate receptor appears to be critically involved in the rewarding properties of other drugs of abuse, and in the development of physical dependence to nicotine and cannabinoids (Trigo et al., 2010).

Cannabinoid System. Cannabinoid-opiate interactions are gaining more attention in current concepts of addiction and reward mechanisms (Robledo, 2010), including the substrates for nicotine (Maldonado and Berrendero, 2010) and alcohol (López-Moreno et al., 2010) addiction. As discussed by Parolaro and coworkers (2010), there are three primary aspects relevant to this model: (1) cannabinoids can release opioid peptides and opioids can release endocannabinoids; (2) when receptors for these two systems are both located on the same cells, there is evidence for direct receptor-receptor interaction; and (3) there is an interaction between their intracellular pathways. For example, activation of either of these two systems produces a similar degree of relapse to alcohol in animal models of alcohol addiction. The cannabinoid-opioid relationship in the reward system might also differ from their interaction within other systems, such as the pain pathways.

There is also a lot of overlap between cannabis abuse and alcohol abuse. These drugs are both central nervous system depressants and produce similar behavioral reactions, such as ataxia, feelings of intoxication, motor impairments, memory problems, sleep disruption, and other neuropsychological deficits. They also show cross-tolerance with each other to some of these effects. Pava and Woodward (2012) present a comprehensive review of the interactions between alcohol (ethanol) and the endocannabinoid (EC) system, describing the changes in the EC receptors produced by chronic alcohol consumption.

New Directions

Vaccines are another promising therapy for relapse prevention. The approach works by stimulating the production of drug-specific antibodies (to nicotine, opiates, cocaine, or amphetamine). If the drug of abuse is still used, the antibodies bind to the drug molecules in the blood and prevent them from crossing the blood-brain barrier, thereby blocking the euphoria produced in the brain and presumably decreasing further use. Progress has been most advanced with respect to vaccines for nicotine (see Chapter 6) and cocaine addiction (see Chapter 7), and most recently, heroin (see Chapter 10). With regard to THC, the molecule is too hard to access. Alcohol molecules themselves are too small to attach to the protein that would be necessary to deliver the immunity. However, a drug that blocks the gene that produces the alcohol-metabolizing enzyme in the liver (aldehyde dehydrogenase) is being developed. Essentially, this substance would produce a very unpleasant reaction, basically a hangover, if alcohol were taken.

Some novel approaches have come from related areas of research. For example, the overlap between drug stimuli and natural stimuli in the reward system suggests that substances that affect eating might also affect drug use. One agent is GLP-1, a glucagon-like peptide, which is released from the GI tract in response to food and is involved in the regulation of eating. An agonist drug, exenatide (Ex-4), that stimulates the GLP-1 receptor, is currently used in the treatment of diabetes. By acting on the glucagon receptor, the drug appears to reduce the rewarding effect of highly palatable food. Realizing the similarity to drug reward, researchers gave the drug to mice and found that it seemed to reduce the rewarding effect of cocaine (Graham et al., 2013).

Another novel approach, derived from other areas of behavioral treatment, is the possibility of treating addiction by administering deep brain stimulation (DBS). Luigjes and colleagues (2012) review the current evidence from animal and human studies that support this modality for refractory addiction. The primary question is: which brain area would be most effective? The authors support the NAc as the most promising site for human trials, although other locations, notably the medial prefrontal cortex, have not been extensively investigated.

Neuroscientists have begun to recognize the implications of an impaired prefrontal cortex, which regulates long-term planning, decision making, and moral judgment. Researchers are now searching for ways to make these prefrontal systems more resilient. These approaches raise a question: Is drug use the cause of users' prefrontal problems, or do they have preexisting defects that make them susceptible to addiction? After all, a lot of people might be able to use drugs in a socially controlled manner, but only a certain percentage actually go on to become addicted. Perhaps part of the reason is that such people lack prefrontal-mediated control over behavior. In the protected environment of a rehabilitation center, drugs and other cues associated with drug taking are eliminated and stressful situations that suppress prefrontal activity are minimized. This environment, as much as any medication, provides the context in which prefrontal cortex function can be strengthened. Finally, religion has long been shown to have a strong inverse association with drug addiction. Some religious rituals have been found to provoke enhanced activity in prefrontal regions. It may be that the original insight behind Alcoholics Anonymous, of allowing oneself to be guided by a higher power, has a biological substrate in the frontal lobe (Schnabel, 2009).

STUDY QUESTIONS

1. What types of drug abuse problems are currently of most concern, that is, which drugs and which populations?

2. Is a propensity for abusing drugs caused by a psychopathological process in the user, or is it a property of the particular drug?

3. What is the neurobiological mechanism that underlies the behavioral reinforcing properties of abused drugs?

4. How does chronic drug use eventually become addiction?

5. What types of receptor-based approaches to the pharmacotherapy of drug abuse have been developed?

6. How has our understanding of the neurobiology of addiction guided efforts to find new therapies?

REFERENCES

Abulseoud, O. A., et al. (2012). "Ceftriaxone Upregulates the Glutamate Transporter in Medial Prefrontal Cortex and Blocks Reinstatement of Methamphetamine Seeking in a Condition Place Preference Paradigm." *Brain Research* 1456: 14–21.

American Psychiatric Association. (2000). *Diagnostic and Statistical Manual of Mental Disorders*, 4th ed., text revision (DSM-IV-TR). Washington, DC: American Psychiatric Association.

American Psychiatric Association. (2013). *Diagnostic and Statistical Manual of Mental Disorders*, 5th ed. (DSM-5). Washington, DC: American Psychiatric Association.

Bock, R., et al. (2013). "Strengthening the Accumbal Indirect Pathway Promotes Resilience to Compulsive Cocaine Use." *Nature Neuroscience* 16: 632–638.

Brodie, J. D., et al. (2009). "Randomized, Double-Blind, Placebo-Controlled Trial of Vigabatrin for the Treatment of Cocaine Dependence in Mexican Parolees." *American Journal of Psychiatry* 166: 1269–1277.

Brown, R. M., et al. (2012). "mGlu5 Receptor Functional Interactions and Addiction." *Frontiers in Pharmacology* 3: 1–9, article 84.

Cai, Y.-Q., et al. (2013). "Central Amygdala GluA1 Facilitates Associative Learning of Opioid Reward." *The Journal of Neuroscience* 33: 1577–1588.

Chen, B. T., et al. (2013). "Rescuing the Cocaine-Induced Prefrontal Cortex Hypoactivity Prevents Compulsive Cocaine Seeking." *Nature* 496: 359–362.

Cleva, R. M., and Olive, M. F. (2012). "Metabotropic Glutamate Receptors and Drug Addiction." *Wiley Interdisciplinary Reviews: Membrane Transport and Signaling* 1:281–295.

Cooper, Z. D., et al. (2012). "Glial Modulators: A Novel Pharmacological Approach to Altering the Behavioral Effects of Abused Substances." *Expert Opinion on Investigational Drugs* 21: 169–178.

Cousins, M. S., et al. (2002). "GABA B Receptor Agonists for the Treatment of Drug Addiction: A Review of Recent Findings." *Drug and Alcohol Dependence* 65: 209–220.

Damez-Werno, D., et al. (2012). "Drug Experience Epigenetically Primes *Fosb* Gene Inducibility in Rat Nucleus Accumbens." *The Journal of Neuroscience* 2: 10267–10272.

Dean, O., et al. (2011). "N-Acetylcysteine in Psychiatry: Current Therapeutic Evidence and Potential Mechanisms of Action." *Journal of Psychiatry and Neuroscience* 36: 78–86.

Duncan, J. R., and Lawrence, A. J. (2012). "The Role of Metabotropic Glutamate Receptors in Addiction: Evidence from Preclinical Models." *Pharmacology Biochemistry and Behavior* 100: 811–824.

Durazzo, T. C., et al. (2011). "Cortical Thickness, Surface Area, and Volume of the Brain Reward System in Alcohol Dependence: Relationships to Relapse and Extended Abstinence." *Alcoholism: Clinical and Experimental Research (ACER)* 35: 1187–1200.

Feltenstein, M. W., et al. (2007). "Aripiprazole Blocks Reinstatement of Cocaine Seeking in an Animal Model of Relapse." *Biological Psychiatry* 61: 582–590.

Fowler, J. S., et al. (2007). "Imaging the Addicted Human Brain." *Addiction Science & Clinical Practice* 3: 4–16 (NIH Publication No. 07-6171).

Gaval-Cruz, M., and Weinshenker, D. (2009). "Mechanisms of Disulfiram-Induced Cocaine Abstinence: Antabuse and Cocaine Relapse." *Molecular Interventions* 9: 175–187.

Graham, D. L., et al. (2013). "GLP-1 Analog Attenuates Cocaine Reward." *Molecular Psychiatry* 18: 961–962.

Haass-Koffler, C. L., and Bartlett, S. E. (2012). "Stress and Addiction: Contribution of the Corticotropin Releasing Factor (CRF) System in Neuroplasticity." *Frontiers in Molecular Neuroscience* 5: 1–13, article 91.

Hammond, S., et al. (2013). "D-serine Facilitates the Effectiveness of Extinction to Reduce Drug-Primed Reinstatement of Cocaine-Induced Conditioned Place Preference." *Neuropharmacology* 64: 464–471.

Heberlein, A., et al. (2011). "Serum Levels of BDNF Are Associated with Craving in Opiate-Dependent Patients." *Journal of Psychopharmacology* 25: 1480–1484.

Herin, D. V., et al. (2010). "Agonist-Like Pharmacotherapy for Stimulant Dependence: Preclinical, Human Laboratory, and Clinical Studies." *Annals of the New York Academy of Sciences* 1187: 76–100.

Jayaram-Lindström, N., et al. (2008). "Naltrexone for the Treatment of Amphetamine Dependence: A Randomized, Placebo-Controlled Trial." *American Journal of Psychiatry* 165: 1442–1448.

Johnson, B. A., et al. (2007) "Topiramate for Treating Alcohol Dependence: A Randomized Controlled Trial." *Journal of the American Medical Association* 298: 1641–1651.

Kalivas, P. W., et al. (2006). "Animal Models and Brain Circuits in Drug Addiction." *Molecular Interventions* 6: 339–344.

Kalivas, P. W. (2009). "The Glutamate Homeostasis Hypothesis of Addiction." *Nature Reviews Neuroscience* 10: 561–572.

Kalivas, P. W., and Volkow, N. D. (2011). "New Medications for Drug Addiction Hiding in Glutamatergic Neuroplasticity." *Molecular Psychiatry* 16: 974–986.

Kupchik, Y. M., et al. (2012). "The Effect of N-Acetylcysteine in the Nucleus Accumbens on Neurotransmission and Relapse to Cocaine." *Biological Psychiatry* 71: 978–986.

Li, X., et al. (2013). "Metabotropic glutamate 7(mGlu 7) Receptor: A Target for Medication Development for the Treatment of Cocaine Dependence." *Neuropharmacology* 66: 12–23.

Lingford-Hughes, A. R., et al. (2004). "Evidence-Based Guidelines for the Pharmacological Management of Substance Misuse, Addiction and Comorbidity." *Journal of Psychopharmacology* 18: 293–335.

López-Moreno, J. A., et al. (2010). "Functional Interactions Between Endogenous Cannabinoid and Opioid Systems: Focus on Alcohol, Genetics and Drug-Addicted Behaviors." *Current Drug Targets* 11: 406–428.

Luigjes, J., et al. (2012). "Deep Brain Stimulation in Addiction: A Review of Potential Brain Targets." *Molecular Psychiatry* 17: 572–583.

Madsen, H. B., et al. (2012). "Neuroplasticity in Addiction: Cellular and Transcriptional Perspectives." *Frontiers in Molecular Neuroscience* 5: 1–16, article 99.

Mahler, S. V., et al. (2012). "Modafinil Attenuates Reinstatement of Cocaine Seeking: Role for Cystine-Glutamate Exchange and Metabotropic Glutamate Receptors." *Addiction Biology* doi: 10.1111/j.1369-1600.2012.00506.x.

Maldonado R., and Berrendero, F. (2010). "Endogenous Cannabinoid and Opioid Systems and Their Role in Nicotine Addiction." *Current Drug Targets* 11: 440–449.

Mameli, M., and Lüscher, C. (2011). "Synaptic Plasticity and Addiction: Learning Mechanisms Gone Awry." *Neuropharmacology* 61: 1052–1059.

Mason, B. J., and Heyser, C. J. (2010). "The Neurobiology, Clinical Efficacy and Safety of Acamprosate in the Treatment of Alcohol Dependence." *Expert Opinion on Drug Safety* 9: 177–188.

Maze, I., et al. (2013). "Histone Regulation in the CNS: Basic Principles of Epigenetic Plasticity." *Neuropsychopharmacology* 38: 3–22.

Moore, L. D., et al. (2013). "DNA Methylation and Its Basic Function." *Neuropsychopharmacology* 38: 23–38.

Muzyk, A. J., et al. (2012). "Defining the Role of Baclofen for the Treatment of Alcohol Dependence: A Systematic Review of the Evidence." *CNS Drugs* 26: 69–78.

Myers, K. M, and Carlezon, W. A., Jr. (2012). "D-Cycloserine Effects on Extinction of Conditioned Responses to Drug-Related Cues." *Biological Psychiatry* 71: 947–955.

Nestler, E. (2005). "Is There a Common Molecular Pathway for Addiction?" *Nature Neuroscience* 8: 1445–1449.

Nestler, E. J., and Malenka, R. C. (2004). "The Addicted Brain." *Scientific American* 290: 78–85.

Novak, M. (2010). "Incentive Learning Underlying Cocaine-Seeking Requires mGluR5 Receptors Located on Dopamine D1 Receptor-Expressing Neurons." *The Journal of Neuroscience* 30: 11973–11982.

Nutt, D., and Lingford-Hughes, A (2008). "Addiction: The Clinical Interface." *British Journal of Pharmacology* 154: 397–405.

Olds, J., and Milner, P. (1954). "Positive Reinforcement Produced by Electrical Stimulation of Septal Area and Other Regions of Rat Brain." *Journal of Comparative and Physiological Psychology* 47: 419–427.

Olive, M. F., et al. (2012). "Glutamatergic Medications for the Treatment of Drug and Behavioral Addictions." *Pharmacology, Biochemistry and Behavior* 100: 801–810.

Parolaro, D., et al. (2010). "Cellular Mechanisms Underlying the Interaction Between Cannabinoid and Opiate System." *Current Drug Targets* 11: 393–405.

Pava, M. J., and Woodward, J. J. (2012). "A Review of the Interactions Between Alcohol and the Endocannabinoid System: Implications for Alcohol Dependence and Future Directions for Research." *Alcohol* 46: 185–204.

Pettinati, H. M., et al. (2006). "The Status of Naltrexone in the Treatment of Alcohol Dependence: Specific Effects on Heavy Drinking." *Journal of Clinical Psychopharmacology* 26: 610–625.

Pettinati, N. M., et al. (2013). "Current Status of Co-Occurring Mood and Substance Use Disorders: A New Therapeutic Target." *American Journal of Psychiatry* 170: 23–30.

Pierce, R. C., and Kumaresan, V. (2006). "The Mesolimbic Dopamine System: The Final Common Pathway for the Reinforcing Effect of Drugs of Abuse?" *Neuroscience and Biobehavioral Reviews* 30: 215–238.

Pierce, R. C., et al. (2012). "Rational Development of Addiction Pharmacotherapies: Successes, Failures, and Prospects." *Cold Spring Harbor Perspectives in Medicine* 2: a012880.

Pitchers, K. K., et al. (2013)."Natural and Drug Rewards Act on Common Neural Plasticity Mechanisms with ΔFosB as a Key Mediator." *The Journal of Neuroscience* 33: 3434–3442.

Preti, A. (2007). "New Developments in the Pharmacotherapy of Cocaine Abuse." *Addiction Biology* 12: 133–151.

Riegel, A. C., and Kalivas, P. W. (2010). "Lack of Inhibition Leads to Abuse." *Nature* 463: 743–744.

Robison, A. J., and Nestler, E. J. (2011). "Transcriptional and Epigenetic Mechanisms of Addiction." *Nature Reviews Neuroscience* 12: 623–637.

Robledo, P. (2010). "Cannabinoids, Opioids and NMDA: Neuropsychological Interactions Related to Addiction." *Current Drug Targets* 11: 429–439.

Schnabel, J. (2009). "Rethinking Rehab." *Nature* 458: 25–27.

Sofuoglu, M., et al. (2013). "Cognitive Enhancement as a Treatment for Drug Addictions." *Neuropharmacology* 64: 452–463.

Sofuoglu, M., and Kosten, T. R. (2006). "Emerging Pharmacological Strategies in the Fight Against Cocaine Addiction." *Expert Opinion on Emerging Drugs* 11: 91–98.

Steensland, P., et al. (2007). "Varenicline, an a_4b_2 Nicotinic Acetylcholine Receptor Partial Agonist, Selectively Decreases Ethanol Consumption and Seeking." *Proceedings of the National Academy of Sciences USA* 104: 12518–12523.

Tamir, D. I., and Mitchell, J. P. (2012). "Disclosing Information About the Self is Intrinsically Rewarding." *Proceedings of the National Academy of Sciences USA* 109: 8038-8043.

Tiihonen, J., et al. (2007). "A Comparison of Aripiprazole, Methylphenidate, and Placebo for Amphetamine Dependence." *American Journal of Psychiatry* 164: 160–162.

Tiihonen, J., et al. (2012). "Naltrexone Implant for the Treatment of Polydrug Dependence: A Randomized Controlled Trial." *American Journal of Psychiatry* 169: 531–536.

Trigo, J. M., et al. (2010). "The Endogenous Opioid System: A Common Substrate in Drug Addiction." *Drug and Alcohol Dependence* 108: 183–194.

Volkow, N. D., et al. (1997). "Relationship Between Subjective Effects of Cocaine and Dopamine Transporter Occupancy." *Nature* 386: 827–830.

Volkow, N. D., et al. (2004). "The Addicted Human Brain Viewed in the Light of Imaging Studies: Brain Circuits and Treatment Strategies." *Neuropharmacology* 47, Supplement 1: 3–13.

Volkow, N. D., et al. (2011). "Addiction: Beyond Dopamine Reward Circuitry." *Proceedings of the National Academy of Sciences* 108: 15037–15042.

Wang, W.-S., et al. (2012). "Extinction of Aversive Memories Associated with Morphine Withdrawal Requires ERK-Mediated Epigenetic Regulation of Brain-Derived Neurotrophic Factor Transcription in the Rat Ventromedial Prefrontal Cortex." *The Journal of Neuroscience* 32: 13763–13775.

Wong, C. C. Y., et al. (2011). "Drugs and Addiction: An Introduction to Epigenetics." *Addiction* 106: 480–489.

Yadid, G., et al. (2012). "Modulation of Mood States as a Major Factor in Relapse to Substance Use." *Frontiers in Molecular Neuroscience* 5: 1–5, article 81.

Chapter 5

Ethyl Alcohol and the Inhalants of Abuse

ETHYL ALCOHOL

Ethyl alcohol (ethanol) is a psychoactive drug that is similar in most respects to all the other sedative-hypnotic compounds that will be discussed in Chapter 13. The main differences from classical sedative-hypnotics (e.g., benzodiazepines) are twofold: ethanol is used primarily for recreational rather than medical purposes and ethanol has unique kinetics of metabolism that separates it from most other drugs. Ethyl alcohol is not merely a recreational beverage; it is a drug that, like any other psychoactive agent, affects the brain and behavior. Therefore, in discussing alcohol, we need to address its basic pharmacology (pharmacokinetics and pharmacodynamics) as well as its side effects, teratogenic effects, and toxicities. In addition, because alcohol ingestion is widely associated with drug dependence, treatment of alcohol dependence must be addressed.

Pharmacokinetics of Alcohol

Alcohol, taken orally, is rapidly and completely absorbed, both in the stomach and the upper intestine. This applies to all alcoholic beverages, including beer, fortified beers, wine, and hard liquors; hard liquors as well as high alcohol-containing beers are fortified to alcohol levels beyond those achievable with fermentation.

Absorption

Ethyl alcohol is a very simple molecule, found in 12 percent to 15 percent concentrations in wines, about 5 percent in beers (as much as 7 percent to 10 percent in some "microbrews," and as high as 10 percent to 12 percent in 16- and 24-ounce cans of fortified beverages). In "hard" liquors, alcohol is present in concentrations of 40 to 50 percent. In the latter, concentration is usually expressed as alcohol "proof," which is twice the percent concentration (for example, 80 proof = 40 percent ethanol). The appendix at the end of this chapter addresses the amount of alcohol that is present in representative forms of alcohol-containing beverages.

Alcohol diffuses easily across all biological membranes. Thus, after it is drunk, alcohol is rapidly and completely absorbed from the entire gastrointestinal tract, although most is absorbed from the upper intestine because of its large surface area. The time from the last drink to maximal concentration in blood ranges from 15 to 60 minutes. In a person with an empty stomach, approximately 20 percent of a single dose of alcohol is absorbed directly from the stomach, usually quite rapidly. The remaining 80 percent is absorbed rapidly and completely from the upper intestine; the only limiting factor is the time it takes to empty the stomach.

In persons who have undergone gastric bypass surgery for morbid obesity, the stomach and most of the upper intestine are bypassed. Interestingly, in such persons alcohol absorption occurs in the lower intestine and, in the absence of an alcohol-metabolizing enzyme normally in the stomach and upper intestine (described below), the lower intestine adapts to the presence of alcohol by slowly adapting to its presence and eventually absorbing alcohol very readily. Indeed, post-gastric-bypass patients have much higher peak blood alcohol concentrations (BAC) after ingesting alcohol and they require more time to become sober (Woodard et al. 2011). Such increases have not been observed in patients who have undergone gastric banding instead of a complete gastric bypass (Suzuki et al., 2012). These unexpected increases in BAC have been linked to potential increases in alcohol use disorders in gastric bypass patients (King et al., 2012).

Distribution

After absorption, alcohol is evenly distributed throughout all body fluids and tissues. The blood-brain barrier is freely permeable to alcohol. When alcohol appears in the blood and reaches a person's brain, it crosses the blood-brain barrier almost immediately. Alcohol is also freely distributed across the placenta and easily enters the brain of a developing fetus. Fetal blood alcohol levels are essentially the same as those of the drinking mother.

Metabolism and Excretion

Approximately 95 percent of the alcohol a person ingests is enzymatically metabolized by the enzyme *alcohol dehydrogenase* (ADH). The other 5 percent is excreted unchanged; mainly through the lungs.[1] Very small amounts of alcohol are excreted in the urine.

About 85 percent of the metabolism of alcohol occurs in the liver by ADH enzyme. Up to 15 percent of alcohol metabolism is carried out by a *gastric* ADH enzyme, located in the lining of the stomach, which can decrease the blood level of alcohol by about

---

[1] Small amounts of alcohol are excreted from the body through the lungs; most of us are familiar with "alcohol breath." This excretion forms the basis for the breath analysis test because alcohol equilibrates rapidly across the membranes of the lung. In the "breathalyzer" test, a ratio of 1:2,300 exists between alcohol in inhaled air and alcohol in venous blood. The blood alcohol concentration is easily extrapolated from alcohol concentration in the expired air.

15 percent, obviously attenuating alcohol's systemic toxicity. Rapid gastric emptying (as by drinking on an empty stomach, or by having had bariatric surgery) reduces the time that alcohol is susceptible to gastric metabolism and results in increased blood levels. Drinking on a full stomach retains alcohol in the stomach, increases its exposure to gastric ADH, and reduces the resulting peak blood level of the drug.

It is well recognized that whenever women and men consume comparable amounts of alcohol (after correction for differences in body weight), women have higher blood ethanol concentrations than men. The reasons appear to be threefold:

1. Women have about 50 percent less gastric metabolism of alcohol than men because women, whether alcoholic or nonalcoholic, have a lower level of gastric ADH enzyme. Because the gastric enzyme metabolizes about 15 percent of ingested alcohol, the blood alcohol concentration is increased by about 7 percent over that in a male drinking the same weight-adjusted amount of alcohol.

2. Men may have a greater ratio of muscle to fat than do women. Men thus have a larger vascular compartment (fat has little blood supply). Therefore, alcohol is somewhat more diluted in men, again decreasing blood alcohol levels in men compared to women.

3. Women, with higher body fat than men (fat contains little alcohol), concentrate alcohol in plasma, drink for drink, more than men, raising the apparent blood level.

The metabolism of alcohol by ADH is only the first step in a normal three-step metabolic process involved in the breakdown of alcohol (Figure 5.1):

1. Alcohol dehydrogenase functions to convert alcohol to acetaldehyde. A coenzyme called *nicotinamide adenine dinucleotide* (NAD) is required for the activity of this enzyme. The availability of NAD is the rate-limiting step in this reaction; enough is present so that the maximum amount of alcohol that can be metabolized in 24 hours is about 170 grams.

2. The enzyme ADH converts acetaldehyde to acetic acid. The drug *disulfiram* (Antabuse) irreversibly inhibits this enzyme and is one possible treatment for alcoholism.

3. Acetic acid is broken down into carbon dioxide and water, thus releasing energy (calories).

The average person metabolizes about 10 to 14 milliliters of 100 percent alcohol per hour, independent of the blood level of alcohol. This rate is fairly constant for different people.[2] Figure 5.2 illustrates the rate of alcohol elimination for a group of 48 healthy men administered a standard dose of ethanol. Here, the blood alcohol concentration falls at a rate of about 0.011 and 0.015 grams%/hour.[3] It takes an adult 1 hour to metabolize the amount of alcohol that is contained in a 1-ounce glass of 80 proof (40 percent) whiskey, a 4-ounce glass of 12 percent wine, a 12-ounce bottle of 5 percent beer, or a 6-ounce glass of 8 to 10 percent microbrew or fortified beer. Commercially poured

[2] In biochemical terms, this is called zero-order metabolism. Virtually all other drugs are metabolized by first-order metabolism, which means that the amount of drug metabolized per unit time depends on the amount (or concentration) of drug in blood. Perhaps zero-order metabolism occurs because the amount of enzyme (or a cofactor required for activity of the enzyme) is limited and becomes saturated with only small amounts of alcohol in the body.

[3] Grams% is the number of grams of ethanol that would be contained in 100 milliliters of blood.

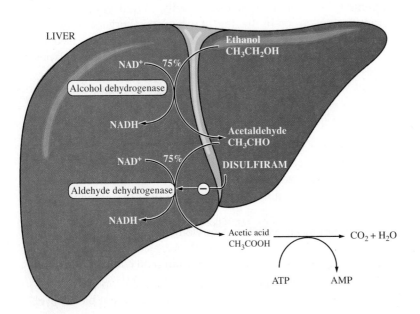

FIGURE 5.1   Metabolism of ethanol. Ethanol is oxidized by the enzyme alcohol dehydrogenase using NAD (nicotinamide adenine dinucleotide) as a cofactor to form acetaldehyde. A second oxidative step converts acetaldehyde to acetic acid, which, in turn, is broken down to carbon dioxide and water. The first step involving alcohol dehydrogenase is the rate-limiting step. The drug disulfiram (Antabuse) blocks the second step by blocking the activity of aldehyde dehydrogenase. ATP = adenosine phosphate; AMP = adenosine monophosphate.

(for example, by bartenders) alcoholic drinks usually exceed these amounts by about 50 percent; similar variation occurs in home-poured drinks.

Consumption of 4 to 5 ounces of wine, 12 ounces of 5 percent beer, or 1.0 to 1.5 ounces of 80 proof whiskey per hour would keep the blood levels of alcohol in a person fairly constant. If a person ingests more alcohol in any given hour than is metabolized, his or her blood concentrations increase. Consequently, there is a limit to the amount of alcohol a person can consume in an hour without becoming drunk. The appendix at the end of this chapter expands on the topic of drink equivalents.

Such kinetics allow not only estimation of BAC after drinking a known amount of alcoholic beverage, but also estimation of the fall in blood concentration over time after drinking ceases. The following may serve to explain the relationship between the amounts of alcohol consumed, the resulting BAC, and the impairment of motor and intellectual functioning (here, driving ability): today, all states have set a BAC of 0.08 grams% as intoxication, and a person who drives with a BAC above this amount can be charged with driving while under the influence of alcohol. Thus, one might assume that a level of 0.07 grams% is acceptable but a level of 0.09 grams% is not. However, the behavioral effects of alcohol are not all or none; alcohol (like all sedatives) progressively

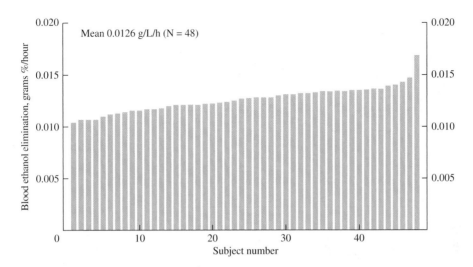

FIGURE 5.2   Individual variations in the elimination rate of ethanol as measured in 48 healthy males after they drank 0.68 gram of ethanol per kilogram of body weight. Neat whisky was ingested on an empty stomach. Values are expressed as grams of alcohol metabolized per liter of blood per hour. If expressed as grams%, 0.10 g/L/h would equate to a 0.01 grams% per hour fall in blood concentration; 0.15 g/L/hr would equal a 0.015 grams% per hour fall in blood concentration. [Reproduced data from A. W. Jones, "Disposition and Fate of Ethanol in the Body." In J. C. Garriott, ed., *Medical-Legal Aspects of Alcohol*, 4th ed. Tucson, AZ: Lawyers & Judges Publishing Company, 2003, p. 73, Figure 3.9.]

impairs a person's ability to function. Thus, the 0.08 grams% blood level is only a legally established, arbitrary value. A person whose BAC is under 0.08 grams% yet functions with impairment detrimental to operation of a motor vehicle can still suffer criminal penalties. Driving ability is minimally impaired at a BAC of 0.01 grams%, but at 0.04 to 0.08 grams%, a driver has increasingly impaired judgment and reactions and becomes less inhibited. As a result, the risk of an accident quadruples. The deterioration of a person's driving ability continues at a BAC of 0.10 to 0.14 grams%, leading to a sixfold to sevenfold increase in the risk of having an accident. At 0.15 grams% and higher, a person is 25 times more likely to become involved in a serious accident. Recognizing that over 100 countries on six continents have BAC limits set at 0.05 grams% or lower, the National Traffic Safety Board in April 2013 recommended to states that they lower the BAC content that constitutes drunken driving to the 0.05 grams% level. This likely will become very controversial over the coming years.

Figure 5.3 illustrates the correlation between the number of drink equivalents imbibed, gender, body weight, and the resulting blood alcohol concentration. First choose the correct chart (male or female). Then find the number that is closest to your body weight in pounds. Look down the left column to find the number of drinks consumed. BAC is found by matching body weight with number of drinks ingested. Then note that BAC falls about 0.015 grams% every hour from the time that the first drink was ingested. From the total number of drinks ingested, subtract the amount of alcohol that has been metabolized from the number of hours since drinking began (remember that

Blood Alcohol Concentration – A Guide

One drink equals 1 ounce of 80 proof alcohol; 12-ounce bottle of beer; 2 ounces of 20% wine; 3 ounces of 12% wine.

Men

Drinks	Body weight (pounds) Approximate blood alcohol percentage (grams%)								
	100	120	140	160	180	200	220	240	
0	.00	.00	.00	.00	.00	.00	.00	.00	Only safe driving limit
1	.04	.03	.03	.02	.02	.02	.02	.02	Impairment begins
2	.08	.06	.05	.05	.04	.04	.03	.03	Driving skills significantly affected
3	.11	.09	.08	.07	.06	.06	.05	.05	
4	.15	.12	.11	.09	.08	.08	.07	.06	Possible criminal penalties
5	.19	.16	.13	.12	.11	.09	.09	.08	
6	.23	.19	.16	.14	.13	.11	.10	.09	
7	.26	.22	.19	.16	.15	.13	.12	.11	Legally intoxicated
8	.30	.25	.21	.19	.17	.15	.14	.13	
9	.34	.28	.24	.21	.19	.17	.15	.14	
10	.38	.31	.27	.23	.21	.19	.17	.16	Criminal penalties

Alcohol is "burned up" by the body at .015 grams% per hour, as follows:

Number of hours since starting first drink   1   2   3   4   5   6
Percent alcohol burned up   .015 .030 .045 .060 .075 .090

Calculate BAC
Example:
180 lb. man? – 6 drinks in 4 hours
BAC = .130 grams% on chart
Subtract .060 grams% metabolized in 4 hours
BAC = .070 grams% – DRIVING IMPAIRED

Women

Drinks	Body weight (pounds) Approximate blood alcohol percentage (grams%)									
	90	100	120	140	160	180	200	220	240	
0	.00	.00	.00	.00	.00	.00	.00	.00	.00	Only safe driving limit
1	.05	.05	.04	.03	.03	.03	.02	.02	.02	Impairment begins
2	.10	.09	.08	.07	.06	.05	.05	.04	.04	Driving skills significantly affected
3	.15	.14	.11	.10	.09	.08	.07	.06	.06	
4	.20	.18	.15	.13	.11	.10	.09	.08	.08	
5	.25	.23	.19	.16	.14	.13	.11	.10	.09	Criminal penalties
6	.30	.27	.23	.19	.17	.15	.14	.12	.11	
7	.35	.32	.27	.23	.20	.18	.16	.14	.13	Legally intoxicated
8	.40	.36	.30	.26	.23	.20	.18	.17	.15	
9	.45	.41	.34	.29	.26	.23	.20	.19	.17	
10	.51	.45	.38	.32	.28	.25	.23	.21	.19	Criminal penalties

Alcohol is "burned up" by the body at .015 grams% per hour, as follows:

Number of hours since starting first drink   1   2   3   4   5   6
Percent alcohol burned up   .015 .030 .045 .060 .075 .090

Calculate BAC
Example:
140 lb woman – 6 drinks in 4 hours
BAC = .190 grams% on chart
Subtract .060 grams% metabolized in 4 hours
BAC = .130 grams% – LEGALLY INTOXICATED

FIGURE 5.3 Relation between blood alcohol concentration, body weight, and the number of drinks ingested for men and women. See text for details.

approximately 1 drink equivalent is metabolized in 1 hour). The final figure is the approximate BAC. By calculating this number, the degree to which driving ability is impaired can be predicted.

Some agencies and organizations have even more stringent BAC standards than the states. For example, Federal Department of Transportation regulations prohibit truck drivers from driving at 0.04 grams% and airline pilots from flying at 0.02 grams% after 8 hours of abstinence.

Factors that may alter the predictable rate of metabolism of alcohol are usually not of major clinical significance. However two such factors should be briefly mentioned. First, with long-term use, alcohol can induce drug-metabolizing enzymes in the liver, increasing the liver's rate of metabolizing alcohol (and so inducing *tolerance*) as well as its rate of metabolizing other compounds that are similar to alcohol (termed *cross-tolerance*). Second, as discussed above, ADH enzyme (termed *ADH1*) usually is responsible for alcohol metabolism, in chronic alcohol use, in very high (toxic) blood levels, and in persons with alcohol-induced liver failure, a variant of ADH1 enzyme (termed either *ADH3* or *ADH1C*) is produced as the liver becomes incapable of metabolizing alcohol by ADH (Haseba and Ohno, 2010). This enzyme variant may help persons with potentially fatal blood alcohol levels to survive toxic levels of alcohol. Protective effects of this enzyme variant appear most prominently in Asian persons (Li et al., 2012).

Finally, biological markers that detect alcohol use even when BAC levels are reported as zero have been recently developed. Because alcohol is cleared fairly rapidly from the body, these biomarkers detect minor metabolites of alcohol and are usually positive for about 80 hours following drinking. Such biomarkers are proving to be valuable tools to improve verification of abstention in alcohol-dependent persons (Dahl et al., 2011; Albermann et al., 2012). These minor metabolites include ethyl glucuronide and ethyl sulfate. The ethyl glucuronide and ethyl sulfate comprise about 0.02 and 0.010 percent of the ethanol dose, but they can be reliably detected in blood, urine, and hair samples. Such testing is now being widely used in programs where abstinence from alcohol is required. False positives can be obtained when one has used alcohol-containing products such as mouthwashes (Reisfield et al., 2011a) or hand sanitizers (Reisfield et al., 2011b).

Pharmacodynamics

Identifying the mechanism of the action of alcohol continues to be difficult. For many years, it was presumed that alcohol acted through a general depressant action on nerve membranes and synapses. Because it is both water-soluble and lipid-soluble, ethanol dissolves into all body tissues. This property led to a unitary hypothesis of action—that the drug dissolves in nerve membranes, distorting, disorganizing, or "perturbing" the membrane, similar to the action of general anesthetics (see Chapter 13). The result is a nonspecific and indirect depression of neuronal function. This mechanism would account for the nonspecific and generalized depressant behavioral effects of the drug. The hypothesis, however, does not explain the evidence that alcohol may disturb both the synaptic activity of various neurotransmitters, especially major excitatory (glutamate) and inhibitory (GABA) systems, and various intracellular transduction processes that modulate memory, cognitive performance, and motor performance.

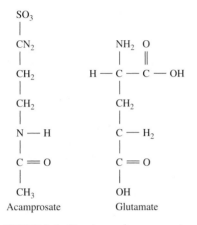

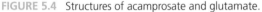

Acamprosate   Glutamate

FIGURE 5.4   Structures of acamprosate and glutamate.

Glutamate Receptors

Ethanol is a potent inhibitor of the function of the NMDA subtype of glutamate receptors and glutamate receptor-mediated synaptic plasticity (Moykkynen and Korpi, 2012). Ethanol disrupts glutaminergic neurotransmission by depressing the responsiveness of NMDA receptors to released glutamate. This ethanol inhibition of glutamate receptors, however, seems to be restricted to certain brain areas such as the hippocampus, amygdala, and striatum and requires fairly high concentrations of the drug. This action may serve to explain consequences of severe alcohol intoxication such as seen in impairments of motor performance and memory.

This attenuation of glutamate responsiveness may be exacerbated by alcohol's known enhancement of inhibitory GABA neurotransmission. With chronic alcohol intake and persistent glutaminergic suppression, there is a compensatory up regulation of NMDA receptors. Thus, on removal of ethanol's inhibitory effect (as would occur during alcohol withdrawal), these excess excitatory receptors would result in withdrawal signs, including seizures. Excess glutamate release during withdrawal may also be responsible for excitatory neuronal nerve damage and loss (Heinz et al., 2009).

The drug *acamprosate*, a structural analogue of glutamate (Figure 5.4), is an anticraving drug used to maintain abstinence in alcohol-dependent patients, an action thought to be produced by interaction with glutaminergic NMDA receptors, attenuating neuronal hyperexcitability induced by chronic alcohol ingestion and withdrawal (Mann et al., 2008). The use of acamprosate in the treatment of alcoholism is discussed later in this chapter.

GABA Receptors

Ethanol activates the GABA-mediated increase in chloride ion flows, resulting in neuronal inhibition. The behavioral results of this inhibition include sedation, muscle relaxation, and inhibition of cognitive and motor skills. A GABAergic antianxiety effect is indicated by the fact that low doses of ethanol reduce both panic and the anxiety surrounding panic. This lends support to the view that drinking by those with panic disorder, stress, and anxiety is reinforced by this GABAergic agonistic effect. Thus, the use of alcohol to self-medicate one's panic or anxiety may contribute to the high rate of co-occurring alcohol use disorders with these other conditions.

Ethanol and stress may interact such that GABA-mediated inhibition may lead to activation of opioid receptors that in turn influences the behavior rewarding associated with the activation of dopaminergic neurons (Boehm et al., 2002). Ethanol binds to a different subunit on the $GABA_A$ receptor than do other GABA agonists (Strac et al., 2012). Chronic exposure seems to involve changes in intracellular mRNA, suggesting that chronic alcoholism can affect gene expression. As a result of the GABAergic agonistic action, the activity of other transmitter systems is affected. The abuse potential of alcohol follows from the ultimate effect of augmenting dopamine neurotransmitter systems, particularly the dopaminergic projection from the ventral tegmental area to the nucleus accumbens, amygdala, and to the frontal cortex (Roberto et al., 2010; Marty and Spigelman, 2012). This action is an indirect effect rather than a direct action exerted on dopamine-secreting neurons.

Opioid Receptors

A dysfunctional brain opioid system may be involved in heavy alcohol drinking and alcohol dependence. Ethanol may induce opioid release, which in turn triggers dopamine release in the brain reward system, especially the nucleus accumbens and orbitofrontal cortex (Mitchell et al., 2012). Administration of *naltrexone* (ReVia, Vivatrol) blocks opioid receptors and may reduce alcohol craving. Naltrexone is approved by the Food and Drug Administration (FDA) for the treatment of alcohol dependence; its use in treating alcohol dependence is discussed later in this chapter.

Robson and coworkers (2012) recently discussed the role of sigma-1 receptors (a subclass of opioid receptors) as targets for the development of pharmacotherapies for alcohol and substance abuse and dependence. Indeed, sigma-1 receptors appear to modulate the effects of alcohol and other drugs of abuse on neurotransmission, gene regulation, and neuroplasticity.

Serotonin Receptors

There is some literature and increasing emphasis on the role of serotonin in the actions of alcohol and as a mediator of alcohol reward, preference, dependence, and craving (Sari et al., 2011). Chronic alcohol consumption results in augmentation of serotonergic activity and serotonin dysfunction has been postulated to play a role in the pathogenesis of some types of alcoholism. Today, emphasis is on the role of serotonin $5-HT_2$ and $5-HT_3$ receptors in the central effects of ethanol; these receptors are located on dopaminergic neurons in the nucleus accumbens. Serotonin reuptake-inhibiting antidepressants such as *sertraline* (Zoloft) (see Chapter 12) reduce alcohol consumption in individuals who are considered to be at a lower risk for drinking excessively, or have a lower severity of the disorder. Serotonin receptors appear to be involved in impulsivity, a core behavior that contributes to the vulnerability to addiction and relapse (Kirby et al., 2011).

Cannabinoid Receptors

Within the past few years, important information has been gathered on the probable role of cannabinoid receptors (see Chapter 9) in the actions of alcohol, especially in postwithdrawal cravings and in the relapse to drinking. Chronic ingestion of ethanol stimulates the formation of the endogenous neurotransmitter for cannabinoid receptors, a substance called *anandamide*. This neurotransmitter activates the cannabinoid receptors and, with continued ethanol ingestion, eventually leads to down regulation of these receptors. Removal of ethanol by cessation of drinking leads to a hyperactive endocannabinoid reaction, which appears to result in a craving for alcohol and a return to drinking. As will be discussed in Chapter 9, blockade of cannabinoid receptors leads to loss of desire to self-administer alcohol and other drugs of compulsive abuse. As reviewed recently by Pava and Woodward (2012), stimulation of cannabinoid receptors contributes to the motivational and reinforcing properties of alcohol and, conversely, chronic consumption of alcohol alters the functioning of the endogenous cannabinoid system.

Therefore, it now appears that ethanol and cannabinoid agonists (for example, tetrahydrocannabinol in marijuana) activate the same reward system. Down regulation of cannabinoid receptors may be involved in the development of tolerance to and dependence on ethanol, and an active response from cannabinoid receptors after alcohol detoxification may lead to alcohol craving and eventual compulsion to relapse.

Pharmacological Effects

The graded, reversible depression of behavior, mental functioning, and cognition is the primary pharmacological effect of alcohol (Oscar-Berman and Marinkovic, 2007). Respiration is transiently stimulated at low doses, but as blood concentrations of alcohol increase, respiration becomes progressively depressed; at toxic doses, respiration ceases, causing death. Alcohol is also anticonvulsant, although it is not clinically used for this purpose. On the other hand, withdrawal from alcohol ingestion is accompanied by a prolonged period of hyperexcitability, and seizures can occur; seizure activity peaks approximately 8 to 12 hours after the last drink.

In the central nervous system (CNS), the effects of alcohol are additive with those of other sedative-hypnotic compounds, resulting in more sedation and greater impairment of motor and cognitive abilities. Other sedatives (especially the benzodiazepines) and marijuana are the sedative-hypnotic drugs most frequently combined with alcohol, and they increase its deleterious effects on motor and intellectual skills (for example, driving ability) as well as alertness. Patients suffering from insomnia find alcohol to be an effective hypnotic agent, although the short duration of action of alcohol can lead to early morning wakenings and insomnia.

Alcohol also affects the circulation and the heart. Alcohol dilates the blood vessels in the skin, producing a warm flush and a decrease in body temperature. Thus, it is pointless and possibly dangerous to drink alcohol to keep warm when one is exposed to cold weather. Long-term use of high doses of alcohol is associated with diseases of the heart muscle, which can result in heart failure. However, *low* doses of alcohol consumed daily (up to 2 drink equivalents per day for men and 0.5 to 1.0 daily drink equivalent for women) *reduce* the risk of coronary artery disease and peripheral artery disease. This protective effect on blood vessels occurs because of an alcohol-induced increase in high-density lipoprotein in blood, with a corresponding decrease in low-density lipoprotein.[4]

---

[4] The higher the concentration of high-density lipoprotein and the lower the concentration of low-density lipoprotein, the lower the incidence of development of arteriosclerosis and occlusive vascular disease.

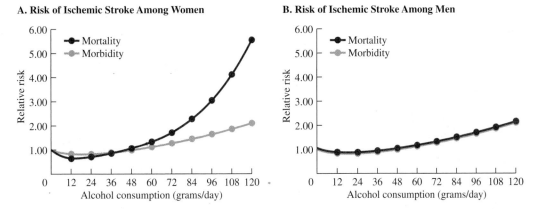

A. Risk of Ischemic Stroke Among Women

B. Risk of Ischemic Stroke Among Men

FIGURE 5.5   Dose-response relationship between daily alcohol consumption and the risk of ischemic stroke in women (A) and men (B). Data for hemorrhagic stroke is very similar. Note the slightly decreased risk at doses of about12–24 grams of alcohol daily. This equates to about 1–2 drink equivalents daily. Higher daily doses associated with increased risk. [Data from Patra et al., 2010, "Alcohol Consumption and the Risk of Morbidity and Mortality for Different Stroke Types—A Systematic Review and Meta-Analysis," *BMC Public Health 10: 258,* Figure 7.]

Unfortunately, the cardioprotective effect of low doses of alcohol is lost on people who also smoke cigarettes or who are binge drinkers[5] (Ruidavets et al., 2010).

Light to moderate doses of alcohol have also been shown to reduce the incidence of strokes, especially in women (Figures 5.5). The mechanisms responsible for the protective effect of low doses of alcohol on stroke appear to involve increases in (protective) high-density cholesterol and an aspirinlike decrease in platelet aggregation.

Alcohol (like all depressant drugs) is not an aphrodisiac. The behavioral disinhibition induced by low doses of alcohol may appear to cause some loss of restraint, but alcohol depresses body function and interferes with sexual performance. As Shakespeare wrote in *Macbeth*: "It provokes the desire, but it takes away the performance."

Psychological Effects

The short-term psychological and behavioral effects of alcohol are primarily related to a mixture of stimulant and depressant effects of low doses of the drug in the CNS. Figure 5.6 correlates the effects of alcohol with levels of the drug measured in the blood. The behavioral reaction to disinhibition, which occurs at low doses, is largely determined by the person, his or her mental expectations, and the environment in which drinking occurs. In one setting a person may become relaxed and euphoric; in another, withdrawn or violent. Mental expectations and the physical setting become progressively less important at increasing doses because the sedative effects increase and behavioral activity decreases.

---

[5] Binge drinking defined as more than 5 drink equivalents within 2 hours (by men) or more than 4 drink equivalents within 2 hours (women).

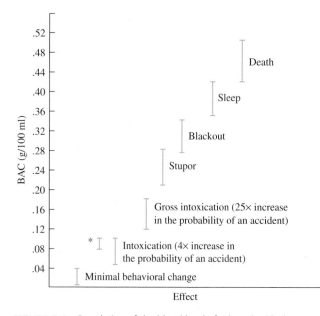

FIGURE 5.6   Correlation of the blood level of ethanol with degrees of intoxication. The legal level of intoxication (*) varies according to state law; the range of BAC values is shown. BAC = blood alcohol concentration.

As doses increase, a person may still function (although with less coordination) and attempt to drive or otherwise endanger self and others. Perceptual speed is an important component of task performance and is markedly impaired by ethanol. At BAC values of about 0.05 to 0.09 grams%, some common clinical symptoms are increased sociability and talkativeness; decreased inhibitions; diminution of attention, judgment, and control; slowed information processing; and loss of efficiency in critical performance testing. As the BAC increases, the drinker becomes progressively more incapacitated. Memory, concentration, and insight are progressively dulled and lost, even though one may remain in a state of wakefulness.

Alcohol intoxication, with its resulting disinhibition, plays a major role in a large percentage of violent crimes, including battery, rape, sexual assault, and certain kinds of deviant behaviors. Indeed, there is a dose-related increase in aggressive responsiveness applicable to both males and females (Duke et al., 2011). Alcohol is implicated in more than half of all homicides and assaults; about 40 percent of violent offenders in jail were drinking at the time of the offense for which they were incarcerated. Many of these offenses probably would not have occurred if the offender, the victim, or both had not been intoxicated. Martin and Bryant (2001) studied how alcohol use by men affects intimate-partner violence. They stated that alcohol intoxication may contribute to aggressive and criminal behavior through its mediating effects on the physiological, cognitive, affective, or behavioral functioning of the drinker. Through effects on the GABA system, alcohol reduces anxiety about the consequences of aggressive behavior. Through dopaminergic activation, impulse control is reduced, which increases the likelihood of aggression. Through glutamate depression, cognitive functioning is impaired, reducing the drinker's ability to find peaceful (nonviolent) solutions to difficult situations. Many drinkers develop a type of "alcohol myopia," defined as shortsightedness in which superficially understood, immediate aspects of experience have a disproportionate influence on behavior and emotion (Giancola et al., 2011). Cognitive and attentional deficits cause a focus on the present, reduce fear and anxiety, and impair problem-solving ability. Finally, alcohol use increases concerns with power and dominance, which are linked to male violence generally and to intimate-partner interactions in particular. The effect can be an inappropriate sense of mastery, control, or power.

Did You Know?

Alcohol Is Directly Related to Four of the Top Ten Offenses in the United States

According to data from the national Uniform Crime Reporting (UCR) Program, of the estimated 12,408,899 arrests made in the United States in 2011, the highest number were for drug abuse violations, and driving under the influence. However, as seen in the chart below, alcohol is involved in at least three of these categories, namely, disorderly conduct, drunkenness and liquor laws and contributes to other offenses, such as assaults and vandalism.

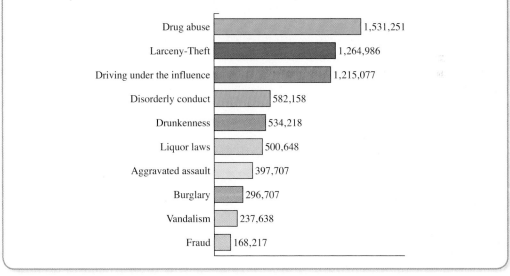

More than 50 percent of all motor vehicle highway accidents are alcohol related, a number that has changed little in 20 years. More than 10 million people in the United States currently suffer the consequences of their alcohol abuse, which include arrests, traffic accidents, occupational injuries, violence, and health and occupational losses. This number does not include the 10 million people considered to be alcohol dependent (and suffering their own negative consequences). About 10 percent of our society is personally afflicted with (or suffers the consequences of) another's alcohol use. Untreated alcohol problems lead to death, disability, and $185 billion each year in avoidable health, business, and criminal justice costs.

Did You Know?

Designated Drivers Don't Always Abstain

Maybe you had better call that cab after all: a new study found that 35 percent of designated drivers had drunk alcohol and most had blood-alcohol levels high enough to impair their driving. More than 1,000 bar patrons in the downtown restaurant and bar district of a major university town in the southeast were interviewed and breath-tested. Of the designated drivers who had consumed alcohol, half recorded a blood-alcohol level higher than .05 percent —a recently recommended threshold to be considered driving under the influence.

The researchers recruited patrons as they left bars between 10 P.M. and 2:30 A.M. across six Friday nights before home football games in the fall of 2011. The mean age of the 1,071 people who agreed to be tested was 28. Most were white male college students, while 10 percent were Hispanic, 6 percent were Asian, and 4 percent were African American.

Some research suggests that designated drivers might drink because the group did not consider who would drive before they started drinking. There is no universally accepted definition of a designated driver.

Although most U.S. researchers say drivers should completely abstain, international researchers have discovered that designated drivers believe that they can drink as long as their blood-alcohol level remains below the legal limit. It is interesting to note that the U.S. limit is much higher than it is in most other countries. Denmark, Finland, and Greece use the .05 level; Russia and Sweden set the limit at .02; and Japan has a zero percent tolerance.

Noel and colleagues (2001) studied 30 detoxified male alcoholics (with matched controls) to assess "frontal lobe" or "executive" functioning and the vulnerability of the frontal lobes to alcohol abuse. In all tests of executive function, nondrinking alcoholics performed poorly compared with controls. The researchers stated:

> Chronic alcohol consumption is associated with severe executive function deficits, still present after a protracted period of alcohol abstinence. This supports the idea that cognitive deficit in detoxified, sober alcoholics is due, at least partly, to frontal lobe dysfunction. (p. 1152)

Furthermore:

> These findings could have important implications, particularly concerning relapse. Since drug use is largely controlled by automatic processes, executive functions are needed to block this and maintain abstinence. Thus, the existence of persistent executive function deficits could affect the capacity to maintain abstinence. (p. 1152)

Persistent alcohol use harms adolescents. Brown and coworkers (2000) studied alcohol-dependent adolescents (who developed dependency in early adolescence) and found that recent detoxification was associated with poor visuospatial functioning (as might be expected), whereas alcohol withdrawal early in life was associated with persistence of poor retrieval of verbal and nonverbal information. This finding reflects long-term effects on working memory.

Long-term effects of alcohol may also involve many different organs of a person's body. Long-term ingestion of only moderate amounts of alcohol seems to produce few physiological alterations. As noted earlier, low to moderate doses can even be protective to the heart and vascular system. On the downside, long-term ingestion of larger amounts of alcohol leads to a variety of serious neurological, mental, and physical disorders. For example, monthly binge drinking in midlife is an independent risk factor, doubling the risk of long-term cognitive impairments later in life (Jyri et al., 2010). Alcohol is high in calories but has little nutritional value; consumption of a high-alcohol diet (and little else!) slowly leads to vitamin deficiencies and nutritional diseases, which may result in physical deterioration. Alcohol abuse has been suggested as the most common cause of vitamin and trace element deficiencies in adults.

Did You Know?

Rejected, Male Fruit Flies Turn to Alcohol

It has long been known that mice, rats, and monkeys drink more after periods of isolation; the same is true of mice that are bullied or are victims of aggression.

To test the relationship between stress and alcohol in fruit flies, researchers let one group of male flies mate freely with available virgin females. Another group of male flies had the opposite experience: the females they mingled with had already mated, and were unreceptive to further relations. After four days, the flies in both groups fed in glass tubes outfitted with four straws, two providing a regular diet of yeast and sugar and two containing yeast, sugar, and 15 percent alcohol. Like many people, fruit flies as a rule will develop a taste for alcohol and, in time, a preference for the 15 percent solution. But the rejected flies drank a lot more on average, supping from the spiked mixture about 70 percent of the time, compared with about 50 percent for their sexually sated peers.

The researchers conducted several additional experiments to rule out other explanations. The flies were apparently using the alcohol as a way to compensate for their frustrated desire. Apparently some aspects of the brain's reward system have not changed much during evolution!

Effects on Memory Formation. Alcohol's effects on memory range from mild deficits to alcohol-induced blackouts. These blackouts are of two types: *fragmentary* blackouts (where bits and pieces are remembered and much is not encoded) and *en* bloc, where nothing is remembered. Blackouts occasionally begin to occur at BACs in excess of about 0.14 grams%, becoming more complete at BACs of 0.25 to 0.30 grams%

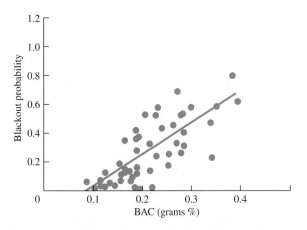

FIGURE 5.7   Probability of blackouts as a function of the blood alcohol concentration (BAC) (grams%, or grams per 100 cc whole blood). [Data from Perry et al., 2006, Figure 2, page 898.]

(White et al., 2004). Perry and coworkers (2006) presented a dose-response curve for alcohol-induced blackouts (Figure 5.7). The probability of experiencing blackout at BACs below 0.2 grams% is about 20%. At a BAC of about 0.28–0.3 grams%, the probability of a blackout is 50% or higher. Gender, drinking experience, drinking without eating, the rate at which alcohol is ingested, and gulping of alcohol all predict blackout at lower BACs. Also, some persons may have an inherent neurobiological vulnerability to alcohol-induced memory impairments due to alcohol's effects on contextual memory processes (Wetherill et al., 2012a, 2012b). Of importance is that during a blackout one is still awake and is capable of engaging in complicated and potentially hazardous activities, which often lead to adverse legal consequences. During a blackout, one performs acts (e.g., driving, engaging in sexual activity, etc.) without having memory of having done so.

The mechanism responsible for a blackout is usually ascribed to alcohol-induced suppression of transcription of memory protein formation from genetic material (DNA). In other words, alcohol appears to block memory protein formation that is essential for the formation of long-term encoding of memory (Gold, 2008). Indeed, with maintenance of the awake state, these BACs "disrupt limbic areas to prevent consolidation of encoded stimuli into lasting memory traces" (Hartzler and Fromme, 2003, p. 547).

This state is closely related to organic dementia in which severe cognitive dysfunction occurs (Lee et al., 2009). Finally, Tokuda and coworkers (2011) postulate that at very high concentrations of ethanol, memory production in hippocampal neurons (and presumably cognitive functions) may be inhibited through a process called neurosteroidogenesis. Such research is in its infancy.

In summary, ethanol inhibits cognitive functioning and produces blackouts by suppressing production of memory proteins in the hippocampus, blocks glutaminergic NMDA receptors, and may produce neurosteroids that interfere with memory consolidation.

Tolerance and Dependence

The patterns and mechanisms for the development of tolerance to, physical dependence on, and psychological dependence on alcohol are similar to those for other CNS depressants. The extent of tolerance depends on the amount, pattern, and extent of alcohol ingestion. People who ingest alcohol only intermittently on sprees or more regularly but in moderation develop little or no tolerance. People who regularly ingest large amounts of alcohol develop marked tolerance. The tolerance is of three types:

1. *Metabolic tolerance,* whereby the liver increases its amount of drug-metabolizing enzyme. This type accounts for at most 25 percent of the tolerance to alcohol.

2. *Tissue, or functional, tolerance,* whereby neurons in the brain adapt to the amount of drug present. Drinkers who develop this type of tolerance characteristically display blood alcohol levels about twice those of nontolerant drinkers at a similar level of behavioral intoxication. Note, however, that despite behavioral adaptation, impairments in cognitive function are similar at similar blood levels in both tolerant and nontolerant drinkers. In other words, at a BAC of 0.15 grams%, both tolerant and nontolerant drinkers display marked deficits in insight, judgment, cognition, and other executive functions. The tolerant person may just *appear* less intoxicated.

3. *Associative, contingent, or homeostatic tolerance.* A variety of environmental manipulations can counter the effects of ethanol, and counterresponses are a possible mechanism of tolerance.

After physical dependence develops, withdrawal of alcohol results in a period of rebound hyperexcitability within hours that may eventually lead to convulsions. Alcohol abuse is one of the most common causes of adult-onset seizures; seizures occur in about 10 percent of adults during alcohol withdrawal. Alcohol withdrawal seizures are a life-threatening consequence of alcohol cessation in alcoholics. The period of seizure activity is relatively short, usually 6 hours or less, but seizures can be very severe. Blocking seizure activity during withdrawal is a major goal of detoxification and usually involves two classes of agents: the benzodiazepines and the anticonvulsants. A "kindling" model of alcohol withdrawal seizures suggests that repeated alcohol withdrawals may lead to an increase in the severity of subsequent withdrawals and a greater likelihood of withdrawal seizures with each detoxification. Indeed, the number of detoxifications is an important variable in the predisposition to withdrawal seizures. Using this concept, Malcolm and coworkers (2000) postulated that repeated detoxifications might also cause neurobehavioral alterations that in turn may affect alcohol craving. Patients who had experienced multiple detoxifications had higher scores on tests that measure obsessive thoughts about alcohol, drink urges, and drinking behaviors. Thus, recurrent detoxifications may lead to increased rates of relapse due to a "kindling" of behaviors and thoughts leading to a compulsion to return to drinking. The researchers added that the kindling effect persists despite treatment with benzodiazepines or other traditional sedative-hypnotic drugs. In fact, the medical management of alcohol detoxification may be better achieved with anticonvulsant "mood stabilizers" (see Chapter 14) than with benzodiazepines (Becker et al., 2006; Martinotti et al., 2010).

In addition to withdrawal seizures and cravings, the alcohol withdrawal syndrome can consist of a period of tremulousness, with hallucinations, psychomotor agitation, confusion and disorientation, sleep disorders, and a variety of associated discomforts. This syndrome is sometimes referred to as *delirium tremens* (DTs).

Side Effects and Toxicity

Many side effects and toxicities associated with alcohol have already been mentioned; following is a summary and expansion. In acute use, a *reversible drug-induced dementia* is produced. This syndrome is manifested as a clouded sensorium with disorientation, impaired insight and judgment, anterograde amnesia (blackouts), and diminished intellectual capabilities.

With increasing doses (or blood levels) of alcohol, a person's affect may become labile, with emotional outbursts precipitated by otherwise innocuous events. With higher doses of alcohol, delusions and hallucinations may occur. In social situations, these alterations result in unpredictable states of disinhibition (drunkenness), alterations in driving performance, and uncoordinated motor behavior. As stated earlier, only at very high doses (perhaps at BACs of 0.4 grams% and greater) is consciousness lost and a state of "anesthesia" with immobilization occurs. At this point, respiration becomes shallow and death can result.

Liver damage is a serious long-term physiological consequence of excessive alcohol consumption. Irreversible changes in both the structure and the function of the liver are common. For example, ethanol produces active oxidants during its metabolism by hepatocytes, which results in oxidative stress on liver cells. The significance of alcohol-induced liver dysfunction is illustrated by the fact that 75 percent of all deaths attributed to alcoholism are caused by cirrhosis of the liver, and cirrhosis is the seventh most common cause of death in the United States.

Long-term alcohol ingestion may irreversibly cause the *destruction of nerve cells*, producing a permanent brain syndrome with dementia (Korsakoff's syndrome). More subtle and persistent cognitive deficits may be present whether or not a diagnosis of Korsakoff's syndrome is made. This condition is termed *alcohol dementia*, and it can involve long-term problems with memory, learning, and other cognitive skills. The *digestive system* may also be affected. *Pancreatitis* (inflammation of the pancreas) and *chronic gastritis* (inflammation of the stomach), with the development of peptic ulcers, may occur.

A great deal of epidemiological evidence now shows that chronic excessive alcohol consumption is a major risk factor for *cancer* in humans. Schutze and coworkers (2011) stated that 10 percent of total cancers in men and 3 percent of total cancers in women were attributable to alcohol. Digestive and liver cancers were most prominently associated with alcohol. Consuming more than two drinks daily for men and one drink daily for women accounted for much of the alcohol-attributable cancers. Although ethanol alone may not be strongly carcinogenic, it appears to be a cocarcinogen, or a tumor promoter. For example, the risk of head and neck cancers for heavy drinkers who also smoke cigarettes is 6 to 15 times greater than for those who abstain from both. The risk of throat cancer is 44 times greater for heavy users of both alcohol and tobacco than for nonusers.

Ethanol may increase the risk for breast cancer, with about 5 percent of such cancers attributable to alcohol. In adolescent females, a correlation has been reported between increasing alcohol use and benign breast disease (Liu et al., 2012).

Teratogenic Effects

For years we have known that alcohol is both a physical and a behavioral teratogen. Drug-induced alterations occur in brain structure and/or function. *Fetal alcohol syndrome* (FAS) is a devastating developmental disorder that occurs in the offspring of mothers who have high blood levels of alcohol during critical stages of fetal development; it affects as many as 30 percent to 50 percent of infants born to alcoholic women. Clearly, a relatively large number of otherwise biologically normal infants may be irreversibly damaged by maternal alcohol abuse during pregnancy, and alcohol abuse during pregnancy appears to be the most frequent known teratogenic cause of mental retardation.

Sayal and coworkers (2009) noted that binge drinking even in the absence of regular ingestion of alcohol increased the risk of child mental health problems, primarily related to hyperactivity and inattention problems. Kot-Leibovich and Fainsod (2009) noted that alcohol competes with the biosynthesis of retinoic acid, which is required for normal brain development. Because subtle intellectual and behavioral effects of low-level alcohol consumption may go unnoticed, no safe level of alcohol intake during pregnancy has been established and there is no threshold level of alcohol ingestion that triggers fetal alcohol syndrome (Feldman et al., 2012). Features of the full fetal alcohol syndrome include the following:

- CNS dysfunction, including low intelligence and microcephaly (reduced cranial circumference), mental retardation, and behavioral abnormalities (often presenting as hyperactivity and difficulty with social integration)
- Retarded body growth rate (fetal growth retardation)
- Facial abnormalities (short palpebral fissures, short nose, wide-set eyes, and small cheekbones)
- Other anatomical abnormalities (for example, congenital heart defects and malformed eyes and ears).

In the United States, an estimated 2.6 million infants are born annually following significant in utero alcohol exposure. Many display the full features of FAS, and about 1 newborn out of every 100 live births displays a lesser degree of damage, termed *fetal alcohol effects*, perhaps more correctly termed *alcohol-related neurodevelopmental disorder* (ARND). Taken together, the combined rate of FAS and ARND is estimated to be at least 9 per 1,000 live births. Alcohol ingestion is thus the third leading cause of birth defects with associated mental retardation; it is the only one that is preventable.

Perhaps a new term should be coined to encompass the full spectrum of fetal damage that can follow ingestion of ethanol by pregnant women. "Fetal alcohol spectrum disorder" would include both fetal alcohol syndrome and fetal alcohol effects, covering that gray area between infants with facial abnormalities and infants with "milder" effects, such as hyperactivity and aggressive behaviors.

Although the structural abnormalities and growth retardation of FAS are well described, the behavioral and cognitive effects of alcohol exposure are less appreciated. Intelligence (IQ), attention, learning, memory, language, and motor and visuospatial activities are affected and subject to impairment in children prenatally exposed to varying amounts of alcohol (Sayal et al., 2009). Sensory problems can also be present, involving ocular, auditory, vestibular, and speech and language development. Medina (2011) discusses alcohol-induced learning and memory disorders in offspring of women who drank through the third trimester of pregnancy. This is a period during which the fetal brain goes through a period of fast growth ("brain growth spurt") and neurons are more susceptible to alcohol exposure. Here, depression of synaptogenesis and interference with brain "wiring" may lead to persistent deficits in neuronal plasticity.

Carmichael and coworkers (1997) had earlier studied a cohort of 500 children, 250 of whom were born to "heavier" drinkers who typically drank at "social drinking levels." The other 250 children were born to infrequent drinkers and abstainers. There were significant alcohol-related differences in behavioral and learning difficulties during adolescence. Exposure to alcohol during pregnancy was associated "with a profile of adolescent antisocial behavior, school problems, and self-perceived learning difficulties" (Carmichael et al., 1997, p. 1187). Thus, brain function can be markedly affected in offspring of alcohol-drinking mothers in the absence of the observable structural abnormalities.

In a study in Finland, Autti-Ramo (2000) followed 70 children with fetal alcohol exposure (42 with recognized cognitive and other deficits, 10 with physical growth restrictions only, and 18 classified as normal). They were assessed at age 12 for psychosocial well-being. The longer the alcohol exposure during pregnancy, the more likely the child was to have significant cognitive and social impairments. Of the 42 children with early recognition of cognitive deficits, 29 (69 percent) were in permanent foster or institutional care. Even among the children in the normal and growth-restricted groups, 10 (36 percent) were temporarily or permanently in alternative care. Behavioral problems were significant. Thus, alcohol exposure in utero can be associated with social disadvantages, including alternative care and behavioral problems.

Baer and coworkers (2003) reported results of a 21-year longitudinal study in which they followed offspring of 500 women who, in 1974–1975, drank during their pregnancy (30 percent were binge drinkers). Offspring of two women displayed FAS, and 31 offspring were identified as having components of ARND. When these offspring attained the age of 21, 11 percent of their mothers and 21 percent of their fathers were identified as having had a history of alcohol problems. The offspring of mothers who were binge drinkers during pregnancy exhibited three times the likelihood of at least mild alcohol dependence than did offspring of mothers who did not drink alcohol during their pregnancy (14.1 percent versus 4.5 percent).

The prevention of FAS and ARND obviously involves abstinence from alcohol by women who are, plan to become, or are capable of becoming pregnant. Screening questionnaires may be effective in helping to protect not only the unborn infant but also the long-term health of the mother. Because alcohol screening can effectively identify women and infants at risk, it is recommended for women during prenatal visits. Here, the five "Ps" might be useful. This attempts to recognize problems with alcohol or drugs by identifying comments from (1) **P**arents, (2) **P**eers, (3) **P**artner, (4) before **P**regnancy occurred, and (5) use in **P**art of the month while pregnant.

Alcoholism and Its Pharmacological Treatment

Why is it necessary to recognize alcoholism as a major medical problem? Schuckit (2009) stated:

> Alcohol dependence and alcohol abuse or harmful use cause substantial morbidity and mortality. Alcohol-use disorders are associated with depressive episodes, severe anxiety, insomnia, suicide, and abuse of other drugs. Continued heavy alcohol use also shortens the onset of heart disease, stroke, cancers, and liver cirrhosis by affecting the cardiovascular, gastrointestinal, and immune systems. Heavy drinking can also cause mild anterograde amnesias, temporary cognitive deficits, sleep problems, and peripheral neuropathy; cause gastrointestinal problems; decrease bone density and production of blood cells; and cause fetal alcohol syndrome. Alcohol-use disorders complicate assessment and treatment of other medical and psychiatric problems. (p. 492)

The recognition of alcoholism as a multifaceted disease and behavioral process is relatively recent. In 1935, Alcoholics Anonymous was founded on a *moral model* of alcoholism; it offered a spiritual and behavioral framework for understanding, accepting, and recovering from the compulsion to use alcohol. In the late 1950s, the American Medical Association recognized the syndrome of alcoholism as an illness. In the mid-1970s, alcoholism was redefined as a *chronic, progressive, and potentially fatal disease*. In 1992, the description was expanded as follows:

> Alcoholism is a primary, chronic disease with genetic, psychosocial, and environmental factors influencing its development and manifestations. The disease is often progressive and fatal. It is characterized by impaired control over drinking, preoccupation with the drug alcohol, use of alcohol despite adverse consequences, and distortions in thinking, most notably denial. Each of these symptoms may be continuous or periodic. (Morse and Flavin, 1992, p. 1012)

In this definition, "adverse consequences" involve impairments in physical health, psychological functioning, interpersonal functioning, and occupational functioning as well as legal, financial, and spiritual problems. "Denial" refers broadly to a range of psychological maneuvers that decrease awareness of the fact that alcohol use is the cause of problems rather than a solution to problems. Denial becomes an integral part of the disease and is nearly always a major obstacle to recovery.

As with other addictions, alcoholism is characterized as a chronically relapsing condition. It contributes to the risk of bodily harm, relationship troubles, problems in meeting obligations, and run-ins with the law. Consequently, the therapeutic goal is the development of safe, clinically effective medications that promote high adherence rates and prevent relapse. These drugs can then be used in conjunction with psychosocial approaches. Efficacy of combination therapy is currently the subject of a large government-sponsored study called COMBINE (Combining Medications and Behavioral Interventions for Alcoholism) (Gueorguieva et al., 2012; Prisciandaro et al., 2012).

It is now obvious that the *age of onset* of drinking behaviors markedly affects long-term outcomes and societal functioning. Heavy users of alcohol at early ages have, as might be predicted, the poorest outcomes as adults. Heavy drinking as early as age 13 predicts a high risk for subsequent alcohol dependency, low levels of academic achievement, and poor interactions in family and social activities. Binge drinking at age 15 and continuing through age 18 results in an even higher rate of alcohol dependency.

Rohde and coworkers (2001) followed a large cohort of adolescents (14 to 18 years old) through age 24. Approximately three-quarters of the adolescents at initial interview had tried alcohol; those who drank often consumed large quantities of alcohol. Problematic alcohol use occurred in 23 percent. Of the latter group, 80 percent had some form of comorbidity with alcohol use: increased rates of depression, disruptive behavior, drug use disorders, and daily tobacco use. By age 24, problem-drinking adolescents exhibited increased rates of substance abuse disorders, depression, and antisocial and borderline personality disorders. Therefore, excessive alcohol use in early adolescence is not a benign condition that resolves over time.

In many cases, alcohol may (at least at first) be ingested in an attempt at *self-medication* of psychological distress. A person who, before drinking alcohol, experiences anxiety, depression, bipolar, or other responsive psychological disorders may find the symptomatology alleviated by ethanol. This relief then leads to unregulated and unmonitored drug ingestion (the drug is not taken under a physician's supervision). Either the positive reinforcing effects of the drug or drinking to avoid the unpleasantness of withdrawal then trap the person. Goodwin and Gabrielli (1997) stated that 30 percent to 50 percent of alcoholics meet criteria for major depression, 33 percent have a coexisting anxiety disorder, many have antisocial personalities, some are schizophrenic, and many (36 percent) are addicted to other drugs. Some, if not many, alcoholics may have first used alcohol and become psychologically dependent on the drug as a self-prescribed medication to treat their primary disorder.

Lapham and coworkers (2001) studied psychiatric diagnoses in over 1,000 males and females aged 23 to 54 convicted of driving while impaired. Eighty-five percent of female and 91 percent of male offenders reported a lifetime alcohol use disorder; 32 percent of female and 38 percent of male offenders had a drug use disorder. Fifty percent of female and 33 percent of male offenders had at least one additional psychiatric disorder, mainly posttraumatic stress disorder or major depression. We obviously need to implement treatment interventions for these offenders.

As many as 38 percent of alcohol-dependent patients demonstrate impulse-control problems. The co-occurrence of pathologic gambling (one type of impulse-control disorder) was associated with a younger age of onset of alcohol dependence, a higher number of detoxifications, and a longer duration of dependence. Both alcohol dependence and pathologic gambling are pleasure-seeking dependencies, and alcohol use may provide much the same reinforcement as gambling. Frye and Salloum (2006) discuss the co-occurrence of alcoholism and bipolar disorder. An overwhelmingly positive association exists between alcohol use disorder and personality disorders, especially antisocial, histrionic, and dependent disorders (Grant et al., 2004). Finally, as many as 31 percent of heavy drinkers over the age of 12 years, are using illicit drugs. *Dual diagnosis* (or *comorbid illness*) must always be considered with alcohol use disorders (Tiet and Mausbach, 2007).[6]

Dawson and coworkers (2007) studied the relationship between early-onset drinking (age 14 or younger) and life stressors. They found that initiation of drinking at age 14 or

---

[6]For additional information on co-occurring disorders, see www.samhsa.gov/co-occurring/.

younger increased the association between the number of stressors and the average daily volume of alcohol ingested. Early-onset drinking thus appears to increase stress-reactive alcohol consumption. In other words, early-onset ethanol drinkers are more likely to use alcohol as a "stress reducer" than are drinkers who begin drinking at a later age.

Kushner and coworkers (Kushner et al., 2011, 2012; Menary et al., 2011) discussed the comorbidity of current anxiety disorders and the development of alcoholism. About 50 percent of persons being treated for alcoholism have a co-occurring anxiety or depressive ("internalizing") disorder. Self-medication for one's anxiety holds that drinking behavior is negatively reinforced when alcohol temporarily reduces anxiety and the resulting escalation of drinking increases the risk for the development of anxiety disorders. Further, persons with anxiety disorders transition from regular drinking to alcohol dependence more rapidly than do persons without anxiety disorders. Pharmacological treatment of co-occurring alcoholism and anxiety is difficult. Few studies have investigated this important area. Perhaps combining pharmacotherapy for alcoholism (discussed below) and relatively nonaddicting anxiolytics (anticonvulsants such as pregabalin or topiramate) and/or atypical antipsychotics (such as quetiapine) may be helpful. Benzodiazepine anxiolytics (see Chapter 13) are problematic because their use is time-limited due to the development of tolerance. Also, alcohol and benzodiazepines are additive in their pharmacological effects.

Alcoholism is a major public health problem. Of the 160 million Americans who are old enough to drink legally, 112 million do so. As many as 14 million Americans may have serious alcohol problems, and about half that number are considered to be alcoholic. Alcoholism costs about 100,000 American lives each year and in excess of $166 billion annually in direct and indirect health and societal costs.

In 2005, the National Institute on Alcohol Abuse and Alcoholism published a clinician's guide asking all clinicians and mental health workers to screen for alcohol use patterns that place a person at risk for alcohol-related problems. This guide, titled *Helping Patients Who Drink Too Much,* was updated in 2007 (National Institute on Alcohol Abuse and Alcoholism, 2007). Men who drink 5 or more standard drinks in a day (or 15 or more per week) and women who drink 4 or more in a day (or 8 or more per week) are at increased risk for alcohol-related problems. The guide asks practitioners to utilize a simple, single question prescreen: "Do you sometimes drink beer, wine, or other alcoholic beverages?" A "yes" answer leads to two additional questions to determine the weekly average number of drinks ingested as well as a maladaptive pattern of alcohol use. This guide can be downloaded at www.niaaa.nih.gov and is discussed at length by Willenbring et al. (2009). Treatments for alcohol dependence, both psychological and pharmacologic, are cost-effective (Popova et al., 2011). Schuckit (2009) stated:

> Treatment can include motivational interviewing to help people to evaluate their situations, brief interventions to facilitate more healthy behaviors, detoxification to address withdrawal symptoms, cognitive-behavioral therapies to avoid relapse, and judicious use of drugs to diminish cravings or discourage relapses. (p. 492)

Pharmacotherapies for Alcohol Abuse and Dependence

Because alcoholism involves the ingestion of alcohol, eliminating such ingestion is an obvious therapeutic strategy. Achieving success, however, is an extremely difficult task.

Almost 20 years ago Vaillant (1996) performed a remarkable 50-year follow-up of two cohorts of men who began abusing alcohol at an early age. One group consisted of university undergraduates; the second consisted of nondelinquent inner-city adolescents. By 60 years of age, 18 percent of the college alcohol abusers had died, 11 percent were abstinent, 11 percent were controlled drinkers, and 60 percent were still abusing alcohol. By 60 years of age, 28 percent of the inner-city alcohol abusers had died, 30 percent were abstinent, 12 percent were controlled drinkers, and 30 percent were still abusing alcohol. Because alcohol abuse after age 60 can be devastating, the greater levels of abuse by college-educated males need to be addressed. The ideal goals of pharmacotherapy for alcohol dependence and abuse include the following:

- Reversal of the acute pharmacologic effects of alcohol
- Treatment and prevention of withdrawal symptoms and complications
- Maintenance of abstinence, prevention of relapse, or reduction in the number of active drinking days with agents that decrease craving for alcohol or the loss of control over drinking or make it unpleasant to ingest alcohol
- Treatment of coexisting psychiatric disorders that complicate recovery
- Limitation of neuronal injury during detoxification by blocking withdrawal-induced glutaminergic activation and glutamate receptor up regulation

Can any of these goals be met? First, at this time, no agent can reverse the acute pharmacologic effects of alcohol. Some feel that *caffeine* can antagonize alcohol intoxication and increase alertness. Caffeine, however, does not reverse the intoxicating effects of alcohol. As a behavioral stimulant, caffeine can only increase activity, not reverse the motor, cognitive, or other dysfunctions induced by alcohol. Therefore, acute alcohol intoxication is usually treated with supportive care and a quiet environment to protect both the intoxicated person and others placed at risk of injury.

Pharmacotherapies are available for several goals of therapy:

- To treat and prevent withdrawal symptoms, including withdrawal convulsions
- To reduce consumption of and cravings for alcohol
- To prevent relapse to drinking behaviors
- To treat complications in alcohol-dependent people who are decreasing or discontinuing alcohol consumption
- To treat associated psychiatric problems
- To reduce glutamate release and glutamate receptor up regulation with subsequent neuronal damage

Medications can effectively prevent and treat the symptoms, seizures, and DTs associated with withdrawal. In addition, several classes of medications are available to help address and treat the psychiatric comorbidities observed in alcohol-dependent people. However, pharmacological agents are much less effective in reducing the rates of relapse to renewed drinking.

The FDA has approved four medications specifically for the treatment of alcohol dependence (oral naltrexone, acamprosate, injectable long-acting naltrexone, and disulfiram). Early research into *cannabinoid receptor antagonists* demonstrated very good efficacy in reducing drinking behaviors, but use was limited by adverse side effects that include anxiety reactions as well as major depression with melancholic features and even suicides (deMattos et al., 2009).

In addition to the above four medications approved specifically by the FDA for the treatment of alcohol dependence, other psychotropic agents are used to treat comorbid disorders often found in patients with alcohol dependence. Several of these have also been shown to reduce certain drinking behaviors (Clapp, 2012). Such agents include certain mood-stabilizing anticonvulsants (which have efficacy as detoxification and antirelapse agents), the alpha-1 adrenergic antagonists such as prazosin (Minipress), the atypical antipsychotic drugs quetiapine (Seroquel) and aripiprazole (Abilify), and several of the antidepressants.

Pharmacotherapies for Management of Alcohol Withdrawal

At its simplest, if ingesting alcohol reduces glutamate activity and increases GABA activity in the brain, alcohol withdrawal results in the opposite: reduced GABA activity and increased glutamate activity. These changes result in uncontrolled excitation (excitotoxicity) that can damage neurons as well as having long-term effects on cognitive functioning. The major therapeutic goal of managing acute alcohol withdrawal or detoxification is to prevent uncontrolled excitation by either reducing glutamate activity or increasing GABA activity. Classically this has been achieved through use of either benzodiazepines (see Chapter 13) or anticonvulsant medications (see Chapter 14).

Benzodiazepines. A recent review (Amato et al., 2011) noted that benzodiazepines, especially chlordiazepoxide (Librium), was efficacious for the prevention of alcohol withdrawal seizures. However, their use is restricted to only a few days or perhaps a month because of the potential for developing physical dependence on these drugs.

Increasing GABA activity is the mechanism underlying this classical use. It may not seem logical to substitute one potentially addictive drug (a benzodiazepine) for another (ethanol). Here is the explanation: the short duration of the action of alcohol and its narrow range of safety make it an extremely dangerous drug from which to withdraw. When alcohol ingestion is stopped, withdrawal symptoms begin within a few hours. Substituting a long-acting drug prevents or suppresses the withdrawal symptoms. The longer-acting benzodiazepine is then either maintained at a level low enough to allow the person to function or is withdrawn gradually. Preferred drugs are the benzodiazepines with long-acting active metabolites—chlordiazepoxide (Librium) or diazepam (Valium). Acute seizure activity can be controlled with the faster-onset, shorter-acting benzodiazepine lorazepam. The pharmacology of the benzodiazepines is discussed in Chapter 13.

Anticonvulsant Mood Stabilizers. The benzodiazepines have important limitations when used for the treatment of alcohol withdrawal: sedation, psychomotor impairments, additive interactions with alcohol, and the potential for abuse and dependence. Because seizures are common in acute alcohol withdrawal, use of an antiepileptic drug seems intuitively appropriate. Although older anticonvulsants have significant limitations that can be deleterious in alcoholics (contributing to liver and pancreatic problems, for example), they have historically been demonstrated to be effective. Examples include carbamazepine (Tegretol) and valproic acid (Depakote); their use, however, is limited by adverse effects on the liver. Newer anticonvulsants are much less liver-toxic and include gabapentin (Neurontin), pregabalin (Lyrica), oxcarbazepine (Trileptal), lamotrigine (Lamictal), and topiramate (Topamax). Leggio and coworkers (2008) reviewed such use; Guglielmo and coworkers (2012) recently studied the efficacy of pregabalin for alcohol withdrawal syndrome. Rubio and coworkers (2006) and Krupitsky and coworkers (2007) reported on the efficacy of lamotrigine (Lamictal) to improve mood, decrease alcohol craving, and decrease alcohol consumption while reducing glutamate release and presumably exerting "brain protection" during alcohol withdrawal in patients with alcoholism. The pharmacology of anticonvulsants is presented in Chapter 14, where they are discussed as mood stabilizers for the treatment of bipolar disorder.

Pharmacotherapies to Help Maintain Abstinence and Prevent Relapse

As noted above, four FDA-approved drugs are available to decrease daily consumption of ethanol and prevent clinical relapse to continued drinking. These and several other medications will be discussed here. Most of these drugs have only modest effects and are of limited use.

Alcohol-Sensitizing Drug. Disulfiram (Antabuse), available for over 60 years, is intended to deter a patient from drinking alcohol by producing an aversive reaction if the patient drinks. Disulfiram alters the metabolism of alcohol by inhibiting a liver enzyme needed to metabolize alcohol. By doing so, a chemical called *acetaldehyde* accumulates. If the patient ingests alcohol within several days of taking this "aversive drug," the accumulation results in an acetaldehyde syndrome, characterized by flushing, throbbing headache, nausea, vomiting, chest pain, and other miserable symptoms. If taken daily, disulfiram can result in total abstinence in many patients. However, controlled trials of disulfiram therapy to reduce alcohol consumption have been disappointing (Elbreder et al., 2010). Acute disulfiram reactions can be both a mental and physical challenge to the patient, involving often quite severe cardiovascular stress (Manasco et al., 2012).

Opioid Antagonists. Naltrexone, an opioid antagonist (see Chapter 10), was approved in oral formulation (as *ReVia*) by the FDA in 1984 for use in the treatment of alcohol dependence to reduce the craving for alcohol, even though the effect is small (Hackl-Herrwerth et al., 2010). The hypothesis of action is that the reinforcing properties of alcohol involve the opioid system; blockade of the opioid system by naltrexone should reduce craving by reducing the positive reinforcement associated with alcohol use, blocking the rewards of alcohol or stabilizing systems dysregulated by chronic alcohol intake (Garbutt, 2009). Initial studies with naltrexone were encouraging; however, subsequent studies determined that the efficacy of orally administered naltrexone in the prevention of alcohol relapse is much more modest. On average, oral naltrexone reduces heavy drinking by 17 percent and drinking days by 4 percent; it does not increase abstinence from alcohol.

In 2006, naltrexone (as *Vivitrol)* was FDA-approved as a once-a-month depot inject-able, intended to treat opioid (narcotic)-dependent patients, removing the euphoric effect should opioids be taken. It has also been found to have some efficacy in reducing relapse and prolonging abstinence in patients with alcohol dependence. While overall reductions in heavy drinking only amount to about 25 percent (at a cost of about $1,200 per injec-tion versus $85 for the tablet form), who, if anyone, may benefit from this formulation is unclear. Because naltrexone is a blocker of opioid receptors, it is an antagonist of opi-oid medications. If opioids are present in blood, opioid withdrawal will be precipitated. Conversely, in patients taking naltrexone, opioids will be ineffective as pain relievers.

Some research has been done with a naltrexone derivative called nalmefene (Revex) for treatment of alcohol dependence. The drug is currently available only in immediate-acting injectable formulation intended for reversal of opioid toxicity. In a preclinical European study of nalmefene *tablets,* taken each day of perceived alcohol craving (*as needed*), resulted in a modest decrease of heavy drinking days (compared with placebo) over the 6-month trial period (Mann et al., 2013). Dropout rates were quite high. The authors concluded that while total abstinence is a desirable goal, reduction in consumption may be a viable alterna-tive in many patients who cannot attain abstinence or who are not yet capable of doing so.

Acamprosate.   Acamprosate (Campral) was approved by the FDA in 1984 for use in the treatment of alcoholism, as it has been in many other countries. Acamprosate was the first pharmacologic agent specifically designed to maintain abstinence in ethanol-dependent people after detoxification. Acamprosate is thought to exert both a GABA-agonistic action at GABA receptors and an inhibitory action at glutaminer-gic NMDA receptors. It appears to act in the CNS to restore the normal activity of glutaminergic neurotransmission altered by chronic alcohol exposure (Mason and Heyser, 2010). Acamprosate is poorly absorbed orally and therefore is given in rela-tively high doses (about 2 grams per day). It has a half-life of about 18 hours and is excreted unchanged by the kidneys; it is not metabolized before excretion.

In early human studies, acamprosate was thought to be about three times as effec-tive as placebo, with drinking frequency reduced by 30 percent to 50 percent. Today, it is thought perhaps to be comparable to naltrexone, with efficacy increased by adding the drug to established, abstinence-based, cognitive-behavioral rehabilitation programs or by combining the drug with naltrexone. In both situations, naltrexone and acamprosate, although less than impressive individually, can be effective when used together and/or added to intensive psychotherapies. Coadministration of acamprosate and naltrexone significantly increased the rate and extent of absorption of acamprosate, as indicated by a 33 percent increase in acamprosate blood level and a 33 percent reduction in time to peak blood level. Acamprosate did not affect the pharmacokinetics of naltrexone. Thus, when using the two drugs in combination, the dose of acamprosate, although poorly absorbed orally, can be reduced by 33 percent. Used alone in the treatment of alcohol de-pendence, acamprosate has had limited efficacy (Rosner et al., 2010). This relative lack of efficacy was verified in the COMBINE study discussed later.

Dopaminergic Drugs.   *Dopaminergic drugs,* such as *bupropion* (Wellbutrin), have theoretical use in maintaining abstinence because (1) the positive reinforcement associated with alcohol appears to involve the dopaminergic reward system; (2) withdrawal may be accompanied by hypofunction of this reward system; and (3) depression is often comorbid with alcohol dependency. Because bupropion acts as an antidepressant at least partly through a dopaminergic action, patients with co-morbid depression and alcohol dependence might be candidates for treatment with this drug. Bupropion is commonly used as a part of smoking-cessation strategies. When such strategies are employed in patients with alcohol dependence, craving for cigarettes is reduced and precipitation of increased drinking does not appear to happen (Karam-Hage et al., 2011).

Serotonergic Drugs. *Serotonergic drugs* have been studied as agents for treating alcohol dependence. The research follows from the concept that there may be a relationship between serotonin function and alcohol consumption. In addition, different subtypes of alcoholics may be differentiated by the type or complexity of their serotonin dysfunction (Pettinati et al., 2003). Beyond excessive drinking, behaviors that are indicators of serotonin dysregulation include depression, anxiety, impulsiveness, and early-onset drinking. The major serotoninergic drugs that have been studied in alcoholism are the selective serotonin reuptake inhibitors (SSRIs), such as *fluoxetine* (Prozac) and *sertraline* (Zoloft) and the serotonin 5-HT$_{1A}$ agonist, *buspirone* (BuSpar) (discussed in Chapter 12).

These drugs are used for treating depression and anxiety disorders. SSRIs have also been evaluated for treating alcohol dependence, especially when alcoholic patients exhibit comorbid depression or anxiety. In general, SSRIs reduce patients' depressive symptoms, but have little efficacy in reducing these patients' drinking patterns. Recently, Pettinati and coworkers (2010) studied the combination of sertraline (an SSRI) and naltrexone in 170 depressed, alcohol-dependent patients. Patients also received weekly cognitive-behavioral therapy. In a 14-week trial, the combination was successful in producing abstinence from alcohol in a greater number of patients (53 percent) than either drug alone (about 23 percent to 27 percent) or placebo (23 percent). There was also a strong trend for major reductions in depressive symptomatology. Buspirone appears to be less effective (Kenna, 2010), being no more effective than placebo. Research continues into subtypes of alcoholics, especially age-of-onset subtypes who may be differentially sensitive to SSRIs (Kranzler et al., 2012).

Nicotinic Mechanism. Chapter 6 discusses a new treatment for cigarette (nicotine) dependence. Varenicline (Chantix) is a "partial nicotinic agonist," reducing the reinforcing effect of nicotine. Crunelle and coworkers (2010) reported that it reduces alcohol consumption, at least in rats. Early data indicate that it reduces the rate of relapse in people with alcohol dependence (Steensland et al., 2007; McKee et al., 2009). More should be forthcoming in this interesting area.

Baclofen. Baclofen (Lioresal) has been available since the late 1970s for the treatment of neuromuscular spasticity. It is an agonist of a specific subtype of GABA receptor, the GABA(b) receptor, modulating the GABA-glutamate balance. Studies during the late 1970s showed some efficacy in treating alcoholism. More recent studies produced mixed results, but very high doses (100–200 mg daily) have efficacy in reducing craving and promoting abstinence from alcohol (Gorsane et al., 2012; Muzyk et al., 2012; Pastor et al., 2012; Rigal et al., 2012). Baclofen may also be useful in alcohol withdrawal syndrome (Lyon et al., 2011), although this study needs verification.

Topiramate. Topiramate is an FDA-approved anticonvulsant. Today, it is generally considered to be a part of standard treatment for alcoholism (Florez et al., 2011; Paparrigopoulos et al., 2011). Topiramate is useful in alcohol withdrawal syndrome (serving as an anticonvulsant) and in long-term treatment of alcoholism as an anxiolytic, antirelapse agent, and antianger medication. Because it is not an aversion agent, treatment can begin while a patient is still drinking and continue through withdrawal and maintenance (Johnson and Ait-Daoud, 2011). The most prominent side effect of topiramate is cognitive dysfunction (see Chapter 14). However, this adverse side effect is more than offset by the improvements in cognition seen as a consequence of alcohol withdrawal (Likhitsathian et al., 2012). DeSousa (2010) compares topiramate with other anticonvulsants for use in the treatment of alcoholism.

Quetiapine and Aripiprazole. Quetiapine (Seroquel) and aripiprazole (Abilify) are atypical antipsychotic drugs with prominent antidepressant and antianxiety properties. They have both been tried in the treatment of alcoholism with variable results (Litten et al., 2012; Moallem and Ray, 2012;). It is too soon to conclude that either is clinically useful.

COMBINE Study

Treatment for alcohol dependence may include medications, behavioral therapies, or both. To understand how combining these treatments may impact effectiveness, a large, placebo-controlled study (1,383 recently alcohol-abstinent volunteers in 11 treatment sites) was designed—the Combined Pharmacotherapies and Behavioral Interventions for Alcohol Dependence, or COMBINE, study. In different combinations, two medications (oral naltrexone and acamprosate) and two behavioral interventions (medical management, or MM, and combined behavioral intervention, or CBI) were employed.

All treatment groups showed substantial reductions in drinking (Anton et al., 2006). Unexpectedly, acamprosate showed no evidence of efficacy. MM with naltrexone, CBI, or both fared better than placebo on drinking outcomes (percent days abstinent from alcohol and time to first heavy drinking day). Anton and coworkers (2006) concluded "naltrexone with MM could be delivered in health care settings, thus serving alcohol-dependent patients who might otherwise not receive treatment" (p. 2003).

In a 2008 update, Zarkin and coworkers performed a cost-benefit analysis and concluded:

> Focusing only on effectiveness, MM-naltrexone-acamprosate therapy is not significantly better than MM-naltrexone therapy. However, considering cost and cost-effectiveness, MM-naltrexone-acamprosate therapy may be a better choice, depending on whether the cost of incremental increase in effectiveness is justified by the decision maker. (p. 1214)

More recent studies (Gueorguieva et al., 2011, 2012) have added little to the previous COMBINE results.

Pharmacotherapies to Help Treat Comorbid Psychological Conditions

Relapse to drinking behaviors and untreated comorbid psychological disorders are closely intertwined. Addictive behaviors and cravings as well as affective psychopathology (anxiety, depression, irritability, anger, insomnia, and so on) involve complex and poorly understood interactions among the opioid, dopaminergic, and serotonergic systems. Opioid and dopaminergic systems are probably involved in mechanisms of craving, and serotonergic dysfunction is at a minimum involved in affective dysregulation.

When alcohol abuse and aggressive behaviors occur comorbidly, with or without abuse of other drugs, psychosocial and behavioral therapies are essential. Pharmacological treatments are not (and probably never will be) effective without the addition of intensive psychological therapies in all their various forms. In the treatment of affective disorders that occur comborbidly with alcohol dependence, antidepressants may be useful. Anticonvulsant mood stabilizers (drugs such as pregabalin or topiramate) may be of use in the control of emotional states such as anger, aggression, insomnia, and emotional outbursts.

INHALANTS OF ABUSE

Inhalants are breathable chemical vapors that produce psychoactive (mind-altering) effects. They are among the most toxic and lethal of substances that can be abused.[7] Inhalant abuse (also known as *huffing, sniffing,* or *bagging*) is the intentional inhalation of a volatile substance for the purposes of achieving an altered mental state (Williams et al., 2007). Although other abused substances can be inhaled (for example, nicotine, THC, cocaine, methamphetamine), the term *inhalants* is used to describe a variety of substances whose main common characteristic is that they are rarely, if ever, taken by any route other than inhalation. A variety of products commonplace in the home and the workplace contain substances that can be inhaled. A few were developed as general anesthetics; examples include nitrous oxide and halothane. These anesthetics were never meant to be used to achieve a "recreational" intoxicating effect. Likewise, other agents were developed for home and industrial use and were never intended to be used to affect the mind. Household inhalants include such products as nail polish remover, spray paint, glues, lighter fluid, hair and deodorant sprays, cleaning fluids, and pressurized whipped cream. Common industrial agents include gasoline, dry cleaning fluids, helium, paint thinner, and paint remover. Table 5.1 lists many of the commonly encountered inhalants of abuse.

Not included in Table 5.1 are the *nitrites,* a special class of inhalants. Although other inhalants are used to alter mood, the nitrites are used primarily as sexual enhancers. Formerly, one nitrite (amyl nitrite) was used to dilate veins and reduce the workload of the heart; it relieved chest pain associated with coronary artery disease. Today, amyl nitrite is infrequently used for this purpose. Other nitrites (isobutyl nitrite and butyl nitrite) are sold as video head cleaners, leather cleaners, and so on. These nitrites produce vasodilatation and a "flush" with reduction in blood pressure that is claimed to increase sexual satisfaction.

Inhalant abuse disproportionately affects young people. Nearly 20 percent of children in middle school and high school have experimented with inhaled substances.

---

[7] See www.inhalants.com, sponsored by the National Inhalant Prevention Coalition.

TABLE 5.1 Chemicals commonly found in inhalants

	Inhalant	Chemical
Adhesives	Airplane glue	Toluene, ethyl acetate
	Other glues	Hexane, toluene, methyl chloride, acetone, methyl ethyl ketone, methyl butyl ketone
	Special cements	Trichloroethylene, tetrachloroethylene
Aerosols	Spray paint	Butane, propane (U.S.), fluorocarbons, toluene, hydrocarbons, "Texas shoe shine" (a spray containing toluene)
	Hair spray	Butane, propane (U.S.), CFCs
	Deodorant, air freshener	Butane, propane (U.S.), CFCs
	Analgesic spray	Chlorofluorocarbons (CFCs)
	Asthma spray	Chlorofluorocarbons (CFCs)
	Fabric spray	Butane, trichloroethane
	PC cleaner	Dimethyl ether, hydrofluorocarbons
Anesthetics	Gas	Nitrous oxide
	Liquid	Halothane, enflurane
	Local	Ethyl chloride
Cleaning agents	Dry cleaning	Tetrachloroethylene, trichloroethane
	Spot remover	Xylene, petroleum distillates, chlorohydrocarbons
	Degreaser	Tetrachloroethylene, trichloroethane, trichloroethylene
Solvents and gases	Nail polish remover	Acetone, ethyl acetate
	Paint remover	Toluene, methyl chloride, methanol acetone, ethyl acetate
	Paint thinner	Petroleum distillates, esters, acetone
	Correction fluid and thinner	Trichloroethylene, trichloroethane
	Fuel gas	Butane, isopropane
	Lighter fluid	Butane, isopropane
	Fire extinguisher	Bromochlorodifluoromethane
Aerosol whipped cream canisters		Nitrous oxide
"Room odorizers"	Locker Room, Rush, poppers	Isoamyl, isobutyl, isopropyl or butyl nitrate (now illegal), cyclohexyl

Inhalants are frequently the first mind-altering drugs used by children, occasionally as young as 3 or 4 years of age. Inhalant abuse reaches its peak at some point during the seventh to ninth grades, with eighth graders regularly showing the highest rates of abuse. Inhalants are popular with youth because of peer influence, low cost, availability, and rapid onset of effect. When inhaled, they produce euphoria, delirium, intoxication, and alterations in mental status, resembling alcohol intoxication or a "light" state of general anesthesia. Users are usually not aware of the potentially serious health consequences that can result. Especially in children, inhalant abuse is an underrecognized form of substance abuse with significant morbidity and mortality.

Why Inhalants Are Abused and Who Abuses Them

Inhalant abuse goes back at least a hundred years, when ether, nitrous oxide, and chloroform were introduced into medicine as general anesthetics. Concomitant with their discovery as anesthetics was their discovery as intoxicating agents, leading to nitrous oxide and ether parties. Today, helium inhalation is common, with toxicity and even deaths resulting from displacement by helium of oxygen from the lungs. The Substance Abuse and Mental Health Services Administration (SAMHSA) reported that more 12 year-olds have used inhalants than have used marijuana, cocaine, and hallucinogens combined (6.7 percent lifetime use at age 12 compared with 5 percent nonmedical abuse of prescription drugs, 1.4 percent use of marijuana, 0.7 percent use of hallucinogens, and 0.1 percent use of cocaine). Howard and coworkers (2011) noted that more than 22 million Americans age 12 and older have used inhalants, and every year more than 750,000 use inhalants for the first time. They termed such use "the forgotten epidemic."

A few users continue their abuse of inhalants into adulthood, usually as part of a polysubstance abuse pattern. Patterns of abuse resemble patterns seen in abuse of other types of substances: there are experimenters, intermittent users, and chronic abusers. The majority of young inhalant abusers do not view such abuse as being risky (Perron and Howard, 2008), although about 20 percent of abusers will develop an inhalant substance abuse disorder (Perron et al., 2009).

Consequences of Acute Use of Inhalants

Acute consequences of inhalant use are generally divided into several types of toxicity:

- Acute hypoxic injury resulting from gaseous displacement of oxygen from one's lungs and subsequently the brain
- Acute intoxication, similar to alcohol intoxication, with resultant injury from motor vehicle and other accidents
- Medical emergencies such as cardiac arrhythmias leading to "sudden sniffing deaths"

Acute *hypoxia* follows from the replacement of oxygen in the lungs by gases such as nitrous oxide from whipping cream cans or "whippets." Reduced oxygen levels in the lungs lead to reduced oxygenation in the blood and hence in the brain. Similar effects can also follow from inhalation of helium, an inert gas often used to fill party balloons. By such displacement and the resulting hypoxia, helium can cause disorientation, blackouts, and even death. The nitrous oxide not only displaces oxygen in the lungs, but its absorption leads to an anesthetic state with disorientation, confusion, and sleep. If not administered together with oxygen (as with an anesthetic gas machine), severe hypoxia and death can result.

Acute *intoxication* is a syndrome consisting of dizziness, incoordination, slurred speech, euphoria, lethargy, slowed reflexes, slowed thinking and movement, tremor, blurred vision, stupor or coma, generalized muscle weakness, and involuntary eye movements similar to alcohol intoxication (Howard et al., 2011). This obviously impairs driving abilities.

The so-called *sudden sniffing death syndrome* can even occur in first-time users. Here, volatile hydrocarbons sensitize the heart to serious arrhythmias produced by the sudden surge of adrenalin that occurs when a person is startled or becomes excited during intoxication. This kind of episode can occur during initial experimentation or during any episode of abuse. Indeed, *sudden sniffing death syndrome* may account for 50 percent of fatalities from acute intoxication.

Therefore, although death is relatively rare during acute intoxication, when it does occur, it usually follows from lack of oxygen to the brain (anoxia), cardiac arrhythmias, or trauma. Gasoline fuels accounted for 46 percent of acute fatalities. Butane and propane sniffing is also associated with "sudden sniffing death" due to production of rapid-onset, potentially fatal cardiac arrhythmias. Currently, helium inhalation is increasingly being reported as responsible for hypoxia-associated fatalities. Alper and coworkers (2008) discuss toluene inhalation (glue sniffing) and sudden deaths.

Long-Term Consequences of Chronic Inhalant Abuse

Most inhalants produce intoxication that lasts only a few minutes. If one survives the experience, usually little damage is caused, unless hypoxia or arrhythmias occur. With *chronic abuse* of inhalants, serious complications can include peripheral and central nervous system dysfunction including peripheral neuropathies and encephalopathy, liver and/or kidney failure, dementia, loss of cognitive and other higher functions due to damage to the cerebellum, gait disturbances, loss of coordination, neurological disorders such as parkinsonism, and loss of muscle strength (Lubman et al., 2008; Dingwall and Cairney, 2011; Howard et al., 2011). Certainly, when abuse occurs in young persons, such CNS damage result in long-term or even permanent intellectual impairment.

Toluene is a common ingredient in a number of the substances sought out for inhalant abuse, apparently for its euphorigenic, hallucinogenic, and behaviorally rewarding effects. Indeed, toluene is taken up into and activates the central reward centers, including the mesolimbic dopaminergic reward centers and the frontal cortex. This may account for acute rewarding effects. Long-term, however, neurotoxicity is prominent, especially cerebellar degeneration, encephalopathy, and dementia. Peripheral toxicities include renal (kidney) and liver dysfunction.

Inhalant misuse during pregnancy is associated with significant risks to the developing fetus as inhalants readily cross the placental barrier; maternal hypoxia can also damage the fetus. Bowen (2011) has termed this "fetal solvent syndrome."

Many people who abuse inhalants for prolonged periods over many days feel a strong need to continue abusing them, implying compulsive abuse. A mild withdrawal syndrome can follow long-term abuse, perhaps similar to withdrawal from any of many sedative-hypnotic drugs. Long-term inhalant abusers exhibit symptoms including weight loss, muscle weakness, disorientation, incoordination, irritability, depression, and neurocognitive deficits.

Treatment of acute inhalant intoxication is primarily supportive with the administration of supplemental oxygen. Treatment of chronic inhalant abuse is much more difficult. Results of a survey of 550 drug treatment program directors indicate that most inhalant abusers have a pessimistic attitude about the treatment effectiveness and hopes for long-term recovery (Beauvais et al., 2002). The surveyed directors perceived that a great deal of neurological damage results from inhalant use and that education, preventive efforts, and treatments are inadequate. Early identification of abusers and rapid intervention are essential in preventing both short-term and long-term consequences.

Treatment programs that specialize in inhalant dependence are almost nonexistent, despite desperate need (Konghom et al., 2010). Standard approaches are generally ineffective for inhalant abusers because of the need for long-term detoxification and adverse effects on cognitive function. Talk therapies are inappropriate for many patients with neurological dysfunction, and the short attention span and poor impulse control of many patients make group therapy a poor choice as well. Instead, special treatment approaches for habitual users might include the following:

- Detoxification
- Medical and neurological evaluation
- Neurocognitive assessment
- Neurocognitive rehabilitation for patients who are impaired
- Academic programs to ensure participation in school
- Team approach with medical, neurological, psychological, occupational, psychomotor rehabilitation, and educational components
- Occupational and physical therapy where indicated
- Restriction or elimination of access to inhalable substances
- Aftercare that takes easy availability of inhalants into account, as well as residual cognitive impairment and poor social functioning

The best treatment is prevention. It must include everyone involved in a child's life: parents, educators, school nurses, school bus drivers, school cafeteria workers, and any other adults in the child's world.

STUDY QUESTIONS

1. Pharmacologically, what is ethyl alcohol?
2. Describe the metabolism of alcohol. What enzymes are involved? What drug blocks one of these enzymes?
3. How do women and men differ in their metabolism of alcohol?

4. How does the kinetics of alcohol metabolism differ from that of most other drugs?

5. How long does it take for an adult to metabolize the alcohol in a 1-ounce glass of 80 proof whiskey? A 4-ounce glass of wine? A 12-ounce bottle of beer? A pint of 7 percent microbrew?

6. What BAC is defined in most states as "intoxication"?

7. Describe what effects alcohol exerts on the CNS.

8. Why might a person who has developed a physical dependence on alcohol be treated with a benzodiazepine as a substitute for the alcohol?

9. Summarize some of the drugs and techniques used in treating alcoholism. What medications might be used to ameliorate alcohol withdrawal? Discuss in terms of the COMBINE report.

10. Describe the disease concept of alcoholism. Discuss the comorbidity of alcohol dependence with other psychological disorders.

11. Describe some of the fetal effects of alcohol. Is there a "safe" level of drinking during pregnancy?

12. Summarize some of the problems associated with both acute and chronic inhalant abuse.

REFERENCES

Albermann, M. C., et al. (2012). "Preliminary Investigations on Ethyl Glucuronide and Ethyl Sulfate Cutoffs for Detecting Alcohol Consumption on the Basis of an Ingestion Experiment and on Data from Withdrawal Treatment." *International Journal of Legal Medicine* 126: 757–764.

Alper, A. T., et al. (2008). "Glue (Toluene) Abuse: Increased QT Dispersion and Relation with Unexplained Syncope." *Inhalation Toxicology* 20: 37–41.

Amato, L., et al. (2011). "Efficacy and Safety of Pharmacological Interventions for the Treatment of the Alcohol Withdrawal Syndrome." *Cochrane Database of Systematic Reviews* June 15; 6: CD008537.

Anton, R. F., et al. (2006). "Combined Pharmacotherapies and Behavioral Interventions for Alcohol Dependence: The COMBINE Study: A Randomized Controlled Trial." *Journal of the American Medical Association* 295: 2003–2017.

Autti-Ramo, I. (2000). "Twelve-Year Follow-Up of Children Exposed to Alcohol in Utero." *Developmental Medicine and Child Neurology* 42: 406–411.

Baer, J. S., et al. (2003). "A 21-Year Longitudinal Analysis of the Effects of Prenatal Alcohol Exposure on Young Adult Drinking." *Archives of General Psychiatry* 60: 377–385.

Beauvais, F., et al. (2002). "A Survey of Attitudes Among Drug Use Treatment Providers Toward the Treatment of Inhalant Users." *Substance Use and Abuse* 37: 1391–1410.

Becker, H. C., et al. (2006). "Pregabalin Is Effective Against Behavioral and Electrographic Seizures During Alcohol Withdrawal." *Alcohol and Alcoholism* 24: 399–406.

Boehm, S. L., et al. (2002). "Ventral Tegmental Area Region Governs GABA(B) Receptor Modulation of Ethanol-Stimulated Activity in Mice." *Neuroscience* 115: 185–200.

Bowen, S. E. (2011). "Two Serious and Challenging Medical Complications Associated with Volatile Substance Misuse: Sudden Sniffing Death and Fetal Solvent Syndrome." *Substance Use and Misuse* 46, Supplement 1: 68–72.

Brown, S. A., et al. (2000). "Neurocognitive Functioning of Adolescents: Effects of Protracted Alcohol Use." *Alcoholism: Clinical and Experimental Research* 24: 164–171.

Carmichael, H., et al. (1997). "Association of Prenatal Alcohol Exposure with Behavioral and Learning Problems in Early Adolescence." *Journal of the American Academy of Child and Adolescent Psychiatry* 36: 1187–1194.

Clapp, P. (2012). "Current Progress in Pharmacological Treatment Strategies for Alcohol Dependence." *Expert Reviews in Clinical Pharmacology* 5: 427–435.

Crunelle, C. L., et al. (2010). "The Nicotinic Acetylcholine Receptor Partial Agonist Varenicline and the Treatment of Drug Dependence: A Review." *European Neuropsychopharmacology* 20: 69–79.

Dahl, H., et al. (2011). "Urinary Ethyl Glucuronide and Ethyl Sulfate Testing for Recent Drinking in Alcohol-Dependent Outpatients Treated with Acamprosate or Placebo." *Alcohol and Alcoholism* 46: 553–557.

Dawson, D. A., et al. (2007). "Impact of Age at First Drink on Stress-Reactive Drinking." *Alcoholism: Clinical and Experimental Research* 31: 69–77.

deMattos, V. B., et al. (2009). "Melancholic Features Related to Rimonabant." *General Hospital Psychiatry* 31: 583–585.

DeSousa, A. (2010). "The Role of Topiramate and Other Anticonvulsants in the Treatment of Alcohol Dependence: A Clinical Review." *CNS & Neurological Disorders—Drug Targets* 9: 45–49.

Dingwall, K. M., and Cairney, S. (2011). "Recovery from Central Nervous System Changes Following Volatile Substance Misuse." *Substance Use and Misuse* 46 (Supplement 1): 73–83.

Duke, A. A., et al. (2011). "Alcohol Dose and Aggression: Another Reason Why Drinking More Is a Bad Idea." *Journal of Studies on Alcohol and Drugs* 72: 34–43.

Elbreder, M. F., et al. (2010). "The Use of Disulfiram for Alcohol-Dependent Patients and Duration of Outpatient Treatment." *European Archives of Psychiatry and Clinical Neuroscience* 260: 191–195.

Feldman, H. S., et al. (2012). "Prenatal Alcohol Exposure Patterns and Alcohol-Related Birth Defects and Growth Abnormalities: A Prospective Study." *Alcoholism: Clinical & Experimental Research* 36: 670–676.

Florez, G., et al. (2011). "Topiramate for the Treatment of Alcohol Dependence: Comparison with Naltrexone." *European Addiction Research* 17: 29–36.

Frye, M. A., and Salloum, I. M. (2006). "Bipolar Disorder and Comorbid Alcoholism: Prevalence Rate and Treatment Considerations." *Bipolar Disorder* 8: 677–685.

Garbutt, J. C. (2009). "The State of Pharmacotherapy for the Treatment of Alcohol Dependence." *Journal of Substance Abuse Treatment* 36: S15–S23.

Giancola, P. R., et al. (2011). "Alcohol, Violence, and the Alcohol Myopia Model: Preliminary Findings and Implications for Prevention." *Addictive Behaviors* 36: 1019–1022.

Gold, P. E. (2008). "Protein Synthesis Inhibition and Memory: Formation vs Amnesia." *Neurobiology of Learning and Memory* 89: 201–211.

Goodwin, D. W., and Gabrielli, W. F. (1997). "Alcohol: Clinical Aspects." In J. H. Lowinson, P. Ruiz, R. B. Millman, and J. G. Langrod, eds. *Substance Abuse: A Comprehensive Textbook*, 3rd ed. (pp. 142–148). Baltimore: Williams & Wilkins.

Gorsane, M. A., et al. (2012). "Is Baclofen a Revolutionary Medication in Alcohol Addiction Management? Review and Recent Updates." *Substance Abuse* 33: 336–349.

Grant, B. F., et al. (2004). "Co-Occurence of 12-Month Alcohol and Drug Use Disorders and Personality Disorders in the United States." *Archives of General Psychiatry* 61: 361–368.

Gueorguieva, R., et al. (2011). "Baseline Trajectories of Drinking Moderate Acamprosate and Naltrexone Effects in the COMBINE Study." *Alcoholism: Clinical and Experimental Research* 35: 523–531.

Gueorguieva, R., et al. (2012). "Baseline Trajectories of Heavy Drinking and Their Effects on Postrandomization Drinking in the COMBINE Study: Empirically Derived Predictors of Drinking Outcomes During Treatment." *Alcohol* 46: 121–131.

Guglielmo, R., et al. (2012). "Pregabalin for Alcohol Dependence: A Critical Review of the Literature." *Advances in Therapeutics* 29: 947–957.

Hackl-Herrwerth, R. S., et al. (2010). "Opioid Antagonists for Alcohol Dependence." *Cochrane Database of Systematic Reviews* 12: CD001867.

Hartzler, B., and Fromme, K. (2003). "Fragmentary and En Bloc Blackouts: Similarity and Distinction Among Episodes of Alcohol-Induced Memory Loss." *Journal of Studies on Alcohol* 64: 547–550.

Haseba, T., and Ohno, Y. (2010). "A New View of Alcohol Metabolism and Alcoholism—Role of the High-*Km* Class III Alcohol Dehydrogenase (ADH3)." *International Journal of Environmental Research and Public Health* 7: 1076–1092.

Heinz, A., et al. (2009). "Identifying the Neural Circuitry of Alcohol Craving and Relapse Vulnerability." *Addiction Biology* 14: 108–118.

Howard, M. O., et al. (2011). "Inhalant Use and Inhalant Use Disorders in the United States." *Addiction Science & Clinical Practice* 6: 18–31.

Johnson, B. A., and Ait-Daoud, N. (2011). "Topiramate in the New Generation of Drugs: Efficacy in the Treatment of Alcoholic Patients." *Current Pharmaceutical Design* 16: 2103–2112.

Jyri, J., et al. (2010). "Midlife Alcohol Consumption and Later Risk of Cognitive Impairment: A Twin Follow-up Study." *Journal of Alzheimer's Disease* 22: 939–948.

Karam-Hage, M., et al. (2011). "Bupropion-SR for Smoking Cessation in Early Recovery from Alcohol Dependence: A Placebo-Controlled, Double-Blind Study." *American Journal of Drug and Alcohol Abuse* 37: 487–490.

Kenna, G. A. (2010). "Medications Acting on the Serotonergic System for the Treatment of Alcohol Dependent Patients." *Current Pharmaceutical Design* 16: 2126–2135.

King, W. C., et al. (2012). "Prevalence of Alcohol Use Disorders Before and After Bariatric Surgery." *Journal of the American Medical Association* 307: 2516–2525.

Kirby, L. G., et al. (2011). "Contributions of Serotonin in Addiction Vulnerability." *Neuropharmacology* 61: 421–432.

Konghom, S., et al. (2010). "Treatment for Inhalant Dependence and Abuse." *Cochrane Database of Systematic Reviews* December 8 (12): CD007537.

Kot-Leibovich, H., and Fainsod, A. (2009): "Ethanol Induces Embryonic Malformations by Competing for Retinaldehyde Dehydrogenase Activity During Vertebrate Gastrulation." *Disease Models and Mechanisms* 2: 295–305.

Kranzler, H. R., et al. (2012). "Comparison of Alcoholism Subtypes as Moderators of the Response to Sertraline Treatment." *Alcoholism: Clinical and Experimental Research* 36: 509–516.

Krupitsky, E. M., et al. (2007). "Antiglutamatergic Strategies for Ethanol Detoxification: Comparison with Placebo and Diazepam." *Alcoholism: Clinical and Experimental Research* 31: 604–611.

Kushner, M. G., et al. (2011). "Vulnerability to the Rapid ("Telescoped") Development of Alcohol Dependence in Individuals with Anxiety Disorder." *Journal of Studies on Alcohol and Drugs* 72: 1019–1027.

Kushner, M. G., et al. (2012). "Alcohol Dependence Is Related to Overall Internalizing Psychopathology Load Rather than to Particular Internalizing Disorders: Evidence from a National Sample." *Alcoholism: Clinical and Experimental Research* 36: 325–331.

Lapham, S. C., et al. (2001). "Prevalence of Psychiatric Disorders Among Persons Convicted of Driving While Impaired." *Archives of General Psychiatry* 58: 943–949.

Lee, H., et al. (2009). "Alcohol-Induced Blackout." *International Journal of Environmental Research and Public Health* 6: 2783–2792.

Leggio, L., et al. (2008). "New Developments for the Pharmacological Treatment of Alcohol Withdrawal Syndrome. A Focus on Non-Benzodiazepine GABA-ergic Medications." *Progress in Neuro-Psychopharmacology and Biological Psychiatry* 32: 1106–1117.

Li, D., et al. (2012). "Further Clarification of the Contribution of the ADH1C Gene to Vulnerability of Alcoholism and Selected Liver Diseases." *Human Genetics* 131: 1361–1374.

Likhitsathian, S., et al. (2012). "Cognitive Changes in Topiramate-Treated Patients with Alcoholism: A 12-Week Prospective Study in Patients Recently Detoxified." *Psychiatry and Clinical Neurosciences* 66: 235–241.

Litten, R. Z., et al. (2012). "A Double-Blind, Placebo-Controlled Trial to Assess the Efficacy of Quetiapine Fumarate XR in Very Heavy-Drinking Alcohol-Dependent Patients." *Alcoholism: Clinical and Experimental Research* 36: 406-416.

Liu, Y., et al. (2012). "Intakes of Alcohol and Folate During Adolescence and Risk of Proliferative Benign Breast Disease." *Pediatrics* 129: e1192–e1198.

Lubman, D. I., et al. (2008). "Inhalant Abuse Among Adolescents: Neurobiological Considerations." *British Journal of Pharmacology* 154: 316–326.

Lyon, J. E., et al. (2011). "Treating Alcohol Withdrawal with Oral Baclofen: A Randomized, Double-Blind, Placebo-Controlled Trial." *Journal of Hospital Medicine* 6: 469–474.

Malcolm, R., et al. (2000). "Recurrent Detoxification May Elevate Alcohol Craving as Measured by the Obsessive Compulsive Drinking Scale." *Alcohol* 20: 181–185.

Manasco, A., et al. (2012). "Alcohol Withdrawal." *Southern Medical Journal* 105: 607–612.

Mann, K., et al. (2008). "Acamprosate: Recent Findings and Future Research Directions. *Alcoholism: Clinical and Experimental Research* 32: 1105–1110.

Mann, K., et al. (2013). "Extending the Treatment Options in Alcohol Dependence: A Randomized Controlled Study of As-Needed Nalmefene." *Biological Psychiatry* 73: 706–713.

Martin, S. E., and Bryant, K. (2001). "Gender Differences in the Association of Alcohol Intoxication and Illicit Drug Abuse Among Persons Arrested for Violent and Property Offenses." *Journal of Substance Abuse* 3: 563–581.

Martinotti, G., et al. (2010). "Pregabalin, Tiapride and Lorazepam in Alcohol Withdrawal Syndrome: A Multi-Centre, Randomized, Single-Blind Comparison Trial." *Addiction* 105: 288–299.

Marty, V. N., and Spigelman, I. (2012). "Effects of Alcohol on the Membrane Excitability and Synaptic Transmission of Medium Spiny Neurons in the Nucleus Accumbens." *Alcohol* 46: 317–327.

Mason, B. J., and Heyser, C. J. (2010). "The Neurobiology, Clinical Efficacy and Safety of Acamprosate in the Treatment of Alcohol Dependence." *Expert Opinion on Drug Safety* 9: 177–188.

McKee, S. A., et al. (2009). "Varenicline Reduces Alcohol Self-Administration in Heavy-Drinking Smokers." *Biological Psychiatry* 66: 185–190.

Medina, A. E. (2011). "Fetal Alcohol Spectrum Disorders and Abnormal Neuronal Plasticity." *The Neuroscientist* 17: 274–287.

Menary, K. R., et al. (2011). "The Prevalence and Clinical Implications of Self-Medication among Individuals with Anxiety Disorders." *Journal of Anxiety Disorders* 25: 335–339.

Mitchell, J. M., et al. (2012). "Alcohol Consumption Induces Endogenous Opioid Release in the Human Orbitofrontal Cortex and Nucleus Accumbens." *Science Translational Medicine* 11 January 4: 116ra6.

Moallem, N., and Ray, L. A. (2012). "Quetiapine Improves Response Inhibition in Alcohol-Dependent Patients: A Placebo-Controlled Pilot Study." *Pharmacology Biochemistry and Behavior* 100: 490–493.

Morse, R. M., and Flavin, D. K. (1992). "The Definition of Alcoholism." *Journal of the American Medical Association* 268: 1012–1014.

Moykkynen, T., and Korpi, E. R. (2012). "Acute Effects of Ethanol on Glutamate Receptors." *Basic Clinical Pharmacology and Toxicology* 111: 4–13.

Muzyk, A. J., et al. (2012). "Defining the Role of Baclofen for the Treatment of Alcohol Dependence: A Systematic Review of the Evidence." *CNS Drugs* 26: 69–78.

National Institute on Alcohol Abuse and Alcoholism. (2007). "Helping Patients Who Drink Too Much." NIAAA Publications Distribution Center, P. O. Box 10686, Rockville, MD 20849-0686. Downloadable at www.niaaa.nih.gov.

Noel, X., et al. (2001). "Supervisory Attentional System in Nonamnestic Alcoholic Men." *Archives of General Psychiatry* 58: 1152–1158.

Oscar-Berman, M., and Marinkovic, K. (2007): "Alcohol: Effects on Neurobehavioral Functions and the Brain." *Neuropsychology Review* 17: 239–257.

Paparrigopoulos, T., et al. (2011). "Treatment of Alcohol Dependence with Low-Dose Topiramate: An Open-Label Controlled Study." *BMC Psychiatry* 11: 41.

Pastor, A., et al. (2012). "High Dose Baclofen for Treatment-Resistant Alcohol Dependence." *Journal of Clinical Psychopharmacology* 32: 266–268.

Pava, M. J., and Woodward, J. J. (2012). "A Review of the Interactions between Alcohol and the Endocannabinoid System: Implications for Alcohol Dependence and Future Directions for Research." *Alcohol* 46: 185–204.

Perron, B. E., and Howard, M. O. (2008). "Perceived Risk of Harm and Intentions of Future Inhalant Use Among Adolescent Inhalant Users." *Drug and Alcohol Dependence* 97: 185–189.

Perron, B. E., et al. (2009). "Prevalence, Timing, and Predictors of Transitions from Inhalant Use to Inhalant Use Disorders." *Drug and Alcohol Dependence* 100: 277–284.

Perry, P. J., et al. (2006). "The Association of Alcohol-Induced Blackouts and Grayouts to Blood Alcohol Concentrations." *Journal of Forensic Science* 51: 896–899.

Pettinati, H. M., et al. (2003). "The Status of Serotonin-Selective Pharmacotherapy in the Treatment of Alcohol Dependence." *Recent Developments in Alcoholism* 16: 247–262.

Pettinati, H. M., et al. (2010). "A Double-Blind, Placebo-Controlled Trial that Combines Sertraline and Naltrexone for Treating Co-Occurring Depression and Alcohol Dependence." *American Journal of Psychiatry* 167: 668–675.

Popova, S., et al. (2011). "A Literature Review of Cost-Benefit Analysis for the Treatment of Alcohol Dependence." *International Journal of Environmental Research and Public Health* 8: 3351–3364.

Prisciandaro, J. J., et al. (2012). "Simultaneous Modeling of the Impact on Alcohol Consumption and Quality of Life in the COMBINE Study: A Coupled Hidden Markov Analysis." *Alcoholism: Clinical and Experimental Research* 36: 2141–2149.

Reisfield, G. M., et al. (2011a). "Ethyl Glucuronide, Ethyl Sulfate, and Ethanol in Urine after Intensive Exposure to High Ethanol Content Mouthwash." *Journal of Analytical Toxicology* 35: 264–268.

Reisfield, G. M., et al. (2011b). "Ethyl Glucuronide, Ethyl Sulfate, and Ethanol in Urine after Sustained Exposure to an Ethanol-Based Hand Sanitizer." *Journal of Analytical Toxicology* 35: 85–91.

Rigal, L., et al. (2012). "Abstinence and 'Low-Risk' Consumption 1 Year after the Initiation of High-Dose Baclofen: A Retrospective Study among "High-Risk" Drinkers." *Alcohol and Alcoholism* 47: 439–442.

Roberto, M., et al. (2010). "The Endocannabinoid System Tonically Regulates Inhibitory Transmission and Depresses the Effect of Ethanol in Central Amygdala." *Neuropsychopharmacology* 35: 1962–1972.

Robson, M. J., et al. (2012). "Sigma-1 Receptors: Potential Targets for the Treatment of Substance Abuse." *Current Pharmaceutical Design* 18: 902–919.

Rohde, P., et al. (2001). "Natural Course of Alcohol Use Disorders from Adolescence to Young Adulthood." *Journal of the American Academy of Child and Adolescent Psychiatry* 40: 83–90.

Rosner, S., et al. (2010). "Acamprosate for Alcohol Dependent Patients." *Cochrane Database of Systematic Reviews* 9: CD004332.

Rubio, G., et al. (2006). "Effects of Lamotrigine in Patients with Bipolar Disorder and Alcohol Dependence." *Bipolar Disorder* 8: 289–293.

Ruidavets, J.-B., et al. (2010). "Patterns of Alcohol Consumption and Ischemic Heart Disease in Culturally Divergent Countries: The Prospective Epidemiological Study of Myocardial Infarction (PRIME)." *British Medical Journal (BMC)* November 23: 341; c6077.

Sari, Y., et al. (2011). "Role of the Serotonergic System in Alcohol Dependence: From Animal Models to Clinics." *Progress in Molecular Biology and Translational Sciences* 98: 401–443.

Sayal, K., et al. (2009). "Binge Pattern of Alcohol Consumption During Pregnancy and Childhood Mental Health Outcomes: Longitudinal Population-Based Study." *Pediatrics* 123: e289–e296.

Schuckit, M. A. (2009). "Alcohol-Use Disorders." *Lancet* 373: 492–501.

Schutze, M., et al. (2011). "Alcohol Attributable Burden of Incidence of Cancer in Eight European Countries Based on Results from Prospective Cohort Study." *BMC* 342:d1584

Steensland, P., et al. (2007). "Varenicline, an α4β2 Nicotinic Acetylcholine Receptor Partial Agonist, Selectively Decreases Ethanol Consumption and Seeking." *Proceedings of the National Academy of Sciences* 104: 12518–12523.

Strac, D. S., et al. (2012). "The GABAA Receptor Alpha-2 Subunit Gene (GABARA2) Is Associated with Alcohol-Related Behavior." *BMC Pharmacology and Toxicology* 13(Supplement 1): A8.

Suzuki, J., et al. (2012). "Alcohol Use Disorders After Bariatric Surgery." *Obesity Surgery* 22: 201–207.

Tiet, Q. Q., and Mausbach, B. (2007). "Treatments for Patients with Dual Diagnosis: A Review." *Alcoholism: Clinical and Experimental Research* 31: 513–536.

Tokuda, K., et al. (2011). "Ethanol Enhances Neurosteroidogenesis in Hippocampal Pyramidal Neurons by Paradoxical NMDA Receptor Activation." *Journal of Neurosciemce* 31: 9905–9909.

Vaillant, G. E. (1996). "A Long-Term Follow-Up of Male Alcohol Abuse." *Archives of General Psychiatry* 53: 243–249.

Wetherill, R. R., et al. (2012a). "Acute Alcohol Effects on Contextual Memory BOLD Response: Differences Based on Fragmentary Blackout History." *Alcoholism: Clinical and Experimental Research* 36: 1108–1115.

Wetherill, R. R., et al. (2012b). "Subjective Perceptions Associated with the Ascending and Descending Slopes of Breath Alcohol Exposure Vary with Recent Drinking History." *Alcoholism: Clinical and Experimental Research* 36: 1150–1157.

White, A. M., et al. (2004). "Experiential Aspects of Alcohol-Induced Blackouts Among College Students." *American Journal of Drug and Alcohol Abuse* 30: 205–224.

Willenbring, M. L., et al. (2009). "Helping Patients Who Drink Too Much: An Evidence-Based Guide for Primary Care Physicians." *American Family Physician* 80: 44–50.

Williams, J. F., et al. (2007). "Inhalant Abuse." *Pediatrics* 119: 1009–1017.

Woodard, G. A. (2011). "Impaired Alcohol Metabolism After Gastric Bypass Surgery: A Case-Crossover Trial." *Journal of the American College of Surgeons* 212: 209–214.

Zarkin, G. A., et al. (2008). "Cost and Cost-Effectiveness of the COMBINE Study in Alcohol-Dependent Patients." *Archives of General Psychiatry* 65: 1214–1221.

What Is a Drink?
How Much Alcohol Is in Your Drink?

One drink equivalent is the amount of alcohol that contains 10 cubic centimeters (1/3 ounce) of 100 percent ethanol. This is the amount of ethanol that the body metabolizes in 1 hour and that reduces the blood alcohol concentration (BAC) by 0.015 grams%.

This amount of alcohol is contained in about 1 to 1.5 ounces of 40 percent (80 proof) liquor, 4 ounces of 12 percent wine, or a 12-ounce bottle of 5 percent beer.

In the table below, typical alcoholic beverages are converted to their calculated drink equivalents.

If you consume	You have consumed about
One 12-oz Budweiser (5% alcohol)	1.5 drink equivalents
One 6-pack of 12-oz Budweiser	9 drink equivalents
Short case (12 bottles) of 12-oz Budweiser	18 drink equivalents
One 16-oz Budweiser	1.9 (about 2) drink equivalents
One 24-oz Budweiser	3 drink equivalents
One 40-oz Budweiser	5 drink equivalents
One 12-oz Bud Light (4.2%)	1.25 drink equivalents
One 12-oz Bud-Ice (5.5%)	1.9 (almost 2) drink equivalents
One 16-oz Old English 800 (8%)	3.8 (almost 4) drink equivalents
One 40-oz Old English 800	9 drink equivalents
Two 40-oz Old English 800	18 drink equivalents (2/3 pint of whiskey)
One 16-oz Rainier Ale (7.2%)	3.5 drink equivalents
One 40-oz St. Ides Malt (7.3%)	8 drink equivalents
One 16-oz microbrew (5% to 7%)	2.2 to 3.4 drink equivalents
One 64-oz pitcher of microbrew	9.5 to 13 drink equivalents
One 12-oz Hornsby Draft Cider (6%)	2 drink equivalents
One 16-oz barley wine (10%)	4.8 drink equivalents
One 12-oz Zima cooler (4.6%)	1.6 drink equivalents
One 12-oz Mike's Hard Lemonade (5%)	1.8 drink equivalents

Comments

Budweiser and the other brand names are used for illustration only. Other beers are similar, with modest differences. Their alcohol concentration may or may not be listed on the label or package. Coors beer, another popular beer, is 4.9 percent alcohol; Coors Light is 4.2 percent. Busch beer is 4.5 percent; Henri Weinhard Private Reserve is 4.6 percent; Red Dog is 5 percent alcohol.

Ice beers are made by slightly freezing the brew and removing some of the ice, increasing the alcohol content. Most are 5.9 percent alcohol (12-oz bottle = 2 drink equivalents).

Wine coolers are classified as malt beverages and have alcohol contents from 4.6 percent to 7 percent. They are considered to be 1.5 to 2 drink equivalents per bottle.

A tavern can sell beer, ale, and malt liquor up to 14 percent alcohol, hard cider up to 10 percent alcohol, and wine up to 14 percent alcohol. Taverns and pubs often serve beer and ale in pitchers that contain from 60 to 72 ounces. If the pitcher contains regular draft beer at about 5 percent alcohol, a 64-ounce pitcher contains about 9.5 drink equivalents of ethanol.

Chapter 6

Caffeine and Nicotine

CAFFEINE

Caffeine is the most widely consumed psychoactive drug in the world; in the United States, it is consumed daily by 80 percent or more of the adult population (Childs and deWit, 2012). It belongs to a family of substances, called xanthines, that also includes theophylline and theobromine. These substances stimulate the central nervous system, act on the kidneys to produce diuresis (urine), stimulate cardiac muscle, and relax smooth muscle.

Caffeine occurs naturally in the coffee bean (*Coffea arabica*, from Arabia), the tea leaf (*Thea sinensis* from China), the kola nut (*Cola nitida* from West Africa), and the cocoa bean (*Theobroma cacao*, from Mexico). (In 1688 the Dutch began the cultivation of coffee on the island of Java. It is this association with coffee production that led to the nickname "Java" for a good cup of coffee!) The reason why caffeine is found in so many plants is not known for certain, but it is speculated that it serves as a pesticide, because caffeine is toxic to the larva of several insects.

In addition to these organic sources, caffeine is often added to soft drinks, bottled water, candies, and medications (Table 6.1). In particular, since the introduction of the energy drink Red Bull (in Austria in 1987 and the United States in 1997), many other brands of energy drinks have been marketed, containing about 80 milligrams of caffeine per serving, with a range of 50 milligrams to 550 milligrams per can or bottle, although the caffeine content may not be listed on the label (Ishak et al., 2012; Sepkowitz, 2013; see Torpy and Livingston, 2013, for a table of caffeine content in energy drinks and other beverages). Store shelves will soon see a new product category alongside the Red Bulls and the mini bottles of energy shot drinks, called caffeine mist. Caffeine mist products come in a small tube—which resembles an asthma inhaler—and give you a shot of caffeine when you inhale them. Aero Shot Pure Energy, the first caffeine mist product to be available to consumers, gives a 100-milligram

TABLE 6.1 Caffeine content in beverages, foods, and medicines	
Tea (6 oz.)	
Black tea	25–110 mg
Oolong tea	12–55 mg
Green tea	8–16 mg
Coffee (8 oz.)	
Brewed	135–150 mg
Instant	60–100 mg
Decaffeinated	1–25 mg
Sodas (12 oz.)	
Coke	46 mg
Pepsi	38 mg
Jolt	59 mg
Mountain Dew	52 mg
Surge	52.5 mg
Other	
Chocolate bar (50 gm)	20 mg
Cocoa (5 oz.)	2–20 mg
Hot chocolate (220 ml)	4 mg
Vivarin (1 tablet)	200 mg
Espresso drinks	
Latte	70 mg

shot of caffeine and is recommended to be used no more than three times per day. Assorted B vitamins are also delivered with the mist. In contrast, the average cup of coffee contains about 135 milligrams[1] and among regular caffeine users daily intake averages between 200 and 500 milligrams, correlating with two to five cups of coffee daily. Currently, regulatory agencies impose no restrictions on the sale or use of caffeine, nor is the human consumption of caffeine-containing beverages commonly considered to be drug abuse. Recent increases in the consumption of, and adverse reactions to, energy drinks, may change this situation. Concerns about energy drinks have increased since the report of 18 deaths possibly related to these products. Sales from these drinks increased by almost 17 percent in 2011, at a cost of almost $9 billion in the United States ($37 billion globally). Ironically, over 100 years ago, in 1911, the FDA seized 40 kegs and 20 barrels of Coca-Cola syrup because the caffeine was

---

[1] The caffeine content of one cup of coffee varies widely. One hundred milligrams is often used as an average. However, among popular "gourmet" coffees, one company's coffee averages 200 milligrams per 8 fluid ounces. Thus, a 12-ounce cup of black coffee has 300 milligrams; the 16-ounce "grande" has 400 milligrams. Mixed coffee drinks have less caffeine because of added milk or flavorings. Another company's coffee averages 80 to 90 milligrams; the coffee of a third company has 100 to 125 milligrams of caffeine per 8 ounces.

considered a significant health hazard. By that time the cocaine and alcohol had already been removed. The case dragged on for years until Coca-Cola eventually reduced the amount of caffeine and the legal action was dropped (Sepkowitz, 2013).

Pharmacokinetics

Taken orally, caffeine is rapidly and completely absorbed. Significant blood levels are reached after oral ingestion in 15 to 20 minutes and 99 percent is taken up within 45 minutes (Persad, 2011). Caffeine is soluble in both water and oil, therefore it is equally distributed throughout the body and the brain, and, like all psychoactive drugs, freely crosses the placenta to the fetus.

The liver metabolizes most caffeine into active stimulants, such as theophylline and theobromine, before the kidneys excrete it. Only about 2 percent to 3 percent of the drug is excreted in the urine unchanged (Persad, 2011). Caffeine's half-life of elimination varies from about 2.5 hours to 10 hours (Magkos and Kavouras, 2005) and is extended by alcohol and other medications, in infants, women taking oral contraceptives, pregnant women, the elderly, and patients with chronic liver disease. Conversely, in cigarette smokers, caffeine's half-life is shortened; however, when smoking is terminated, caffeine's half-life increases. The reduced metabolism of caffeine can increase plasma caffeine levels and may contribute to cigarette withdrawal symptoms in heavy coffee drinkers, particularly because caffeine can induce or intensify anxiety disorders, such as panic disorder (Lambert et al., 2006).

The structure and metabolism of caffeine are shown in Figure 6.1. The two major metabolites of caffeine, theophylline and paraxanthine, behave similarly to caffeine; a third

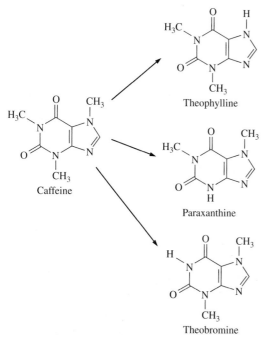

FIGURE 6.1   Metabolism of caffeine to three endproducts.

metabolite, theobromine, does not. Caffeine is metabolized by the CYP-1A2 subgroup of hepatic drug-metabolizing enzymes. Certain selective serotonin reuptake inhibitor (SSRI) antidepressants, such as fluoxetine and fluvoxamine (see Chapter 12), are potent inhibitors of CYP-1A2, and people taking these antidepressants can exhibit unexpected toxicity or intolerance to caffeine as plasma levels of caffeine rise, including de novo production of "caffeinism" (defined in the next section) with severe anxiety reactions.

Pharmacological Effects

There is mounting evidence that the world's most widely used stimulant has a variety of positive effects, on both mental and physiological processes. In fact, a recent large study found that people who drank four to five cups of coffee a day reduced their overall risk of death by 12 percent (in men) to 16 percent (in women) (Freedman et al., 2012). While these beneficial actions are perhaps a welcome contrast to the frequent warnings about the dangers of many foods and medicines, it is important to maintain a balanced view. There is concern in regard to the adverse effects of increasing consumption of caffeine, especially by young people using energy drinks, particularly when combined with alcohol, such as in bars (Red Bull and vodka), premixed (Four Loco), mixed individually, or drunk separately (Howland and Rohsenow, 2013).

Beneficial Effects of Caffeine

In spite of the fact that caffeine consumption can transiently raise blood pressure when caffeine is taken in coffee, the blood pressure elevations are small and long-term risks may be mitigated by compensatory actions. Coffee beans contain antioxidant compounds and coffee consumption has been associated with reduced concentrations of inflammatory markers (Natella et al., 2007; Montagnana et al., 2012). Moderate coffee intake was found to be associated with a lower risk for coronary heart disease as far out as 10 years (Wu et al., 2009), and new data suggest that an average of two cups a day actually protects against heart failure (Mostofsky et al., 2012).

According to one review, drinking between one and six cups of coffee a day also cut stroke risk by 17 percent (Larsson and Orsini, 2011). And although the effect of coffee on stroke risk in those with cardiovascular disease (CVD) may be increased, one review reported that one to three cups a day might protect against ischemic stroke in the general population (D'Elia et al., 2012).

While caffeine dilates coronary arteries, it exerts an opposite effect on cerebral blood vessels; it constricts these vessels, thus decreasing blood flow to the brain by about 30 percent and reducing pressure within the brain. This action can produce striking relief from headaches, especially migraines, and is the reason why it is an ingredient in some analgesics.

Regular coffee drinking has been shown to improve glucose metabolism, insulin secretion, and significantly reduce risk for type 2 diabetes (Huxley et al., 2009; Floegel et al., 2012). A statistical correlation between high consumption of black tea and low prevalence of type 2 diabetes across 50 countries has also been reported (Beresniak et al., 2012). Preliminary data also showed that overweight patients treated with unroasted coffee beans in supplement form lost an average of 17 pounds over 22 weeks. The authors speculated that the weight loss may be due in part to coffee containing chlorogenic acid, a plant compound with antioxidant properties thought to reduce glucose absorption (Vinson et al., 2012; but see below).

Did You Know?

Lab Experiments Question Effectiveness of Green Coffee Bean Weight-Loss Supplements

A major ingredient in green coffee bean dietary supplements—often touted as "miracle" weight-loss products—does not prevent weight gain in obese laboratory mice fed a high-fat diet when given at higher doses. That's the conclusion of a first-of-its-kind study published in the American Chemical Society's *Journal of Agricultural and Food Chemistry*. Evidence from past studies shows that coffee drinkers have a lower risk of obesity, high blood pressure, type 2 diabetes, and other disorders collectively termed the "metabolic syndrome." Chlorogenic acid (CGA), one coffee polyphenol, is the main ingredient in scores of dietary supplements promoted as weight-loss products. However, mice fed a high-fat diet and mice on a high-fat diet plus CGA gained the same amount of weight. The CGA mice, however, were more likely to develop disorders that often lead to type 2 diabetes. They also accumulated fat inside the cells in their livers.

Evidence suggests that moderate to heavy coffee consumption (three to six cups a day, across studies) can reduce the risk for numerous cancers, including endometrial (Je et al., 2011), prostate (Wilson et al., 2011), head and neck (Galeone et al., 2010), basal cell carcinoma (Song et al., 2012), and estrogen-receptor–negative breast cancer (Li et al., 2011). These protective effects are believed to be at least partially due to coffee's antioxidant and antimutagenic properties (Je et al., 2011; Turati et al., 2011). Other reported benefits include protection against liver diseases (Molloy et al., 2012), decreased risk for gout (Choi et al., 2007), and a possible antimicrobial effect (Matheson et al., 2011).

Numerous studies, including six large prospective studies, have supported a protective effect of caffeine against Parkinson's disease (PD) in both men and women (James et al., 2011; Liu et al., 2012). It does not matter if the caffeine is in coffee or tea, but decaffeinated coffee is not effective. Furthermore, no study has ever found that coffee increases the risk of PD. Evidence also suggests that daily coffee/caffeine ingestion during middle age and old age decreases the risk of Alzheimer's disease (AD). One hypothesis for this action is that caffeine increases blood levels of a growth factor called granulocyte colony stimulating factor (GCSF), which is very low in patients with Alzheimer's disease. Caffeinated coffee produces an increase in GCSF blood levels, and this substance has been shown to improve memory in laboratory animals (Cao et al., 2012). Regardless of the mechanism, and, although there is not a great deal of data, the evidence suggests that overall coffee and tea drinkers may experience less cognitive decline as they age (Arab et al., 2013).

Of course, it is not clear whether the consumption promotes cognition, or vice versa. However, it has been reported that honeybees, given caffeine paired with sugar water, were three times more likely to remember a learned floral scent after 24 hours than bees given just the sugar water. Caffeine occurs naturally in the nectar of Coffea and Citrus plant species, and it may be that the caffeine in their nectar improves the likelihood that their pollen will be distributed (Wright et al., 2013)!

Coffee consumption might also benefit mental health (Lucas et al., 2011). Women who drank two to four cups of coffee per day had a 15 percent to 20 percent decreased risk for depression compared with those who drank less than one cup per week. There was no association with depression and decaffeinated coffee. This is perhaps not surprising, because caffeine is a psychostimulant, and is usually taken because of its activation of mood and behavior. At low doses, caffeine increases subjective arousal and physical endurance, improves concentration, elevates mood, and enhances performance on simple motor (such as driving simulation) and cognitive tasks, especially monotonous tasks (Smith et al., 2013). Fatigue is reduced and the need for sleep is delayed (Childs and deWit, 2012). Energy drinks also improve performance on laboratory tasks of memory and cognition. However, it is not yet clear whether this effect is due to the caffeine alone, or the fact that these drinks also contain a lot of sugar (glucose) (Ishak et al., 2012). In a rare study of "real world" conditions, it was found that long-haul truckers who reported that they used caffeinated drinks to stay awake had a 63 percent reduced likelihood of crashing compared with drivers who did not take caffeinated products (Sharwood et al., 2013).

Other physiological actions of caffeine include bronchial relaxation (an antiasthmatic effect), increased secretion of gastric acid, and increased urine output (although this may become tolerant in habitual users).

Adverse Effects of Caffeine

Most people adjust, or titrate, their intake of caffeine to achieve the beneficial effects while minimizing undesirable effects. Heavy consumption of coffee (12 or more cups per day, or 1.5 grams of caffeine) can cause agitation, anxiety, tremors, rapid breathing, and insomnia. The lethal dose of caffeine is about 10 grams, although ingestion in a short period of time of only 3 grams might be fatal; a blood level of 80 micrograms or more is considered potentially lethal (Sepkowitz, 2013). There are documented cases of seizures and deaths associated with caffeine consumption in energy drinks (and caffeine pills), which may be exacerbated by sleep deprivation (Ishak et al., 2012; Szpak and Allen, 2012). The number of people seeking emergency treatment after energy drink consumption has doubled during the past 4 years, from about 10,000 to about 20,000. In a recent survey of combat soldiers, about 45 percent reported consuming at least one energy drink a day (14 percent used three or more and stated that they had problems staying awake on duty) (Toblin et al., 2012). The Food and Drug Administration limits caffeine content in soft drinks, but energy drinks do not always fit into that classification and, depending on the manufacturer, may be categorized as dietary supplements, because they contain "natural" substances such as ginkgo or other herbs, which are not regulated by the FDA.

People with anxiety disorders, such as panic and social anxiety disorder, tend to be sensitive to the anxiogenic properties of caffeine, especially if they usually avoid caffeinated products and do not develop a tolerance to caffeine's effect, but high doses can produce anxiety even in healthy persons. The wide variability in sensitivity to the anxiogenic effect of caffeine may be due to differences in caffeine metabolism or in the amount of adenosine receptors through which caffeine exerts its effects (discussed below) (Childs and deWit, 2012).

Caffeinism is a clinical syndrome produced by the overuse or overdoses of caffeine. Central nervous system (CNS) symptoms include increases in anxiety, agitation, and insomnia as well as mood changes. Peripheral symptoms include tachycardia, hypertension, cardiac arrhythmias, and gastrointestinal disturbances. Caffeinism is usually dose related, with doses higher than about 500 to 1000 milligrams (1 gram, or five to ten cups of coffee) causing the most unpleasant effects. After prolonged or high doses, caffeine can produce psychosis in otherwise healthy people, especially during periods of increased stress, and worsen this condition in people with schizophrenia (Crowe et al., 2011; Persad, 2011; Childs and deWit, 2012). Cessation of caffeine ingestion resolves these symptoms.

There is also some controversy in regard to the practical benefit obtained from the use of caffeine to increase alertness. While frequent consumers may feel more alert after consumption, evidence suggests that this may be due to the reversal of acute withdrawal effects (Rodgers et al., 2010). In this study, medium/high caffeine consumers given placebo reported a decrease in alertness and an increase in headache, which was not reported by the group that got caffeine. After caffeine was administered, the alertness of these subjects was no different than that of non/low users who received a placebo. This indicates that caffeine brings caffeine users back to "normal."

Perhaps the most concerning adverse effect of caffeine is its effect on sleep, and the consequences of the combined use of energy drinks and alcohol on alertness and risky behavior. Although caffeine reduces fatigue and improves attention, it disturbs sleep. Even when taken during the day, and certainly before bedtime, caffeine may impair the duration and quality of sleep and cause repeated awakenings (Childs and deWit, 2012). Ishak et al. (2012) describe a study in which 67 percent of a college student population consumed energy drinks to stay awake, 65 percent consumed to increase energy, and 54 percent to mix it with alcohol. Those who mixed their energy drinks with alcohol in a social setting had more drinks ($\geq$ 3) per sitting compared to those who only consumed them to stay awake or increase energy. While caffeine can reduce some of the motor impairment, sedation, and intoxication produced by alcohol (Childs and deWit, 2012), which is why it is added to alcohol, it also increases sexually risky behaviors, marijuana use, fighting, prescription drug abuse, alcohol abuse, and cigarette smoking (Ishak, 2012). The fact that caffeine enhances alcohol tolerance and can counteract some symptoms of a hangover may also contribute to subsequent alcohol dependence (Childs and deWit, 2012). Drinks containing both caffeine and alcohol were considered dangerous by the FDA in 2010, because the caffeine masked some of the cues that people used to tell if they were intoxicated. However, a growing number of foods with caffeine are being marketed and the FDA is going to start investigating their safety. This reaction followed the introduction of a caffeinated gum by Wrigley, called Alert Energy Gum, in April 2013. Each piece contains about 40 milligrams of caffeine. This follows the recent addition of 50 milligrams of caffeine to Jelly Belly "Extreme Sport Beans" and the caffeine added to Arma Energy Snx trail mix, chips, and other products.

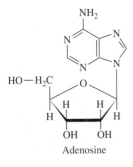

FIGURE 6.2 Structure of adenosine. Note the similarity of adenosine to caffeine (shown in Figure 6.1).

Mechanism of Action

Caffeine acts primarily by blocking all subtypes of adenosine receptors, A_1, A_{2A}, A_3, and A_{2B}. The structure of adenosine is shown in Figure 6.2. Because caffeine is an adenosine antagonist, its pharmacological effects indicate that adenosine receptors are tonically stimulated by adenosine (Magkos and Kavouras, 2005). Adenosine is a *neuromodulator* that influences the release of several neurotransmitters in the CNS. There do not appear to be discrete adenosinergic pathways in the CNS; rather, adenosinergic neurons form a diffuse system. Adenosine levels usually increase during the day and exert a sleep-inducing effect in the brain. By blocking adenosine receptors, caffeine promotes wakefulness.

The positive stimulatory effects of caffeine appear to be due in large measure to blockade of the adenosine receptors that stimulate GABAergic neurons of inhibitory pathways to the dopaminergic reward system of the striatum. Therefore, caffeine may produce its behavioral effects by removing the negative modulatory effects of adenosine from dopamine receptors, thus indirectly stimulating dopaminergic activity. Caffeine does not induce a release of dopamine in the nucleus accumbens; it leads to a release of dopamine in the prefrontal cortex, which is consistent with the drug's alerting effects and mild behavioral reinforcing properties. Besides adenosine antagonism, caffeine and other xanthines have other biological actions: they inhibit phosphodiesterases (PDEs) and promote calcium release from storage sites within neurons (Ribeiro and Sebastião, 2010).

Reproductive Effects

Is caffeine safe during pregnancy? Caffeine, the most widely used psychotropic drug in the world, is consumed by at least 75 percent of pregnant women, but whether it is safe to ingest during pregnancy is an unresolved issue. As early as 1980, the U.S. Food and Drug Administration cautioned pregnant women to minimize their intake of caffeine. Recent reports have explored the connection between caffeine intake and rates of miscarriage (Pollack et al., 2010), fetal growth restriction (CARE Study Group, 2008), birth weight, and length of gestation (Jahanfar and Sharifah, 2009). In general, while data are limited and controversial, caffeine, at least in reasonable doses, seems to cause a modest degree of fetal growth restriction (Figure 6.3) and in very large doses may slightly increase the risk of miscarriage. In contrast to earlier reports, a recent large epidemiological study found caffeine intake

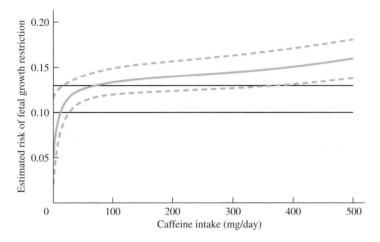

FIGURE 6.3 Relation between the risk of fetal growth restriction and caffeine intake (milligrams per day) during pregnancy. The graph is restricted to less than 500 mg/day (about five cups of coffee) for clarity. Thin horizontal lines mark the average risk of fetal growth restriction (10 percent) and average risk in a study cohort (13 percent). The solid curve represents the average, with 95 percent confidence levels shown above and below it by the dashed curves. [Data from CARE Study Group, 2008, Figure 1.]

(200 to 300 milligrams per day) was consistently associated with decreased birth weight and increased odds of being small for gestational weight (Sengpiel et al., 2013). Caffeine itself does not appear to be a human teratogen, nor does it appear to affect the course of normal labor and delivery (Brent et al., 2011). However, one recent study found that adult offspring of mice that had been treated with caffeine while pregnant did have some neurological abnormalities, cognitive deficits, and increased susceptibility to seizures (Silva et al., 2013). Current U.S. recommendations generally advise that pregnant women limit daily intake to about 200 milligrams or less (300 milligrams per day per the World Health Organization).

Tolerance and Dependence

Chronic use of caffeine, even in regular daily doses as low as 100 milligrams, is associated with habituation and tolerance, and discontinuation may produce low-grade withdrawal symptoms. Because tolerance and dependence can occur rapidly, even after low doses, most habitual users are probably physically dependent to some degree. People who drink a great deal of coffee complain of headache (the most common symptom), drowsiness, fatigue, and a generally negative mood state on withdrawal. Impaired intellectual and motor performance, difficulty with concentration, and drug (caffeine) craving are also reported. Withdrawal symptoms typically begin slowly, maximize after one or two days, and cease within a few days; readministration of caffeine rapidly relieves withdrawal symptoms.

The current manual of psychological disorders, the DSM-5 (American Psychiatric Association, 2013) proposes criteria for four Caffeine-Related Disorders: (1) caffeine intoxication, (2) caffeine withdrawal, (3) other caffeine-induced disorders, and (4) unspecified caffeine-related disorder.

NICOTINE
Epidemiology and Public Policy

Nicotine is one of the three most widely used psychoactive drugs in our society, along with caffeine and ethyl alcohol. Despite the fact that nicotine has no therapeutic applications in medicine, its widespread use and its well-defined toxicity give it immense importance. Tobacco use continues to be the leading cause of preventable death and disease in the United States (Rigotti, 2012; Schroeder, 2013), responsible for nearly half-a-million deaths annually. Tobacco use in the United States has declined during the last 60 years, but remains stuck at about 20 percent of all adults (25.2 percent for any tobacco; 19.5 percent for smoking) (King et al., 2012), although people are smoking less, and rates are much lower in those 45 years and older (Agaku et al., 2012). As in the past, rates are higher among the poor, the least educated, and those with mental health or substance abuse disorders. Moreover, for the first time the data show that women are now as likely to die from tobacco-related disease as men (Schroeder, 2013).

According to the Centers for Disease Control and Prevention, total consumption of all combustible tobacco decreased by 27.5 percent from 2000 to 2011. However, while consumption of cigarettes decreased 32.8 percent, consumption of loose tobacco and cigars *increased* 123.1 percent over the same period. The data suggest that certain smokers have switched from cigarettes to other combustible tobacco products, most notably since a 2009 increase in the federal tobacco excise tax that created tax disparities between product types (Tynan et al., 2012). That year the FDA was granted authority to regulate tobacco products. The Tobacco Control Act became law on June 22, 2009. It gave the FDA authority to regulate the manufacture, distribution, and marketing of tobacco products to protect the public's health. An important provision of this law is that in developing regulations, the FDA must consider the effects on both users and nonusers. This differs from the standard role of the FDA in evaluating safety and effectiveness. A comprehensive review of the scope of this new authority, and developments since the policy was initiated, is provided by Husten and Deyton (2013); similar discussions of tobacco control in Asia (Mackay et al., 2013) and Europe (Britton and Bogdanovica, 2013) make up this series of updates. So many applications for products, or modifications, were then submitted for review, that hundreds are still not on the market.

A 2012 Surgeon General's report (Preventing Tobacco Use Among Youth and Young Adults, http://www.cdc.gov/tobacco/data_statistics/sgr/2012/) found that youths and young adults had even higher rates of cigar use and simultaneous use of multiple tobacco products. The increasing popularity of *hookah* is especially concerning. Hookah use, also known as shisa, narghile, or waterpipe, consists of smoking substances through a waterpipe such that the smoke passes through the water and is cooled before inhalation. Originating in northern Africa and southwest Asia it is a tradition at least four centuries old, although recently it is most popular among adult men in Middle Eastern countries (Brockman et al., 2012). However, hookah smoking is spreading worldwide; in the United States, adolescents and young adults are increasingly adopting this habit, with estimates of 15 percent to 41 percent of college undergraduates using hookahs. In their survey, Brockman and colleagues (2012) reported lifetime hookah use by 27.8 percent of college students, 51.7 percent of them male. Most, 78 percent, reported smoking only tobacco, but 12 percent reported smoking marijuana and 10 percent reported smoking both. Apparently, many hookah smokers believe it is less harmful and addictive than smoking cigarettes. Studies so far show that this is not the case, and that both short- and long-term effects of waterpipe tobacco smoking are just as harmful (Hakim et al., 2011).

Many tobacco products on the market are developed especially to appeal to youth. Some cigarette-sized cigars contain candy and fruit flavoring, such as strawberry and grape. Currently, there is even an ongoing application to the FDA, from the 22nd Century Group, Inc., of two new cigarette brands, "BRAND A." a very low nicotine (VLN) cigarette (lower than any current brand), and "BRAND B," a cigarette with the lowest tar-to-nicotine ratio.

The newest smokeless tobacco products do not require users to spit, and others dissolve like mints. Young people find these products appealing in part because they can be used without detection at school or other places where smoking is banned (2012 Surgeon General's Report, cited earlier). These preparations are useful in smoke-free areas; are discreet; and do not emit any odor or secondhand smoke. They range in nicotine content from less than 1 milligram to about 4 milligrams of drug; brands include Ariva, Stonewall, Camel Strips, Camel Sticks, and Camel Orbs.

The importance of smoking prevention in youth was reinforced by several reports concerning the long-term consequences of early-onset smoking. Not surprisingly, high rates of smoking initiation during adolescence was not only associated with high lung cancer mortality decades later, but at a younger age than would normally be expected (Funatogawa et al., 2012; Whitley et al., 2012).

Did You Know?

Tobacco Laws for Youth May Reduce Adult Smoking

States with more restrictive limits on teens purchasing tobacco have lower adult smoking rates, especially among women. And compared with states with less restrictive limits, they also tend to have fewer adult heavy smokers. Data come from an ongoing National Cancer Institute survey that monitors smoking behavior in all 50 states. Information was gathered from 1998 to 2007 from 105,519 individuals aged 18 to 34. In states with enforcement policies, not only did 17-year-olds have more difficulty purchasing cigarettes, but when they reached their 20s or 30s, they were less likely to smoke. It was estimated that if all states had effective policies in place, it would reduce the prevalence of smoking by about 14 percent and the rates of heavy smoking by 29 percent. The four most effective restrictions included those on cigarette vending machines, in which the machines were either eliminated or housed in locations inaccessible to those under 18; identification requirements for purchasing cigarettes; restrictions on repackaging cigarettes so that 5 or 10 could be sold at a time, rather than an entire 20-cigarette pack; and prohibiting distribution of free cigarettes at public events. Interestingly, policies to restrict youth access to tobacco had a big impact on women but did not seem to influence smoking rates in men.

While nearly 70 percent of adults who smoke report wanting to quit, and more than 50 percent reported making an attempt to stop in the year before they were questioned, only a little over 6 percent were successful (Malarcher et al., 2011). However, in those who succeed, the benefits of quitting can be dramatic. Life expectancy can increase on average from 10 to 4 years in those who quit between 25 years and 64 years of age, respectively (Schroeder, 2013). Moreover, the cardiovascular benefits of quitting are not reduced even if those who quit subsequently gained weight (at least if they did not have diabetes) (Clair et al., 2013).

One creative public health approach to smoking cessation proposes requiring a license for people who want to use tobacco products. This would consist of a smart card, designed to limit access and promote cessation, by setting daily limits and providing financial incentives. Arguments for and against this approach can be found in Chapman (2012).

Aside from the decisions of individual smokers, public policies continue to support cessation. Comprehensive smoke-free laws are gradually spreading across the nation's largest cities. While only one city, San Jose, California, had such a law in 2002, by October of 2012, 30 cities were covered by a local law banning smoking in all indoor private workplaces, bars, and restaurants (Hopkins et al., 2012). In March 2013, the University of Pennsylvania announced that beginning in July, it would no longer hire tobacco users to work in its health care system; this was accompanied by two articles that presented opposing views about the ethics of denying employment to people who smoke (Asch et al., 2013; Schmidt et al., 2013). On the other hand, according to an annual report from several public health organizations, only a small portion, about $460 million, of the $25.7 billion from taxes and the tobacco settlement funds awarded in 1998, is expected to be applied to tobacco prevention and treatment in 2013 (Coalition Report, 2012).

Pharmacokinetics

Although more than 4,000 compounds are released by burning cigarette tobacco, nicotine is the primary addictive substance, and is responsible for tobacco dependence. The other compounds produce the adverse, long-term cardiovascular, pulmonary, and carcinogenic effects of cigarettes.

Nicotine is readily absorbed from every site on or in the body, including the lungs, buccal and nasal mucosa, skin, and gastrointestinal tract. Easy and complete absorption promotes the recreational abuse of smoked or chewed tobacco as well as its therapeutic use in treating nicotine dependency, in chewing gums, nasal sprays, transdermal skin patches, and smokeless inhalers.

Nicotine is suspended in cigarette smoke in the form of minute particles (tars), and is quickly absorbed into the bloodstream from the lungs when the smoke is inhaled, although absorption is much slower than once thought and arterial concentrations of nicotine rise rather slowly. It is likely that blood rapidly saturates with nicotine, and blood leaving the lungs (to the left side of the heart) can carry only a modest amount of drug. Thus, the arterial concentration rises slowly, even though blood carried to the brain at the initiation of smoking is nearly saturated with nicotine, accounting for the early "rush" perceived with the first cigarette.

The average cigarette contains about 8 to 10 milligrams (mg) of nicotine, but only about 20 percent to 25 percent of that amount enters the bloodstream. Because a cigarette is typically smoked in ten puffs and within 5 minutes, the average smoker will absorb 1 to 2 mg of nicotine, but absorption can range from 0.5 to 3 mg. In a typical day, the average smoker absorbs anywhere from 20 to 40 mg.

The lethal dose for the average adult is about 60 mg. A smoker can readily avoid acute toxicity because inhalation as a route of administration offers exceptional controllability of the dose. By controlling the frequency of breaths, the depth of inhalation, the time the smoke is held in the lungs, and the total number of cigarettes smoked, the smoker regulates the rate of drug intake and controls the blood level of nicotine.

Characteristically, smokers wake in the morning in a state of nicotine deficiency, will smoke one or more cigarettes fairly rapidly to achieve a blood level of about 15 milligrams per liter and continue smoking through the day to maintain this level. The elimination half-life of nicotine in a chronic smoker is about 2 hours, necessitating frequent administration of the drug to avoid withdrawal symptoms or drug craving. When nicotine is administered in the form of snuff, chewing tobacco, or gum, blood levels of nicotine are comparable to the levels achieved by smoking.

The liver metabolizes approximately 80 percent to 90 percent of the nicotine, primarily by the CYP-2A6 enzyme. People in whom the CYP-2A6 enzyme is absent (or inhibited by certain drugs) have higher blood levels of nicotine and lower levels of its metabolite. However, the constituents of tobacco smoke also induce hepatic enzymes CYP1A1, 1A2, and possibly 2E1, which are involved in the metabolism of many hormones and drugs (such as caffeine, estrogen, some antidepressants, and other psychotropic agents) (Fankhauser, 2013). As a result, smoking may reduce levels of these medications and smoking cessation may increase blood levels, especially in moderate or heavy smokers (ten or more cigarettes a day).

The primary metabolite of nicotine is *cotinine* (Figure 6.4); this substance serves as a marker of both tobacco use and exposure to environmental smoke and is often used to measure tobacco consumption in laboratory experiments. There is some evidence that although cotinine itself is nonaddictive, and has no cardiovascular effects in humans, it might have some anxiolytic and cognitive benefits (Moran, 2012).

Mechanism of Action

Nicotine exerts virtually all its CNS and peripheral effects by activating specific acetylcholine receptors (nicotinic receptors; nAChRs). These are divided into two groups: muscle receptors, found on skeletal (voluntary) muscles, and neuronal receptors, located throughout

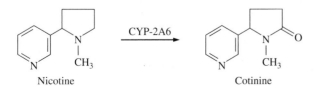

FIGURE 6.4   Structures of nicotine and its metabolite cotinine.

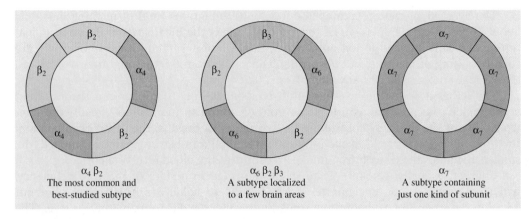

FIGURE 6.5 Diagram of the most common subtypes of the receptor for acetylcholine. [http://www.drugabuse.gov/news-events/nida-notes/2009/12/studies-link-family-genes-to-nicotine-addiction]

the peripheral and central nervous systems. Neuronal nicotinic receptors are composed of five subunits arranged around a central pore (which is termed a pentameric arrangement), like segments of an orange (see Chapter 1). A dozen proteins, labeled $\alpha_{2\text{-}10}$ and $\beta_{2\text{-}4}$, serve as subunits in nACh receptors. The most abundant and widely distributed nACh subunit proteins in the brain are the α_4 and β_2 subunits. Animal and human imaging studies have shown that nACh receptors consisting of two α_4 and three β_2 subunits are critical for the rewarding effects of nicotine (Figure 6.5). Because nicotine stimulates these receptors, it is classified as an agonist. However, while stimulation occurs at low doses, at high doses nicotine can block the receptors, so it has a biphasic action. In addition, within the time it takes to finish smoking a single cigarette, these nicotinic receptors become desensitized, that is, they temporarily do not respond to nicotine, or acetylcholine. During the day tolerance develops as nicotine builds up in the smoker's body, but this is lost overnight when the user is not smoking, which contributes to the powerful effect of the first cigarette of the day.

Pharmacological Effects

The diverse effects of nicotine are a result of widespread actions on receptors throughout the brain and body. Nicotine exerts powerful effects on the central and peripheral nervous systems, which influence the heart, respiratory and neuroendocrine function, and numerous other physiological processes.

Effects on the Brain

In the CNS, nAChRs are widely distributed and may be located on the presynaptic nerve terminals of dopamine-, acetylcholine-, and glutamate-secreting neurons, where their activation, either directly or indirectly, facilitates the release of these and other transmitters, such as serotonin.

The rewarding effect of the drug is believed to be due to the fact that nicotine increases dopamine levels in the mesocorticolimbic reward system involving the ventral tegmentum, nucleus accumbens, and forebrain (see Chapter 1 and Chapter 4). This may occur in three ways: first, nicotinic receptors on the VTA dopamine neurons directly cause dopamine release from these neurons onto the nucleus accumbens. Second, nicotine causes glutamate to be released onto VTA neurons, from glutamate neurons originating in the frontal cortex (see Chapter 4). Glutamate then stimulates the VTA neurons to release dopamine. Third, nicotine desensitizes nicotinic receptors that are on GABA neurons in the VTA. These receptors are normally stimulated by Ach to release GABA onto VTA dopamine neurons, and GABA normally inhibits dopamine release. When nicotine desensitizes the nAChRs, less GABA is released; the VTA is less inhibited and releases more dopamine. Moreover, it has recently been reported that, in laboratory animals, repeated periods of exposure to and subsequent withdrawal from nicotine increased its rewarding value, and also upregulated nicotinic brain receptors. It was speculated that this phenomenon might be one reason why smokers relapse frequently (Hilario et al., 2012).

Nicotine-induced release of acetylcholine may improve cognitive performance, and may also be responsible for the arousal effects commonly seen with smoking. However, early reports of improved cognitive function in humans were criticized because most of the studies were conducted with people who smoked. Very few studies have looked at nicotine's effect on memory performance in normal *nonsmokers*. There is some evidence for improvement of working memory in nonsmokers, but only under specific experimental conditions. However, one study did find that nicotine patches improved some aspects of attention in nonsmokers who had no pre-existing cognitive impairments (Levin et al., 2006). Such outcomes have raised interest in the development of nicotinic drugs as "cognitive enhancers," which might be beneficial in treating Alzheimer's disease. So far, data obtained in studies with nicotine in AD patients show conflicting results in regard to cognitive improvement. Nevertheless, research into the therapeutic possibilities of nicotinic drugs continues; a recent study reported that AD patients taking the highest dose of a selective, partial agonist of alpha-7 nicotinic receptors preserved cognitive function relative to placebo-treated patients (Hilts et al., 2012).

The fact that smoking rates are exceptionally high in schizophrenia patients (and other types of mental illness, Prochaska, 2011) prompted studies of cognitive performance and nicotine in this population; again, results are inconsistent. Studies with adults who have ADHD are slightly more positive in supporting a cognitive effect from nicotine, which is consistent with the high rate of smoking in this population. There is stronger evidence suggesting a protective role for nicotine receptors in Parkinson's disease; as with caffeine, tobacco smoking is associated with a reduced likelihood of PD (Quik et al., 2012).

Several reports indicate a relationship between smoking and depression. Past research had concluded that depressed smokers are unwilling to quit or unable to quit, and that smoking cessation caused or worsened depressive symptoms. It has been argued, however, that the evidence does not clearly support this interpretation (Lembke et al., 2007). At least 25 percent of nonhospitalized psychiatric patients with a diagnosis of a depressive disorder are willing to try to quit smoking. Past history of depression, and even depressive symptoms at the start of smoking cessation treatment, do not consistently reduce quit rates. Depressed smokers may be more likely to experience depression with smoking cessation than nondepressed smokers, but the data are equivocal. This effect may be relevant to the fact that acute withdrawal (8 hours) from heavy smoking (25 or more cigarettes a day) in nondepressed people increased levels of monoamine oxidase-A, the enzyme that metabolizes epinephrine, dopamine, and serotonin (Bacher et al., 2011). This could contribute to the relapse risk after smoking cessation in depressed patients. In fact, transdermal nicotine patches have been shown to improve mood in nonsmoking depressed patients (Salin-Pascual et al., 1996; McClernon et al., 2006). Evidence also suggests that smoking may be more cognitively effective in depressed patients who smoke compared with those who are not smokers (Caldirola et al., 2013).

Acute Effects on the Body

In the peripheral nervous system, nicotine causes an increase in blood pressure, heart rate, and cardiac contractility, release of epinephrine (adrenaline) from the adrenal glands, and an increase in the activity of the gastrointestinal tract.

In nonatherosclerotic coronary arteries, nicotine produces vasodilation, increasing blood flow to meet the increased oxygen demand of the heart muscle. In atherosclerotic coronary arteries (which cannot dilate), however, cardiac ischemia can result when the oxygen supply fails to meet the oxygen demand created by the drug's cardiac stimulation. This occurrence can precipitate angina or myocardial infarction (heart attack).

In the early stages of smoking, nicotine causes nausea and vomiting by stimulating both the vomiting center in the brain stem and the sensory receptors in the stomach. Tolerance to this effect develops rapidly. Nicotine also reduces weight gain, probably by reducing appetite and altering taste bud sensitivity. Stomach secretions are inhibited but bowel activity is stimulated; in people with little tobacco tolerance, the drug is a laxative. Nicotine stimulates the hypothalamus to release a hormone, antidiuretic hormone, which causes fluid retention. The activity of afferent nerve fibers coming from the muscles is reduced by nicotine, leading to a decrease in muscle tone. This action may be involved (at least partially) in the relaxation a person may experience as a result of smoking.

Tolerance and Dependence

While some of the acute effects wane, there is little tolerance to the primary rewarding effects of nicotine. On the other hand, nicotine clearly induces both physiological and psychological dependence in a majority of smokers. As early as 1988, the Surgeon General of the United States (U.S. Department of Health and Human Services, 1988) concluded that tobacco use is addictive, that nicotine was the substance in tobacco that causes addiction, and that nicotine addiction was pharmacologically as powerful as addiction to other drugs, such as heroin and cocaine.

A well-defined withdrawal syndrome has been delineated which is alleviated by nicotine replacement. Abstinence symptoms include a severe craving for nicotine, irritability, anxiety, anger, difficulty in concentrating, restlessness, impatience, increased appetite, weight gain, and insomnia. Symptoms usually begin within about 2 hours after the last use of tobacco, peak within 24 to 48 hours and gradually decline over the next 10 days to several weeks. Mild depression (dysphoria and anhedonia) and increased appetite may persist for months. In one study, smoking cessation produced a mean increase in body weight of 4 to 5 kg after 12 months of abstinence, although most weight was gained in the first 3 months (Aubin et al., 2012). The difficulty in handling cigarette dependence is illustrated by the fact that cigarette smokers who seek treatment for other drug and alcohol problems often find it harder to quit cigarette smoking than to give up the other drugs. Even Sigmund Freud continued his cigar habit (20 per day) until death, in spite of an endless series of operations for mouth and jaw cancer (his jaw was eventually totally removed), persistent heart problems that were exacerbated by smoking, and numerous attempts at quitting.

Unlike other drugs that produce physical dependence, the severity of tobacco withdrawal does not seem to be related to the dose (heavy or light amount of smoking), the duration of the habit, previous attempts at quitting, sex, age, education, or alcohol and caffeine use (McKim and Hancock, 2013). On the other hand, there is some evidence that genetic factors play a role in the development of dependence, specifically in the probability of smoking 20 or more cigarettes daily, in earlier and faster onset of heavy smoking, and in the likelihood of relapse after quitting (Belsky et al., 2013).

Toxicity

Both the acute pharmacological effects and the withdrawal signs seen on cessation of smoking result from the nicotine in tobacco. The tar in tobacco is mainly responsible for the diseases associated with long-term tobacco use. Of the nearly half-a-million premature deaths each year in the United States from tobacco use, about 19 percent are caused by noncancerous lung diseases, about 26 percent are caused by lung cancer, 7 percent are caused by cancers of other body organs, and more than 45 percent from heart and vascular diseases. A person who smokes two packs of cigarettes a day for 20 years loses about 13 or 14 years of his or her life.

Cardiovascular Disease

The carbon monoxide in smoke decreases the amount of oxygen delivered to the heart muscle, while nicotine increases the amount of work the heart must do (by increasing the heart rate and blood pressure). Both carbon monoxide and nicotine increase the incidence of atherosclerosis (narrowing) and thrombosis (clotting) in the coronary arteries. These three actions (among others) seem to underlie the dramatic increase in the risk of death from coronary heart disease in smokers compared to nonsmokers (Teo et al., 2006). Cigarette smokers manifest a 50 percent increase in the progression of atherosclerosis when compared with people who have never smoked.

Besides the coronary arteries, atherosclerosis occurs in other arteries as well, most notably the aorta (in the abdomen), the carotid arteries (in the neck), and the femoral and other arteries of the legs. Cigarette-induced occlusion of these vessels blocks the blood flow to important body organs and results in ischemic damage, strokes, and other disorders. Analysis of data from the Nurses Health Study showed that the risk of sudden cardiac death was higher in women who smoked, and greatest for those who smoked the most. However, in women who quit smoking for 20 years or more this risk dropped to the level of those who never smoked, compared to current smokers (Sandhu et al., 2012).

Pulmonary Disease

When tobacco smoke is inhaled, tar and ash are deposited on the moist membranes through which oxygen and carbon dioxide have to cross to and from the blood. Eventually these toxins overcome the processes by which pollutants are removed and destroyed in the lung. This leaves the lung more susceptible to infections and other toxic damage. Chronic smoking results in difficulty in breathing, wheezing, chest pain, lung congestion, and increased susceptibility to infections of the respiratory tract. Cigarette smoking impairs ventilation and greatly increases the risk of emphysema (a form of irreversible lung damage). Smoke exposure also reduces the efficacy of the immune defense mechanisms in the lungs.

Cancer

Although nicotine itself is not carcinogenic, the relationship between smoking and cancer is now beyond question. Cigarette smoke contains diverse carcinogens and cigarette smoking is the major cause of lung cancer in both men and women. Smoking is also a major cause of cancers of the mouth, voice box, and throat. Concomitant alcohol ingestion greatly increases the incidence of these problems. In addition, cigarette smoking is a primary cause of bladder cancer and pancreatic cancer, and it increases the risk of cancer of the uterine cervix twofold.

In addition to these disorders, smoking promotes many other illnesses. Among hormonal effects, smoking contributes to the development of insulin resistance and type 2 diabetes. It has several effects on the visual system: it increases the risk of cataract formation and a condition called Graves' ophthalmopathy (Kapoor and Jones, 2005), an autoimmune disease associated with too much thyroid activation, in which the eyes bulge because of swelling and inflammation. Smoking also causes premature aging of the skin (at least partly because of blood vessel constriction) and current smokers have a greater risk of developing cutaneous squamous cell cancer compared to nonsmokers (Leonardi-Bee et al., 2012).

The FDA has established a list of 93 harmful and potentially harmful constituents (HPHCs) that tobacco companies will eventually be required to report for every regulated tobacco product sold in the United States. All HPHCs included on the list cause or may cause serious health problems including cancer, lung disease, and addiction to tobacco products. The complete list includes ammonia, formaldehyde, nicotine, nitrosamines, carbon monoxide, and other toxins (http://www.fda.gov/downloads/tobaccoproducts/guidancecomplianceregulatoryinformation/ucm297981.pdf).

Effects of Passive Smoke

Many nonsmokers are exposed to the toxic agents in cigarette smoke by inhaling the exhaled smoke of smokers. This is called "environmental tobacco smoke (ETS)," "secondhand smoke," or "passive smoking." The first Surgeon General's report recognizing the health consequences of being exposed to the smoke of cigarettes smoked by other people was released in 1986 (U.S. Department of Health and Human Services, 1986). In 1993 the Environmental Protection Agency classified secondhand smoke as a Class A carcinogen. Twenty years after the first, a second Surgeon General's report (U.S. Department of Health and Human Services, 2006), documented that in 2005, exposure to secondhand smoke killed more than 3,000 adult nonsmokers from lung cancer, 46,000 adult nonsmokers from coronary heart disease, and 430 newborns from sudden infant death syndrome. Secondhand smoke exposure has even been found to increase the risk of psychiatric disorders in adults (Hamer et al., 2010). Recent analyses of 1995, 1996, and 2001 survey data in England found a significant relationship between exposure to passive smoking and increasing risk of chronic obstructive pulmonary disease (COPD), such as emphysema (Jordan et al., 2012). Similarly, the risk of clogged arteries from secondhand smoke is greater than that from other heart disease risk factors, such as high cholesterol, diabetes, or hypertension (Hecht et al., 2013).

In 2011 the first global assessment published data from 2004 across 192 countries and concluded that secondhand smoke accounted for about 1 percent, or about 603,000 deaths worldwide. This included about 281,000 women; women are at least 50 percent more likely to be exposed to secondhand smoke than men (Öberg et al., 2011). Of particular concern, 165,000 children were estimated to have died from smoke-related respiratory infections, mostly in Southeast Asia and Africa. Children whose parents smoke had a higher risk of sudden infant death syndrome, ear infections, pneumonia, bronchitis, and asthma. Data from the National Health and Nutrition Examination Surveys from 2003 through 2010 of children ages 6 to 19 who had been diagnosed with asthma showed that 53 percent had cotinine in their blood. Smoke exposure increased doctor visits, disturbed sleep, and impaired physical activity (Akinbami et al., 2012). Prenatal exposure has also been found to increase subsequent psychiatric problems in offspring of smokers (Ekblad et al., 2010). Unfortunately, more than two-thirds of parents who smoke did not have a no-smoking policy in their cars, although 57 percent of smoking parents had such a policy in the home (Nabi-Burza et al., 2012). There is even evidence that children who are exposed to secondhand smoke are more likely to start smoking themselves than children who are not exposed to passive smoke (Doweicko, 2012).

Effects During Pregnancy

Cigarette smoking produces a two- to threefold increase in being small for gestational age (SGA) or being born preterm (McCowan et al., 2009). Even women exposed to passive smoke inhalation have low-birth-weight children. In fact, when a smoking ban was introduced in northern Belgium, gradually over successive years (2006, 2007, and 2010), there was a statistical decrease in the rate of preterm births. The rate dropped the most during the last phases, when smoking was banned in restaurants and in bars selling food (Cox et al., 2013).

These risks can be reversed if smoking is stopped early in pregnancy. Also, the weight of a smoker's SGA offspring usually becomes normal at about 18 months of age.

Cigarette smoking reduces oxygen delivery to the developing fetus, causing a variable degree of fetal hypoxia. This condition may underlie the reported increases in irritability and increased muscle tone in the neonate (Stroud et al., 2009) and even longer-term intellectual and physical deficiencies (Abbott and Winzer-Serhan, 2012).

Smoking cessation programs designed to reduce smoking behaviors and nicotine dependence during pregnancy offer special challenges (Oncken and Kranzler, 2009), because the safety of pharmacological interventions (bupropion, nicotine replacement therapies, varenicline) has not been established. Therefore, psychosocial interventions should likely be the first treatment option for pregnant smokers.

Pharmacological Therapies for Nicotine Dependence

Nicotine Replacement Therapies

As noted above, while most smokers say they want to quit, only a small percent are successful. Nevertheless, even minimal interventions, such as having their doctor ask about their willingness to quit (or asking them not to start smoking in the first place, Patnode et al., 2013) will increase the likelihood of successful cessation, or will reduce initiation of smoking. One nonpharmacological approach to help patients quit smoking has been called the Five "As": Ask, Advise, Assess, Assist, and Arrange (Rigotti, 2002). Moreover, it does not matter whether cessation occurs by a gradual reduction in the number of cigarettes smoked, or by quitting abruptly with no prior decrease, the quit rates are the same (Lindson-Hawley et al., 2012).

However, as nicotine dependence gradually became recognized during the 1990s, a variety of pharmacological treatments were developed to "reduce the harm" of smoking, with the presumed goal of promoting cessation. These are sometimes referred to as PREPs, potentially reduced exposure products, developed as a means of tobacco harm reduction (THR).

These products can be divided into two categories. The first consists of *nicotine replacement therapies* (NRTs). These products are available in different flavors, which the FDA prohibits in regular cigarettes. NRTs include nicotine-containing gum, lozenges, transdermal patches, nasal sprays, inhalers, dissolvable tobacco (fine-grained tobacco formed into pellets, strips, or toothpick-size "sticks" that dissolve in the mouth), mouth spray (Hansson et al., 2012), and sublingual products, referred to as "snus." Snus consist of moist powdered tobacco sold as small mesh pouches, which are placed behind the upper lip, not chewed, and held in the mouth for about 30 minutes, then discarded. The amount of tobacco delivered is comparable to what is absorbed from smoking cigarettes. While the use of oral tobacco in general is linked to cancers of the mouth, head, and neck, the data so far do not show an excess of oral or lung cancer in snus users. (Nonmalignant oral lesions and dental caries are caused by snus, but disappear when use stops; Foulds et al., 2003.) However, there is increasing evidence that snus are a risk factor for pancreatic cancer (Luo et al., 2007). Evidence shows that the increase in the use of snus in Sweden was associated with a decrease in cigarette smoking and an overall reduction in tobacco-caused illness (Foulds et al., 2003).

Perhaps the most controversial product in the PREP category is the electronic (e) cigarette (EC). Invented only 20 years ago, in 1993, by a Chinese pharmacist, Hon Lik, and patented in 2003, the EC is rapidly gaining attention. More than twice as many adult smokers used them in 2011 (about 21 percent) as in 2010 (King et al., 2013). The e-cigarette has no tobacco. Instead, users add drops of liquid nicotine to the battery-powered device, which delivers a propylene glycol/nicotine vapor that is inhaled. This formulation seems to be more appealing to smokers than other NRTs; ECs are cheaper, and may allow for more precise nicotine control. Because ECs contain no tobacco, until recently the Food and Drug Administration (FDA) did not regulate them. A court decision changed that and the FDA expects soon to propose regulation of ECs under the Family Smoking Prevention and Tobacco Control Act (2009).

Laboratory studies suggest that e-cigarettes may be safer than tobacco products because they essentially do not contain nonnicotinic toxic substances and they do not produce secondhand smoke. ECs also have the advantage of providing the behavioral stimuli that is often conditioned to smoking—the physical act of holding a cigarette, and inhaling and exhaling a vapor. However, the presence of diethylene glycol, a toxic chemical found in antifreeze, raises safety concerns. Users can also modify the apparatus to produce more vapor, increase the amount of nicotine, or add other ingredients besides nicotine. Currently, there is a wide variation in the amount of nicotine, even in different samples of the same product. Most important, even if quality control is improved, the question is whether the EC will be used as an effective method of smoking cessation, or a more socially acceptable means of getting more people addicted (or a way to add more nicotine to current smoking). Initial studies show that even when the amount of nicotine delivered is low, ECs can reduce the craving for cigarettes, and may motivate quitting, but more research on this issue is needed (Odum et al., 2012; Wagener et al., 2012).

The objective of NRTs is to replace smoking cigarettes as a source of the nicotine with one of the approved alternatives. Then the dose of nicotine in the replacement product can be slowly reduced and ultimately eliminated. Nicotine gum, patches, and lozenges are currently available over the counter (OTC), which usually makes them the first choice of smokers who want to quit; inhalers, sprays, and other cessation medications require a prescription. Plasma nicotine levels of the patch, a cigarette, gum, and nasal spray are shown in Figure 6.6. It is important to avoid smoking while using NRTs, and

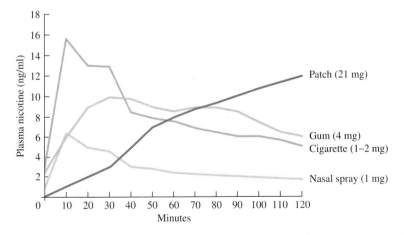

FIGURE 6.6 Plasma nicotine levels after a smoker has smoked a cigarette, received nicotine nasal spray, begun chewing nicotine gum, or applied a nicotine patch. The amount of nicotine in each product is shown in parentheses. The pattern produced by use of a nicotine inhaler (not shown) is similar to that for nicotine gum. [Data from Rigotti, 2002, Figure 2, p. 510.]

psychological counseling in conjunction can be useful. Burghardt and Ellingrod (2012) describe clinical applications for the therapeutic use of NRTs.

The second category of medications used for smoking cessation consists of drugs not considered to be NRTs, although they may act on the nicotinic receptor. Currently, these include antidepressants, primarily bupropion (Zyban), *partial nicotine receptor agonists,* such as varenicline (trade name Chantix), dianicline and cytosine (trade name Tabex), and tobacco vaccines.

In their review, Hughes and coworkers (2007) concluded that the antidepressants bupropion (Wellbutrin, Zyban) and nortriptyline (Pamelor) double a person's chances of giving up smoking and have an acceptable rate of side effects. SSRI antidepressants such as fluoxetine (Prozac) are not effective. Of the two, bupropion is the most studied and most widely used. Bupropion delays smoking relapse and also results in less weight gain. Interestingly, bupropion and nortriptyline appear to work equally well in both depressed and nondepressed smokers; this suggests that these drugs help smokers quit in some way other than through their action as antidepressants. Because low concentrations of bupropion may act as an antagonist at a certain subtype of nicotinic receptor, this pharmacological property may contribute to the smoking cessation effect (Slemmer et al., 2000).

Partial Nicotinic Agonists

In late 2006, a new approach to treating nicotine dependence was introduced. Varenicline (Chantix; Figure 6.7 and Figure 6.8) (Jorenby et al., 2006) and two other drugs, cytisine (West et al., 2011) and dianicline (Tonstad et al., 2011) are pharmacologically classified as *partial nicotine receptor agonists.* By partially stimulating the receptor they reduce withdrawal symptoms but block access of nicotine to the receptor. Continued smoking is less satisfying, and may help the person to quit and maintain abstinence. Because nicotine indirectly induces the release of dopamine (which produces its stimulant and reinforcing action), these drugs also enable a low-level release of dopamine (Zierler-Brown and Kyle, 2007).

Although initial reports were positive, subsequent outcomes were less impressive. Dianicline was not very effective in promoting abstinence and is no longer under development. Cytisine is an unusual compound (West et al., 2011). It is extracted from the seeds

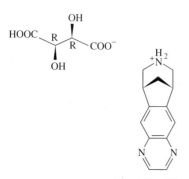

Varenicline (Chantix)

FIGURE 6.7   Structure of varenicline, illustrated as the commercially available tartrate salt Chantix.

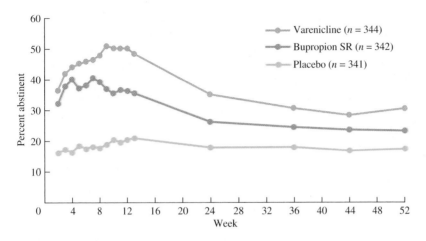

FIGURE 6.8   Percentage of smokers maintaining abstinence over a 52-week period of treatment with varenicline (1 milligram twice daily), bupropion-SR, (150 milligrams twice daily), or placebo. [Data from Jorenby et al., 2006, Figure 3, p. 60.]

of Cytisus laborinum (Golden Rain acacia), was first marketed in Bulgaria in 1964, and has been available in former socialist countries for over 40 years (brand name Tabex); it is not available in the United States. Cytisine results were very modest. In one clinical trial, 8.4 percent of cytosine and 2.4 percent of placebo patients were abstinent after 12 months.

Most information about these products comes from studies of varenicline. According to one comparison, varenicline increases the chances of long-term smoking cessation by two to three times, when compared with no other medication, and more patients quit successfully with varenicline than bupropion (Figure 6.8; Garrison and Dugan, 2009; Cahill et al., 2012). However, varenicline is not more effective than NRT (Prochazka and Caverly, 2012). And, unlike with bupropion, NRT is not indicated with varenicline because nicotine might overcome the partial block caused by varenicline.

Side effects include nausea and other gastrointestinal symptoms (Leung et al., 2011). While one review found a significantly increased risk of serious cardiovascular events with varenicline (Singh et al., 2011), another review did not (Prochaska and Hilton, 2012). However, in 2008, serious neuropsychiatric disturbances in mood (depression), agitation, hostility, suicidal ideation, and suicide were reported in people who had begun to use varenicline. In July 2009 the FDA required the manufacturer to add a black box warning highlighting these risks. A similar warning was required of bupropion. The next year, Moore and colleagues (2010) published 26 cases of "inexplicable and unprovoked" aggression/violence associated with varenicline in people with no prior history of such behavior. In contrast to these reports, two large governmental studies released by the FDA concluded that smokers using varenicline were no more likely to be hospitalized for a psychiatric event than those using the nicotine patch (Meyer et al., 2013). But Moore and colleagues (2011) have argued that hospitalizations may not be a sufficient measure, and countered that, out of 3,249 case reports of suicidal behavior or depression between

1998 and 2010 that were linked to smoking cessation products, 2,925 were associated with varenicline, 229 with bupropion, and 95 with the nicotine patch. Interestingly, in one study concerning alcohol in healthy volunteers, varenicline was also found to increase dysphoria, regardless of whether the participant took the drug with alcohol or a placebo drink (Childs et al., 2012).

Concerns about side effects may be moot if varenicline turns out not to be very effective. One small group study, funded by the manufacturer, found no difference in psychological side effects between varenicline and placebo, but the rates of abstinence were low (29 percent and 18 percent for varenicline and placebo, respectively) and did not differ between the groups (Garza et al., 2011). On the other hand, some studies have provided evidence that perhaps varenicline would be more effective if given for a longer period of time (3 or 4 weeks instead of just 1 week) before attempting smoking cessation (Hajek et al., 2011; Ashare et al., 2012; Cinciripini et al., 2013). Moreover, other studies have broadened the population for which varenicline treatment might be useful: it has been reported to be effective in helping smokeless tobacco users quit (Fagerström et al., 2010) in patients with schizophrenia or schizoaffective disorder (Williams et al., 2012) and even in patients with depression (reported by the manufacturer, Pfizer, in 2012).

Unfortunately, the long-term prognosis for smoking abstinence remains poor. Alpert and colleagues (2013) found that NRT products were no better in preventing relapse, even when used in conjunction with counseling, than no treatment. These authors argue that public health policies, based on mass-media campaigns and no-smoking laws, are more effective in the long-term. Even in combination, drugs and counseling to help patients stop smoking, while doubling the odds of success relative to no intervention, still rarely exceeds a 20 percent success rate (Ong, 2012).

Vaccine Therapy

A nicotine vaccine (similar to a cocaine vaccine; see Chapter 7) is one novel approach. Nicotine itself is a nonimmunogenic molecule and must be conjugated (attached) to a carrier protein to induce antibodies. The idea is that, once bound to antibodies, nicotine cannot cross the blood-brain barrier. This reduces its rewarding effect, which should promote abstinence. However, a vaccine does not reduce the drug craving; it only blocks the drug's access to the brain.

Currently, two products, NicVAX and NIC002 (formerly NicQbeta) have been sufficiently tested. Results have been disappointing; none of the included studies detected a statistically significant difference in long-term cessation between participants receiving vaccine and those receiving placebo (Hartman-Boyce et al., 2012; Raupach et al., 2012). Essentially, only those participants who had high antibody titers had high quit rates (Figure 6.9). Nevertheless, even smokers who were not trying to quit showed a 40 percent decrease in smoking, a reported decrease in craving, and associated decreases in brain nicotine, after a short-term vaccine treatment (Esterlis et al., 2013).

It is recognized that the problem with these standard vaccines is that they directly deliver the nicotine antibodies, which only last a few weeks and must be repeatedly injected. However, a new type of vaccine has recently been developed, based on a novel mechanism. In this case, the genetic instructions for producing the antibody are incorporated into a virus, which is then programmed to imbed itself into the nucleus

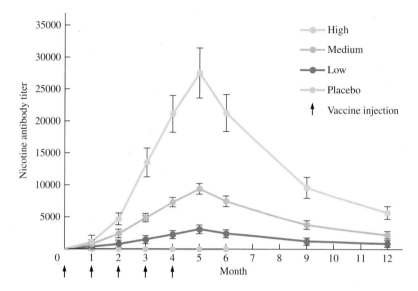

FIGURE 6.9 Antibody titers in subjects who received four injections of NicQbeta vaccine (upper three traces) in 229 persons or placebo vaccine (lowest trace) in 111 persons, administered intramuscularly at 1-month intervals. Active vaccine produced antibodies in all subjects but was clinically effective only in persons who developed high vaccine titers. Note that titers reached maximal levels about one month following the last injection and declined thereafter. [Data from Cornuz et al., 2008, Figure 3, p. e2547.]

of liver cells. The liver cells then "read" the genetic instructions and start making the antibodies. Studies in mice have shown this approach to be very effective, and development is continuing. Essentially, if it works in humans, smokers will get no pleasure from smoking (Hicks et al., 2012). Fahim and colleagues review the current status of nicotine vaccines (Fahim et al., 2013).

Other antitobacco approaches have been explored. Evidence linking a hyperactive endogenous cannabinoid system to addictions suggested that the novel cannabis receptor antagonist, surinabant, might be an effective drug for smoking cessation. However, one study found no difference between surinabant and placebo (Tonstad and Aubin, 2012).

Interestingly, some exciting results have been reported for an unusual agent. Fibrate medications (such as clobigrate or Atromid-S) are currently used to lower triglyceride levels and increase HDL (good cholesterol) levels. One recent study, conducted in laboratory animals, found that fibrate treatment prevented naïve animals from taking nicotine, decreased nicotine use in experienced animals, and protected against relapse in previously addicted animals. If fibrates have the same effect in humans, they might be an effective way to treat tobacco addiction and reduce the risk of cardiovascular disease and death from smoking. Because fibrate medications are already FDA approved for humans, clinical trials and any treatment based on this work might be quickly implemented (Panlilio et al., 2012).

One of the most unusual observations in regard to nicotine addiction was a report several years ago that some patients who were smokers, and who had experienced a stroke in a part of the brain called the insular cortex, had lost their desire to smoke. These patients were able to quit easily one day after surgery and did not have an urge to resume smoking. The involvement of this site in nicotine addiction has since been supported by experiments in rats, which have shown the phenomenon to be specific to the insular region (Pushparaj et al., 2013). Although unexpected, this accidental discovery may lead to new approaches to treating this difficult addiction.

STUDY QUESTIONS

1. Describe the mechanism of action of caffeine. How does this mechanism explain the clinical effects of the drug?

2. What are the positive and negative effects of caffeine?

3. Discuss the political, health, and economic issues related to tobacco. Should the FDA regulate nicotine as a drug? Should tobacco be banned?

4. What are the psychoactive effects of nicotine? How do they contribute to cigarette dependence?

5. Discuss the clinical uses and limitations of nicotine replacement devices. How might their efficacy be boosted?

6. Compare and contrast the pharmacotherapeutic options for smoking cessation.

REFERENCES

Abbott, L. C., and Winzer-Serhan, U. H. (2012). "Smoking During Pregnancy: Lessons Learned from Epidemiological Studies and Experimental Studies Using Animal Models." *Critical Reviews in Toxicology* 42: 279–303.

Agaku, I., et al. (2012). "Current Cigarette Smoking Among Adults—United States, 2011." *Morbidity & Mortality Weekly Report* 61: 889–894.

Akinbami, L. J., et al. (2012). "Impact of Tobacco Smoke Exposure on Children Ages 6–19 Years with Asthma in the US, 2003–2010." *Pediatric Academic Societies* Abstract 4340.2.

Alpert, H., et al. (2013). "A Prospective Cohort Study Challenging the Effectiveness of Population-Based Medical Intervention for Smoking Cessation." *Tobacco Control* 22: 32–37.

American Psychiatric Association. (2013). *Diagnostic and Statistical Manual of Mental Disorders* (5th ed.). Arlington, VA: American Psychiatric Publishing.

Arab, L., et al. (2013). "Epidemiologic Evidence of a Relationship Between Tea, Coffee, or Caffeine Consumption and Cognitive Decline." *Advances in Nutrition* 4: 115–122.

Asch, D. A., et al. (2013). "Conflicts and Compromises in Not Hiring Smokers." *New England Journal of Medicine* 368: 1369–1371.

Ashare, R. L., et al. (2012). "Effects of 21 Days of Varenicline Versus Placebo on Smoking Behaviors and Urges Among Non-Treatment Seeking Smokers." *Journal of Psychopharmacology* 26: 1383–1390.

Aubin, H. J., et al. (2012). "Weight Gain in Smokers After Quitting Cigarettes: Meta-Analysis." *British Medical Journal* 345: e4439.

Bacher, I., et al. (2011). "Monoamine Oxidase A Binding in the Prefrontal and Anterior Cingulate Cortices During Acute Withdrawal from Heavy Cigarette Smoking." *Archives of General Psychiatry* 68: 817–826.

Belsky, A., et al. (2013). "Polygenetic Risk and the Developmental Progression to Heavy, Persistent Smoking and Nicotine Dependence: Evidence from a 4-Decade Longitudinal Study." *Journal of the American Medical Association Psychiatry* 70: 534–542.

Beresniak, A., et al. (2012). "Relationships Between Black Tea Consumption and Key Health Indicators in the World: An Ecological Study." *British Medical Journal Open* 2: e000648.

Brent, R. L., et al. (2011). "Evaluation of the Reproductive and Developmental Risks of Caffeine." *Birth Defects Research (Part B)* 92: 152–187.

Britton, J., and Bogdanovica, I. (2013). "Tobacco Control Efforts in Europe." *Lancet* 381: 1588–1595.

Brockman, L. N., et al. (2012). "Hookah's New Popularity Among US College Students: A Pilot Study of the Characteristics of Hookah Smokers and Their Facebook Displays." *British Medical Journal Open* 2: e001709.

Burghardt, K., and Ellingrod, V. L. (2012). "Smoking Cessation: What to Tell Patients About Over-the-Counter Treatments." *Current Psychiatry* 11: 43–47.

Cahill, K., et al. (2012). "Nicotine Receptor Partial Agonists for Smoking Cessation." *Cochrane Database of Systematic Reviews* 4: CD006103.

Caldirola, D., et al. (2013). "Effects of Cigarette Smoking on Neuropsychological Performance in Mood Disorders: A Comparison Between Smoking and Nonsmoking Inpatients." *Journal of Clinical Psychiatry* 74: e130–e136.

Cao, C., et al. (2012). "High Blood Caffeine Levels in MCI Linked to Lack of Progression to Dementia." *Journal of Alzheimer's Disease* 30: 559–572.

CARE Study Group. (2008). "Maternal Caffeine Intake During Pregnancy and Risk of Fetal Growth Restriction: A Large Prospective Observational Study." *British Medical Journal* 337: a2332.

Chapman, S. (2012). "The Case for a Smoker's License." *PLoS Medicine* 9: e1001342.

Childs, E., and deWit, H. (2012). "Potential Mental Risks." In Yi-Fang Chu, ed., *Coffee: Emerging Health Effects and Disease Prevention*, pp. 293–306. Hoboken, NJ: John Wiley & Sons.

Childs, E., et al. (2012). "Varenicline Potentiates Alcohol-Induced Negative Subjective Responses and Offsets Impaired Eye Movements." *Alcohol and Clinical Experimental Research* 36: 906–914.

Choi, H. K., et al. (2007). "Coffee Consumption and Risk of Incident Gout in Men: A Prospective Study." *Arthritis & Rheumatism* 56: 2049–2055.

Cinciripini, P. M., et al. (2013). "Effects of Varenicline and Bupropion Sustained-Release Use Plus Intensive Smoking Cessation Counseling on Prolonged Abstinence from Smoking and on Depression, Negative Affect, and Other Symptoms of Nicotine Withdrawal." *Journal of the American Medical Association Psychiatry* 70: 522–533.

Clair, C., et al. (2013). "Association of Smoking Cessation and Weight Change with Cardiovascular Disease Among Adults with and without Diabetes." *Journal of the American Medical Association.* 309: 1014–1021.

Cornuz, J., et al. (2008). "A Vaccine Against Nicotine for Smoking Cessation: A Randomized Controlled Trial." *PLoS One* 3: e2547.

Coalition Report (2012). "A Broken Promise to Our Children: The 1998 State Tobacco Settlement 13 Years Later." Robert Wood Johnson Foundation. (http://www.issuelab.org/resource/broken _promise_to_our_children_the_1998_state_tobacco_settlement_13_years_later).

Cox, B., et al. (2013). "Impact of a Stepwise Introduction of Smoke-Free Legislation on the Rate of Preterm Births: Analysis of Routinely Collected Birth Data." *British Medical Journal* 346: f441.

Crowe, S. F., et al. (2011). "The Effect of Caffeine and Stress on Auditory Hallucinations in a Non-Clinical Sample." *Personality and Individual Differences* 50: 626

D'Elia, L., et al. (2012). "Moderate Coffee Consumption Is Associated with Lower Risk of Stroke: Meta-Analysis of Prospective Studies." *Journal of Hypertension* 30 (e-Supplement A): e107.

Doweiko, H. E. (2012). *Concepts of Chemical Dependency,* 8th ed. Belmont, CA: Brooks/Cole.

Ekblad, M., et al. (2010). "The Effect of Prenatal Smoking Exposure on Adolescents' Use of Psychiatric Drugs." *Pediatric Academic Societies,* Abstract 4401.56.

Esterlis, I., et al. (2013). "Effect of a Nicotine Vaccine on Nicotine Binding to β_2 *- Nicotinic Acetylcholine Receptors *In Vivo* in Human Tobacco Smokers." *American Journal of Psychiatry* 170: 399–407.

Fagerström, K., et al. (2010). "Stopping Smokeless Tobacco with Varenicline: Randomized Double-Blind Placebo Controlled Trial." *British Medical Journal* 341: c6549.

Fahim, R. E., et al. (2013). "Therapeutic Vaccines Against Tobacco Addiction." *Expert Review of Vaccines* 12: 333–342.

Fankhauser, M. P. (2013). "Drug Interactions with Tobacco Smoke: Implications for Patient Care." *Current Psychiatry* 12: 12–16.

Floegel, A., et al. (2012). "Coffee Consumption and Risk of Chronic Disease in the European Prospective Investigation into Cancer and Nutrition (EPIC) →Germany Study." *American Journal of Clinical Nutrition* 95: 901–908.

Foulds, J., et al. (2003). "Effect of Smokeless Tobacco (snus) on Smoking and Public Health in Sweden." *Tobacco Control* 12: 349–359.

Freedman, N. D., et al. (2012). "Association of Coffee Drinking with Total and Cause-Specific Mortality." *New England Journal of Medicine* 366: 1891–1904.

Funatogawa, I., et al. (2012). "Impacts of Early Smoking Initiation: Long-term Trends of Lung Cancer Mortality and Smoking Initiation from Repeated Cross-Sectional Surveys in Great Britain." *British Medical Journal Open* 2:e001676.

Galeone, C., et al. (2010). "Coffee and Tea Intake and Risk of Head and Neck Cancer: Pooled Analysis in the International Head and Neck Cancer Epidemiology Consortium." *Cancer Epidemiology, Biomarkers & Prevention* 19: 1723–1736.

Garrison, G. D., and Dugan, S. E. (2009). "Varenicline: A First-Line Treatment Option for Smoking Cessation." *Clinical Therapeutics* 31: 463–491.

Garza, D., et al. (2011). "A Double-Blind Randomized Placebo-Controlled Pilot Study of Neuropsychiatric Adverse Events in Abstinent Smokers Treated with Varenicline or Placebo." *Biological Psychiatry* 69: 1075.

Hajek, P., et al. (2011). "Use of Varenicline for 4 Weeks Before Quitting Smoking: Decrease in Ad Lib Smoking and Increase in Smoking Cessation Rates." *Archives of Internal Medicine* 171: 770–777.

Hakim, F., et al. (2011). "The Acute Effects of Water-Pipe Smoking on the Cardiorespiratory System." *Chest* 139: 775–781.

Hamer, M., et al. (2010). "Objectively Assessed Secondhand Smoke Exposure and Mental Health in Adults." *Archives of General Psychiatry* 67: 850–855.

Hansson, A., et al. (2012). "Effects of Nicotine Mouth Spray on Urges to Smoke, a Randomized Clinical Trial." *British Medical Journal* 2: e001618.

Hartman-Boyce, J., et al. (2012). "Nicotine Vaccines for Smoking Cessation." *Cochrane Database Systems Review* 8: CD007072.

Hecht, H. S., et al. (2013). "Secondhand Tobacco Smoke in Never Smokers Is a Significant Risk Factor for Coronary Artery Calcification." Abstract 13-A-12975-ACC.

Hicks, M. J., et al. (2012). "AAV-Directed Persistent Expression of a Gene Encoding Anti-Nicotine Antibody for Smoking Cessation." *Science Translational Medicine* 4: 140ra87.

Hilario, M. R. F., et al. (2012). "Reward Sensitization: Effects of Repeated Nicotine Exposure and Withdrawal in Mice." *Neuropsychopharmacology* 37: 2661–2670.

Hilts, D., et al. (2012). "EVP-6124, a Selective Alpha-7 Partial Agonist, Has Positive Effects on Cognition and Clinical Function in Mild to Moderate Alzheimer's Disease Patients: Results of a Six-Month, Double-Blind, Placebo Controlled, Dose Ranging Study." *Alzheimer's Association International Conference* Abstract O4-12-04.

Hopkins, M., et al. (2012). "Comprehensive Smoke-Free Laws—50 Largest U. S. Cities, 2000 and 2012." *Morbidity and Mortality Weekly Report* 61: 914–917.

Howland, J., and Rohsenow, D. H. (2013). "Risks of Energy Drinks Mixed with Alcohol." *Journal of the American Medical Association* 309: 245–246.

Hughes, J. R., et al. (2007). "Antidepressants for Smoking Cessation." *Cochrane Database of Systematic Reviews*, Issue 1, CD000031.

Husten, C. G., and Deyton, L. R. (2013). "Understanding the Tobacco Control Act: Efforts by the US Food and Drug Administration to Make Tobacco-Related Morbidity and Mortality Part of the USA's Past, Not Its Future." *Lancet* 381: 1570–1580.

Huxley, R., et al. (2009). "Coffee, Decaffeinated Coffee, and Tea Consumption in Relation to Incident Type 2 Diabetes Mellitus: A Systematic Review with Meta-Analysis." *Archives of Internal Medicine* 169: 2053–2063.

Ishak, W. W., et al. (2012). "Energy Drinks: Psychological Effects and Impact on Well-Being and Quality of Life—A Literature Review." *Innovations in Clinical Neuroscience* 9: 25–34.

Jahanfar, S., and Sharifah, H. (2009). "Effects of Restricted Caffeine Intake by Mother on Fetal, Neonatal and Pregnancy Outcome." *Cochrane Database of Systematic Reviews* 15: CD006965.

James, J. E., et al., (2011). "The Putative Neuroprotective Effects of Caffeine." *Journal of Caffeine Research* 1: 91–96.

Je, Y., et al. (2011). "A Prospective Cohort Study of Coffee Consumption and Risk of Endometrial Cancer Over a 26-Year Follow-Up." *Cancer Epidemiology Biomarkers and Prevention* 20: 1–9.

Jordan, R. E., et al. (2012). "Passive Smoking and Chronic Obstructive Pulmonary Disease: Cross-Sectional Analysis of Data from the Health Survey for England." *British Medical Journal Open* 2: e000153.

Jorenby, D. E., et al. (2006). "Efficacy of Varenicline, an $\alpha_4\beta_2$ Nicotinic Acetylcholine Receptor Partial Agonist, vs Placebo or Sustained-Release Bupropion for Smoking Cessation: A Randomized Controlled Trial." *Journal of the American Medical Association* 296: 56–63.

Kapoor, D., and Jones, T. H. (2005). "Smoking and Hormones in Health and Endocrine Disorders." *European Journal of Endocrinology* 152: 491–499.

King, B. A., et al. (2012). "Current Tobacco Use Among Adults in the United States: Findings from the National Adult Tobacco Survey." *American Journal of Public Health* 102: e93–100.

King, B. A., et al. (2013). "Awareness and Ever Use of Electronic Cigarettes Among U. S. Adults, 2010–2011." *Nicotine and Tobacco Research* PMID: 23449421.

Lambert, R. A., et al. (2006). "A Pragmatic, Unblinded, Randomized, Controlled Trial Comparing an Occupational Therapy-Led Lifestyle Approach and Routine GP Care for Panic Disorder Treatment in Primary Care." *Journal of Affective Disorders* 99: 63–71.

Larsson, S. C., and Orsini, N. (2011). "Coffee Consumption and Risk of Stroke: A Dose-Response Meta-Analysis of Prospective Studies." *American Journal of Epidemiology* 174: 993–1001.

Lembke, A., et al. (2007). "Depression and Smoking Cessation: Does the Evidence Support Psychiatric Practice?" *Neuropsychiatric Disease and Treatment* 3: 487–493.

Leonardi-Bee, J., et al. (2012). "Smoking and the Risk of Nonmelanoma Skin Cancer: Systematic Review and Meta-Analysis." *Archives of Dermatology* 148: 939–946.

Leung, L. K., et al. (2011). "Gastrointestinal Adverse Effects of Varenicline at Maintenance Dose: A Meta-Analysis." *BMC Clinical Pharmacology* 11: 15.

Levin, E. D., et al. (2006). "Nicotinic Effects on Cognitive Function: Behavioral Characterization, Pharmacological Specification, and Anatomic Localization." *Psychopharmacology* 184: 523–539.

Li, J., et al. (2011). "Coffee Consumption Modifies Risk of Estrogen-Receptor Negative Breast Cancer." *Breast Cancer Research* 13: R49.

Lindson-Hawley, N., et al. (2012). "Reduction Versus Abrupt Cessation in Smokers Who Want to Quit." Cochrane Database System Review 11:CD008033.

Liu, R., et al. (2012). "Caffeine Intake, Smoking and Risk of Parkinson Disease in Men and Women." *American Journal of Epidemiology* 175: 1200–1207.

Lucas, M., et al. (2011). "Coffee, Caffeine, and Risk of Depression Among Women." *Archives of Internal Medicine* 171: 1571–1578.

Luo, J., et al. (2007)."Oral Use of Swedish Moist Snuff (Snus) and Risk for Cancer of the Mouth, Lung, and Pancreas in Male Construction Workers: A Retrospective Cohort Study." *Lancet* 369: 2015–2020.

Mackay, J., et al. (2013). "Tobacco Control in Asia." *Lancet* 381: 1581–1587.

Magkos, F., and Kavouras, S. A. (2005). "Caffeine Use in Sports, Pharmacokinetics in Man, and Cellular Mechanisms of Action." *Critical Reviews in Food Science and Nutrition* 45: 535–562.

Malarcher, A., et al. (2011). "Quitting Smoking Among Adults—United States 2001–2010." *Morbidity and Mortality Weekly Report* 60: 1513–1519.

Matheson, E. M., et al. (2011)."Tea and Coffee Consumption and MRSA Nasal Carriage." *Annals of Family Medicine* 9: 299–304.

McClernon, F. J., et al. (2006)."Transdermal Nicotine Attenuates Depression Symptoms in Nonsmokers: A Double-Blind, Placebo-Controlled Trial." *Psychopharmacology* 189: 125–133.

McCowan, L. M. E., et al. (2009). "Spontaneous Preterm Birth and Small for Gestational Age Infants in Women Who Stop Smoking Early in Pregnancy: Prospective Cohort Study." *British Medical Journal* 338: b1081.

McKim, W. A., and Hancock, S. (2013). *Drugs and Behavior,* 7th ed. Saddle River, NJ: Pearson Prentice Hall.

Meyer, T. E., et al. (2013). "Neuropsychiatric Events in Varenicline and Nicotine Replacement Patch Users in the Military Health System." *Addiction* 108: 203–210.

Molloy, J. W., et al. (2012). "Association of Coffee and Caffeine Consumption with Fatty Liver Disease, Nonalcoholic Steatohepatitis, and Degree of Hepatic Fibrosis." *Hepatology* 55: 429–436.

Montagnana, M., et al. (2012). "Coffee Intake and Cardiovascular Disease: Virtue Does Not Take Center Stage." *Seminars in Thrombosis and Hemostasis* 38:164–177.

Moore, T. J., et al. (2010). "Thoughts and Acts of Aggression/Violence Toward Others Reported in Association with Varenicline." *The Annals of Pharmacotherapy* 44: 1389–1394.

Moore, T. J., et al. (2011). "Suicidal Behavior and Depression in Smoking Cessation Treatments." *PLoS One* 6: e27016.

Moran, V. E. (2012). "Cotinine: Beyond That Expected, More Than a Biomarker of Tobacco Consumption." *Frontiers in Pharmacology* 3: 173.

Mostofsky, E., et al. (2012). "Habitual Coffee Consumption and Risk of Heart Failure: A Dose-Response Meta-Analysis." *Circulation: Heart Failure* 5: 401–405.

Nabi-Burza, E., et al. (2012). "Parents Smoking in Their Cars with Children Present." *Pediatrics* 130: e1471–e1478

Natella, F., et al. (2007). "Coffee Drinking Induces Incorporation of Phenolic Acids Into LDL and Increases the Resistance of LDL to Ex Vivo Oxidation in Humans." *American Journal of Clinical Nutrition* 86: 604–609.

Öberg, M., et al. (2011). "Worldwide Burden of Disease from Exposure to Second-Hand Smoke: A Retrospective Analysis of Data from 192 Countries." *Lancet* 377: 139–146.

Odum, l. E., et al. (2012). "Electronic Cigarettes: Do They Have a Role in Smoking Cessation?" *Journal of Pharmacy Practice* 25: 611–614.

Oncken, C. A., and Kranzler, H. R. (2009). "What Do We Know About the Role of Pharmacotherapy for Smoking Cessation Before or During Pregnancy?" *Nicotine and Tobacco Research* 11: 1265–1273.

Ong, M. (2012). "Smoking Cessation and Alcoholism." *American College of Physicians*. The ACP Internal Medicine 2012 Conference Session: 852-276.

Panlilio, L. V., et al. (2012). "Novel Use of a Lipid-Lowering Fibrate Medication to Prevent Nicotine Reward and Relapse: Preclinical Findings." *Neuropsychopharmacology* 37: 1838–1847.

Patnode, C., et al. (2013). "Primary Care-Relevant Interventions for Tobacco Use Prevention and Cessation in Children and Adolescents: A Systematic Evidence Review for the U. S. Preventive Services Task Force." *Annals of Internal Medicine* 158: 253–260.

Persad, L. A. B. (2011). "Energy Drinks and the Neurophysiological Impact of Caffeine." *Frontiers in Neuroscience* 5: 1–8.

Pollack, A. Z., et al. (2010). "Caffeine Consumption and Miscarriage: A Prospective Cohort Study." *Fertility and Sterility* 93: 304–306.

Prochaska, J. J. (2011). "Smoking and Mental Illness—Breaking the Link." *The New England Journal of Medicine* 365: 196–198.

Prochaska, J. J., and Hilton, J. F. (2012). "Risk of Cardiovascular Serious Adverse Events Associated with Varenicline Use for Tobacco Cessation: Systematic Review and Meta-Analysis. *British Medical Journal* 344: e2856.

Prochazka, A. V., and Caverly, T. J. (2012). "Review: Varenicline Is Better Than Bupropion but Not Nicotine Patch for Smoking Abstinence in Adults." *Annals of Internal Medicine* 157: JC3–7.

Pushparaj, A., et al. (2013). "Electrical Stimulation of the Insular Region Attenuates Nicotine-Taking and Nicotine-Seeking Behaviors." *Neuropsychopharmacology* 38: 690–698.

Quik, M., et al. (2012). "Nicotine as a Potential Neuroprotective Agent for Parkinson's Disease." *Movement Disorders* 27: 947–957.

Raupach, T., et al. (2012). "Nicotine Vaccines to Assist with Smoking Cessation: Current Status of Research." *Drugs* 72: e1–16.

Ribeiro, J. A., and Sebastião, A. M. (2010). "Caffeine and Adenosine." *Journal of Alzheimer's Disease* 20: Suppl. 1: S3–15.

Rigotti, N. A. (2002). "Treatment of Tobacco Use and Dependence." *New England Journal of Medicine* 346: 506–512.

Rigotti, N. A. (2012). "Strategies to Help a Smoker Who Is Struggling to Quit." *Journal of the American Medical Association* 308: 1573–1580.

Rodgers, P. J., et al. (2010). "Association of the Anxiogenic and Alerting Effects of Caffeine with ADORA2A and ADORA1 Polymorphisms and Habitual Level of Caffeine Consumption." *Neuropsychopharmacology* 35: 1973–1983.

Salin-Pascual, R. J., et al. (1996). "Antidepressant Effect of Transdermal Nicotine Patches in Nonsmoking Patients with Major Depression." *Journal of Clinical Psychiatry* 57: 387–389.

Sandhu, R., et al. (2012). "Smoking, Smoking Cessation and Risk of Sudden Cardiac Death in Women." *Circulation: Arrhythmia and Electrophysiology* 5: 1091–1097.

Schmidt, H., et al. (2013). "The Ethics of Not Hiring Smokers." *New England Journal of Medicine* 368: 1369–1371.

Schroeder, S. A. (2013). "New Evidence That Cigarette Smoking Remains the Most Important Health Hazard." *New England Journal of Medicine* 368: 389–390.

Sengpiel, V., et al. (2013). "Maternal Caffeine Intake During Pregnancy Is Associated with Birth Weight but Not with Gestational Length: Results from a Large Prospective Observational Study." *BMC Medicine* 11: 42.

Sepkowitz, K. A. (2013). "Energy Drinks and Caffeine-Related Adverse Events." *Journal of the American Medical Association* 309: 243–244.

Sharwood, L. N., et al. (2013). "Use of Caffeinated Substances and Risk of Crashes in Long Distance Drivers of Commercial Vehicles: Case-Control Study." *British Medical Journal* 346: f1140.

Silva, C. G., et al. (2013). "Adenosine ReceptorAntagonists Including Caffeine Alter Fetal Brain Development in Mice." *Science Translational Medicine* 5: 197ra104.

Singh, S., et al. (2011). "Risk of Serious Adverse Cardiovascular Events Associated with Varenicline: A Systematic Review and Meta-Analysis." *Canadian Medical Association Journal* 183: 1359–1366.

Slemmer, J. E., et al. (2000). "Bupropion Is a Nicotinic Antagonist." *The Journal of Pharmacology and Experimental Therapeutics* 295: 321–327.

Smith, A. P., et al. (2013). "Acute Effects of Caffeine on Attention: A Comparison of Non-Consumers and Withdrawn Consumers." *Journal of Psychopharmacology* 27: 77–83.

Song, F., et al. (2012). "Increased Caffeine Intake Is Associated with Reduced Risk of Basal Cell Carcinoma of the Skin." *Cancer Research* 72: 3282–3289.

Stroud, L. R., et al. (2009). "Maternal Smoking During Pregnancy and Neonatal Behavior: A Large-Scale Community Study." *Pediatrics* 123: e842–e848.

Szpak, A., and Allen, D. (2012). "A Case of Acute Suicidality Following Excessive Caffeine Intake." *Journal of Psychopharmacology* 26: 1502–1510.

Teo, K. K., et al. (2006). "Tobacco Use and Risk of Myocardial Infarction in 52 Countries in the INTERHEART Study: A Case-Controlled Study." *Lancet* 368: 642–658.

Toblin, R. L., et al. (2012). "Energy Drink Consumption and Its Association with Sleep Problems Among U.S. Service Members on a Combat Deployment—Afghanistan, 2010." *Morbidity and Mortality Weekly Report* 61: 895–898.

Tonstad, S., et al. (2011). "Dianicline, a Novel $\alpha_4\beta_2$ Nicotinic Acetylcholine Receptor Partial Agonist, for Smoking Cessation: A Randomized Placebo-Controlled Clinical Trial." *Nicotine Tobacco Research* 13: 1–6.

Tonstad, S., and Aubin, H.-J. (2012). "Efficacy of a Dose Range of Surinabant, a Cannabinoid Receptor Blocker, for Smoking Cessation: A Randomized Controlled Clinical Trial." *Journal of Psychopharmacology* 26: 1003–1009.

Torpy, J. M., and Livingston, P. H. (2013). "Energy Drinks." *Journal of the American Medical Association* 309: 297.

Turati, F., et al. (2011). "Coffee and Cancers of the Upper Digestive and Respiratory Tracts: Meta-Analyses of Observational Studies." *Annals of Oncology* 22: 536–544.

Tynan, M. A., et al. (2012). "Consumption of Cigarettes and Combustible Tobacco—United States, 2000–2011." *Morbidity and Mortality Weekly Report* 61: 565–569.

U.S. Department of Health and Human Services. (1986). "The Health Consequences of Involuntary Smoking: A Report of the Surgeon General." Centers for Disease Control and Prevention, Office of Smoking and Health. U.S. Government Printing Office. www.cdc.gov/tobacco.

U.S. Department of Health and Human Services. (1988). "The Health Consequences of Smoking—Nicotine Addiction: A Report of the Surgeon General." Centers for Disease Control and Prevention, Office of Smoking and Health. U.S. Government Printing Office. www.cdc.gov/tobacco.

U.S. Department of Health and Human Services. (2006). "The Health Consequences of Involuntary Exposure to Tobacco Smoke: A Report of the Surgeon General." Centers for Disease Control and Prevention, Office of Smoking and Health. U.S. Government Printing Office. www.cdc.gov/tobacco.

U.S. Department of Health and Human Services. (2012). "Preventing Tobacco Use Among Youth and Young Adults: A Report of the Surgeon General." Centers for Disease Control and Prevention, Office of Smoking and Health. U.S. Government Printing Office. www.cdc.gov/tobacco.

Vinson, J. A., et al. (2012). "Randomized Double-Blind Placebo-Controlled Crossover Study to Evaluate the Efficacy and Safety of a Green Coffee Bean Extract in Overweight Subjects." Program and Abstracts of the 243rd American Chemical Society National Meeting and Exposition; March 25–29, 2012; San Diego, California. Abstract 92.

Wagener, T. L., et al. (2012). "Electronic Cigarettes: Achieving a Balanced Perspective." *Addiction* 107: 1545–1555.

West, R., et al. (2011). "Placebo-Controlled Trial of Cytisine for Smoking Cessation." *The New England Journal of Medicine* 365: 1193–1200.

Whitley, E., et al. (2012). "Association of Cigarette Smoking from Adolescence to Middle-Age with Later Total and Cardiovascular Disease Mortality: The Harvard Alumni Health Study." *Journal of the American College of Cardiology* 60: 1839–1840.

Williams, J. M., et al. (2012). "A Randomized, Double-Blind, Placebo-Controlled Study Evaluating the Safety and Efficacy of Varenicline for Smoking Cessation in Patients with Schizophrenia or Schizoaffective Disorder." *Journal of Clinical Psychiatry* 73: 654–660.

Wilson, K. M., et al. (2011). "Coffee Consumption and Prostate Cancer Risk and Progression in the Health Professionals Follow-up Study." *Journal of the National Cancer Institute* 103: 876–884.

Wright, G. A., et al. (2013). "Caffeine in Floral Nectar Enhances a Pollinator's Memory of Reward." 339: 1202–1204.

Wu, J. N., et al. (2009). "Coffee Consumption and Risk of Coronary Heart Diseases: A Meta-Analysis of 21 Prospective Cohort Studies." *International Journal of Cardiology* 137: 216–225.

Zierler-Brown, S. L., and Kyle, J. A. (2007). "Oral Varenicline for Smoking Cessation." *Annals of Pharmacotherapy* 41: 95–99.

Chapter 7

Cocaine, the Amphetamines, and Other Psychostimulants

The psychostimulants are drugs that exert their behavioral effects by augmenting the action of the monoamine (biogenic amine) neurotransmitters, the most important of which is dopamine. Sometimes these drugs are referred to as sympathomimetics, because they activate the transmitters that stimulate the sympathetic nervous system and mimic sympathetic arousal.

In addition to cocaine and amphetamines (including methamphetamine), the psychostimulants include the naturally occurring plant products, such as ephedrine and cathinone, as well as the synthetic drugs methylphenidate and modafinil (and its active isomer, armodafinil). Although these latter substances have approved medical uses, this chapter primarily concerns their recreational use as drugs of abuse.

COCAINE

History

Cocaine is derived from the leaves of the *Erythroxylon coca* plant, grown in the high altitude of the Peruvian and Bolivian Andes of South America. It has been suggested that this substance may have arisen naturally because it is toxic to insects that eat the leaves of the plant, and therefore protects it from damage. Nevertheless, at least 5,000 years ago, humans discovered the psychoactive properties of the plant, and its ability to reduce fatigue, thirst, and hunger was appreciated for many centuries by the indigenous Indian population. In fact, the practice of chewing the leaves or brewing a tea from the leaves persists today. When chewed, the leaves are usually mixed with lime (often from sea shells), which interacts with saliva to release the cocaine and reduce its bitter taste, resulting in a daily dose of about 200 milligrams. When the Incas conquered the region in about the tenth century, they adopted it as a sacred substance, restricted to the priests and nobility for special ceremonies. When the Spanish conquered the Incas in the sixteenth century, they initially banned coca use, but then realized how useful it was as a form of money and as a way of increasing the productivity of the native workers.

The Spanish sent samples of the plant to Europe, where eventually Carl Linnaeus classified it in its own family (Erythroxylaceae), and the most important species was named *Erythroxylon coca* by Jean-Baptise Lamarck. However, the Europeans were unaware of the psychoactive properties of the plant, perhaps because its potency deteriorated during the long trip from South America to Europe. It was not until 1857 (or 1859) that the compound was isolated and named cocaine by the chemist Albert Nieman, who noted its anesthetic effect on his tongue.

Cocaine soon became very popular as an additive to drinks and elixirs, most famously when added to wine by Angelo Mariani in 1863. This product, Vin Mariani, was extremely successful and was endorsed by a long list of celebrities including presidents, kings, and even the Pope. In the United States, a Georgia pharmacist, John Pemberton, developed a similar product called "French Wine of Cola, Ideal Tonic." However, when the city of Atlanta prohibited alcohol he changed the formulation, removing alcohol, adding soda water, and combining the coca (about 60 milligrams in 8 ounces) with syrup of the kola nut, containing 2 percent caffeine. This drink, named Coca-Cola, was promoted as a health drink, and is one reason why soda fountains in the United States were located in drug stores, that is, with other medicinal products.

At the same time, the introduction of the syringe and hypodermic needle prompted many attempts to use cocaine to produce local anesthesia for surgery. Perhaps the first medical report of cocaine's local anesthetic action was made in 1880,[1] and cocaine became widely used for topical anesthesia, spinal anesthesia, and nerve blocks from about 1884 until about 1918, when procaine (Novocaine) was developed as the first synthetic local anesthetic. Procaine is devoid of psychological and dependence-producing effects.

In 1884, Sigmund Freud advocated the use of cocaine to treat depression and to alleviate chronic fatigue. He described cocaine as a marvelous drug with the ability even to cure opioid (morphine and heroin) addiction. While using cocaine to relieve his own depression, Freud described the drug as inducing exhilaration and lasting euphoria that was no different from the normal euphoria of the healthy person. Unfortunately, he did not immediately perceive its side effects—tolerance, dependence, a state of psychosis, and withdrawal depression. But eventually, in his later writings, Freud called cocaine the "third scourge" of humanity, after alcohol and heroin.

Around the end of the nineteenth century in the United States there were no restrictions on the sale or consumption of cocaine and it became popular with writers and other artists. Robert Louis Stevenson is said to have conceived of Dr. Jekyll and Mr.

---

[1] At that time, no other anesthetics (general or local) had been discovered. Surgery was limited to brief procedures conducted without anesthetic or with the patient under alcohol intoxication.

Hyde with cocaine in mind, and some of the behavioral effects of the drug were exhibited by Sir Arthur Conan Doyle's character Sherlock Holmes, under the supervision of his companion, Dr. Watson. In the late 1800s, however, concern about cocaine's toxicities increased, with several hundred reports of cocaine intoxication and several reported deaths. About 1910, President Taft proclaimed cocaine to be "Public Enemy Number One", and in 1914 the Harrison Narcotic Act banned the incorporation of cocaine into patent medicines and beverages. With enforcement of the Narcotic Act, cocaine use decreased during the 1930s, largely replaced by the newly available amphetamines, which were cheaper and produced longer-lasting yet similar effects. Cocaine all but disappeared until the late 1960s, when tight federal restrictions on their distribution raised the cost of amphetamines, once again making cocaine attractive.

In the 1980s, a new epidemic of cocaine use began with the widespread availability of crack cocaine, intended for use by inhalation (smoking) rather than injection. This cocaine epidemic continues today, although the relatively inexpensive and widely available methamphetamine is currently more commonly encountered. With the increased availability of lower-cost methamphetamine, the number of cocaine users has stabilized (Doweicko, 2012; Levinthal, 2012; McKim and Hancock, 2013).

Forms of Cocaine

The leaf of *E. coca* contains about 1 percent cocaine. When the leaves are soaked and mashed, cocaine is extracted in the form of coca paste (60 percent to 80 percent cocaine). Coca paste is usually treated with hydrochloric acid to form the less potent, water-soluble salt *cocaine hydrochloride* before it is exported. The powdered hydrochloride salt can be absorbed through the nasal mucosa (snorted, i. e., by nasal insufflation) and, because this salt form is water soluble, it can be injected intravenously. However, in the hydrochloride form, cocaine decomposes when it is heated and is destroyed at the temperature of smoke, making it unsuitable for use by inhalation. In contrast, cocaine base, also known as *freebase* or *crack cocaine*, is insoluble in water but is soluble in alcohol, acetone, or ether. Heating the freebase converts cocaine to a stable vapor that can be inhaled, but this process can be dangerous and there is considerable risk of fire or an explosion. However, when cocaine freebase is smoked, the drug may reach the brain within less than 10 seconds, with as much as 60 percent to 90 percent reaching the general circulation. Because of this very potent, addictive characteristic, it was appreciated that it might be very profitable to offer a safer smokeable form of cocaine. This product, called "crack," is essentially cocaine base that is prepared for smoking before it is sold to the user. In illicit factories, cocaine hydrochloride is mixed with baking soda and water and heated until cocaine crystals precipitate. The name *crack* is derived from the sound of the crystals popping when smoked. (Interestingly, this is a variant of the method used by the Incas. By mixing the coca leaves with lime, they made saliva more basic, which enhanced absorption.)

Cocaine hydrochloride ("crystal" or "snow"), when snorted as a line of drug, provides a dose of about 25 milligrams; a user might sniff about 50 to 100 milligrams of drug at a time. The smoking of crack cocaine yields average doses in the range of 250 milligrams to 1 gram (Table 7.1).

TABLE 7.1 Pharmacokinetics of cocaine administration

Administration		Initial onset of action (sec)	Duration of "high" (min)	Average acute dose (mg)	Peak plasma levels (ng/ml)	Purity (%)	Bioavailability (% absorbed)
Route	Mode						
Oral	Coca leaf chewing	300–600	45–90	20–50	150	0.5–1	25
Oral	Cocaine HCl	600–1800		100–200	150–200	20–80	20–30
Intranasal	Snorting cocaine HCl	120–180	30–45	5–30	150	20–80	20–30
Intravenous	Cocaine HCl	30–45	10–20	25–50	300–400	10–100	100
				>200	1000–1500		
Smoking	Coca paste	8–10	5–10	60–250	300–800	40–85	6–32
	Free base	8–10	5–10	250–1000	800–900	90–100	6–32
	Crack	8–10	5–10	250–1000	?	50–95	6–32

From M. S. Gold, "Cocaine (and Crack): Clinical Aspects," in J. H. Lowinson, P. Ruiz, R. B. Millman, and J. G. Langrod, eds., *Substance Abuse: A Comprehensive Textbook,* 3rd ed. (Baltimore: Williams & Wilkins, 1997), p. 185.

Pharmacokinetics

Absorption

Cocaine is absorbed from all sites of application, including mucous membranes, the stomach, and the lungs. Table 7.1 presents some pharmacokinetic data for common methods of administration. Cocaine hydrochloride crosses the mucosal membranes poorly because the drug is a potent vasoconstrictor (one of its defining pharmacological actions), constricting blood vessels and limiting its own absorption. In addition, anywhere from 70 to 80 percent of the amount absorbed may be biotransformed by the liver before it reaches the brain. As a consequence, only about 20 to 30 percent of the snorted drug is absorbed through the nasal mucosa into blood. When cocaine base is vaporized and smoked absorption is rapid and quite complete; effects begin within seconds and peak at 5 minutes. Intravenous injection of cocaine hydrochloride bypasses all the barriers to absorption, placing the total dose of drug immediately into the bloodstream. The 30- to 60-second delay in onset of action simply reflects the time it takes the drug to travel from the site of injection through the pulmonary circulation and into the brain.

Distribution

Cocaine penetrates the brain rapidly; initial brain concentrations far exceed the concentrations in plasma. After it penetrates the brain, cocaine is rapidly redistributed to other tissues. Cocaine freely crosses the placental barrier, achieving levels in the fetus equal to those in the mother.

Metabolism and Excretion

Cocaine has a biological half-life in plasma of only about 50 minutes; enzymes located both in plasma and in the liver rapidly and almost completely metabolize it. Butyrylcholinesterase is the major enzyme for metabolizing cocaine in humans. Although cocaine is rapidly removed from plasma, it is more slowly removed from the brain, in which it can be detected for 8 or more hours after initial use. Urine can test positive for cocaine for up to 12 hours. The major metabolite of cocaine is the inactive compound *benzoylecgonine* (BE) (see Figure 7.1), which can be detected in the urine for about 48 hours and much longer (up to 2 weeks) in chronic users, and forms the primary basis of drug testing for cocaine use. The persistence of BE in urine implies that high-dose, long-term users might accumulate drug in their body tissues. Cocaine and BE can also be detected in hair for several months; hair closest to the scalp took 3 to 4 months to become negative (Garcia-Bournissen et al., 2009).

There is an important metabolic interaction between cocaine and ethanol. In people who use cocaine and concurrently drink alcohol, the liver enzymes that metabolize the two drugs produce a unique ethyl ester of benzoylecgonine. This metabolite (called *cocaethylene*) (see Figure 7.1) is pharmacologically as active as cocaine in blocking the presynaptic dopamine reuptake transporter (see below), potentiating the euphoric effect of cocaine, increasing the risk of dual dependency, and increasing the severity of withdrawal with chronic use (Bunney et al., 2001). Cocaethylene is actually more toxic than cocaine, as it is a potent calcium channel blocker in the heart, and exacerbates cocaine's toxicity (Farooq et al., 2009). The half-life of cocaethylene is about 150 minutes, outlasting cocaine in the body.

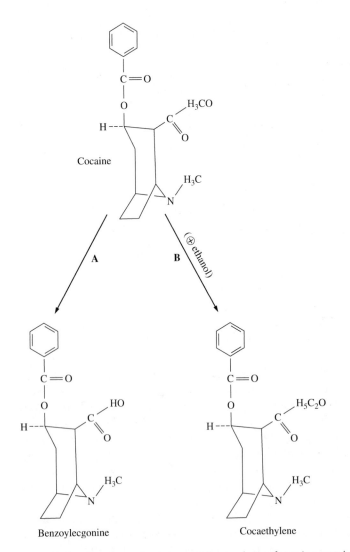

FIGURE 7.1 Structures of cocaine and the products of cocaine metabolism.
A. Normal metabolism to benzoylecognine. **B.** Metabolism to the abnormal, active metabolite cocaethylene, formed from the interaction between cocaine and alcohol. Cocaethylene is the ethyl ester of benzoylecognine.

Mechanism of Action

> ### Did You Know?
>
> #### Skin Reactions to Adulterated Cocaine
>
> The U.S. Department of Justice has reported that up to 70 percent of cocaine in the United States is contaminated with the drug levamisole, which is cheap, widely available, and commonly used for deworming livestock. Levamisole had been prescribed for humans in the past but was discontinued after patients developed side effects similar to those found in the cocaine users. There are recent reports of patients who developed purple-colored patches of necrotic skin on their ears, nose, cheeks, and other parts of their body and, in some instances, suffered permanent scarring after they had used cocaine. Twenty-three cases were recently described, with symptoms of fever, body aches, and sore throats, in addition to necrotic lesions (Vagi et al., 2013).
>
>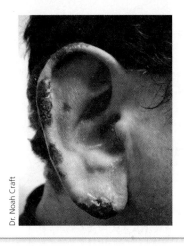
>
> Dr. Noah Craft

Pharmacologically, cocaine has three prominent actions that account for virtually all its physiological and psychological effects; cocaine is the only drug that possesses these three characteristics: it is a potent *local anesthetic*; it is a *vasoconstrictor*, strongly constricting blood vessels and raising blood pressure; and it is a powerful *psychostimulant*. Its vasoconstrictive and cardiac depressant actions contribute to severe cardiovascular and cerebrovascular toxicities (Phillips et al., 2009), while the stimulant action is responsible for its addictive potency.

Cocaine blocks the reuptake of all the monoamine neurotransmitters, although most of its effects appear to be due to the blockade of dopamine reuptake (see Figure 7.2). Blockade of the dopamine transporter markedly increases the levels of dopamine within the synaptic cleft. Increased dopamine levels in the nucleus accumbens (NAc) and other components of the dopaminergic reward system seem to be responsible for the euphoric effects of the drug (see Chapter 4). Brain imaging studies suggest that at least 47 percent of the transporters must be blocked for cocaine to produce the "high" and that the doses of cocaine commonly abused block about 60 to 77 percent of dopamine transporters.

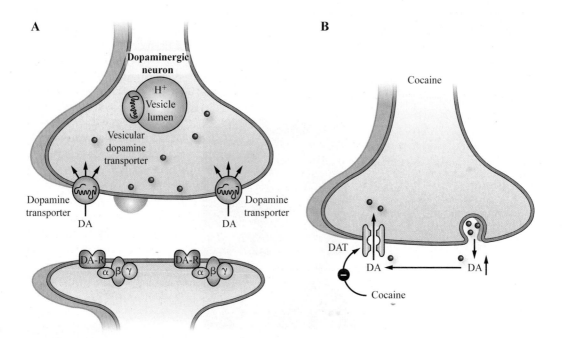

FIGURE 7.2   Dopamine nerve terminal and transporter proteins involved in the active uptake of dopamine (DA). **A.** Two transporters are shown. The first is a vesicular DA transporter (VMAT) located in the cytoplasm of the presynaptic neuron, bound to DA-containing storage vesicles. This transporter carries DA from the cytoplasm into storage. The second type of DA transporter (the DAT) is found on the synaptic membrane of the presynaptic neuron and functions to transport DA from the synaptic cleft into the presynaptic nerve terminal, recycling the transmitter and ending the process of synaptic transmission. **B.** It is the DAT that is blocked by cocaine, prolonging the action of DA in the synaptic cleft. [Adapted after Katzung et al., 2009, Figure 32-5, p. 732/e1547.]

Pharmacological Effects in Human Beings

Because the psychostimulants activate the sympathetic nervous system, they produce the characteristic physiological effects of an increased heart rate, blood pressure, vasodilation, and bronchodilation. (In fact, as discussed below, this last action was a primary reason for the development of amphetamine.) Body temperature rises, pupils dilate, blood glucose increases, and blood flow to the muscles increases. Subjective effects of low doses of cocaine (25 to 75 milligrams) include increased energy and alertness, with a decrease in fatigue, increased libido, and a general feeling of euphoria or elevation of mood. Appetite is reduced, activity increases, and sleep is prevented. If snorted, there may first be a numbing sensation (termed the *freeze*); if injected or inhaled the euphoric effect is so rapid, it is called the *rush*. The typical duration of the positive feelings may be 10 to 20 minutes, followed by a mild depression, called the *letdown*, or *comedown* (McKim and Hancock, 2013). Tolerance to the euphoric effects of cocaine develops rapidly, and this can result in continuous cycles of cocaine use, known as "coke runs," lasting for hours. Tolerance may cause the user to switch from the intranasal route to a method that provides a more intense euphoric rush, namely, inhalation or injection.

As the dose of cocaine or its duration of use increases, all the effects are intensified. Higher blood levels may elicit agitation, impulsiveness, anxiety, suspiciousness or outright paranoia, and a toxic, paranoid psychosis, which is indistinguishable from true paranoid schizophrenia. One disturbing symptom of cocaine-induced psychosis may be the sensation of bugs crawling around under the skin, a phenomenon called *formication*, from the Latin word *formica*, meaning "ant." A stereotyped, compulsive, repetitive pattern of behavior may occur (although it is more common among amphetamine users), in which the user becomes absorbed in taking apart and putting together objects, such as a bike or a computer—or in otherwise aversive activity, such as cleaning an apartment. During this behavior users may not eat or drink or even go to the bathroom, and they may become annoyed if interrupted. Associated physiological toxicity may result in cardiac arrhythmias, convulsions, strokes, and lethal cardiorespiratory arrest. A high prevalence of cardiac damage has been seen in heavy cocaine users (with an average of 12 years use and an average daily amount of 5.5 grams). Even without overt symptoms, cardiac imaging showed structural damage, fibrosis, and edema in most users, 48 hours after their last dose (Aquaro et al., 2011). Complications can occur during prolonged use or with single use. Indeed, the cardiac side effects comprise the single greatest cause of premature deaths due to cocaine (Phillips et al., 2009). According to a presentation at the meeting of the American Heart Association (Kozor et al., 2012), chronic cocaine users have an increase in aortic stiffening, higher systolic blood pressure, and greater thickness of the heart's left ventricle. The lead researcher of the study called it ". . . the perfect heart attack drug."

When the acute effects wear off, depression, dysphoria, anxiety, somnolence, and drug craving follow the CNS activation. Although using cocaine may heighten sexual interest, and high doses (injected or smoked) are sometimes described as orgasmic, cocaine is not an aphrodisiac. Sexual dysfunction is common in heavy users, because they lose interest in interpersonal and sexual interactions. Dependence on cocaine can produce brain damage. Ersche and colleagues (2011) scanned the brains of 120 people,

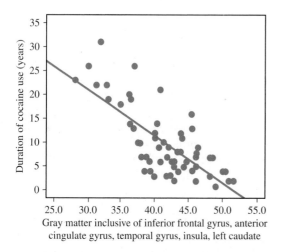

FIGURE 7.3 A graph of brain regions demonstrating a significant association between the decrease in gray matter volume and duration of cocaine use. Individuals who had been using cocaine for longer periods of time had greater extent of gray matter volume reduction in the anterior and middle cingulate gyrus, middle frontal cortex (orbital part), rectus gyrus, supplementary motor area, superior temporal gyrus, insula, cerebellum and in the left caudate ($r = -0.75$, $P < 0.001$). [Ersche et al., 2011, Figure 2, p. 2019.]

half of whom were cocaine dependent. Not only was there widespread loss of gray matter (neurons), the decrease was related to the duration of the cocaine abuse. That is, the longer they had been abusing the drug, the greater the loss of gray matter (Figure 7.3) and the volume of the reduction was associated with greater compulsion to take cocaine.

With or without alcohol, cocaine plays a role in fatal automobile crashes. The mechanisms probably involve visual deficits, alterations in judgment, incoordination, and feeling of power. Finally, in cocaine-positive emergency room patients, 24 percent of chief complaints were related to violent trauma, and an autopsy study found that the most common cause of death among cocaine-positive patients (37 percent) was violent injury (Walton et al., 2009).

An acutely toxic dose of cocaine has been estimated to be about 2 milligrams per kilogram of body weight. Thus, 150 milligrams of cocaine is a toxic one-time dose for a 150-pound (70-kilogram) person. Serious physiological toxicity follows higher doses.

Comorbidity

Cocaine-dependent people are typically young (12- to 39-years of age), male, and dependent on at least three drugs. They tend to have coexisting psychopathology (30 percent have anxiety disorders, 67 percent suffer from clinical depression, and 25 percent exhibit paranoia). Other comorbidities include bipolar disorder, antisocial personality disorder, posttraumatic stress disorder, and attention deficit/hyperactivity disorder (Kaye et al., 2013). Intravenous drug users often take cocaine and heroin together in a mixture known as a *speedball*. The heroin reduces the jitteriness and hypervigilence caused by the cocaine, while the cocaine reduces the sleepiness caused by the heroin. Probably more than half of people treated for cocaine abuse are also alcoholic, and the rate of alcoholism in the families of cocaine addicts is high.

Cocaine and Pregnancy

Cocaine rapidly crosses the placenta and a higher concentration occurs in the fetus; cocaine, benzoylecgonine, and norcocaine are stored in the uterine wall and the placental membrane and, by diffusion, provide continuous drug delivery to the amniotic fluid (De Giovanni and Marchetti, 2012). It is well established that cocaine use in pregnant women causes low birth weight, reduces intrauterine growth, and results in decreased head circumference (Gouin et al., 2011). Cocaine use during the early months of pregnancy can cause spontaneous abortion, probably due to an increase in maternal plasma norepinephrine, which increases uterine contractility, constricts placental vessels, and decreases blood flow to the fetus. It is more common with cocaine binging than with regular use. Congenital anomalies have been reported to occur in up to 40 percent of infants exposed to cocaine in utero, particularly brain malformation and cardiovascular abnormalities. Withdrawal symptoms may occur in about one-third of babies born to cocaine-using mothers. These include seizures, lethargy, hyperactive reflexes, vomiting, diarrhea, high-pitched cry, and restlessness. Such babies have a harder time feeding and are more likely to be sick in their first year of life. Prenatal cocaine exposure may impair attentiveness and emotional expressivity in offspring, producing a condition that resembles attention deficit hyperactivity disorder (Thompson et al., 2009). Although one study found that intrauterine cocaine was not a strong predictor of adolescent delinquent behaviors (Gerteis et al., 2011), another group of researchers reported that adolescents between the ages of 14 and 17 exposed to cocaine in utero, had lower gray matter volume in brain regions involved in emotion, reward, memory, and executive function compared with nonexposed adolescents. Amazingly, each 1 milliliter decrease in gray matter volume increased the probability of initiating substance use by more than 69 percent to 83 percent (Rando et al., 2013).

In addition to the direct effect of the drug, cocaine use during pregnancy is a major risk factor for infant neglect and abuse. Prenatal care is often poor, tobacco and alcohol use is prevalent, and cocaine significantly suppresses maternal appetite, which contributes to poor maternal and fetal nutrition (Keegan et al., 2010). Many negative effects of cocaine on offspring are due to psychiatric problems of the mothers, which may be mediated by depression. Cocaine-using mothers are less attentive and interactive with their infants during the first 6 months. As the number of environmental risk factors (depression, domestic abuse, psychiatric symptoms, absence of significant other) increases, a substance-abusing mother may be overwhelmed and have little time for effective parenting. High levels of cocaine use are strongly associated with failure to maintain custody of children due to neglect and/or abuse (Nephew and Febo, 2012).

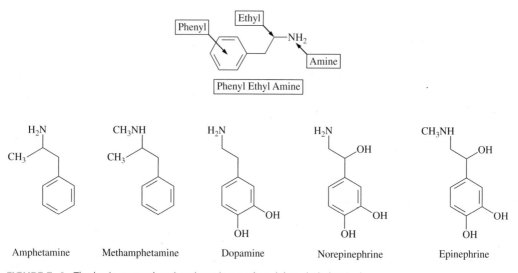

FIGURE 7. 4 The basic sympathomimetic amine nucleus (phenylethylamine), the neurotransmitters dopamine, norepinephrine and epinephrine, and the structures of amphetamine and methamphetamine.

AMPHETAMINES

Like cocaine, the amphetamines (Figure 7.4) produce a variety of sympathomimetic effects on both the CNS and the autonomic nervous system.[2] The amphetamine molecule has two isomers. The more potent one is dextroamphetamine, or d-amphetamine (Dexedrine, DextroStat); the less potent is the levo- or l-amphetamine isomer. The two isomers are combined in the medication Adderall, approved for treatment of ADHD (see Chapter 15). A modified version of d-amphetamine is formed by substituting CH_3 (called a methyl group) for the H at one end, producing methamphetamine (see Figure 7.4). This change allows the drug to cross the blood-brain barrier much faster. It is methamphetamine that is the most abused form of this drug in the last few years.

[2] The *autonomic nervous system* (ANS) is frequently called the visceral nervous system because it regulates and maintains the homeostasis of the body's internal organs. It controls the function of the heart, the flow of blood, and the functioning of the digestive tract, and it regulates other internal functions that are essential for maintaining the balance necessary for life. The ANS comprises two subdivisions—the *sympathetic* and the *parasympathetic*. The function of the parasympathetic nervous system can be viewed as maintaining our "vegetative" functions, while the sympathetic nervous system handles the body's reaction to stress, fear, and other responses that demand an immediate alerting response. Neurotransmitters in the sympathetic division of the ANS include epinephrine (adrenaline), norepinephrine, and dopamine.

History

Amphetamine was synthesized in 1887 by the Romanian chemist Lazard Edeleanu in Berlin, Germany, who named the compound phenylisopropylamine. It was one of a series of compounds related to the substance ephedrine, which itself had been isolated from the plant ma-huang that same year by Nagayoshi Nagai. However, the actions of amphetamine were not studied until 1910, when the pharmacologists Barger and Dale wrote about its effects. But, at that time there was no therapeutic use for amphetamine, therefore it was not developed further. The related compound, methamphetamine, was first synthesized from ephedrine in Japan in 1918 by the chemist Akira Ogata.

In 1924, ephedrine's structure was determined and it was found to have an effect similar to our transmitter epinephrine. Epinephrine was already being used to treat asthma, but it was short-lived and had to be injected. Ephedrine was better because it could be taken orally and was longer-lasting. However, being a natural plant product, there were concerns that supplies would run out, and there was intense effort to find an alternative.

The pioneer psychopharmacologist Gordon Alles in search of an artificial replacement for ephedrine remembered amphetamine, resynthesized it and tested it on himself and suggested amphetamine would be a cheaper alternative.

From 1933 or 1934 the pharmaceutical firm Smith, Kline and French began selling the volatile base form of amphetamine as an inhaler under the trade name Benzedrine, useful as a decongestant, particularly for treating asthma. But the ampule formulation was easily usable for nonmedical purposes and the drug began to be abused.

During World War II, the United States, Germany, and Japan gave amphetamines to their soldiers to fight battle fatigue and enhance performance. Hitler was said to be addicted to amphetamine. Between 1935 and 1946, a list of 39 conditions for which amphetamines could be used in treatment included schizophrenia, morphine addiction, tobacco smoking, head injury, radiation sickness, hypotension, seasickness, severe hiccups, and caffeine dependence. In 1935, amphetamine was found to be effective in promoting wakefulness, for the treatment of the neurological disorder of *narcolepsy*, and in 1937 it was first reported to have a "calming" effect on hyperactive children. Large-scale abuse (usually oral ingestion of amphetamine tablets) began in the late 1940s, primarily by students and truck drivers to maintain wakefulness, temporarily increase alertness, and delay sleep. In the 1960s, amphetamines were also used as diet pills and as antidepressants. However, their anorexic and antidepressant actions become tolerant within weeks, and they are no longer approved for those uses. Today, legitimate use is largely restricted to the clinical treatment of ADHD and occasionally in the treatment of narcolepsy.

In the late 1960s the abuse pattern changed with the advent of injectable forms of the drug. During the next decades there was an epidemic of abuse (especially in Japan) that saw the appearance of the "speed freak"—users who took IV doses continuously for days.

After decades of reported abuse the FDA restricted amphetamine to prescription use in 1965, but nonmedical use remained widespread. Amphetamine became a Schedule II drug under the Controlled Substances Act in 1971. Eventually the epidemic receded for several reasons. First, users saw the dangers of compulsive use, and this understanding was expressed in the phrase "speed kills." Second, at the same time, the government exerted pressure on drug companies to decrease their legal production of the drug; medical use was inhibited and unethical physicians prosecuted. Third, more effective and legal medical alternatives to depression were discovered. And fourth, cocaine reappeared. During the 1970s and 1980s more people could afford cocaine. In 1974, 5 million people said they had tried it; by 1985, 25 million people had done so. Although cocaine use began leveling off in the mid 1980s, it rose again after "crack" appeared—the smokeable version of cocaine. And then, in the mid-1990s, amphetamine abuse resurfaced, becoming even more of a scourge when the smokeable form of methamphetamine, "ice," was developed.

Pharmacokinetics of Amphetamine Compared with Cocaine

Most of the pharmacokinetic differences between cocaine and amphetamine are minor. Both are very lipid soluble and well absorbed from all sites in the body. Amphetamine has a longer duration of effect than cocaine. The half-life of cocaine is short, 30 to 90 minutes, which promotes repeated use. Enzymes in the plasma and liver rapidly and almost completely metabolize cocaine. Amphetamines' half-life is in hours. Taken repeatedly, levels will accumulate and metabolites may be active. Cocaine is less potent orally and 60 percent as potent IV as amphetamine. Cocaine is a local anesthetic but amphetamine is not.

Mechanism of Action

Similar to cocaine, amphetamine modifies the action of dopamine and norepinephrine in the brain (see Figure 7.5). However, amphetamine does this in several ways. At low doses (1) it binds to the presynaptic membrane of dopaminergic neurons and induces the release of dopamine from the nerve terminal; (2) it interacts with dopamine-containing synaptic storage vesicles, releasing free dopamine into the nerve terminal; (3) it binds to the dopamine reuptake transporter, causing it to not only block reuptake, but to act in reverse and transport free dopamine out of the nerve terminal; and (4) at high doses, amphetamine binds to monoamine oxidase (MAO) in dopaminergic neurons and prevents the degradation of dopamine, leaving free dopamine in the nerve terminal. High-dose amphetamine has a similar effect on noradrenergic neurons; it can induce the release of norepinephrine into the synaptic cleft and inhibit the norepinephrine reuptake transporter.

Pharmacological Effects

Both cocaine and amphetamine have the net effect of increasing the amount of dopamine available (although through different mechanisms), therefore cocaine abusers have difficulty distinguishing between the subjective effects of 8 to 10 milligrams of cocaine and 10 milligrams of dextroamphetamine when the doses are administered intravenously.

Pharmacological responses to amphetamines vary with the specific drug, the dose, and the route of administration. In general, with amphetamine itself, effects may be categorized as those produced by low to moderate doses (5 to 50 milligrams), usually administered orally, and those observed at high doses (more than approximately 100 milligrams) often administered intravenously. These dose ranges are not the same for all amphetamines. For example, dextroamphetamine is three to four times more potent than amphetamine; low to moderate doses range from 2.5 to 20 milligrams, while high doses are 50 milligrams or more. Amphetamine metabolites are excreted in the urine and are detectable for up to 48 hours. Methamphetamine is even more potent, although

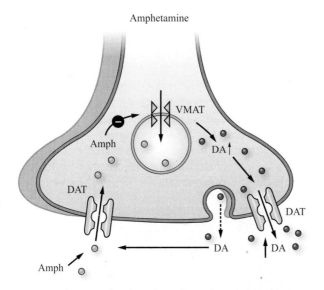

FIGURE 7.5 Mechanism of action of amphetamine on dopamine nerve terminals. Amphetamine blocks the dopamine (DA) transporter (DAT), preventing reuptake of DA. Amphetamine is also taken up into the terminal by the DAT, where it interferes with the DA transporter of the synaptic vesicles (VMAT). This depletes the vesicles, and increases DA levels in the cytoplasm of the terminal. As a result, the direction of the DAT reverses, which means more DA is released into the synaptic cleft. Not shown is an additional effect of amphetamine, a weak block of the enzyme MAO. Amphetamine also has comparable effects on the norepinephrine transporter (NET) [Adapted after Katzung, et al., 2009, Figure 32-5, p. 732/e1547.]

methamphetamine-dependent people who have developed a tolerance to the drug take massive doses.

At low doses, all amphetamines increase blood pressure and heart rate, relax bronchial muscle, and produce a variety of other actions that follow from the body's alerting response. In the CNS, amphetamine is a potent stimulant, producing alertness, euphoria, excitement, wakefulness, a reduced sense of fatigue, loss of appetite, increased mood, motor and speech activity, and a feeling of power. Interestingly, some subjective effects of amphetamine, such as "arousal" and "euphoria," are related to personality traits, such as "impulsivity" (Kirkpatrick et al., 2013). During short-duration, high-intensity activity, such as an athletic competition, performance may be enhanced despite impairment of dexterity and fine motor skills.

At moderate doses (20 to 50 milligrams), additional effects of amphetamines include stimulation of respiration, slight tremors, restlessness, and a greater increase in motor activity, insomnia, and agitation. As doses increase, this reaction is accompanied by the worsening or de novo production of anxiety disorders, possibly progressing from restlessness and nonspecific anxiety to obsessive behaviors, panic disorders, paranoia, and eventually a paranoid psychosis.

Did You Know?

Two-and-a-Half Years of Meth Abuse

One of the most striking effects of meth is the change in the physical appearance of meth users. Because meth causes the blood vessels to constrict, it cuts off the steady flow of blood to all parts of the body. Heavy usage can weaken and destroy these vessels, causing tissues to become prone to damage and inhibiting the body's ability to repair itself. Acne appears, sores take longer to heal, and the skin loses its luster and elasticity. Some users are covered in small sores, the result of obsessive skin-picking brought on by the hallucination of having bugs crawling beneath the skin, a disorder known as formication.

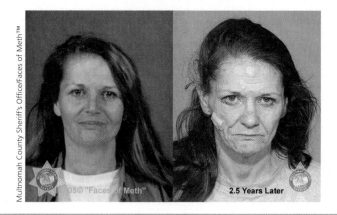

Multnomah County Sheriff's Office/Faces of Meth™

05© "Faces of Meth"   2.5 Years Later

Chronic high doses produce additional effects. Stereotypical behaviors include continual, purposeless, repetitive acts; sudden outbursts of aggression and violence; paranoid delusions; and severe anorexia. Weight loss, skin sores, infections from neglected health care, and a variety of other consequences occur both because of the drug itself and because of poor eating habits, lack of sleep, or the use of unsterile equipment for intravenous injections. Most high-dose users show a progressive deterioration in their social, personal, and occupational affairs.

The toxic dose of amphetamine varies widely. Severe reactions can occur even from low doses (20 to 30 milligrams). On the other hand, people who have not developed tolerance have survived doses of 400 to 500 milligrams. Even larger doses are tolerated by chronic users. The slogan "speed kills" refers not only to a direct fatal effect of single doses of amphetamine but also to the deteriorating mental and physical condition of the addicted user.

Methamphetamine

It has been estimated that 35 percent of methamphetamine (MA) in the United States comes from clandestine laboratories (Talbert et al., 2012). It is easily synthesized from readily obtainable chemicals, including pseudoephedrine. Methamphetamine was originally an approved drug, effective in the treatment of ADHD. Today, however, it is rarely used legitimately and has clearly demonstrated neurotoxicity.

Like cocaine hydrochloride, methamphetamine (the hydrochloride salt) is broken down at temperatures required for smoking. However, when converted to its crystalline form, MA can be effectively vaporized and inhaled in smoke, and is also known as ice, speed, crystal, crank, and go, with considerable overlap in nomenclature with other amphetamines except for "ice," which refers to the smokeable form. Thus, ice is to methamphetamine as crack is to cocaine: the crystalline, smokeable form of the parent compound. However, unlike cocaine, methamphetamine has an extremely long half-life (about 12 hours), resulting in an intense, persistent drug action.

Pharmacokinetics

Smoking ice results in its near-immediate absorption into plasma, with additional absorption continuing over the next 4 hours. The blood level then progressively declines. The biological half-life of MA is more than 11 hours. After distribution to the brain, about 60 percent of the methamphetamine is slowly metabolized in the liver, and the end products are excreted through the kidneys, along with unmetabolized MA (about 40 percent is excreted unchanged) and small amounts of its pharmacologically active metabolite, amphetamine.

Did You Know?

Meth Mouth

Users with "meth mouth" have blackened, stained, or rotting teeth, which often cannot be saved, even among young or short-term users. The exact causes of "meth mouth" are not fully understood. Various reports have attributed the decay to the corrosive effects of the chemicals found in the drug, such as anhydrous ammonia (found in fertilizers), red phosphorus (found on matchboxes), and lithium (found in batteries), which when smoked or snorted might erode the tooth's protective enamel coating; however, it is more likely that this degree of tooth decay is brought on by a combination of side effects from a meth high. The drug causes the salivary glands to dry out, which allows the mouth's acids to eat away at the tooth enamel, causing cavities. Teeth are further damaged when users obsessively grind them, binge on sugary food and drinks, and neglect to brush or floss for long periods of time.

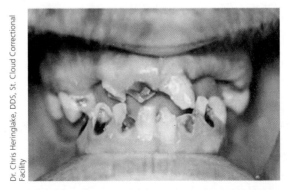

Dr. Chris Heringlake, DDS, St. Cloud Correctional Facility

Neurotoxicity

Methamphetamine produces acute delusional and psychotic behavior. Psychotic symptoms in one study were just over five times more likely to occur during episodes of methamphetamine use. The risk was dose-dependent and doubled if the addict also used marijuana or alcohol (McKetin et al., 2013).

Methamphetamine users are at risk for various types of cardiac toxicity, such as strokes, heart attack, and tears of the aorta (aortic dissection) (Westover and Nakonezny, 2010).

Neurotoxicity includes damage to serotonin and dopamine nerve terminals, neuronal death, and replacement with astroglial and microglial cells in the brain (Sekine et al., 2008; Cadet and Krasnova, 2009). Dopaminergic defects have been associated with slower motor function and memory deficits, perhaps with predisposition to future development of neurodegenerative disorders such as Parkinson's disease (Callaghan et al., 2012).

Thompson and coworkers (2004) first identified the structural defects in the human brain associated with chronic methamphetamine abuse (Figure 7.6). The authors noted an 11 percent reduction in gray matter (neurons), a 7 percent *increase* in white matter volume

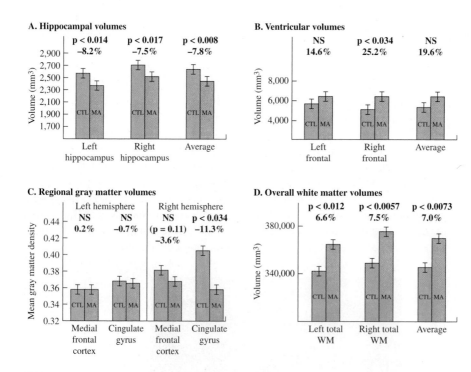

FIGURE 7.6 Comparison of brain structure volumes in methamphetamine abusers (MA) and healthy control persons (CTL). Mean values and mean percentage gains/losses (percent) are shown for the volumes of the hippocampus (**A**), ventricles (**B**), total cerebral gray matter (**C**), and white matter (**D**). In general, hippocampal and gray matter volumes decrease and are compensated for by increases in ventricle and white matter volumes. NS = nonsignificant increase/decrease. The hippocampal volume deficits correlate with word recall (memory) performance. [Modified data from Thompson et al. (2004), Figure 3, p. 6032.]

(due to inflammation), and a 20 percent increase in ventricular (fluid chamber) volumes. These data indicate neuronal loss with scar replacement (white matter) and compensatory increase in ventricle size. In brief, the limbic region, involved in drug craving, reward, mood, and emotion, lost 11 percent of its tissue. "The cells are dead and gone," Dr. Thompson stated. Addicts were depressed, anxious, and unable to concentrate. The 8 percent tissue loss in the hippocampus, the brain's center for making new memories, was comparable to the brain deficits in early Alzheimer's. The MA addicts also performed significantly worse on memory tests than healthy people of the same age. Nevertheless, whether or not abuse causes cognitive decline in humans is not certain and the evidence is mixed. Overall, most of the data argues for intellectual decline for some duration in some users (Dean et al., 2013).

The molecular basis of this neurotoxic effect includes "oxidative stress (metabolic activation), activation of genetically-based transcription factors, DNA damage, excitotoxicity, blood-brain barrier (BBB) breakdown, glial cell activation, and neuronal degeneration" (Cadet and Krasnova, 2009, p. 101). Acute and chronic methamphetamine "induces robust, widespread, but structure-specific leakage of the BBB, acute glial cell activation, and increased water content (edema), which are related to drug-induced brain hyperthermia (elevated temperature)" (Kiyatkin and Sharma, 2009, p. 65). The "leaky" BBB ultimately increases the migration of reactive oxygen molecules, such as white blood cells into the brain, initiating the neuronal damage. The increased brain temperature produced by MA potentiates these toxic effects (Kiyatkin et al., 2007; Kiyatkin and Sharma, 2012). This same action (and potential for brain injury) is also caused by methamphetamine derivatives, including MDMA (ecstasy) and 5-MeO-DiPT (Foxy) (Nakagawa and Kaneko, 2008; Gouzoulis-Mayfrank and Daumann, 2009).

Effects in Pregnancy

As with cocaine, there is no clear-cut pattern of congenital abnormalities, although infants born to MA-abusing mothers exhibit growth retardation and lower birth weights (Smith et al., 2006), and an increased rate of intracerebral hemorrhage. Sowell and colleagues (2010) reported that brain structures known to be sites of neurotoxicity in adult MA abusers are more vulnerable to prenatal MA exposure than to alcohol exposure and more severe cortical damage is associated with more severe cognitive deficits in offspring. However, although there is some empirical evidence for amphetamine-induced neurotoxicity and neurodevelopmental deficits, the data are scarce, and it is difficult to separate from the other factors of poverty, neglect, and other drug use (Oei et al., 2012; Behnke and Smith, 2013).

Good and colleagues (2010) reported on the demographic variables associated with pregnancy in methamphetamine-using mothers. Half of the users delivered their babies preterm compared to 17 percent of the control population. More of the users had C-sections, uncontrolled high blood pressure, and suffered placental abruption. The team also found that more than two-thirds of the women who had used MA reported fewer than five prenatal care visits, compared to 10 percent of the control women. Six percent of the babies of MA users had low scores on a test designed to measure newborn health, and 4 percent died soon after birth compared to 1 percent of the control group babies. Nearly a quarter of the MA-using women reported being victims of domestic violence while pregnant. Forty percent of the MA-exposed babies were taken from their mothers at least temporarily, to be adopted, placed in Child Protective Services or foster care, or cared for by another person.

The first study of behavioral effects of children born to MA-using mothers was published by LaGasse and colleagues in 2012. They found that at age 3, scores for anxiety, depression, and moodiness were slightly higher in children of MA users, with differences persisting at age 5. The older children who had been exposed to MA also had more aggression and attention problems similar to ADHD (attention deficit hyperactivity disorder). Another recent study found some subtle deficits in children, aged 5.5 years, preexposed to MA in utero, which also suggested a risk for ADHD (Kiblawi et al., 2013).

Dependence and Tolerance

Amphetamines are prone to compulsive abuse, and physical dependence is readily induced. Once drug use is stopped, a person experiences a withdrawal syndrome, although it is less dramatic than the withdrawal associated with either opioids (see Chapter 10) or barbiturates (see Chapter 13). Withdrawal symptoms associated with the amphetamines include increased appetite, weight gain, decreased energy, and increased need for sleep. Patients may develop a voracious appetite and sleep for several days after amphetamines are discontinued. Paranoid symptoms may persist but generally do not develop as a result of withdrawal. However, the patient suddenly discontinuing amphetamine use may develop severe depression and become suicidal. Management of amphetamine withdrawal does not require detoxification, but it does require appropriate and cautious clinical observation of the patient, recognition of depression, and treatment with an appropriate antidepressant drug if clinically necessary. Antipsychotic drugs (see Chapter 11) may be necessary to treat paranoid or psychotic reactions or behaviors (Shoptaw et al., 2009).

Tolerance to the euphoria rapidly develops and can necessitate higher and higher doses, which starts a vicious cycle of drug use and withdrawal. Comer and coworkers (2001) studied the effects of 5 and 10 milligrams of methamphetamine twice daily on nonusers in a controlled setting. Positive feelings toward the drug were experienced only on day 1; on subsequent days, the subjects felt a loss of positive effects and increases in negative feelings (dizziness, nausea, depression, and so on). (For a recent review of methamphetamine, see Panenka et al., 2013.)

NONAMPHETAMINE BEHAVIORAL STIMULANTS

Nonamphetamine stimulants include ephedrine (found in nature in the Chinese herb ma-huang), pseudoephedrine, the herbal substance *khat* (and related drugs such as mephedrone), DMAA, methylphenidate, pemoline, modafinil (Provigil), and armodafinil (Nuvigil).

Ephedrine today has little use in medicine other than IV use in anesthesiology as transient-release epinephrine, a normal adrenal hormone that causes elevations in blood pressure and heart rate. Ephedrine also transiently reduces appetite. Most use of ephedrine has been in herbal medicine, incorporated into herbal and dietary supplements for energy increase and weight loss. Unfortunately, the drug can be toxic or even fatal when combined with other stimulant drugs such as caffeine, and was banned in dietary supplements by the FDA in 2004. Pseudoephedrine is used in cough and cold medicines to relieve nasal congestion. However, as a compound used in the illicit manufacture of methamphetamine, it has been placed under prescription-only restriction.

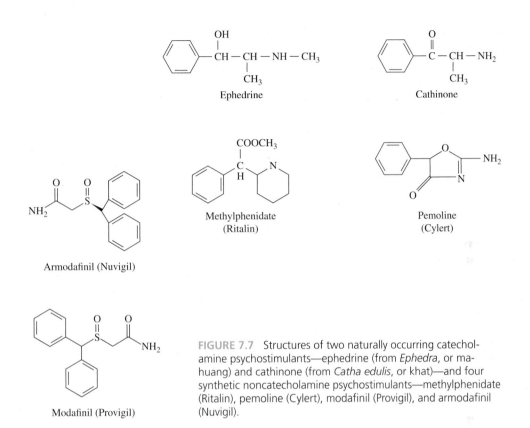

FIGURE 7.7 Structures of two naturally occurring catecholamine psychostimulants—ephedrine (from *Ephedra*, or mahuang) and cathinone (from *Catha edulis*, or khat)—and four synthetic noncatecholamine psychostimulants—methylphenidate (Ritalin), pemoline (Cylert), modafinil (Provigil), and armodafinil (Nuvigil).

Catha edulis is a flowering shrub in East Africa. The leaves and fresh shoots are commonly known as *khat*. Khat can be chewed (like loose tobacco) or brewed as a tea at a daily dose of up to several hundred grams. Khat has stimulant properties and is said to cause excitement, loss of appetite, and euphoria, similar to the effects of amphetamine or cocaine. The active components of khat are cathinone (Figure 7.7) and cathine (closely related in structure). Khat must be used fresh because cathinone, the pharmacologically more active substance, deteriorates within about 48 hours after harvest. The cathine appears to be a mild psychostimulant, comparable to caffeine in potency. Khat is being increasingly encountered as a substance of abuse in the United States and elsewhere; in 2006 there were an estimated 10 million khat users around the world (Rosenbaum et al., 2012).

Synthetic Cathinones ("Bath Salts")

The synthetic cathinones are derivatives of the naturally occurring cathinone betaketone amphetamine analogue, which is why they are sometimes referred to as "bk-amphetamines." Several are now appearing as drugs of abuse (Prosser and Nelson, 2012).

The first synthetic cathinone, methcathinone (*Methylmethcathinone*, *Mephedrone*, also known as 4-methylmethcathinone, or 4-methylephedrone), was produced in 1928, and by 1933 the League of Nations was already raising concerns about its detrimental effects. But it was not until the 1990s that outbreaks occurred globally, eventually reaching the United States around 2009 along with other synthetic cathinones such as methylone and 3,4-methylenedioxypyrovalerone (MDPV). In September of 2011, the Drug Enforcement Administration (DEA) gave notice that it intended to temporarily "schedule" these three drugs—mephedrone, methylone, and MDPV—and methylone was officially classified as a Schedule I drug on April 12, 2013. Legal regulation is difficult because each compound has to be individually banned. Because these agents are "not intended for consumption," the DEA, not the FDA, is the regulating authority (Beaman and Hayes, 2013). These drugs have all been shown to inhibit reuptake of the biogenic amines (serotonin, dopamine, and norepinephrine) and to perhaps release them as well; MDPV may have weaker effects on serotonin than mephedrone and methylone (Baumann et al., 2012). Several routes of exposure are effective, including nasal insufflation, oral ingestion, rectal insertion, and intravenous and intramuscular injection. According to user input, mephedrone and methylone doses are 100 to 200 milligrams orally; effects begin about 30 to 45 minutes after ingestion and last about 2 to 5 hours. MDPV appears more potent, with effects elicited 15 to 30 minutes after a typical oral dose of 10 to 15 milligrams and lasting 2 to 7 hours. In rodent studies, MDPV produced a state similar to MDMA (ecstasy) and MA, although its effects on motor activity and body temperature differed from those two drugs (Fantegrossi et al., 2013). MDPV blocks monoamine transport more potently and more selectively for the catecholamines (dopamine and norepinephrine) than cocaine (Baumann et al., 2013). Users report that these drugs produce sensations of euphoria, heightened alertness, increased energy, talkativeness, and increased libido (Prosser and Nelson, 2012). Medical personnel dealing with intoxicated users report bizarre behaviors similar to those caused by phencyclidine (PCP) (see Chapter 8) and there are some reports of self-mutilation, suicide attempts, and paranoid psychosis. Physical signs are consistent with sympathomimetic effects and toxicity, such as hypertension, tachycardia, hyperthermia, and dehydration. The most commonly reported adverse symptoms include palpitations, headache, chest pain, tremors, insomnia, and paranoia. Mephedrone and MDPV were detected in deaths occurring in the context of bath salt use. Tolerance and dependence have been acknowledged, with 30 percent of mephedrone users reporting tolerance, impaired control, and craving (Rosenbaum et al., 2012). More concerning, there was behavioral evidence in laboratory rats for memory loss after mephedrone use, weeks after the last dose had been given, without any obvious signs of brain damage. This is consistent with some reports of memory impairment in humans (Motbey et al., 2012). No specific antidote is available; acute treatment consists of benzodiazepine for agitation, seizures, and other reactions.

DMAA (1,3-dimethylamylamine or methylhexaneamine) is similar in structure to ephedrine and amphetamine. In 1944 it was patented by Eli Lilly and Company as a nasal decongestant called Forthane, but was withdrawn in the 1970s. In 2004, after the FDA banned the sale of the stimulant ephedra in dietary supplements (because of thousands of adverse event reports), DMAA reappeared. Supplement manufacturers claimed it was a natural component of the geranium plant, which meant the FDA had no jurisdiction. Unlike drugs, which must be proved safe and effective before they are marketed, the FDA does not "approve" supplements; the FDA can only act to ban them after they reach consumers.

In April 2012, the FDA sent letters to ten companies that manufactured and distributed 16 dietary supplements containing DMAA, stating that it is not a "dietary ingredient." DMAA can narrow blood vessels and arteries, which increases blood pressure and leads to shortness of breath, a tightening in the chest, or heart attack. The FDA said it had received 42 adverse event reports on products containing DMAA. The U.S. Army has pulled DMAA supplements from all of its on-base stores after two soldiers' deaths were linked to its use. Several lawsuits regarding DMAA have also been filed. The World Anti-Doping Agency added DMAA to its list of prohibited substances. "Adding a stimulant to someone who already has an accelerated heartbeat and is exercising can have particularly dangerous effects," said Travis Tygart, CEO of the U.S. Anti-Doping Agency. Unfortunately, all of the products listed by the FDA were still available online in May 2012 (Gregory, 2013).

Some manufacturers have removed DMAA from their products, but others have insisted that the product is a natural component of the geranium plant, and is safe when used as directed. Evidence that DMAA is found in geranium plants comes from a single Chinese study published in 1996 in a now defunct journal. But even that study did not actually "find" DMAA in geranium oil; the authors speculated that it was a component but did not do any analyses to confirm that. Since then, at least half a dozen peer-reviewed reports have been unable to confirm the finding, and Armstrong and colleagues (Zhang et al., 2012) have found no detectable DMAA in eight different geranium oils. The American Herbal Products Association now prohibits member companies from labeling DMAA or methylhexaneamine as "geranium" on product labels. And the American Botanical Council does not recognize DMAA as an herbal preparation.

Methylphenidate (Ritalin) (Figure 7.7) is a nonamphetamine behavioral stimulant in which the regular-release formulation has a half-life of 2 to 4 hours. Its primary medical use is in the treatment of ADHD (see Chapter 15). Methylphenidate increases the synaptic concentration of dopamine by blocking the presynaptic dopamine transporter (a cocainelike action) and also perhaps by slightly increasing the release of dopamine (an amphetaminelike or ephedrinelike action). When methylphenidate is injected intravenously, experienced cocaine users report a cocainelike or amphetaminelike rush, an action not usually experienced with oral dosage. At clinically relevant doses, methylphenidate blocks more than 50 percent of the dopamine transporters 60 minutes after oral administration. A slow uptake of methylphenidate into the brain after oral administration accounts for its low level of positive reinforcement effects.

Pemoline (Cylert) is a CNS stimulant structurally dissimilar to either methylphenidate or amphetamine (see Figure 7.7). Its use, for treatment of ADHD, is limited by reports of rare instances of hepatitis, necessitating close monitoring of liver function. Indeed, the risks of pemoline outweigh its usefulness and it has been removed from the market. *Modafinil* (Provigil) (see Figure 7.7) is a nonamphetamine psychostimulant whose primary characteristic is "wakefulness promotion." Its mechanism of action is not well established; it does block dopamine transporters in the human brain in a manner similar to that exerted by cocaine (Volkow et al., 2009), but perhaps less potently (Loland et al., 2012). Modafinil appears to have a lower abuse potential, although this potential should be considered in at-risk populations. A potentially serious skin rash limits its use.

The FDA has approved modafinil for treatment of three disorders: narcolepsy, shift-work sleep disorder, and obstructive sleep apnea with residual excessive sleepiness despite use of a continuous positive airway pressure (CPAP) device. Modafinil has also been used in the treatment of ADHD, although the FDA has not approved it for this use. One recent study did not find it effective for ADHD in adults (Arnold et al., 2012). Although it also had no significant cognitive effects in methamphetamine addicts, except in a test of sustained attention (Dean et al., 2011), it has been used for enhancing cognition even in the absence of a therapeutic diagnosis.[3]

Laboratory investigations of putative cognitive enhancement from modafinil in healthy volunteers have shown consistent but relatively modest benefit. However, the drug increased "motivation," in that participants described feeling more pleasure in performing the experimental tasks (Müller et al., 2013). This effect may have produced the cognitive improvement.

Armodafinil (Nuvigil) is the active (R)-isomer of the racemic drug modafinil. As with citalopram/escitalopram, methylphenidate/dexmethylphenidate, and amphetamine/dextroamphetamine, when an older racemic medicine goes generic and becomes less expensive, a manufacturer can market the active "half" of the drug under a new patent (making it more expensive). That seems to be the situation with armodafinil, making it twice as "potent" as the racemic counterpart (therefore, one uses half of the milligram dosage). Nuvigil is protected by a U.S. patent that expires in 2023. Armodafinil has the same FDA indications as modafinil (Krystal et al., 2010), which can become generic in 2012. Armodafinil is also approved for treatment of sleepiness due to jet lag, a lower dose of 50 to 150 milligrams being recommended.

Pharmacological Treatment of Stimulant Dependency

At the outset, it should be stated that there are no pharmacotherapies for cocaine addiction that have been proven or approved by the Food and Drug Administration (FDA) (Shorter and Kosten, 2011; Haile et al., 2012a). Pharmacological strategies include blocking euphoria, reducing withdrawal and negative mood symptoms (such as depression), and ameliorating craving by enhancing the prefrontal glutaminergic cortical projections that seem to be impaired in drug dependency (discussed in more detail in Chapter 4) (Elkashef and Vocci, 2011; Karila et al., 2011; Elkashef and Montoya, 2012; Olive et al., 2012).

Dopaminergic/Adrenergic Treatment Approaches

The subjective effects and euphoria of cocaine are believed to be due to blockade of the dopamine transporter and consequent buildup and release of dopamine in the reward pathways. However, even a single cocaine dose may cause an upregulation of the transporter that can last as long as a month. This means that, even after acute use, there is a decrease in dopamine molecules in the synapse, which may lead to craving and drug seeking (Zheng and Zhan, 2012a). There is also experimental evidence that low dopamine receptor function is correlated with a greater likelihood of relapse in methamphetamine

---

[3] Drugs considered to be cognitive enhancers are referred to as "neuroenhancers" or "nootropics."

abusers (Wang et al., 2012). Therefore, drugs that are either direct or indirect dopaminergic agonists might replace the drug-induced dopaminergic stimulation and reduce both craving and relapse. An extraordinary number of such drugs have been assessed, but results are not impressive. One review of clinical trials examined three direct dopamine agonists (amantadine, bromocriptine, and L-dopa/Carbidopa) and concluded that none of them were effective for the treatment of cocaine abuse or dependence (Amato et al., 2011). Another study found little benefit for the dopamine agonist, ropinirole, or the antipsychotic, partial dopamine agonist, aripiprazole (Meini et al., 2011). Aripiprazole was also ineffective for the treatment of methamphetamine dependence (Coffin et al., 2013). The antidepressant drug bupropion (Wellbutrin) acts primarily to block the uptake of dopamine, although it also has some effect on norepinephrine. It is approved, as the drug Zyban, for treatment of nicotine addiction. However, it has not shown substantial effectiveness against either cocaine (Shoptaw et al., 2008) or methamphetamine addiction (Elkashef et al., 2008; Heinzerling et al., 2013). The serotonergic antidepressants are also not very effective in this regard (Shorter and Kosten, 2011). Similarly, the sustained release formulation of methylphenidate (Ritalin), which is a well-established stimulant treatment for ADHD, has been investigated in cocaine abusers, with and without comorbid ADHD. Although it appears effective in regard to reducing ADHD symptoms, methylphenidate does not seem to be very useful against cocaine addiction (Grabowski et al., 1997; Haile et al., 2012a). In parallel with the success of "agonist replacement" treatment for nicotine and opioid addiction, amphetamine and methamphetamine have also been tested for treatment of cocaine abuse. Sustained release amphetamine and methamphetamine agents are being studied as possible "replacement" options, but, understandably, only in certain patients who would not be considered at risk for abuse and diversion (Grabowski et al., 2001; Herin et al., 2010; Mariani and Levin, 2012; Rush and Stoops, 2012). Although they might be effective under controlled environmental situations, sustained-release amphetamine and methamphetamine are clearly problematic options for widespread use. The "wakefulness-promoting" drug modafinil (Provigil) has also generated interest, especially because it was shown not to be reinforcing on its own, in cocaine abusers (Vosburg et al., 2010). Unfortunately, it was not effective in reducing either methamphetamine abuse (Anderson et al., 2012) or cocaine abuse (Dackis et al., 2012). Modafinil might be helpful in improving the sleep quality of people undergoing stimulant withdrawal (Shorter and Kosten, 2011). The fact that psychostimulants have noradrenergic effects as well as dopaminergic actions has prompted studies of adrenergic antagonists for cocaine abuse. The α-1 receptor antagonist doxazosin has a long half-life of 22 hours, and has been found to decrease positive subjective effects of cocaine in cocaine-dependent persons who have not sought treatment (Newton et al., 2012), which suggests it may have some therapeutic benefit. Finally, the drug buspirone (Buspar), a nonbenzodiazepine anxiolytic that acts on both serotonin and dopamine, was recently shown to selectively reduce responding for cocaine (but not food) in rhesus monkeys (Mello et al., 2013).

GABAergic/Glutamatergic Treatment Approaches

In addition to the dopaminergic class of possible antiaddiction medicines, the GABA system has received substantial interest. This is derived from the fact that GABA has an inhibitory effect on dopamine release in the brain reward pathways (see Chapter 4).

Unfortunately, because GABA is so widespread within the central nervous system, it has been difficult to develop effective antiaddiction drugs without unacceptable side effects.

Gamma-vinyl-GABA (Vigabatrin, an antiepileptic drug available in Europe) is an irreversible inhibitor of the metabolic enzyme *GABA transaminase*; it increases GABA activity and reduces drug-induced increases in extracellular nucleus accumbens dopamine. Vigabatrin shows anticraving effects against abused drugs, including cocaine (Brodie et al., 2009). Its use is limited by a drug-induced loss of some portion of the visual field (peripheral vision), although one study demonstrated that short-term use of Vigabatrin is less damaging to visual fields than originally thought (Fechtner et al., 2006). Baclofen is a GABA$_B$ receptor agonist, which had shown some signs of efficacy in clinical trials with cocaine abusers. However, subsequent results have been modest, although it may have a place in helping to prevent relapse in severe cocaine addiction (Shorter and Kosten, 2011). Several anticonvulsants, which act to increase GABA levels or to decrease glutamate (or both), have also been evaluated for cocaine addiction. Agents include valproate, tiagabine, topiramate (Elkashef et al., 2012; Johnson et al., 2013), lamotrigine (Brown et al., 2012), and vigabatrin (Somoza et al., 2013). Although in some cases the drugs may affect subjective reports of "drug craving," none of these studies have found significant decreases in cocaine use. In regard to glutamate, the broad effects of this excitatory transmitter make it even more difficult to isolate a drug that would exert a specific antiaddictive action. However, the substance N-acetylcysteine has received some attention because it appears to modulate the presynaptic control of cortical glutamate release (on the reward pathway) that is regulated by the metabotropic glutamate autoreceptor, mGluR2/3 (see Chapter 4). By improving the function of this autoreceptor, N-acetylcysteine may help to reduce glutamate release and thereby decrease drug craving (Amen et al., 2011). Other glutamatergic agents relevant to this approach are also being assessed (Xia et al., 2013).

Disulfiram (Antabuse) is used to treat alcoholism because it blocks the enzyme aldehyde dehydrogenase, which metabolizes alcohol (see Chapter 5). This inhibition causes the metabolite acetaldehyde to build up, which is very unpleasant and produces several noxious symptoms. It has been discovered that disulfiram also blocks the enzyme dopamine-beta-hydroxylase (DBH; DβH), which converts dopamine (DA) to norepinephrine (NE), thereby decreasing the levels of NE relative to DA. In addition, this drug also inhibits enzymes that metabolize cocaine, and has other biochemical actions that have produced conflicting outcomes in both laboratory and clinical experiments that complicate predictions about its antiaddictive actions (Gavel-Cruz and Weinshenker, 2009; Pani et al., 2010). Apparent conflicts in the data might be resolved by a recent clinical study that revealed a bimodal effect of this drug in cocaine users. These investigators found that the effect of disulfiram on cocaine use depended on the dose, relative to body weight. Specifically, participants given 4 milligrams per kilogram of body weight self-administered the smallest amount of cocaine, and those given 2 milligrams per kilogram self-administered the most (Haile et al., 2012b). Currently, a more selective inhibitor of DβH, called nepicastat, is being studied as a possible treatment for cocaine addiction.

Inhibition of the enzyme aldehyde dehydrogenase by another drug, ALDH2i, has also been found to reduce cocaine use and relapse in laboratory animals. Here the mechanism seems to be due to a series of biochemical reactions initiated by antagonism of the enzyme that leads to production of the substance tetrahydropapaveroline. This substance in turn blocks the enzyme tyrosine hydroxylase, which is the first step in dopamine synthesis. As a result, less DA is produced. It is hypothesized that the decrease in dopamine production and release is responsible for suppressing cocaine-seeking behavior in laboratory studies (Yao et al., 2010).

Another agent of current interest is *Tetrahydropalmatine* (THP) an alkaloid found in several different plant species, including the *Corydalis* family and the plant *Stephania rotunda*. These plants have traditional uses in Chinese herbal medicine as treatment for anxious insomnia and chronic pain. The pharmaceutical industry has synthetically produced the more potent enantiomer Levo-tetrahydropalmatine (*l*-THP), which has been marketed worldwide under different brand names as an alternative to anxiolytic and sedative drugs of the benzodiazepine group and analgesics such as opiates. It is also sold as a dietary supplement. *l*-THP has several neurobiological actions: it antagonizes DA_1 and DA_2 receptors and perhaps DA_3 receptors also. It may also block the alpha-1 type of adrenergic receptor and it may modulate $GABA_A$ receptors. In laboratory experiments it reduces cocaine self-administration and relapse (Shorter and Kosten, 2011; Wang and Mantsch, 2012). Currently it is undergoing clinical trials in human cocaine users, with an expected completion date of June 2015.

Several drug combinations have also been assessed in efforts to find effective treatments for stimulant abuse. One example is the medication Prometa, which is a combination of three drugs: the benzodiazepine antagonist flumazenil (for recovery from sedation); the drug gabapentin (Neurontin), believed to reduce glutamate and relieve cravings); and the antihistamine agent hydroxyzine (believed to help manage withdrawal symptoms). In a randomized, double-blind, placebo-controlled 108-day study trial, 120 MA-dependent patients were administered this cocktail. Although drug use declined in the Prometa and placebo groups, there was no difference between them in any measure (Ling et al., 2012).

Another combination that has blocked cocaine use in laboratory animals is that of the opiate antagonist naltrexone and the partial opiate agonist buprenorphine. The concept behind this approach is that chronic cocaine use produces a negative emotional state of stress and a dysphoric mood that is actually mediated by the endogenous opiate dynorphin (see Chapter 10). It remains to be seen if this indirect method of reducing stimulant-induced stress will be useful (Wee et al., 2012a).

Taking a similar approach, Kablinger and colleagues conducted a preliminary study in 45 cocaine-dependent patients of two drugs, *metyrapone*, a drug that blocks the synthesis of the stress hormone cortisol, and the drug *oxazepam*, a benzodiazepine (Kablinger et al., 2012). The combination was well tolerated, and was found to reduce craving and cocaine use.

The more general approach of trying to heal the neural damage produced by stimulant abuse, is also the rationale for an ongoing clinical trial of the drug Ibudilast, for methamphetamine abuse. When individuals first become abstinent from MA, an inflammatory process occurs in brain cells, especially glial cells. By dampening inflammation in glial cells, Ibudilast may preserve glial and other nerve cells during early abstinence. For 18 years in Japan and South Korea, Ibudilast has been used safely in humans as a treatment for asthma and pulmonary and cardiovascular diseases, therefore it is safe to use as a potential treatment for methamphetamine dependence.

The 11 MA addicts in this trial, all paid volunteers, were housed in a hospital unit and not allowed to leave for 3 weeks. They were intravenously injected with methamphetamine while being treated with Ibudilast. Now that the initial results have shown that the combination is safe, the second phase of the study, begun in midsummer, will be a 12-week trial of 140 treatment-seeking human MA addicts. Half the volunteers will take Ibudilast twice a day, and the other half will take a placebo. They will visit the trial unit three times a week for drug-craving monitoring, urine drug screens, and medication adherence monitoring. The results will show if addicts taking Ibudilast have reduced MA cravings and improved sobriety rates. (For a review of Ibudilast, see Rolan et al., 2013.)

Interestingly, in nonhuman laboratory animals, modafinil also showed some protection from the toxic effect of MA on dopamine neurons (Raineri et al., 2012). On the other hand, another compound, citicoline [known as cytidine diphosphate-choline (CDP-Choline) or cytidine 5-diphosphocholine] had no effect on cocaine use or craving (Licata et al., 2011). This agent is a substance found in the biochemical pathways involving choline (used for making acetylcholine). It was hypothesized to be helpful because it has some benefit for treating neuronal damage from stroke or brain injury. Finally, there is evidence that the hormone *oxytocin* modulates behavioral effects of psychostimulants in rodents and might be a possible candidate for treatment of abuse (Carson et al., 2013).

Pharmacokinetic Approaches to Psychostimulant Abuse— Metabolizing Enzymes

One novel approach to addressing cocaine abuse that has recently undergone rapid development is to intercept the drug molecule before it reaches the brain. These pharmacokinetic (PK) methods do not involve direct effects on either transporters or receptors. Rather, this approach counteracts cocaine either by binding to it, as an antibody that prevents it from crossing the blood-brain barrier, or as a cocaine-metabolizing enzyme, which breaks down the drug to inactive metabolites in the plasma, so that only a small amount drug reaches the CNS (Gorelick, 2012). With regard to the antibody method, antibodies can be obtained "actively" through a vaccine, or "passively," with antibodies produced in another host and then administered to the addict-patient. The disadvantage is that "passive" vaccines have a shorter half-life.

With regard to enzymes, the cocaine-metabolizing enzyme can be administered as an exogenous drug therapy, or it can be provided as a gene therapy, which means the person receiving the modified gene can then make the modified enzyme for him- or herself. In the exogenous enzyme approach, two types have been developed: mutations of human butyrylcholinesterase and a bacterial cocaine esterase found in the soil of coca plants. These compounds accelerate cocaine metabolism and antagonize the behavioral and toxic effects of cocaine in animal models. Of these two approaches, the human butyrylcholinesterase mutants show the more immediate promise, as they would not be expected to evoke an immune response in humans. The past decade has seen rapid progress with alteration of human plasma butyrylcholinesterase producing enzymes that destroy cocaine so efficiently that even though the enzyme is restricted to the blood, they prevent or interrupt drug actions in the CNS. During the same time, gene-transfer technology has also been improved such that enzymes can be delivered by endogenous gene transduction at high levels for periods of a year or longer after a single treatment

(Brimijoin and Gao, 2012; Narasimhan et al., 2012; Schindler and Goldberg, 2012; Zheng and Zhan, 2012b).

Cocaine-metabolizing enzymes have one advantage over vaccines and antibodies. At sufficiently high concentrations of cocaine, the antibodies may be saturated, leaving enough of the drug left over to produce the desired effect. In contrast, even if the cocaine-metabolizing enzyme is saturated, it maintains its effectiveness. That is, because it degrades the drug, each enzyme molecule can metabolize many cocaine molecules. One molecule of a currently available enzyme can metabolize 5,700 cocaine molecules a minute (Zheng and Zhan, 2012a).

The short half-life of cocaine might seem to make this approach impractical. However, because the half-life of cocaine is proportional to the dose, the half-life increases and becomes much longer under cocaine overdose conditions, and there is enough time for an enzyme injection to be effective. Furthermore, because the drug is distributed equally in plasma, brain, and heart tissue, metabolism of cocaine molecules in the blood will rapidly cause the molecules in the brain and heart to return to the plasma to maintain equilibrium. Clinical trials of cocaine-metabolizing enzymes are currently in progress for cocaine addiction treatment, and have shown that it is safe and that it reduces many of the positive subjective effects of the drug (Zheng and Zhan, 2012a). Furthermore, the combination of enzyme *and* antibody administration gave an even better blockade of cocaine-induced behavioral stimulation in rodents (Carroll et al., 2012).

Pharmacokinetic Approaches to Psychostimulant Abuse—Vaccines

The cocaine vaccine (termed TA-CD) is a cocaine derivative (succinyl norcocaine) coupled to recombinant cholera toxin B. It is designed to generate drug-specific antibodies that bind to cocaine and prevent it from traveling to the brain from the blood, thereby neutralizing its psychoactive effect (Figure 7.8). The molecules are then broken down by cholinesterases in the blood to inactive metabolites and excreted. The concept is intriguing and promising, but, as with all vaccines, the problems are, first, getting the concentration of antibodies high enough to block any amount of drug that might be used, and, second, compliance—getting the patients to return for the necessary number of injections to produce the required amount of antibody. Patients need to receive five vaccinations over the course of 2 to 3 months, during which time they are vulnerable to relapse. Incentives such as counseling and an escalating payment for successive vaccinations can improve adherence (Stitzer et al., 2010).

The amount of antibody produced predicts clinical effectiveness. Antibody levels of 43 µg/ml or higher resulted in more cocaine-free urine samples than those with levels less than 43 µg/ml. Unfortunately, only 31 percent of the vaccinated cocaine users attained antibody levels greater than 43 µg/ml (Shen et al., 2012), and even those had only 2 months of adequate cocaine blockade. The most common adverse effect was local injection site irritation. Even if the vaccine is successful, a cocaine-dependent person who has these antibodies in the blood may move to another drug or use large amounts of cocaine. Nevertheless, the methodology is improving, and a recent version produced a high amount of antibody, which lasted for about 4 months in laboratory rats (Wee et al., 2012b). This may be one of the first antiaddiction vaccines approved by the FDA for human use.

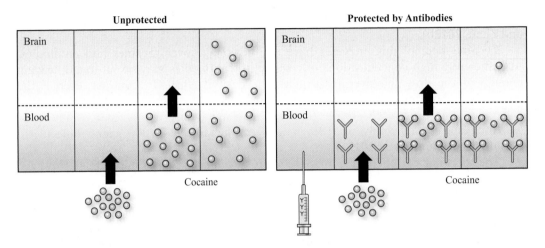

FIGURE 7.8 How the cocaine vaccine works. This pair of diagrams shows the difference between a patient's immune system with and without protection from antibodies against cocaine. In the unprotected immune system (left part of figure), the normal condition, cocaine molecules (circles) enter the bloodstream and then cross unimpeded from the blood into the brain. In the protected immune system (right part of figure), a series of vaccines has stimulated the patient's immune system to produce cocaine antibodies in the blood (Y symbols). They attach to most of the molecules of cocaine and prevent them from reaching the brain. [After http://www.drugabuse.gov/news-events/nida-notes/…/12/cocaine-vaccine-helps-some-reduce-drug-abuse].

Vaccines for use in methamphetamine addiction are also in development, with several laboratories working on specific parameters. One problem is that the methamphetamine molecule is simple, which makes it unnoticeable to the immune system. And, both methamphetamine and its metabolite, amphetamine, also have a long half-life, which makes it difficult for vaccine development. Passive administration of antibodies has already been found to reduce methamphetamine self-administration in rats and to decrease stimulant-induced motor activity. Behavioral assays that are better at measuring the effectiveness of the vaccine are also needed. At present, vaccines capable of producing enough antibody to bind a sufficient amount of drug for a sufficient amount of time are not yet available. However, one new agent, named MH6, is most likely just the beginning of a successful effort to find more effective treatment options for psychostimulant abuse (Miller et al., 2013). Kosten and colleagues (2013) provide a review of current developments in vaccines for cocaine and methamphetamine.

STUDY QUESTIONS

1. Compare and contrast the pharmacological history of cocaine and amphetamine.
2. Compare and contrast the pharmacological effects of cocaine and amphetamine.
3. How do cocaine and amphetamine differ in their mechanism of action?
4. What are the effects of psychostimulants on the fetus?

5. Describe the behavioral consequences of chronic high doses of psychostimulants.

6. What are the neurotoxic effects of methamphetamine on the brain?

7. What are the most common psychostimulants besides cocaine and amphetamine, and how do they differ among themselves?

8. What types of pharmacological approaches have been tried to treat stimulant addiction? How successful are they?

REFERENCES

Amato, L., et al. (2011). "Dopamine Agonists for the Treatment of Cocaine Dependence." *Cochrane Database Systemic Reviews* CD003352. PMID: 22161376.

Amen, S. L., et al. (2011). "Repeated N-Acetyl Cysteine Reduces Cocaine Seeking in Rodents and Craving in Cocaine-Dependent Humans." *Neuropsychopharmacology* 36: 871–878.

Anderson, A. L., et al. (2012). "Modafinil for the Treatment of Methamphetamine Dependence." *Drug and Alcohol Dependence* 120: 135–141.

Aquaro, G. D., et al. (2011). "Silent Myocardial Damage in Cocaine Addicts." *Heart* 97: 2056–2062.

Arnold, V. K., et al. (2012). "A 9-Week, Randomized, Double-Blind, Placebo-Controlled, Parallel-Group, Dose-Finding Study to Evaluate the Efficacy and Safety of Modafinil as Treatment for Adults with ADHD." *Journal of Attention Disorders* Online May 2012: DOI 10.1177/1087054712441969.

Bauman, M. H., et al. (2012). "The Designer Methcathinone Analogs, Mephedrone and Methylone, Are Substrates for Monoamine Transporters in Brain Tissue." *Neuropsychopharmacology* 37: 1192–1203.

Bauman, M. H., et al. (2013). "Powerful Cocaine-Like Actions of 3,4-Methylenedioxypyrovalerone (MDPV), a Principal Constituent of Psychoactive 'Bath Salts' Products." *Neuropsychopharmacology* 38: 552–562.

Beaman, J., and Hayes, E. E. (2013). "Synthetic Cathinones: Signs, Symptoms and Treatment." *Psychiatric Times* April 30: 1–3.

Behnke, M., and Smith, C. (2013). "Prenatal Substance Abuse: Short- and Long-Term Effects on the Exposed Fetus." *Pediatrics* DOI: 10.1542/peds.2012-3931.

Brimijoin, S., and Gao, Y. (2012). "Cocaine Hydrolase Gene Therapy for Cocaine Abuse." *Future Medicinal Chemistry* 4: 151–162.

Brodie, J. D., et al. (2009). "Randomized, Double-Blind, Placebo-Controlled Trial of Vigabatrin for the Treatment of Cocaine Dependence in Mexican Parolees." *American Journal of Psychiatry* 166: 1269–1277.

Brown, E. S., et al. (2012). "A Randomized, Double-Blind, Placebo-Controlled Trial of Lamotrigine Therapy in Bipolar Disorder, Depressed or Mixed Phase and Cocaine Dependence." *Neuropsychopharmacology* 37: 2347–2354.

Bunney, E. B., et al. (2001). "Electrophysiological Effects of Cocaethylene, Cocaine, and Ethanol on Dopaminergic Neurons of the Ventral Tegmental Area." *Journal of Pharmacology and Experimental Therapeutics* 297: 696–703.

Cadet, J. L., and Krasnova, I. N. (2009). "Molecular Basis of Methamphetamine-Induced Neurodegeneration." *International Review of Neurobiology* 88: 101–119.

Callaghan, R. C., et al. (2012). "Increased Risk of Parkinson's Disease in Individuals Hospitalized with Conditions Related to the Use of Methamphetamine or Other Amphetamine-Type Drugs." *Drug and Alcohol Dependence* 120: 35–40.

Carroll, M. E., et al. (2012). "Combined Cocaine Hydrolase Gene Transfer and Anti-Cocaine Vaccine Synergistically Block Cocaine-Induced Locomotion." *PLoS One* 7: e43536.

Carson, D. S., et al. (2013). "A Brief History of Oxytocin and Its Role in Modulating Psychostimulant Effects." *Journal of Psychopharmacology* 27: 231–247.

Coffin, P. O., et al. (2013). "Aripiprazole for the Treatment of Methamphetamine Dependence: A Randomized, Double-Blind, Placebo-Controlled Trial." *Addiction* 108: 751–761.

Comer, S. D., et al. (2001). "Effects of Repeated Oral Methamphetamine Administration in Humans." *Psychopharmacology* 155: 397–404.

Dackis, C. A., et al. (2012). "A Double-Blind, Placebo-Controlled Trial of Modafinil for Cocaine Dependence." *Journal of Substance Abuse Treatment* 43: 303–312.

Dean, A. C., et al. (2011). "Acute Modafinil Effects on Attention and Inhibitory Control in Methamphetamine-Dependent Humans." *Journal of Studies on Alcohol and Drugs* 72: 943–953.

Dean, A. C., et al. (2013). "An Evaluation of the Evidence That Methamphetamine Abuse Causes Cognitive Decline in Humans." *Neuropsychopharmacology* 38: 259–274.

De Giovanni, N., and Marchetti, D. (2012). "Cocaine and Its Metabolites in the Placenta: A Systematic Review of the Literature." *Reproductive Toxicology* 33: 1–14.

Doweiko, H. E. (2012). *Concepts of Chemical Dependency,* 8th ed. Belmont, CA: Brooks/Cole.

Elkashef, A., and Montoya, I. (2012). "Pharmacotherapy of Addiction." *Drug Abuse and Addiction in Medical Illness* Part 1: 107–119.

Elkashef, A., and Vocci, F. (2011). "Pharmacotherapy of Cocaine Addiction." *Addiction Medicine* Part 8: 1017–128.

Elkashef, A. M., et al. (2008). "Bupropion for the Treatment of Methamphetamine Dependence." *Neuropsychopharmacology* 33: 1162–1170.

Elkashef, A. M., et al. (2012). "Topiramate for the Treatment of Methamphetamine Addiction: A Multi-Center Placebo-Controlled Trial." *Addiction* 107: 1297–1306.

Ersche, K. D., et al. (2011). "Abnormal Structure of Frontostriatal Brain Systems Is Associated with Aspects of Impulsivity and Compulsivity in Cocaine Dependence." *Brain* 134: 2013–2024.

Fantegrossi, W. E., et al. (2013). "*In Vivo* Effects of Abused 'Bath Salt' Constituent 3,4-Methylenedioxypyrovalerone (MDPV) in Mice: Drug Discrimination, Thermoregulation, and Locomotor Activity." *Neuropsychopharmacology* 38: 563–573.

Farooq, M. U., et al. (2009). "Neurotoxic and Cardiotoxic Effects of Cocaine and Ethanol." *Journal of Medical Toxicology* 5: 134–138.

Fechtner, R. D., et al. (2006). "Short-Term Treatment of Cocaine and/or Methamphetamine Abuse with Vigabatrin: Ocular Safety Pilot Results." *Archives of Ophthalmology* 124: 1257–1262.

Garcia-Bournissen, F., et al. (2009). "Pharmacokinetics of Disappearance of Cocaine from Hair After Discontinuation of Drug Use." *Forensic Science International* 189: 24–27.

Gaval-Cruz, M., and Weinshenker, D. (2009). "Mechanisms of Disulfiram-Induced Cocaine Abstinence: Antabuse and Cocaine Relapse." *Molecular Interventions* 9: 175–187.

Gerteis, J., et al. (2011). "Are There Effects of Intrauterine Cocaine Exposure on Delinquency During Early Adolescence? A Preliminary Report." *Journal of Developmental and Behavioral Pediatrics* 32: 393–401.

Gold, M. S. (1997). "Cocaine (and Crack): Clinical Aspects." In J. H. Lowinson, P. Ruiz, R. B. Millman, and J. G. Langrod, eds., *Substance Abuse: A Comprehensive Textbook,* 3rd ed. Baltimore: Williams & Wilkins.

Good, M. M., et al. (2010)."Methamphetamine Use During Pregnancy." *Obstetrics & Gynecology* 116: 330–334.

Gorelick, D. A. (2012). "Pharmacokinetic Strategies for Treatment of Drug Overdose and Addiction." *Future Medicinal Chemistry* 4: 227–243.

Gouin, K., et al. (2011). "Effects of Cocaine Use During Pregnancy on Low Birthweight and Preterm Birth: Systematic Review and Metaanalyses." *American Journal of Obstetrics & Gynecology* 204: 340. e1–340.e12.

Gouzoulis-Mayfrank, E., and Daumann, J. (2009). "Neurotoxicity of Drugs of Abuse—The Case of Methylenedioxyamphetamines (MDMA, Ecstasy) and Amphetamines." *Dialogues in Clinical Neuroscience* 11: 305–317.

Grabowski, J., et al. (1997). "Replacement Medication for Cocaine Dependence: Methylphenidate." *Journal of Clinical Psychopharmacology* 17: 485–488.

Grabowski, J., et al. (2001). "Dextroamphetamine for Cocaine-Dependence Treatment: A Double-Blind Randomized Clinical Trial." *Journal of Clinical Psychopharmacology* 21: 522–526.

Gregory, P. J. (2013). "Availability of DMAA Supplements Despite U. S. Food and Drug Administration Action." *JAMA Internal Medicine* 173: 164–165.

Haile, C. N., et al. (2012a). "Pharmacotherapeutics Directed at Deficiencies Associated with Cocaine Dependence: Focus on Dopamine, Norepinephrine and Glutamate." *Pharmacology and Therapeutics* 134: 260–277.

Haile, C. N., et al. (2012b). "The Impact of Disulfiram Treatment on the Reinforcing Effects of Cocaine: A Randomized Clinical Trial." *PLoS One* 7: e47702.

Heinzerling, K. G., et al. (2013). "Pilot Randomized Trial of Bupropion for Adolescent Methamphetamine Abuse/Dependence." *Journal of Adolescent Health* 52: 502–505.

Herin, D. V., et al. (2010). "Agonist-Like Pharmacotherapy for Stimulant Dependence: Preclinical, Human Laboratory, and Clinical Studies." *Annals of the New York Academy of Sciences* 1187: 76–100.

Johnson, B. A., et al. (2013). "Topiramate's Effects on Cocaine-Induced Subjective Mood, Craving and Preference for Money Over Drug Taking." *Addiction Biology* 18: 405–416.

Kablinger, A., et al. (2012). "Effects of the Combination of Metyrapone and Oxazepam on Cocaine Craving and Cocaine Taking: A Double-Blind, Randomized, Placebo-Controlled Pilot Study." *Journal of Psychopharmacology* 26: 973–998.

Karila, L., et al. (2011). "Pharmacological Treatments for Cocaine Dependence: Is There Something New?" *Current Pharmaceutical Design* 17: 1359–1368.

Katzung, B. G., Masters, S. B., and Trevor, A. J. (2009). *Basic and Clinical Pharmacology*, 11th ed. New York: McGraw-Hill.

Kaye, S., et al. (2013). "Attention Deficit Hyperactivity Disorder (ADHD) Among Illicit Psychostimulant Users: A Hidden Disorder?" *Addiction* 108: 923–931.

Keegan, J., et al. (2010). "Addiction in Pregnancy." *Journal of Addictive Diseases* 29: 175–191.

Kiblawi, Z. N., et al. (2013). "The Effect of Prenatal Methamphetamine Exposure on Attention as Assessed by Continuous Performance Tests: Results from the Infant Development, Environment, and Lifestyle Study." *Journal of Developmental Behavioral Pediatrics* 34: 31–37.

Kirkpatrick, M. G., et al. (2013). "Personality and the Acute Subjective Effects of *d*-Amphetamine in Humans." *Journal of Psychopharmacology* 27: 256–264.

Kiyatkin, E. A., and Sharma, H. S. (2009). "Acute Methamphetamine Intoxication: Brain Hyperthermia, Blood-Brain Barrier, Brain Edema, and Morphological Cell Abnormalities." *International Review of Neurobiology* 88: 65–100.

Kiyatkin, E. A., and Sharma, H. S. (2012). "Environmental Conditions Modulate Neurotoxic Effects of Psychomotor Stimulant Drugs of Abuse." *New Perspectives of Central Nervous System Injury and Neuroprotection* 102: 147–171.

Kiyatkin, E. A., et al. (2007). "Brain Edema and Breakdown of the Blood-Brain Barrier During Methamphetamine Intoxication: Critical Role of Brain Hyperthermia." *European Journal of Neuroscience* 26: 1242–1253.

Kosten, T., et al. (2013). "Vaccines Against Stimulants: Cocaine and Methamphetamine." *British Journal of Clinical Pharmacology* DOI: 10.1111/bcp.12115.

Kozor, R., et al. (2012). "Cardiovascular Impact of Cocaine in Regular Asymptomatic Users Assessed by Cardiovascular Magnetic Resonance Imaging." *American Heart Association Scientific Sessions*, November 5, 2012, Los Angeles, CA, Abstract 18163.

Krystal, A. D., et al. (2010). "A Double-Blind, Placebo-Controlled Study of Armodafinil for Excessive Sleepiness in Patients with Treated Obstructive Sleep Apnea and Comorbid Depression." *Journal of Clinical Psychiatry* 71: 32–40.

LaGasse, L. L., et al. (2012). "Prenatal Methamphetamine Exposure and Childhood Behavior Problems at 3 and 5 Years of Age." *Pediatrics* 129: 681–688.

Levinthal, C. F. (2012). *Drugs, Behavior and Modern Society,* 7th ed. New York: Allyn & Bacon.

Licata, S. C., et al. (2011). "Effects of Daily Treatment with Citicoline: A Double-Blind, Placebo-Controlled Study in Cocaine-Dependence Volunteers." *Journal of Addiction Medicine* 5: 57–64.

Ling, W., et al. (2012). "Double-Blind Placebo-Controlled Evaluation of the Prometa Protocol for Methamphetamine Dependence." *Addiction* 107: 361–369.

Loland, C. J., et al. (2012). "R-Modafinil (Armodafinil): A Unique Dopamine Uptake Inhibitor and Potential Medication for Psychostimulant Abuse." *Biological Psychiatry* 72: 405–413.

Mariani, J. J, and Levin, F. R. (2012). "Psychostimulant Treatment of Cocaine Dependence." *Psychiatric Clinics of North America* 35: 425–439.

McKetin, R., et al. (2013). "Dose-Related Psychotic Symptoms in Chronic Methamphetamine Users: Evidence from a Prospective Longitudinal Study." *JAMA Psychiatry* 70: 319–324.

McKim, W. A., and Hancock, S. (2013). *Drugs and Behavior,* 7th ed. Upper Saddle River, NJ: Pearson Prentice Hall.

Meini, M., et al. (2011). "Aripiprazole and Ropinirole Treatment for Cocaine Dependence: Evidence from a Pilot Study." *Current Pharmaceutical Design* 17: 1376–1383.

Mello, N. K., et al. (2013). "Effects of Chronic Buspirone Treatment on Cocaine Self-Administration." *Neuropsychopharmacology* 38: 455–467.

Miller, M. L., et al. (2013). "A Methamphetamine Vaccine Attenuates Methamphetamine-Induced Disruptions in Thermoregulation and Activity in Rats." *Biological Psychiatry* 73: 721–728.

Motbey, C. P., et al. (2012). "Mephedrone in Adolescent Rats: Residual Memory Impairment and Acute but Not Lasting 5-HT Depletion." *PLoS One* 7: e45473 .

Müller, U., et al. (2013). "Effects of Modafinil on Non-Verbal Cognition, Task Enjoyment and Creative Thinking in Healthy Volunteers." *Neuropharmacology* 64: 490–495.

Nakagawa, T., and Kaneko, S. (2008). "Neuropsychotoxicity of Abused Drugs: Molecular and Neural Mechanisms of Neuropsychotoxicity Induced by Methamphetamine, 3,4-Methylenedioxymethamphetamine (Ecstasy) and 5-Methoxy-N,N-Diisopropyltryptamine (Foxy)." *Journal of Pharmaceutical Sciences* 106: 2–8.

Narasimhan, D., et al., (2012). "Bacterial Cocaine Esterase: A Protein-Based Therapy for Cocaine Overdose and Addiction." *Future Medicinal Chemistry* 4: 137–150.

Nephew, B. C., and Febo, M. (2012). "Effects of Cocaine on Maternal Behavior and Neurochemistry." *Current Neuropharmacology* 10: 53–63.

Newton, T. F., et al. (2012). "Noradrenergic α_1 Receptor Antagonist Treatment Attenuates Positive Subjective Effects of Cocaine in Humans: A Randomized Trial." *PLoS One* 7: e30854.

Oei, J. L., et al. (2012). "Amphetamines, the Pregnant Woman and Her Children: A Review." *Journal of Perinatology* 32: 737–747.

Olive, M. F., et al. (2012). "Glutamatergic Medications for the Treatment of Drug and Behavioral Addictions." *Pharmacology Biochemistry and Behavior* 100: 801–810.

Panenka, W. J., et al. (2013). "Methamphetamine Use: A Comprehensive Review of Molecular, Preclinical and Clinical Findings." *Drug and Alcohol Dependence* 129: 167–179.

Pani, P. P., et al. (2010). "Disulfiram for the Treatment of Cocaine Dependence." *Cochrane Database of Systematic Reviews* CD007024.

Phillips, K., et al. (2009). "Cocaine Cardiotoxicity: A Review of the Pathophysiology, Pathology, and Treatment Options." *American Journal of Cardiovascular Drugs* 9: 177–196.

Prosser, J. M., and Nelson, L. S. (2012). "The Toxicology of Bath Salts: A Review of Synthetic Cathinones." *Journal of Medical Toxicology* 8: 33–42.

Raineri, M. (2012). "Modafinil Abrogates Methamphetamine-Induced Neuroinflammation and Apoptotic Effects in the Mouse Striatum." *PLoS One* 7: e46599.

Rando, K., et al. (2013). "Prenatal Cocaine Exposure and Gray Matter Volume in Adolescent Boys and Girls." *Biological Psychiatry* 74: 482–489.

Rolan, P., et al. (2013). "Ibudilast: A Review of Its Pharmacology, Efficacy and Safety In Respiratory and Neurological Disease." *Expert Opinion on Pharmacotherapy* (EOOP-2009-0238.R1).

Rosenbaum, C. D., et al. (2012). "Here Today, Gone Tomorrow . . . and Back Again? A Review of Herbal Marijuana Alternatives (K2, Spice), Synthetic Cathinones (Bath Salts), Kratom, *Salvia Divinorum*, Methoxetamine, and Piperazines." *Journal of Medical Toxicology* 8: 15–32.

Rush, C. R., and Stoops, W. W. (2012). "Agonist Replacement Therapy for Cocaine Dependence: A Translational Review." *Future Medicinal Chemistry* 4: 245–265.

Sekine, Y., et al., (2008). "Methamphetamine Causes Microglial Activation in the Brains of Human Abusers." *Journal of Neuroscience* 28: 5756–5761.

Shen, X. Y., et al. (2012). "Vaccines Against Drug Abuse." *Nature* 91: 60–70.

Shindler, C. W., and Goldberg, S. R. (2012). "Accelerating Cocaine Metabolism as an Approach to the Treatment of Cocaine Abuse and Toxicity." *Future Medicinal Chemistry* 4: 163–175.

Shoptaw, S. J., et al. (2008). "Bupropion Hydrochloride Versus Placebo, in Combination with Cognitive Behavioral Therapy, for the Treatment of Cocaine Abuse/Dependence." *Journal of Addictive Disorders* 27: 13–23.

Shoptaw, S. J., et al. (2009). "Treatment for Amphetamine Psychosis." *Cochrane Database of Systematic Reviews* CD003026.

Shorter, D., and Kosten, T. R. (2011). "Novel Pharmacotherapeutic Treatments for Cocaine Addiction." *BMC Medicine* 9: 119–128.

Smith, L. M., et al. (2006). "The Infant Development, Environment, and Lifestyle Study: Effects of Prenatal Methamphetamine Exposure, Polydrug Exposure, and Poverty on Intrauterine Growth." *Pediatrics* 118: 1149–1156.

Somoza, E. C., et al. (2013). "A Multisite, Double-Blind, Placebo-Controlled Clinical Trial to Evaluate the Safety and Efficacy of Vigabatrin for Treating Cocaine Dependence. *JAMA Psychiatry* April 10: 1–8

Sowell, E. R., et al. (2010). "Differentiating Prenatal Exposure to Methamphetamine and Alcohol versus Alcohol and Not Methamphetamine Using Tensor-Based Brain Morphometry and Discriminant Analysis." *Journal of Neuroscience* 30: 3876–3885.

Stitzer, M. L., et al. (2010). "Drug Users' Adherence to a 6-Month Vaccination Protocol: Effects of Motivational Incentives." *Drug and Alcohol Dependence* 107: 76–79.

Talbert, J., et al. (2012). "Pseudoephedrine Sales and Seizures of Clandestine Methamphetamine Laboratories in Kentucky." *Journal of the American Medical Association* 308: 1524–1526.

Thompson, B. L., et al. (2009). "Prenatal Exposure to Drugs: Effects on Brain Development and Implications for Policy and Education." *Nature Reviews Neuroscience* 10: 303–312.

Thompson, P. M., et al. (2004). "Structural Abnormalities in the Brains of Human Subjects Who Use Methamphetamine." *Journal of Neuroscience* 24: 6028–6036.

Vagi, S. J., et al. (2013). "Passive Multistate Surveillance for Neutropenia After Use of Cocaine or Heroin Possibly Contaminated with Levamisole." *Annals of Emergency Medicine* 61: 468–474.

Volkow, N. D., et al. (2009). "Effects of Modafinil on Dopamine and Dopamine Transporters in the Male Human Brain: Clinical Implications." *Journal of the American Medical Association* 301: 1148–1154.

Vosburg, S. K., et al. (2010). "Modafinil Does Not Serve as a Reinforcer in Cocaine Abusers." *Drug and Alcohol Dependence* 106: 233–236.

Walton, M. A., et al. (2009). "Predictors of Violence Following Emergency Department Visit for Cocaine-Related Chest Pain." *Drug and Alcohol Dependence* 99: 79–88.

Wang, G. J., et al. (2012). "Decreased Dopamine Activity Predicts Relapse in Methamphetamine Abusers." *Molecular Psychiatry* 17: 918–925.

Wang, J. B., and Mantsch, J. R. (2012). "*l*-Tetrahydropalamatine: A Potential New Medication for the Treatment of Cocaine Addiction." *Future Medicinal Chemistry* 4: 177–186.

Wee, S., et al. (2012a). "A Combination of Buprenorphine and Naltrexone Blocks Compulsive Cocaine Intake in Rodents Without Producing Dependence." *Science Translational Medicine* 4: 146ra110.

Wee, S., et al. (2012b). "Novel Cocaine Vaccine Linked to a Disrupted Adenovirus Gene Transfer Vector Blocks Cocaine Psychostimulant and Reinforcing Effects." *Neuropsychopharmacology* 37: 1083–1091.

Westover, A. N., and Nakonezny, P. A. (2010). "Aortic Dissection in Young Adults Who Abuse Amphetamines." *American Heart Journal* 160: 315–321.

Xia, L., et al. (2013). "Metabotropic Glutamate 7 (Mglur7) Receptor: A Target for Medication Development for the Treatment of Cocaine Dependence." *Neuropharmacology* 66: 12–23.

Yao, L., et al. (2010). "Inhibition of Aldehyde Dehydrogenase-2 Suppresses Cocaine Seeking by Generating THP, a Cocaine Use–Dependent Inhibitor of Dopamine Synthesis." *Nature Medicine* 16: 1024–1028.

Zhang, Y., et al. (2012). "1,3-Dimethylamylamine (DMAA) in Supplements and Geranium Products: Natural or Synthetic?" *Drug Testing and Analysis* 4: 986–990.

Zheng, F., and Zhan, C. -G. (2012a). "Are Pharmacokinetic Approaches Feasible for Treatment of Cocaine Addiction and Overdose?" *Future Medicinal Chemistry* 4: 125–128.

Zheng, F., and Zhan, C. -G. (2012b). "Modeling of Pharmacokinetics of Cocaine in Human Reveals the Feasibility for Development of Enzyme Therapies for Drugs of Abuse." *PLoS Computational Biology* 8: e1002610.

Chapter 8

Psychedelic Drugs

This chapter introduces a class of drugs that act on various neurotransmitter pathways in the central nervous system (CNS) to produce hallucinatory perceptual experiences, which may be accompanied by marked changes in cognition and mood. In contrast to other drugs of abuse, many of these drugs are taken specifically to alter subjective states of consciousness, rather than for a direct reinforcing effect. A current term applied to a person who uses these drugs is "psychonaut," to indicate the exploratory nature of the experience. In fact, it is not uncommon for these substances to produce a dysphoric, rather than euphoric, subjective experience. Moreover, unlike their response to classically rewarding drugs, nonhuman animals are less likely to self-administer these drugs, and may sometimes even work to avoid them. Primarily for this reason, there has been less research on these drugs than on drugs considered to have more therapeutic potential.

Because of the unusual, subjective, psychological, and physiological effects they produce, the best term for classifying these drugs has been debated for a long time. The term *hallucinogen* is used because these agents can, in high enough doses, induce hallucinations, defined as *perceptions in the absence of the appropriate sensations*. However, that is somewhat misleading because illusory phenomena and perceptual distortions are more common than are true hallucinations. The term *psychotomimetic* has also been used because of the alleged ability of these drugs to mimic psychoses or induce psychotic states. However, most of these drugs do not produce the same behavioral patterns that are observed in people who experience psychotic episodes. Descriptive terms, such as *phantasticum* or *psychedelic*, have also been used to indicate that these agents all have the ability to alter sensory perception. In this chapter the term *psychedelic* (mind-manifesting), coined by Humphrey Osmond, is used because it allows for more flexibility in grouping together a disparate array of effects into a recognizable syndrome.

Many psychedelic agents occur in nature; others are synthetically produced. Regardless of their origin, most psychedelic drugs act on one of the known neurotransmitter systems.

TABLE 8.1 Classification of psychedelic drugs

ANTICHOLINERGIC PSYCHEDELIC DRUG
  Scopolamine

CATECHOLAMINELIKE PSYCHEDELIC DRUGS
  Mescaline

DOM, MDA, DMA, MDMA (ecstasy), TMA, MDE
  Myristicin, elemicin

SEROTONINLIKE PSYCHEDELIC DRUGS
  Lysergic acid diethylamide (LSD)
  Dimethyltryptamine (DMT), AMT, 5-MeO-DIPT
  Psilocybin, psilocin, bufotenine
  Ololiuqui
  Harmine

GLUTAMINERGIC NMDA RECEPTOR ANTAGONISTS
  Phencyclidine (Sernyl)
  Ketamine (Ketalar)
  Dextromethorphan

OPIOID KAPPA RECEPTOR AGONIST
  Salvinorin A

Similarities in structure, and in neurochemical and psychological effects lead to the major categories of psychedelic drugs (Table 8.1): *anticholinergic, monoaminergic (catecholaminelike* and *serotoninlike), glutaminergic NMDA receptor antagonists* (the two psychedelic anesthetics as well as dextromethorphan), and the *opioid kappa receptor agonist* salvinorin A. Finally, there are some additional substances, derivatives that are related to these compounds, which are described in the respective sections below.

Scopolamine: The Prototype Anticholinergic (ACh) Psychedelic

This class of drugs might more appropriately be called *antimuscarinic*, because they are competitive antagonists of the muscarinic type of ACh receptor (see Chapter 3). The three most common anticholinergics are *scopolamine, atropine*, and *l-hyoscyamine*; *scopolamine* (Figure 8.1) being the classic example of an anticholinergic drug with psychedelic properties. Anticholinergic, muscarinic, blockade produces a constellation of physiological effects, which are described below. Medically, scopolamine is found in some travel-sickness products including motion-sickness-prevention patches.[1] More commonly, exposure

---

[1] Certain medicines also have anticholinergic properties and can cause similar effects. Examples include antihistamines (such as diphenhydramine, or Benadryl), the tricyclic antidepressants (such as imipramine, or Tofranil), and certain medicines used in the treatment of parkinsonism (e.g., Cogentin).

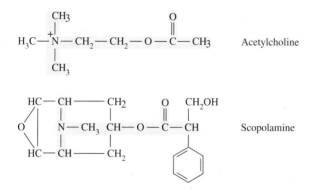

FIGURE 8.1 Structural formulas of acetylcholine (a chemical transmitter) and the anticholinergic psychedelic scopolamine, which acts by blocking acetylcholine receptors. The shaded portion of each molecule illustrates structural similarities, which presumably contribute to receptor fit.

occurs because of the anticholinergic side effects produced by many psychotropic medications, such as antidepressants (see Chapter 12) and antipsychotics (see Chapter 11).

Historical Background

The history of scopolamine is long and colorful (Holzman, 1998). The drug is distributed widely in nature; it is found in especially high concentrations in the plants *Atropa belladonna* (belladonna, or deadly nightshade), *Datura stramonium* (Jamestown weed, jimsonweed, stinkweed, thorn apple, or devil's apple), *Mandragora officinarum* (mandrake), and *Datura inoxia* (moonflower). Both professional and amateur poisoners of the Middle Ages frequently used deadly nightshade as a source of poison. In fact, the plant's name, *Atropa belladonna*, is derived from Atropos, one of the three Fates, who supposedly cut the thread of life. *Belladonna* means "beautiful woman," which refers to the drug's ability to dilate the pupils when it is applied topically to the eyes (eyes with widely dilated pupils were presumably a mark of beauty). Accidental ingestion of berries from *Datura* has even been associated with the incapacitation of whole armies, for example, the defeat of Marc Antony's army in 36 B.C. Ingestion of tea made from this plant was said to have contributed to the defeat of British soldiers by settlers in the rebellion known as Bacon's Revolution near Jamestown, Virginia, in 1676 (hence the name Jamestown weed, or jimson weed).

Scopolamine-containing plants have been used and misused for centuries. For example, the delirium caused by scopolamine may have persuaded certain people that they could fly—associated with the Halloween images of flying witches. Marijuana and opium preparations from the Far East were once fortified with material from *Datura stramonium*. Today, cigarettes made from the leaves of *D. stramonium* and *A. belladonna* are smoked occasionally to induce intoxication. Throughout the world, leaves of plants that contain atropine or scopolamine are still used to prepare intoxicating beverages.

Pharmacological Effects

Scopolamine acts on the peripheral nervous system to produce an anticholinergic syndrome consisting of dry mouth, reduced sweating, dry skin, increased body temperature, dilated pupils, blurred vision, tachycardia, and hypertension. Low doses reaching the CNS produce drowsiness, mild euphoria, profound amnesia, fatigue, mental confusion, dreamless sleep, and loss of attention. Rather than expanding consciousness, awareness, and insight, scopolamine clouds consciousness and produces amnesia. As doses increase, psychiatric symptoms include restlessness, excitement, hallucinations, euphoria, and disorientation (DeFrates et al., 2005). Delirium, that is, mental confusion, may progress to stupor, coma, and respiratory depression. While scopolamine intoxication can convey a sense of excitement and loss of control to the user, the clouding of consciousness and the reduction in memory of the episode render scopolamine rather unattractive as a psychedelic drug. Although historically used as poisons, the margin of safety for these drugs is large and death is usually a result of accidents (wandering into traffic or falling), or of inadvertent ingestion (for example, of the berries by children). There is a classic phrase describing the effects of scopolamine, which states that it makes you "hot as a hare, blind as a bat, dry as a bone, red as a beet, and mad as a hen." Typically, sensorium and psychosis usually clear within 36 to 48 hours. If necessary, the antidote to anticholinergic poisoning is the drug physostigmine, which blocks the enzyme acetylcholinesterase (AChE). AChE metabolizes ACh in the synaptic cleft. By blocking this metabolism, physostigmine may increase the concentration of ACh sufficiently to overcome the lethal effects of scopolamine.

Tolerance to anticholinergics is generally modest and psychological dependence uncommon. Physical dependence can develop, particularly in conjunction with long-term use of medications that have anticholinergic actions or side effects. Withdrawal symptoms include vomiting, excessive sweating and salivation, and general malaise.

Monoaminergic Psychedelics

As the name indicates, these drugs share a neurochemical similarity with the biogenic amine neurotransmitters, serotonin (5-HT), dopamine, and norepinephrine. Examples of the serotonergic category are LSD, psilocybin, and DMT, whereas the catecholamine type includes mescaline and MDMA (ecstasy). Within their respective effective dose ranges, the subjective effects of these drugs are quite similar, although they vary greatly in potency and in duration of action. Essentially, the actions range from amphetaminelike (more stimulatory and less hallucinogenic) to LSD-like (more hallucinatory and less stimulatory). Tolerance usually develops rapidly to the effects of most of these drugs, within three or four successive daily exposures, and they are often cross-tolerant with each other—although not with the drugs in the other psychedelic classes. In addition to sharing many psychological effects, these drugs also produce similar physiological actions, notably sympathomimetic effects such as increases in blood pressure and heart rate, pupil dilation, increased body temperature, tremors, nausea, and other reactions as noted.

Catecholaminergic Psychedelics

A large group of psychedelic drugs are structurally similar to both catecholamine neurotransmitters and the amphetamine stimulants (Figure 8.2). They differ structurally from the normal neurotransmitters by the addition of one or more methoxy ($-OCH_3$)

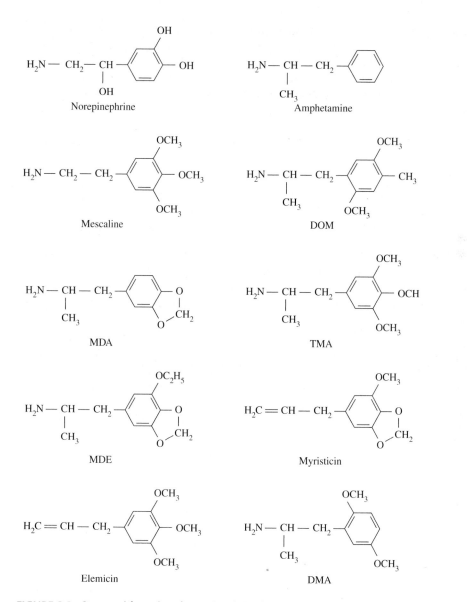

FIGURE 8.2 Structural formulas of norepinephrine (a chemical transmitter), amphetamine, and eight catecholaminelike psychedelic drugs. These eight drugs are structurally related to norepinephrine and are thought to exert their psychedelic actions by altering the transmission of nerve impulses at norepinephrine and serotonin synapses in the brain.

groups to the phenyl ring structure, which confer psychedelic properties in addition to their amphetaminelike psychostimulant properties. Methoxylated amphetamine derivatives include mescaline, DOM (also called STP), MDA, MDE, MDMA (ecstasy), MMDA, DMA, and certain drugs that are obtained from nutmeg (myristicin and elemicin). As a group, these drugs that exhibit a blend of stimulant and hallucinogenic actions have classically been referred to as *entactogens*.

Mescaline

Peyote (*Lophophora williamsii*) is a common plant in the southwestern United States and in Mexico. It is a spineless cactus that has a small crown, or "button," and a long root. When the plant is used for psychedelic purposes, the crown is cut from the cactus and dried into a hard brown disk. This disk, which is frequently referred to as a "mescal button," is later softened in the mouth and swallowed. The psychedelic chemical in the button is mescaline.

Historical Background. The use of peyote extends back perhaps 5,000 years or more in North America; the cactus was used in the religious rites of the Aztecs and other Mexican and North American Indians (el-Seedi et al., 2005). In the eighteenth century the Mescalero Apaches adopted the use of the drug (and provided the origin for the name mescaline) from Mexican Indians who had used it for thousands of years. Currently, peyote is legally available for use in the religious practice of the Native American Church of North America, which was chartered in 1918. Members of this sect regard peyote as sacramental and are exempt from federal criminal penalties for its religious use. The use of peyote for religious purposes is not considered to be abuse, and peyote is seldom abused by members of the Native American Church (Fickenscher et al., 2006).

Pharmacological Effects. Early research on the peyote cactus led in 1896 to the identification of mescaline as its pharmacologically active ingredient. After the chemical structure of mescaline was elucidated in 1918, the compound was produced synthetically. Because of its structural resemblance to norepinephrine, a wide variety of synthetic mescaline derivatives have now been synthesized, and all have methoxy ($-OCH_3$) groups or similar additions on their benzene rings (see Figure 8.2). Methoxylation of the benzene ring apparently adds psychedelic properties to the drug, presumably due to agonist effects at the 5-HT$_{2A}$ receptor.

When taken orally, mescaline is rapidly and completely absorbed, and significant concentrations are usually achieved in the brain within 1 to 2 hours. Between 3.5 and 4 hours after drug intake mescaline produces an acute psychotomimetic state, with prominent effects on the visual system. The effects of a single dose of mescaline persist for approximately 10 hours. The drug does not appear to be metabolized before it is excreted.

The usual oral dose (5 milligrams per kilogram body weight) in the average normal subject causes anxiety, sympathomimetic effects, hyperreflexia of the limbs, tremors, and visual hallucinations that consist of brightly colored lights, geometric designs, animals, and occasionally people; color and space perception is often concomitantly impaired, but otherwise the sensorium is normal and insight is retained.

Synthetic Amphetamine Derivatives

MDMA ("Ecstasy"), and 2C-B, DOM, MDA, DMA, MDE, TMA, AMT, and 5-MeO-DIPT, are structurally related to mescaline and methamphetamine (see Figure 8.2) and, as might be expected, produce similar effects. They have moderate behavioral stimulant effects at low doses, but as with LSD, psychedelic effects dominate as doses increase. These derivatives are considerably more potent and more toxic than mescaline.

MDMA: The Prototype Catecholamine Psychedelic

The German pharmaceutical company E. Merck developed MDMA (methylenedioxy-methamphetamine; "ecstasy") in about 1914, as an appetite suppressant, but this indication was not pursued. In the 1950s, during the Cold War, the United States military tested it on animals as a possible "brainwashing" drug. By the 1970s there was interest in it as a therapeutic aid for patients undergoing psychological treatment and by the 1980s college students started experimenting with the drug. It is most associated with the social phenomenon of the "rave," which usually refers to a large party, with perhaps hundreds of participants, often held in a warehouse or dance hall, and which involves all-night dancing, accompanied by videos and light shows.

MDMA resembles MDA in structure but may be less hallucinogenic. It is a releaser and/or reuptake inhibitor of the monoamines (5-HT, dopamine, and norepinephrine) as well as acetylcholine (Grilly and Salamone, 2012). As with other psychedelic compounds, the psychological experience is not always predictable. Nevertheless, this drug is most commonly associated with reports of "empathy," "insight," "enhanced communication," and transcendent religious experiences. Most frequent adverse reactions are physiological, such as an increase in blood pressure and heart rate, muscle tension and jaw clenching, fatigue, insomnia, sweating, blurred vision, loss of motor coordination, and anxiety. However, when used during periods of intense activity, such as raves, symptoms of a potentially fatal syndrome called malignant hyperthermia may occur. In addition to the hyperthermia, these symptoms include tachycardia, disorientation, dilated pupils, convulsions, rigidity, breakdown of skeletal muscle, kidney failure, cardiac arrhythmias, and death (Hall and Henry, 2006). MDMA-precipitated malignant hyperthermia may be blocked by a drug called dantrolene (Duffy and Ferguson, 2007), and, should an MDMA-intoxicated, hyperthermic patient be taken to an emergency room in time, dantrolene could be lifesaving. (For a recent review of the thermal effects of MDMA in humans see Parrott, 2012.)

Perhaps because tolerance develops rapidly to MDMA, the drug is not conducive to frequent use. In addition to tolerance, other self-reported, long-term effects include the inability to concentrate, depression of mood, and (paradoxically), "feeling more open toward people" (Grilly and Salamone, 2012, p. 332.)

There is concern about MDMA as reports of ecstasy overdoses at dance clubs and raves have increased. At a 2010 New Year's Eve rave in Los Angeles and then 6 months later at events in the San Francisco Bay area, there were an unusual number of emergency room overdose cases. These incidents are indicative of an increase in overall ecstasy use in the community, which is consistent with the increase in the number of people entering drug treatment programs.

More disturbing are the issues raised by chronic MDMA use. Although categorized as a catecholaminelike psychedelic, it has been established that MDMA is a potent and selective serotonin neurotoxin both in animals and in humans (Gouzoulis-Mayfrank and Daumann, 2009; Urban et al., 2012). Even low doses may be neurotoxic, resulting in small but significant effects on brain microvasculature, white matter maturation, and possible axonal damage (deWin et al., 2008). In regard to specific neural structures, there is some evidence that chronic ecstasy use may produce damage to the hippocampus (den Hollander et al., 2012). Brain scans of ten male ecstasy users, mean age 25.4 years, were compared with scans of seven non-drug-using, matched control persons, mean age 21.3 years. The ecstasy users had taken an average of 281 tablets during the last 6.5 years, but were drug free for a mean of 2 months when tested. The hippocampal volume of the ecstasy users was on average 10.5 percent smaller than that of the control group. Even though this might be considered a modest (albeit statistically significant) difference, the fact that all participants were still young adults, and presumably had many more years of life, is disturbing.

Although the behavioral consequences of such damage are not clear, numerous studies in humans have reported that a variety of memory functions are impaired during MDMA intoxication (Kuypers and Ramaekers, 2005, 2007; Kuypers et al., 2011; Grilly and Salamone, 2012, p. 333), including everyday, real-world, memory function (Hadjiefthyvoulou et al., 2011).

While it may not be surprising that acute MDMA intoxication would impair memory, there is some conflict in regard to the important question of whether or not more long-lasting memory impairment is caused by chronic MDMA use. Many studies of this issue have been criticized because they did not determine if the groups of drug users and nonusers had the same initial performance on the memory tasks before drug use began. Wagner and colleagues (2013) addressed this by testing a cohort of new MDMA users between 2006 and 2009, and then following up with a second assessment after 12 months. Of the initial group of 149 individuals, 109 were available 1 year later. Among these, the only illicit drug used by 43 participants was cannabis, while 23 participants used 10 or more pills of MDMA. When tested with various assessments of learning and memory, these two groups differed only on a task involving recall of visual stimuli. However, even this modest degree of cognitive impairment was not seen by Halpern and colleagues (2011), who compared illicit ecstasy users with nonusers on a battery of 15 neuropsychological tests. This study was designed to minimize the defects of other investigations by excluding persons with "significant" lifetime exposure to other illicit drugs or alcohol; requiring that all participants be members of the "rave" subculture; and by testing breath, urine, and hair samples of all participants at the time of evaluation to exclude possible surreptitious substance use. By implementing these measures, they found little evidence of impaired cognitive function.

The issue of whether MDMA produces cognitive deficits is especially relevant because there is interest in its possible therapeutic use. Since 1986, an organization called the Multidisciplinary Association for Psychedelic Studies (MAPS), a nonprofit research group, has tried to get permission to study the therapeutic potential of psychedelic drugs such as ecstasy, as well as cannabis. In 2011, results of the first completed clinical trial were published, which assessed MDMA as a therapeutic addition to psychotherapy

(Mithoefer et al., 2011, 2013). Twenty patients with chronic posttraumatic stress disorder (PTSD) received the psychotherapy over 20 to 30 sessions; 12 patients also received the drug and 8 received placebo, in 2 of these sessions (lasting 8 hours) scheduled a few weeks apart. Two months later, 10 out of 12 patients who had received the drug responded to treatment, while only 2 out of the 8 placebo patients showed improvement. These 12 patients, plus 7 of the initial placebo patients who subsequently chose to take the drug, participated in a long-term follow-up session. After a mean of 45.4 months since the MDMA session, 16 of those 19 maintained their clinical benefit. On the other hand, a subsequent effort to replicate this result, with 12 different patients suffering from treatment-resistant PTSD, did not produce any significant benefit from the drug.

MDMA Related Substances

Occasionally, new MDMA-related drugs emerge. For example, *2,5-dimethoxy-4-propylthiophenethylamine* (Schifano et al., 2005) is known as Blue Mystic, 2C-T-7, T7, Tripstay, and Tweety-Bird Mescaline; *4-bromo-2,5-dimethoxyphenethylamine* is known as 2C-B, Nexus, 2s, Toonies, Bromo, Spectrum, and Venus. These drugs produce hallucinogenic actions with the side effects of nausea, anxiety, panic attacks, and paranoid ideation. A related agent is 4-methylmethcathinone, or mephedrone ("M-smack"), which has been reported to be substituting for MDMA in Europe (Brunt et al., 2011), and is described in Chapter 7. This drug seems to be a cheaper and less-regulated alternative to cocaine and ecstasy, and its use is currently increasing as abuse of other drugs such as heroin, cannabis, and amphetamine decreases. Mephedrone was banned in the United Kingdom in April 2010, and almost immediately an alternative agent, 5,6-methylenedioxy-2-aminoindane or MDAI, took its place. [After the ban, a survey of over 300 clubbers found that users were more likely to add this drug to other agents, rather than replace established drugs (Moore et al., 2013)]. First synthesized in the 1990s by Dr. David Nichols at Purdue University in the United States, MDAI was discovered accidentally during investigations of MDMA, of which it is an analogue. It is a reuptake inhibitor of serotonin, dopamine, and norepinephrine, and also appears to release serotonin as well, although without producing the neurotoxicity associated with MDMA. In low doses, the drugs MDA, MDMA, and MDAI are hallucinogenic, but at higher doses they exert amphetaminelike pharmacological effects. Proponents speak of enhancing the recreational state particularly in regard to entheogenic (spiritual) experiences, a phenomenon common to this class of drugs. In other words, users describe effects similar to those of MDMA (ecstasy)—euphoria, empathy, and intensification of sensory experiences. However, MDAI has also been linked to reports of renal failure, acute respiratory distress, and hepatic failure. Because the first reports of its recreational use are so recent, not appearing until 2011, there is not yet much information about its prevalence and pattern of use (Gallagher et al., 2012).

Another category of drugs used as ecstasy replacement is the piperazines. Piperazine was originally developed as an antihelminthic (a deworming drug), but the amphetamine-like actions were eventually recognized. The best known are 1-benzylpiperazine (BZP), 1-(3-trifluoromethylphenyl)piperazine (TFMPP), and meta-chlorophenylpiperazine (mCPP) (Bossong et al., 2010). BZP was investigated as a potential antidepressant in the early 1970s but was not effective. The first two drugs are often taken together as a combination "party pill." Both enhance the release of catecholamines, particularly of dopamine, from sympathetic nerve terminals. The increased monoamine concentration activates both central and peripheral α- and β-adrenergic postsynaptic receptors. BZP has primarily dopaminergic and noradrenergic actions, but also inhibits serotonin reuptake. TFMPP has more direct serotonin agonist activity and releases 5-HT from neurons (Rosenbaum et al., 2012). There is limited information on the kinetics of these drugs. BZP doses are typically 75 to 150 milligrams, and the effects last about 6 to 8 hours. Because onset of effect may take up to 2 hours, (with peak plasma concentrations reached 60 to 90 minutes after oral administration) users sometimes take multiple doses before experiencing intoxication, which can be dangerous. Both drugs presumably cross the blood-brain barrier. Elimination is essentially complete in 44 hours for BZP (which is excreted unchanged) and 24 hours for TFMPP (which undergoes many metabolic changes). When taken recreationally, low doses cause stimulant effects while hallucinogenic actions predominate at higher doses (Rosenbaum et al., 2012). Commonly reported symptoms include palpitations, QT prolongation, agitation, anxiety, confusion, dizziness, headache, tremor, mydriasis, insomnia, urine retention, and vomiting. Seizures are induced in some patients even at low doses and have been reported up to 8 hours after administration. Severe multiorgan toxicity has been reported, though fatalities have not been recorded conclusively. Supportive care is crucial. Termination of seizures by benzodiazepines alone may be sufficient (Schep et al., 2011).

Meta-chlorophenylpiperazine is a major metabolite of the psychotropic drug trazodone, and may be responsible for some of its side effects, such as headaches and migraines induced many hours after initial consumption; in fact, it has been used for testing potential antimigraine medications. As a recreational substance, mCPP is actually generally considered to be an unpleasant experience and is not desired by drug users. It lacks any reinforcing effects, produces depressive and anxiogenic effects in rodents and humans, and can induce panic attacks in susceptible individuals. It also worsens obsessive-compulsive symptoms in people with the disorder. It is an agonist at practically all serotonergic receptors, and may also block reuptake of and release serotonin. Its potent anorectic effects have prompted the development of selective 5-HT$_{2C}$ receptor agonists for the treatment of obesity.

4-Bromo-2, 5-dimethoxyphenethylamine (2C-B) is a psychoactive analogue of mescaline that is appearing more frequently at raves and club venues. Reported oral doses of about 20 mg produce perceptual effects similar to those of serotonergic agents and positive effects similar to MDMA (Caudevilla-Gálligo et al., 2012).

DOM (dimethoxymethamphetamine) has effects that are similar to those of mescaline; doses of 1 to 6 milligrams produce euphoria, which is followed by a 6- to 8-hour period of hallucinations. DOM is 100 times more potent than mescaline but much less potent than LSD. The use of DOM is associated with a high incidence of overdose (because it is potent and street doses are poorly controlled). Acute toxic reactions are common; they consist of tremors that may eventually lead to convulsive movements, prostration, and even death. Because toxic reactions are common, the use of DOM is not widespread.

MDA (methylenedioxyamphetamine), *DMA* (dimethoxymethylamphetamine), *MDE* (methylenedioxyethylamphetamine), *TMA* (trimethoxyamphetamine), and other structural variations of amphetamine are encountered as "designer psychedelics." MDA is also a metabolite of MDMA, and much of MDMA's effect may be due to the presence of MDA.

In general, the pharmacological effects of these drugs resemble those of mescaline and LSD; they reflect a mix of catecholamine and serotonin interactions. Side effects and toxicities (including fatalities) are similar to those of MDMA. MDA is sometimes represented as MDMA; when this occurs, MDA is more lethal in lower doses and its effects are longer lasting than those of MDMA. Confirmation of the well-established visual effects of MDA was recently obtained from the first human study to be conducted with this drug in over 30 years (Baggott et al., 2010). Consistent with typical anecdotal descriptions, MDA increased self-reports of "mystical" types of hallucinogenic effects, including visual alterations.

AMT and 5-MeO-DIPT. In April 2003, the Drug Enforcement Administration (DEA) designated alpha-methyltryptamine (AMT) and 5-methoxy-diisopropyltryptamine (5-MeO-DIPT, or Foxy) as Schedule I substances under the Controlled Substances Act. This classification for these "new" psychedelics implies high abuse potential with no therapeutic usefulness. Administered orally, both drugs cause hallucinations, mood elevation, nervousness, insomnia, and pupillary dilation. AMT is of slow onset (3 to 4 hours) after oral administration and prolonged duration (12 to 24 hours). It is also a potent reuptake inhibitor of norepinephrine, dopamine, and serotonin (Nagai et al., 2007).

Foxy is of more rapid onset (20 to 30 minutes) and shorter duration (3 to 6 hours). It has been reported to induce an acute confusional state for several hours (Itokawa et al., 2007) and to substitute for MDMA.

Myristicin and Elemicin

Nutmeg and mace are common household spices sometimes abused for their hallucinogenic properties. Myristicin and elemicin, the pharmacologically active ingredients in nutmeg and mace, are responsible for the psychedelic action. Ingestion of large amounts (1 to 2 teaspoons—5 to 15 grams—usually brewed in tea) may, after a delay of 2 to 5 hours, induce feelings of unreality, confusion, disorientation, impending doom, depersonalization, euphoria, visual hallucinations, and acute psychotic reactions. Considering the close structural resemblance of myristicin and elemicin to mescaline (see Figure 8.2), these psychedelic actions are not unexpected. Ingestion of large quantities of nutmeg, however, produces many unpleasant side effects, including vomiting, nausea, and tremors, although deaths are infrequent.

Serotonergic Psychedelics

The predominant serotoninlike psychedelic drugs are *lysergic acid diethylamide* (LSD), *psilocybin* and *psilocin, dimethyltryptamine* (DMT), and *bufotenine* (Figure 8.3). Because of their structural resemblance to one another and to serotonin, it has been presumed that these agents exert their effects through interactions at serotonin 5-HT$_2$ receptors (Geyer and Vollenweider, 2008). Nevertheless, their specific mechanism of action has been difficult to determine. It is generally accepted that the subjective effects are mediated by postsynaptic 5-HT$_2$ receptors. This is consistent with the observation that the

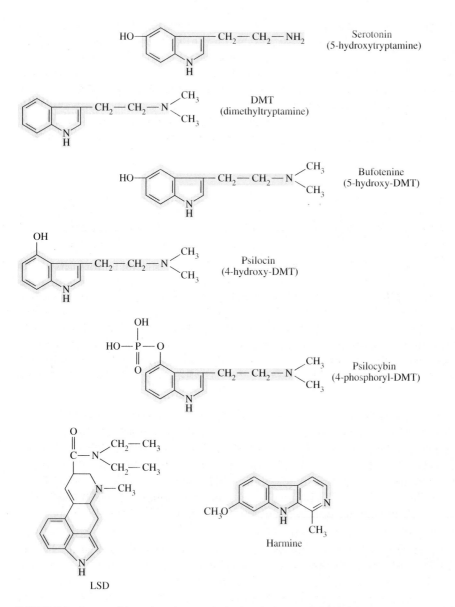

FIGURE 8.3 Structural formulas of serotonin (a chemical transmitter) and six serotoninlike psychedelic drugs. These six drugs are structurally related to serotonin (as indicated by the shading) and are thought to exert their psychedelic actions through alterations of serotonin synapses in the brain. Although LSD is structurally much more complex than serotonin, the basic similarity of the two molecules is apparent.

affinity for these receptors is highly correlated with their hallucinogenic potency in humans, and, with the fact that many, but not all, 5-HT$_2$ antagonists block this effect. Current evidence suggests that 5-HT$_{1A}$, 5-HT$_{2A}$, and 5-HT$_{2C}$ receptor subtypes may all be involved in the hallucinogenic effects, that some of these receptors may be located pre-synaptically and some postsynaptically, and, that, depending on the receptor, some of the drugs may act as agonists, partial agonists, or antagonists (Grilly and Salamone, 2012, p. 326). There is also evidence from nonhuman studies that these drugs exert their hal-lucinogenic effects in the brain by acting on the locus coeruleus and the cerebral cortex.

Lysergic Acid Diethylamide: The Prototype Serotonergic Psychedelic

During the mid-1960s and early 1970s, lysergic acid diethylamide (LSD) became one of the most remarkable and controversial drugs known. In doses that are so small that they might even be considered infinitesimal, LSD induces remarkable psychological changes, enhancing self-awareness and altering internal reality, while causing relatively few altera-tions in the general physiology of the body.

Historical Background. LSD was first synthesized in 1938 by Albert Hofmann, a Swiss chemist, as part of an organized research program to investigate possible therapeutic uses of compounds obtained from ergot, a natural product derived from a fungus (*Claviceps purpurea*). Early pharmacological studies of LSD in animals failed to reveal anything unusual; the psychedelic action was neither sought nor expected. Thus, LSD remained unnoticed until 1943, when Hofmann had an unusual experience:

> In the afternoon of 16 April, 1943, . . . I was seized by a peculiar sensation of vertigo and restlessness. Objects, as well as the shape of my associates in the laboratory, appeared to undergo optical changes. I was unable to concentrate on my work. In a dreamlike state I left for home, where an irresistible urge to lie down overcame me. I drew the curtains and immediately fell into a peculiar state similar to drunkenness, characterized by an exagger-ated imagination. With my eyes closed, fantastic pictures of extraordinary plasticity and intensive color seemed to surge toward me. After two hours, this state gradually wore off. (Hofmann, 1994, p. 80)

Hofmann correctly hypothesized that his experience had resulted from the accidental ingestion of LSD. To confirm that conclusion, he self-administered what seemed to be a minuscule oral dose (only 0.25 milligram). We now know, however, that this dose is about ten times the dose required to induce psychedelic effects in most people. As a result of this miscalculation, his response was quite spectacular:

> After 40 minutes, I noted the following symptoms in my laboratory journal: slight gid-diness, restlessness, difficulty in concentration, visual disturbances, laughing. . . . Later, I lost all count of time. I noticed with dismay that my environment was undergoing progressive changes. My visual field wavered and everything appeared deformed as in a faulty mirror. Space and time became more and more disorganized and I was overcome by a fear that I was going out of my mind. The worst part of it [was] that I was clearly aware of my condition. My power of observation was unimpaired. . . . Occasionally, I felt

as if I were out of my body. I thought I had died. My ego seemed suspended somewhere in space, from where I saw my dead body lying on the sofa. . . . It was particularly striking how acoustic perceptions, such as the noise of water gushing from a tap or the spoken word, were transformed into optical illusions. I then fell asleep and awakened the next morning somewhat tired but otherwise feeling perfectly well. (p. 80)

This description of the sensory distortions elicited by serotonergic psychedelic drugs remains consistent with current reports. Dr. Hoffman died in 2008 at the age of 102.

The first North American study of LSD in humans was conducted in 1949, and during the 1950s large quantities of LSD were distributed to scientists for research purposes. A significant impetus for research was the notion that the effects of LSD might constitute a model for psychosis, which would provide some insight into the biochemical and physiological processes of schizophrenia and its treatment (Passie et al., 2008). However, that was not the case. Drug-induced hallucinations are mostly visual and usually involve distortions of the environment that are generally considered pleasant or neutral. The person taking LSD is very suggestible and concerned about relationships to other people. In contrast, schizophrenic hallucinations are usually auditory, often unpleasant and threatening, and are derived from the user's internal mental state, not from the external environmental context. Schizophrenic patients are not very suggestible and are not greatly affected by interpersonal interactions. People with schizophrenia who have taken LSD acknowledge that it is different from a psychotic experience (Grilly and Salamone, 2012, p. 330).

Some therapists tried LSD as an adjunct to psychotherapy to help patients verbalize their problems and gain some insight into the underlying causes. These investigations reported positive outcomes in people with alcohol or other addictions, in patients dealing with the emotional and physical pain of terminal illnesses, and in people with other psychological problems. Although initial reports were promising, this therapeutic approach died out. Several reasons have been proposed for this lack of follow-up. First, the psychiatric profession did not develop reliable protocols and measures for the consistent therapeutic use of these agents. Second, the dramatic increase in recreational use of the psychedelic drugs in the 1960s, epitomized by the phrase coined by Dr. Timothy Leary, "turn on, tune in, and drop out," led to the perception that such drugs were a public health problem. In 1966, LSD was made illegal and possession was eventually determined to be a felony. By the 1970s, LSD was one of many street drugs and part of the illicit drug culture (Grilly and Salamone, 2012, p. 324). Third, the Central Intelligence Agency (CIA) and other government agencies conducted top-secret experiments between 1953 and throughout the 1970s, in which high doses of potent psychedelic drugs were given to unwitting servicemen as part of research programs prompted by concerns about Cold War enemies. Some of these soldiers eventually sued the United States government, with varied success, for mental or emotional problems they suffered as a result of these involuntary drug exposures. One of the most dramatic cases resulting from those unethical experiments was the case of Frank Olsson, an Army scientist, who died after falling out of a New York hotel window in 1953, 9 days after he was given LSD without his knowledge. His family was told he committed suicide, but in 1975 a commission appointed by President Ford disclosed for the first time that Olsson had been an unwitting drug subject. In 1996, the Manhattan District Attorney's Office opened a homicide investigation, but was unable to bring charges.

As a result of these social and cultural developments, LSD and similar psychedelic drugs were placed in the Schedule I category of abused substances not generally considered useful in a therapeutic context.

Nevertheless, experimentation continued and has culminated in renewed interest in studying possible therapeutic indications of psychedelic drugs. In particular, there has been a resurgence of studies with psilocybin as an adjunct to psychotherapy for depression and end-of-life anxiety in cancer patients, for posttraumatic stress disorder, and for addiction to drugs or alcohol (Bogenschutz and Pommy 2012). Some studies, conducted in healthy persons, have replicated historical descriptions of "mystical experiences" (McLean et al., 2011) and other emotionally positive effects of vivid imagery produced by psilocybin (Carhart-Harris et al., 2012; Studerus et al., 2012). In a small study of 12 patients with anxiety associated with advanced-stage cancer, psilocybin improved anxiety and mood for up to 3 months after administration (Grob et al., 2011). One review of clinical trials for alcoholism concluded that even one dose of LSD, given in conjunction with other treatment, was useful in reducing alcohol misuse (Krebs and Johansen, 2012). It remains to be seen if these reports lead to useful therapeutic approaches. For those interested in learning more about the history and proposed clinical applications, several books have recently been published (Sessa, 2012; Brown, 2013; Roberts, 2013).

Did You Know?

Pont-Saint-Esprit Poisoning: Did the CIA Spread LSD?

On August 16, 1951, postman Leon Armunier was doing his rounds in the southern French town of Pont-Saint-Esprit when he was suddenly overwhelmed by nausea and wild hallucinations.

"It was terrible. I had the sensation of shrinking and shrinking, and the fire and the serpents coiling around my arms," he remembers.

Armunier, now 87, fell off his bike and was taken to the hospital in Avignon. He was put in a straitjacket. He shared a room with three teenagers who had been chained to their beds to keep them under control.

"Some of my friends tried to get out of the window. They were thrashing wildly . . . screaming, and the sound of the metal beds and the jumping up and down . . . the noise was terrible. I'd prefer to die rather than go through that again."

Over the coming days, dozens of other people in the town fell prey to similar symptoms. Doctors at the time concluded that bread at one of the town's bakeries had become contaminated by ergot, a poisonous fungus that occurs naturally on rye.

Biological Warfare

That view remained largely unchallenged until 2009, when an American investigative journalist, Hank Albarelli, revealed a CIA document labeled: "Re: Pont-Saint-Esprit and F. Olson Files. SO Span/France Operation file, inclusive Olson. Intel files. Hand carry to Belin—tell him to see to it that these are buried."

F. Olson is Frank Olson, a CIA scientist who, at the time of the Pont-St-Esprit incident, led research for the agency into the drug LSD. David Belin, meanwhile, was executive director of the Rockefeller Commission created by the White House in 1975 to investigate abuses carried out worldwide by the CIA.

Albarelli believes the Pont-Saint-Esprit and F. Olson Files mentioned in the document would show—if they had not been "buried"—that the CIA was experimenting on the townspeople, by dosing them with LSD.

The conclusion drawn at the time was that one of the town's bakeries, the Roch Briand, was the source of the poisoning. It is possible, Albarelli says, that LSD was put in the bread.

It is well known that biological warfare scientists around the world, including some in Britain, were experimenting with LSD in the early 1950s—a time of conflict in Korea and an escalation of Cold War tensions.

Albarelli says he has found a top secret report issued in 1949 by the research director of the Edgewood Arsenal, where many U.S. government LSD experiments were carried out, which states that the army should do everything possible to launch "field experiments" using the drug.

The local hospital where some of the victims were taken in 1951 has been closed. Using Freedom of Information legislation, Albarelli also got hold of another CIA report from 1954. In it an agent reported his conversation with a representative of the Sandoz chemical company in Switzerland. Sandoz's base, which is just a few hundred kilometers from Pont-Saint-Esprit, was the only place where LSD was being produced at that time. The agent reports that after several drinks, the Sandoz representative abruptly stated: "The Pont-Saint-Esprit 'secret' is that it was not the bread at all. . . . It was not grain ergot."

"Wrong Symptoms"

But American academic Professor Steven Kaplan, who published a book in 2008 on the Pont-Saint-Esprit incident, insists that neither ergot nor LSD could have been responsible.

Ergot contamination would not, he says, have affected only one sack of grain in one bakery, as was claimed here. The outbreak would have been far more widespread. He rules out LSD on the grounds that the symptoms people suffered, though similar, do not quite fit the drug. He also points out that it would not have survived the fierce temperatures of the baker's oven—though Albarelli counters that it could have been added to the bread after baking.

While they disagree on the cause of the hallucinations, on one point Kaplan and Albarelli are united—the need for a French government inquiry to get to the bottom of what really happened in Pont-Saint-Esprit all those years ago.

Pharmacokinetics. LSD is usually taken orally, and it is rapidly absorbed by that route. Usual doses range from about 25 micrograms to more than 300 micrograms. Because the amounts are so small, LSD is often attached to other substances, such as squares of paper, the backs of stamps, or sugar cubes, which can be handled more easily. LSD is absorbed within about 60 minutes, reaching peak blood levels in about 3 hours. It is distributed rapidly and efficiently throughout the body, diffuses easily into the brain, and readily crosses the placenta. The largest amounts of LSD in the body are found in the liver, where the drug is metabolized, before it is excreted, to 2-oxo-3-hydroxy-LSD. The usual duration of action is 6 to 8 hours.

Because of its extreme potency, conventional urine screening tests are inadequate to detect LSD. When the use of LSD is suspected, urine is collected (up to 30 hours after ingestion) and an ultrasensitive radioimmunoassay is performed to verify the presence of the drug.

Physiological Effects. Although the LSD experience is characterized by its psychological effects, subtle physiological changes also occur. The *somatic phase* occurs after absorption of the drug and consists of CNS stimulation and autonomic changes that are predominantly sympathomimetic in nature. A person who takes LSD may experience a slight increase in body temperature; dilation of the pupils; slightly increased heart rate and blood pressure; increased levels of glucose in the blood; and dizziness, drowsiness, nausea, and other effects that, although noticeable, seldom interfere with the psychedelic experience.

LSD has a low level of toxicity; the effective dose is about 50 micrograms, while the lethal dose is about 14,000 micrograms. These figures provide a therapeutic ratio of 280, making the drug a remarkably nonlethal compound; consequently most deaths attributed to LSD result from accidents, homicides, or suicide. The use of LSD during pregnancy is certainly unwise, although a distinct fetal LSD syndrome has not been described.

Psychological Effects. The psychological effects of LSD are intense. Doses of 25 to 50 micrograms produce alterations in perception, thinking, emotion, arousal, and self-image. The *sensory* (or *perceptual*) *phase* is characterized by sensory distortions and pseudohallucinations, which are the effects desired by the drug user. Time is slowed or distorted. Sensory input is intensified with enhanced visualization of previously seen or imagined objects and decreased vigilance and logical thought. Visual alterations are the most characteristic phenomena; they typically include colored lights, distorted perceptions, and vivid and fascinating images and shapes. Colors can be heard and sounds may be seen.

The *psychic phase* signals a maximum drug effect, with changes in mood, disruption of thought processes, altered perception of time, depersonalization, true hallucinations, and psychotic episodes. The loss of boundaries and the fear of fragmentation create a need for a structuring or supporting environment and experienced companions. During the "trip," distressing thoughts and memories can emerge. Mood may be labile, shifting from depression to gaiety, from elation to fear. Tension and anxiety may mount and reach panic proportions. Such an experience is considered a "bad trip."

Tolerance and Dependence. Tolerance of both the psychological and physiological alterations induced by LSD readily and rapidly develops, and cross-tolerance occurs between LSD and other psychedelics. Tolerance is lost within several days after the user stops taking the drug.

Physical dependence on LSD does not develop, even when the drug is used repeatedly for a prolonged period of time. In fact, most heavy users of the drug say that they ceased using LSD because they tired of it, had no further need for it, or had had enough. Even when the drug is discontinued because of concern about bad trips or about physical or mental harm, few withdrawal signs are exhibited. Laboratory animals do not self-administer LSD.

Adverse Reactions and Toxicity. Unpleasant experiences with LSD may involve an uncontrollable drift into confusion, or dissociative, psychotic, or acute panic reactions, perhaps triggered by a reliving of earlier traumatic experiences. One unique characteristic of LSD and related substances is the recurrence, after the immediate effect of the hallucinogen has worn off, of some of the symptoms that appeared during the intoxication. These symptoms are mainly visual and the terms *flashback* and *hallucinogen persisting perception disorder* (HPPD) are used fairly interchangeably. However, a flashback is usually a short-term, nondistressing, spontaneous, recurrent, reversible, and benign condition accompanied by a pleasant affect. In contrast, HPPD is a generally long-term, distressing, spontaneous, recurrent, pervasive, either slowly reversible or irreversible nonbenign condition accompanied by an unpleasant dysphoric affect (Johnson et al., 2008). Although these phenomena can occur without warning, they are most likely to appear just before sleep or when a person enters a dark environment.

Treatment of flashbacks and HPPD has been symptomatic. Case reports note the success of benzodiazepines as well as other drugs, but there is no consensus on appropriate therapy and no specific treatment. Most commonly, an atypical antipsychotic drug with serotonin-2 blocking activity (see Chapter 11) is chosen to treat both acute LSD toxicity and HPPD, although older literature has reported exacerbation of LSD-like panic and visual symptoms.

Other Serotoninlike Hallucinogens

DMT. DMT (dimethyltryptamine) is a short-acting, naturally occurring psychedelic compound that can be synthesized easily and is structurally related to serotonin. DMT produces LSD-like effects in the user, and like LSD it is a partial agonist at 5-HT$_2$ receptors. Widely used throughout much of the world, DMT is an active component of various types of South American plants, such as *Virola calophylla* and *Mimosa hostilis*. Used by itself, DMT is snorted or smoked, often in a marijuana cigarette. After the 30-minute period of effect, the user returns to normal feelings and perceptions—thus the nicknames *lunch-hour drug*, *businessman's lunch*, and *businessman's LSD*.

Interestingly, although DMT is commonly thought to exert its psychedelic effect through action of 5-HT$_{2A}$ receptors, Su and coworkers (2009) demonstrated binding to sigma-1 receptors as a possible mode of action.[2]

In 1994, Strassman and coworkers conducted controlled investigations of DMT in "highly motivated," experienced hallucinogen users. When it was administered intravenously (0.04 to 0.4 milligram per kilogram of body weight), onset of action occurred within 2 minutes and was negligible at 30 minutes. DMT elevated blood pressure, heart rate, and temperature; dilated pupils; and increased body endorphin and hormone levels. The psychedelic threshold dose was 0.2 milligram per kilogram of body weight.

---

[2] Formerly thought to be a type of opioid receptor, the sigma-1 receptor is actually an endoplasmic reticulum protein implicated in neuroprotection, neuronal plasticity, anxiety, and depression (Hashimoto, 2009; Maurice and Su, 2009; Paschos et al., 2009;).

Hallucinogenic effects included a rapidly moving, brightly colored visual display of images. Auditory effects were less common. "Loss of control," associated with a brief but overwhelming "rush," led to a dissociated state, in which euphoria alternated or coexisted with anxiety.

DMT is one of two main ingredients in *ayahuasca* (also called *hoasca*), a psychoactive beverage that, as a tea, has been drunk for centuries in religious, spiritual, and medicinal contexts by Amazon Indians in the rainforests of South America. The other main ingredient is harmine, a substance that is a potent monoamine oxidase, or MAO, inhibitor. Effects have an onset of about 30 to 60 minutes, peak at 1 to 2 hours, and persist for about 3 to 4 hours. In most cases, effects are well tolerated, but disorientation, paranoia, and anxiety may occur. In religious ceremonial use, such reactions are unusual (Gable, 2007).

Bufotenine. Bufotenine (5-hydroxy DMT, or dimethylserotonin), like LSD and DMT, is a potent serotonin agonist hallucinogen with an affinity for several types of serotonin receptors, especially the 5-HT$_{2A}$ receptor. The name bufotenine comes from the name for a toad of the genus *Bufo,* whose skin and glandular secretions supposedly produce hallucinogenic effects when ingested.

After subcutaneous injection into rats, the half-life of bufotenine is about 2 hours, with MAO responsible for metabolism. Bufotenine is not found in the bodies of normal people. However, it can be produced in an alternative and unusual pathway for the metabolic breakdown of serotonin. Indeed, some have attempted to correlate the presence of bufotenine in urine with various psychiatric disorders, although this theory is not generally accepted.

Psilocybin. Psilocybin (4-phosphoryl-DMT) and psilocin (4-hydroxy-DMT) are two psychedelic agents that are found in many species of mushrooms that belong to the genera *Psilocybe, Panaeolus, Copelandia,* and *Conocybe.* As Figure 8.3 shows, the only difference between psilocybin and psilocin is that psilocybin contains a molecule of phosphoric acid. After the mushroom has been ingested, phosphoric acid is enzymatically removed from psilocybin, thus producing psilocin, the active psychedelic agent.

Psilocybin exerts an agonist effect at serotonin 5-HT$_{2A}$ and 5-HT$_{1A}$ receptors, similar to the effects of other serotonin psychedelics, at about 0.25 milligram per kilogram of body weight, when ingested. Psilocybin-containing mushrooms grow throughout much of the world, including the northwestern United States. Psilocin and psilocybin are approximately 1/200th as potent as LSD; their effects peak in about 2 hours and last about 6 to 10 hours. Unlike DMT, psilocin and psilocybin are absorbed effectively when taken orally; the mushrooms are eaten raw to induce psychedelic effects.

There is great variation in the concentration of psilocybin and psilocin among the different species of mushrooms, as well as significant differences among mushrooms of the same species. For example, the usual oral dose of *Psilocybe semilanceata* (liberty caps) may consist of 10 to 40 mushrooms, while the dose for *Psilocybe cyanescens* may be only 2 to 5 mushrooms. Also, some extremely toxic species of mushrooms are not psychoactive, but they bear a superficial resemblance to the mushrooms that contain psilocybin and psilocin. Because the effects of psilocybin so closely resemble those produced by LSD, the "psilocybin" sold illicitly may *be* LSD, and ordinary mushrooms laced with LSD may be sold as "magic mushrooms."

Although the psychedelic effects of *Psilocybe mexicana* are part of Indian folklore, *Psilocybe* intoxication was not described until 1955, when Gordon Wasson, a New York banker, traveled through Mexico. He mingled with native tribes and was allowed to participate in a *Psilocybe* ceremony, during which he consumed the magic mushroom and described his own hallucinatory experience.

Ololiuqui. Ololiuqui is a naturally occurring substance in morning glory seeds that is used by Central and South American Indians as an intoxicant and hallucinogen. The drug is used ritually for spiritual communication, as are extracts of most plants that contain psychedelic drugs. The use of ololiuqui seeds in Central and South America was first described by the sixteenth-century Spanish explorer Francisco Hernandez de Cordoba, who is said to have reported, "When the priests wanted to commune with their Gods, they ate ololiuqui seeds and a thousand visions and satanic hallucinations appeared to them."

The seeds were analyzed in Europe by Albert Hofmann, the discoverer of LSD, who identified several components, one of which was lysergic acid amide (not lysergic acid diethylamide, LSD). The lysergic acid amide that Hofmann identified is approximately one-tenth as active as LSD as a psychoactive agent. However, considering the extreme potency of LSD, lysergic acid amide is still quite potent.

Side effects of ololiuqui include nausea, vomiting, headache, increased blood pressure, dilated pupils, and sleepiness. These side effects are usually quite intense and serve to limit the recreational use of ololiuqui. Ingestion of 100 or more seeds produces sleepiness, distorted perception, hallucinations, and confusion. Flashbacks have been reported, but they are infrequent.

Harmine. Harmine is a psychedelic agent that is obtained from the seeds of *Peganum harmala,* a plant native to the Middle East, and from *Banisteriopsis caapi* of the South American tropics. Intoxication by harmine is usually accompanied by nausea.

Glutaminergic NMDA Receptor Antagonists

Phencyclidine and Ketamine

Phencyclidine (PCP, angel dust) and ketamine ("Special K"), shown in Figure 8.4, are structurally unrelated to other psychedelic drugs. They were first developed as safer surgical anesthetics, because they produce less respiratory depression. This was successful in that, unlike other anesthetics, the lethal dose of PCP is ten times the anesthetic dose, and, at appropriate doses it also reduces pain reactions while maintaining blood pressure and heart rate. Unfortunately however, it was later found that these two drugs also produced a unique psychedelic or dissociative state.

Phencyclidine was developed in 1956 and was briefly used as an anesthetic in humans before being abandoned because of a high incidence of psychiatric reactions, described below, but is still used as a veterinary anesthetic. *Ketamine* (Ketalar), which resembles

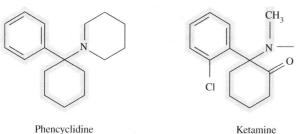

FIGURE 8.4 Structural formulas of the psychedelic anesthetic drugs phencyclidine and ketamine.

Phencyclidine   Ketamine

phencyclidine structurally, was developed shortly after the prominent psychedelic properties of phencyclidine were identified, as a replacement. Introduced in 1960, ketamine induces a phencyclidinelike anesthetic state in low doses, with similar but less severe psychiatric side effects. Ketamine is still used in special situations, such as in pediatric and in veterinary anesthesia, and in the field (where there is limited equipment to counter respiratory depression). It is also occasionally used in patients who cannot tolerate the cardiovascular depressant effects of other anesthetics.

Currently, ketamine has shown some evidence that it might represent a new class of antidepressant. Injections of ketamine appear to produce rapid antidepressant effects in treatment-resistant patients. Unfortunately, so far, even patients who responded repeatedly relapsed within weeks. Nevertheless, research into this possible therapeutic action is ongoing.

In addition to possible antidepressant use, the altered perception, disorganized thought, cognitive dysfunction, suspiciousness, confusion, and lack of cooperation elicited by these drugs resembles both the positive and negative symptoms of a schizophrenic state. In fact, both PCP and ketamine can induce symptoms that are almost indistinguishable from those associated with schizophrenia (Mouri et al., 2007) and they exacerbate psychosis in schizophrenia patients, although infrequent users do not develop schizophrenia. Nevertheless, this phenomenon has led to a glutamatergic model of schizophrenia (see Chapter 11) and experimental evaluation of glutamatergic agents as antipsychotic medications.

Abuse of phencyclidine and ketamine began in the mid-1960s (Wolff and Winstock, 2006) but was not common until the 1990s, when ketamine showed up as an adulterant to ecstasy tablets. Phencyclidine may be sold as crystal, angel dust, hog, PCP, THC, cannabinol, or mescaline. When sold as crystal or angel dust (terms also used for methamphetamine), concentrations vary between 50 percent and 90 percent; when purchased under other names or in concoctions, the amount of PCP falls to between 10 percent and 30 percent; the typical street dose is about 5 milligrams. Phencyclidine can be eaten, snorted, or injected (usually intramuscularly, rarely intravenously), but it is most often smoked, or sprinkled on tobacco, parsley, or marijuana. Ketamine is typically not taken orally because it is metabolized to norketamine, which is less psychedelic and more sedative. Currently, these are increasing in popularity as club drugs.

Pharmacokinetics. When smoked, peak effects occur in about 15 minutes, when about 40 percent of the dose appears in the user's bloodstream. Oral absorption of PCP is slow; maximum blood levels are reached in about 2 hours. The elimination half-life is about 18 hours but ranges from about 11 to about 51 hours. A positive urine assay is assumed to indicate that PCP was used within the previous week. Because false-positive test results are common, a positive assay requires secondary confirmation.

Mechanism of Action. Phencyclidine and ketamine both exert their psychotomimetic, analgesic, and amnestic actions primarily as a result of binding as noncompetitive antagonists of the N-methyl-D-aspartate (NMDA)/glutamate receptors. In addition, these drugs may block acetylcholine receptors, may block dopamine reuptake, induce dopamine release, and act as a partial agonist at dopamine 2 receptors (Morgan and Curran, 2011). These actions prompted the current view that NMDA receptor dysfunction is involved in the pathophysiology of schizophrenia (see Chapter 11).

Phencyclidine and ketamine inhibit NMDA receptors by two mechanisms: (1) blockade of the open channel by occupying a site within the channel in the receptor protein (as discussed earlier for phencyclidine), and (2) reduction in the frequency of NMDA channel opening by binding to a second attachment site on the outside of the receptor protein. As noted, PCP and ketamine are powerful analgesic drugs. The mechanism seems to be twofold: these two drugs (1) block NMDA-glutamate receptors in the spinal cord and (2) activate descending analgesic pathways, pathways that appear to involve norepinephrine and dopamine.

Psychological Effects. Phencyclidine and ketamine are termed "dissociative anesthetics." This means that the analgesia, amnesia, and sensory distortions occur without loss of consciousness. That is, they produce an unresponsive state with intense analgesia and amnesia, although the subject's eyes remain open (with a blank stare) and the subject may even appear to be awake. Phencyclidine in low doses (1 to 5 milligrams) produces mild agitation, euphoria, disinhibition, or excitement in a person who appears to be grossly drunk and exhibits a blank stare. The subject may be rigid and unable to speak. In many cases, however, the subject is communicative but does not respond to pain. At low doses ketamine produces similar effects; distortions of time and space, hallucinations, and mild dissociative effects. Quotes from users describe its effects as "melting into the surroundings," "visual hallucinations," "out-of-body experiences," and "giggliness." At large doses ketamine induces a more severe dissociation referred to as the "k-hole," in which the detachment experienced by users is so intense that their perceptions appear completely divorced from their previous reality (Morgan and Curran, 2011). Subjects may become withdrawn, negativistic, and unable to maintain a cognitive set; they manifest concrete, impoverished, idiosyncratic, and bizarre responses to questions.

High doses induce a state of coma or stupor. However, abusers tend to titrate their dose to maximize the intoxicant effect while attempting to avoid unconsciousness. Blood pressure usually becomes elevated, but respiration does not become depressed. The patient may recover within 2 to 4 hours, although a state of confusion and cognitive poverty may last for 8 to 72 hours. The disruption of sensory input by PCP causes unpredictable, exaggerated, distorted, or violent reactions to environmental stimuli, which may be augmented by PCP-induced analgesia and amnesia. Massive oral overdoses, involving up to

1 gram of street-purchased PCP, result in prolonged periods of stupor or coma followed by a prolonged recovery phase marked by confusion and delusions lasting as long as 2 weeks. In some people, this state of confusion may be followed by a psychosis that lasts from several weeks to a few months.

Side Effects and Toxicity. With regard to lethality, these drugs have a wide margin of safety. For ketamine there have been no adverse outcomes even in medical settings with marked overdoses. Even coughing and swallowing reflexes are maintained. The highest mortality risk comes from accidental death due to dissociation and analgesia, but there is little scientific data available, even on emergency room (ER) presentations of ketamine toxicity. However, one study reported on 233 ER cases (with an average age of 22 years, two-thirds of whom were male) with impaired consciousness in 45 percent; abdominal pain in 21 percent; lower urinary tract symptoms in 12 percent; and dizziness in 12 percent.

On the other hand, ketamine-induced ulcerative colitis of the bladder is a recently identified and potentially severe condition of chronic use. Symptoms include frequency and urgency of urination, incontinence, and sometimes painful passing of blood in the urine. Although it is difficult to get accurate information, there is some evidence that 50 percent of users have sought medical attention for ketamine-induced cystitis. One-third of the cases resolved after cessation of drug use, one-third stabilized, and one-third continued to worsen. Another emerging condition of high-dose ketamine use is water on the kidney (hydronephrosis). In one study, one-third of chronic users also reported "k-cramps," intense abdominal pain associated with bile duct abnormality.

Cognitive impairment occurs in humans even with a single dose, but recreational use is not associated with long-term cognitive impairment, as 1-year-abstinent ex-ketamine users did not show deficits (Morgan and Curran, 2011).

Treatment of Intoxication. Therapy for PCP/ketamine intoxication is aimed at reducing the systemic level of the drug, keeping the patient calm and sedated, and preventing severe adverse medical effects. Sensory inputs should be minimized by placing the intoxicated person in a quiet environment, with physical restraint if necessary to prevent self-injury. Agitation can be reduced with either a benzodiazepine or an atypical antipsychotic. Hyperthermia, hypertension, convulsions, renal failure, and other medical consequences should be treated as necessary. PCP/ketamine-induced psychotic states may be long-lasting, especially in people with a history of schizophrenia.

Tolerance to PCP/ketamine does develop, but gradually; escalation of abused doses may be due to behavioral adaptations that compensate for the disruptive effects of the drug rather than a direct physiological action. The incidence of dependence is not known. A specific withdrawal syndrome has not been described and cravings seem to be the most common symptom.

Methoxetamine

This ketamine analogue first appeared in 2010, and there is not much medical literature as yet. Presumably it acts like ketamine, as a noncompetitive antagonist of the NMDA receptor with dopamine reuptake properties. It is taken orally, inserted rectally, insufflated (snorted), or injected intramuscularly. Doses depend on route of administration: 20 to 100 milligrams orally and 10 to 50 milligrams by intramuscular injection. After insufflation the effect may be delayed, prompting users to take more because they believe the first dose was inadequate. Users have stated that the effects begin in about 5 to 10 minutes after injection and last from 1 to 2 hours, compared with 5 to 7 hours after insufflation. Effects include euphoria, and the perceptual hallucinations typical of ketamine, as well as an "opiatelike" effect. It seems to have less analgesic and anesthetic properties than ketamine, but a longer duration of action (Corazza et al., 2012). Undesirable reactions are primarily gastrointestinal (nausea, vomiting, diarrhea), paranoia and anxiety, tachycardia, and nystagmus. Respiratory depression, reduction of phantom limb pain, and antidepressant effects have also been reported. As with ketamine and PCP, treatment consists of supportive care, benzodiazepines, fluids, and antiemetics as needed (Rosenbaum et al., 2012; Troy, 2013).

Dextromethorphan (DXM)

DXM is a common ingredient in more than 140 varieties of over-the-counter cough suppressants such as various Coricidin products, Robitussin DM, Vicks 44, Tylenol DM, and many others. Recreational ingestion is referred to as roboing, dexing, robo-tripping, or robo-copping. In a recent study in human volunteers, high doses (between 5.7 and 11.4 milligrams /kilogram; Reissig et al., 2012) produced hallucinations that participants identified as being comparable to classic hallucinogens, like psilocybin. However DXM acts through NMDA receptor blockade, an action similar to that of PCP and ketamine. In fact, DXM and its metabolite dextrorphan (DXO) can substitute for PCP and exert PCP-like effects (and the active metabolite DXO may be responsible for many of the high-dose effects of DXM; Miller, 2005). These findings imply that both serotonergic and glutamatergic neurotransmitter systems may be involved in the perceptual, cognitive, and mood-altering effects of many hallucinogenlike compounds including dissociative anesthetics such as ketamine and PCP (Reissig, et al., 2012).

DXM increased blood pressure and heart rate and produced psychological/behavioral activation (such as increased ratings of arousing/stimulating, shaky/jittery, nervous/anxious, restless, and talkative) as well as other somatic effects (light-headedness/dizziness, numbness/tingling, queasiness/feeling sick to the stomach, and headache). DXM also increased ratings of distance from reality, visual effects with eyes open and with eyes closed, restless/fidgety, joy/euphoria/peace, nausea/vomiting, and psychological discomfort. At the maximum dose only, DXM increased ratings of unresponsiveness to questions, anxiety or fearfulness, and confusion/disorientation. Nevertheless, participants also endorsed positive effects in regard to "mysticism" (Reissig et al., 2012). Acute psychotic reactions have occasionally been reported.

Salvinorin A

Salvia divinorum (magic mint, diviner's sage, Sally-D), a member of the mint family of perennial herbs, is a psychoactive plant that has been used for curing and for divination in traditional spiritual practices by the Mazatec peoples of Oaxaca, Mexico, for many centuries (Vortherms and Roth, 2006). Among the various species of *Salvia*, only this plant is known to contain the active hallucinogen, salvinorin A. Generally the leaves of the plant are chewed, or brewed in a tea, but the dried leaves can also be smoked in the manner of marijuana or cocaine freebase. When smoked in doses of 200 to 500 micrograms, *Salvia* has been used as a short-acting (approximately 30 minutes), legal hallucinogen for several years. Ingestion typically does not produce hallucinogenic effects, either because of first-pass metabolism or enzyme breakdown.

In recent years, users of *S. divinorum* have posted videos of themselves under the influence to YouTube, with the mainstream news media occasionally also broadcasting these clips. This agent received much media attention after the singer/actress Miley Cyrus was photographed smoking it, and, the perpetrator of the 2011 Tucson, Arizona, shooting, Jared Loughner, was said to be a long-term user (Rosenbaum et al., 2012).

A compilation of descriptions (from the Internet site Erowid) includes: "Laughter, visions, peace/understanding, experiencing multiple realities/travel to other places or time/contacting other entities/spirits, entering 'realm of the dead,' feeling of being underground, flying, floating, twisting, loss of individuality/connected to a larger 'whole.'" Adverse effects include intense anxiety, dysphoria and confusion, and a hangover with headache and drowsiness for several hours. There are no characteristic physical signs except for some tachycardia and hypertension. But, the drug is often taken with other substances, therefore specific reactions are difficult to determine. Addiction and dependence liability are unknown and there is no recognized antidote for intoxication.

Mechanism of Action

The molecular structure (Figure 8.5), mechanism of action, and perhaps clinical effects of salvinorin A are distinct from other naturally occurring or synthetic hallucinogens (Butelman et al., 2010). Unlike classical hallucinogens, salvinorin A has no action at the serotonin 5-HT$_{2A}$ receptor but is classified as a *kappa opioid agonist*, the first naturally occurring compound known to exhibit such an action (Roth et al., 2002). Laboratory studies in nonhuman animals confirm that salvinorin A's effects differ from 5-HT$_2$ agonists, LSD, psilocybin, THC, NMDA antagonists, and delta or mu opiate agonists, but are similar to the effects of other kappa agonists, and are blocked by kappa antagonists (Addy, 2012). This is unusual because the drug is not *structurally* like other kappa agonists, and because its effects are also similar to those of 5-HT$_{2A}$ agonists (Cunningham et al., 2011; Johnson et al., 2011).

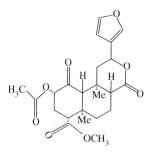

FIGURE 8.5   Structure of salvinorin A, the active drug in *Salvia divinorum*.

Potential Therapeutic Uses of Salvinorum Derivatives

Hanes (2001) reported on one patient with severe depression unrelieved by traditional antidepressant medications. This person obtained *Salvia* through a mail-order house. She chewed two or three leaves at a time three times per week and claimed total remission of depressive symptoms. However, as a kappa agonist, the drug has the potential to induce (rather than relieve) depressive reactions. Braida and coworkers (2009) expand on potential antidepressant and anxiolytic effects of salvinorin A. Historically, *Salvia* preparations have been used to treat gastrointestinal disorders, including diarrhea. Fichna and coworkers (2009) expand on this topic and demonstrate that salvinorin A inhibits colonic contractions and motility through actions on gastric kappa receptors and cannabinoid-2 receptors. The authors postulate use in the treatment of lower intestinal disorders associated with increased intestinal transit and diarrhea. Salvinorin A has therapeutic potential as a treatment for pain, mood and personality disorders, substance abuse, and gastrointestinal disturbances, which suggests that nonalkaloids may be potential options for new, therapeutic, drug development (Cunningham et al., 2011).

STUDY QUESTIONS

1. What is a psychedelic drug?
2. List the major classes of psychedelic drugs presented in this chapter and the respective mechanisms of action that differentiate them.
3. How do the psychedelic drugs differ in their psychological/subjective effects?
4. What therapeutic benefits, if any, have been proposed for the psychedelic hallucinogens?
5. What acute adverse psychological reactions are produced by the various psychedelic drugs?
6. Are there any long-term physical, neurological, or psychological consequences of the psychedelics?
7. How does Salvinorin A differ from other drugs in this category, in its mechanism of action and its psychological effects?

REFERENCES

Addy, P. H. (2012). "Acute and Post-Acute Behavioral and Psychological Effects of Salvinorum A in Humans." *Psychopharmcology* 220: 195–204.

Baggott, M. J., et al. (2010). "Investigating the Mechanisms of Hallucinogen-Induced Visions Using 3,4-Methylenedioxyamphetamine (MDA): A Randomized Controlled Trial in Humans." *PLoS One* 5: e14074.

Bogenschutz, M. P., and Pommy, J. M. (2012). "Therapeutic Mechanisms of Classic Hallucinogens in the Treatment of Addictions: From Indirect Evidence to Testable Hypotheses." *Drug Testing and Analysis* 4: 543–555.

Bossong, M. G., et al. (2010). "mCPP: An Undesired Addition to the Ecstasy Market." *Journal of Psychopharmacology* 24: 1395–1401.

Braida, D., et al. (2009). "Potential Anxiolytic- and Antidepressant-Like Effects of Salvinorin A, the Main Active Ingredient of *Salvia divinorum*, in Rodents." *British Journal of Pharmacology* 157: 844–853.

Brierley, D., and Davidson, C. (2013). "Harmine Augments Electrically Evoked Dopamine Efflux in the Nucleus Accumbens Shell." *Journal of Psychopharmacology* 27: 98–108.

Brown, D. J. (2013). *Psychedelic Drug Research: A Comprehensive Review.* Reality Sandwich Singles http://www.evolver.net/products/psychedelic-drug-research.

Brunt, T. M., et al. (2011). "Instability of the Ecstasy Market and a New Kid on the Block: Mephedrone." *Journal of Psychopharmacology* 25: 1543–1547.

Butelman, E. R., et al. (2010). "The Discriminative Effects of the Kappa-Opioid Hallucinogen Salvinorin A in Nonhuman Primates: Dissociation from Classic Hallucinogen Effects." *Psychopharmacology* 210: 253–262.

Carhart-Harris, R. L., et al. (2012). "Implications for Psychedelic-Assisted Psychotherapy: Functional Magnetic Resonance Imaging with Psilocybin." *British Journal of Psychiatry* 200: 238–244.

Caudevilla-Gálligo, F., et al. (2012). "4-Bromo-2, 5-Dimethoxyphenethylamine (2C-B): Presence in the Recreational Drug Market in Spain, Pattern of Use and Subjective Effects." *Journal of Psychopharmacology* 26: 1026–1035.

Corazza, O., et al. (2012). "Phenomenon of New Drugs on the Internet: The Case of Ketamine Derivative Methoxetamine." *Human Psychopharmacology Clinical and Experimental* 27: 145–149.

Cunningham, C. W., et al. (2011). "Neuropharmacology of the Naturally Occurring κ-Opioid Hallucinogen Salvinorin A." *Pharmacological Reviews* 63: 316–347.

DeFrates, L. J., et al. (2005). "Antimuscarinic Intoxication Resulting from the Ingestion of Moonflower Seeds." *Annals of Pharmacotherapy* 39: 173–176.

den Hollander, B., et al. (2012). "Preliminary Evidence of Hippocampal Damage in Chronic Users of Ecstasy." *Journal of Neurology Neurosurgery and Psychiatry* 83: 83–85.

deWin, M. M. L., et al. (2008). "Sustained Effects of Ecstasy on the Human Brain: A Prospective Neuroimaging Study in Novel Users." *Brain* 131: 2936–2945.

Duffy, M. R., and Ferguson, C. (2007). "Role of Dantrolene in Treatment of Heat Stroke Associated with Ecstasy Ingestion." *British Journal of Anaesthesia* 98: 148–149.

el-Seedi, H. R., et al. (2005). "Prehistoric Peyote Use: Alkaloid Analysis and Radiocarbon Dating of Archaeological Specimens of *Lophophora* from Texas." *Journal of Ethnopharmacology* 101: 238–242.

Fichna, J., et al. (2009). "Salvinorin A Inhibits Colonic Transit and Neurogenic Ion Transport in Mice by Activating Kappa-Opioid and Cannabinoid Receptors." *Neurogastroenterology and Motility* 21: 1326e–1328e.

Fickenscher, A., et al. (2006). "Illicit Peyote Use Among American Indian Adolescents in Substance Abuse Treatment: A Preliminary Investigation." *Substance Use and Misuse* 41: 1139–1154.

Fortunato, J. J., et al. (2009). "Acute Harmine Administration Induces Antidepressant-Like Effects and Increases BDNF Levels in the Rat Hippocampus." *Progress in Neuropsychopharmacology and Biological Psychiatry* 33: 1425–1430.

Gable, R. S. (2007). "Risk Assessment of Ritual Use of Oral Dimethyltryptamine (DMT) and Harmala Alkaloids." *Addiction* 102: 24–34.

Gallagher, C. T., et al. (2012). "5,6-Methylenedioxy-2-aminoindane: From Laboratory Curiosity to 'Legal High.'" *Human Psychopharmacology Clinical and Experimental* 27: 106–112.

Geyer, M. A., and Vollenweider, F. X. (2008). "Serotonin Research: Contributions to Understanding Psychosis." *Trends in Pharmacological Sciences* 29: 445–453.

Gouzoulis-Mayfrank, E., and Daumann, J. (2009). "Neurotoxicity of Drugs of Abuse—The Case of Methylenedioxyamphetamines (MDMA, Ecstasy), and Amphetamines." *Dialogues in Clinical Neuroscience* 11: 305–317.

Grilly, D. M., and Salamone, J. D. (2012). *Drugs, Brain and Behavior.* New York: Pearson.

Grob, C. S., et al. (2011). "Pilot Study of Psilocybin Treatment for Anxiety in Patients with Advanced-Stage Cancer." *Archives of General Psychiatry* 68: 71–78.

Hadjiefthyvoulou, F., et al. (2011). "Everyday and Prospective Memory Deficits in Ecstasy / Polydrug Users." *Journal of Psychopharmacology* 25: 453–464.

Hall, A. P., and Henry, J. A. (2006). "Acute Toxic Effects of 'Ecstasy' (MDMA) and Related Compounds: Overview of Pathophysiology and Clinical Management." *British Journal of Anaesthesia* 96: 678–685.

Halpern, J. H., et al. (2011). "Residual Neurocognitive Features of Long-Term Ecstasy Users with Minimal Exposure to Other Drugs." *Addiction* 106: 777–786.

Hanes, K. R. (2001). "Antidepressant Effects of the Herb *Salvia divinorum:* A Case Report." *Journal of Clinical Psychopharmacology* 21: 634–635.

Hashimoto, K. (2009). "Can the Sigma-1 Receptor Agonist Fluvoxamine Prevent Schizophrenia?" *CNS & Neurological Disorders—Drug Targets* 8: 470–474.

Herraiz, T., et al. (2010). "Beta-Carboline Alkaloids in *Peganum harmala* and Inhibition of Human Monoamine Oxidase (MAO)." *Food and Chemical Toxicology* 48: 839–845.

Hofmann, A. (1994). "Notes and Documents Concerning the Discovery of LSD." *Agents and Actions* 43: 79–81.

Holzman, R. S. (1998). "The Legacy of Atropos, the Fate Who Cut the Thread of Life." *Anesthesiology* 89: 241–249.

Itokawa, M., et al. (2007). "Acute Confusional State After Designer Tryptamine Abuse." *Psychiatry and Clinical Neurosciences* 61: 196–199.

Johnson, M., et al. (2008). "Human Hallucinogen Research: Guidelines for Safety." *Journal of Psychopharmacology* 22: 603–620.

Johnson, M. W., et al. (2011). "Human Psychopharmacology and Dose-Effects of Salvinorin A, a Kappa Opioid Agonist Hallucinogen Present in the Plant *Salvia Divinorum.*" *Drug and Alcohol Dependence* 115: 150–155.

Krebs, T. S., and Johansen, P. O. (2012). "Lysergic Acid Diethylamide (LSD) for Alcoholism: Meta-Analysis of Randomized Controlled Trials." *Journal of Psychopharmacology* 26: 994–1002.

Kuypers, K. P. C., and Ramaekers, J. G. (2005). "Transient Memory Impairment After Acute Dose of 75 mg 3.4-Methylenedioxymethamphetamine." *Journal of Psychopharmacology* 19: 633–639.

Kuypers, K. P. C., and Ramaekers, J. G. (2007). "Acute Dose of MDMA (75 mg) Impairs Spatial Memory for Location but Leaves Contextual Processing of Visuospatial Information Unaffected." *Psychopharmacology* 189: 557–563.

Kuypers, K. P. C., et al. (2011). "MDMA Intoxication and Verbal Memory Performance: A Placebo-Controlled Pharmaco-MRI Study." *Journal of Psychopharmacology* 25: 1053–1061.

Maurice, T., and Su, T. P. (2009). "The Pharmacology of Sigma-1 Receptors." *Pharmacology and Therapeutics* 124: 195–206.

McLean, K., et al. (2011). "Mystical Experiences Occasioned by the Hallucinogen Psilocybin Lead to Increases in the Personality Domain of Openness." *Journal of Psychopharmacology* 25: 1453–1461.

Miller, S. C. (2005). "Dextromethorphan Psychosis, Dependence and Physical Withdrawal." *Addiction Biology* 10: 325–327.

Mithoefer, M. C., et al. (2011). "The Safety and Efficacy of ± 3,4-Methylenedioxymethamphetamine-Assisted Psychotherapy in Subjects with Chronic, Treatment-Resistant Posttraumatic Stress Disorder: The First Randomized Controlled Pilot Study." *Journal of Psychopharmacology* 25: 439–452.

Mithoefer, M. C., et al. (2013). "Durability of Improvement in Post-Traumatic Stress Disorder Symptoms and Absence of Harmful Effects or Drug Dependency After 3,4-Methylenedioxymethamphetamine-

Assisted Psychotherapy: A Prospective Long-Term Follow-Up Study." *Journal of Psychopharmacology* 27: 28–39.

Moore, K., et al. (2013). "Do Novel Psychoactive Substances Displace Established Club Drugs, Supplement Them or Act as Drugs of Initiation: The Relationship Between Mephedrone, Ecstasy and Cocaine." *European Addiction Research* 19: 276–282.

Morgan, C. J. A., and Curran, H. V. (2011). "Ketamine Use: A Review." *Addiction* 107: 27–38.

Mouri, A., et al. (2007). "Phencyclidine Animal Models of Schizophrenia: Approaches from Abnormality of Glutamatergic Neurotransmission and Neurodevelopment." *Neurochemistry International* 51: 173–184.

Nagai, F., et al. (2007). "The Effects of Non-Medically Used Psychoactive Drugs on Monoamine Neurotransmission in Rat Brain." *European Journal of Pharmacology* 559: 132–137.

Parrott, A. C. (2012). "MDMA and Temperature: A Review of the Thermal Effects of 'Ecstasy' in Humans." *Drug and Alcohol Dependence* 121: 1–9.

Paschos, K. A., et al. (2009). "Neuropeptide and Sigma Receptors as Novel Therapeutic Targets for the Pharmacotherapy of Depression." *CNS Drugs* 23: 755–772.

Passie, T., et al. (2008). "The Pharmacology of Lysergic Acid Diethylamide: A Review." *CNS Neuroscience & Therapeutics* 14: 295–314.

Reissig, C. J., et al. (2012). "High Doses of Dextromethorphan, an NMDA Antagonist, Produce Effects Similar to Classic Hallucinogens." *Psychopharmacology* 223: 1–15.

Roberts, T. B. (2013). *The Psychedelic Future of the Mind: How Entheogens Are Enhancing Cognition, Boosting Intelligence, and Raising Values*. South Paris, ME: Park Street Press.

Rosenbaum, C. D., et al. (2012). "Here Today, Gone Tomorrow . . . and Back Again? A Review of Herbal Marijuana Alternatives (K2, Spice), Synthetic Cathinones (Bath Salts), Kratom, *Salvia Divinorum*, Methoxetamine, and Piperazines." *Journal of Medical Toxicology* 8: 15–32.

Roth, B. L., et al. (2002). "Salvinorin A: A Potent Naturally Occurring Nonnitrogenous Opioid Selective Agonist." *Proceedings of the National Academy of Sciences* 99: 11934–11939.

Schep, L. J., et al. (2011). "The Clinical Toxicology of the Designer "Party Pills" Benzylpiperazine and Trifluoromethylphenylpiperazine." *Clinical Toxicology* 49: 131–141.

Schifano, F., et al. (2005). "New Trends in the Cyber and Street Market of Recreational Drugs? The Case of 2C-T-7 ("Blue Mystic")." *Journal of Psychopharmacology* 19: 675–679.

Sessa, B. (2012). *The Psychedelic Renaissance: Reassessing the Role of Psychedelic Drugs in 21st Century Psychiatry and Society*. London: Muswell Hill Press.

Strassman, R. J., et al. (1994). "Dose-Response Study of N, N-Dimethyltryptamine in Humans. II: Subjective Effects and Preliminary Results of a New Rating Scale." *Archives of General Psychiatry* 51: 98–108.

Studerus, E., et al. (2012). "Prediction of Psilocybin Response in Healthy Volunteers." *PLoS One* 7: e30800.

Su, T. P., et al. (2009). "When the Endogenous Hallucinogenic Trace Amine N, N-Dimethyltryptamine Meets the Sigma-1 Receptor." *Science Signaling* 2: pe12.

Troy, J. D. (2013). "New 'Legal' Highs: Kratom and Methoxetamine." *Current Psychiatry* 12: E1–E2.

Urban, N. B. L., et al. (2012). "Sustained Recreational Use of Ecstasy is Associated with Altered Pre- and Postsynaptic Markers of Serotonin Transmission in Neocortical Areas: A PET Study with [^{11}C] DASB and [^{11}C]MDL 100907." *Neuropsychopharmacology* 37: 1465–1473.

Vortherms, T. A., and Roth, B. L. (2006). "Salvinorin A: From Natural Product to Human Therapeutics." *Molecular Interventions* 6: 257–265.

Wagner, D., et al. (2013). "A Prospective Study of Learning, Memory, and Executive Function in New MDMA Users." *Addiction* 108: 136–145.

Wolff, K., and Winstock, A. R. (2006). "Ketamine: From Medicine to Misuse." *CNS Drugs* 20: 199–218.

Cannabis

The hemp plant, cannabis, commonly called marijuana, has such a unique variety of effects that it is placed in a category of its own. It has some stimulatory properties, some sedative actions, it may produce hallucinations, and it can be analgesic. But it is not chemically related to the classical psychostimulants, sedative/hypnotics, hallucinogens, or opiates. Its psychological effects seem to be very malleable. In spite of a long history of medical applications, its therapeutic possibilities, and adverse effects, are just beginning to be experimentally determined. More than any other psychoactive substance, cannabis continues to polarize opinion, and its role in society is still evolving.

Epidemiology

According to most recent estimates, which are understandably difficult to verify in regard to illicit drugs, cannabis is still the most widely used illegal substance in the world, with somewhere between 125 and 203 million users (Degenhardt and Hall, 2012). Data from the National Survey on Drug Use and Health indicate that, in 2011, approximately 3.1 million people in the United States aged 12 or older used a nonalcoholic drug for the first time and that for about 68 percent of them, that drug was marijuana (Figure 9.1). Information from the Substance Abuse and Mental Health Services Administration (SAMHSA) shows that in 2010, about 17.4 million Americans reported cannabis use. According to the National Institute on Drug Abuse annual Monitoring the Future survey, 6.5 percent of high school seniors reported using marijuana daily in 2012, up from 5.1 percent 5 years ago. In fact, only 44 percent of seniors said they saw regular use as harmful, the lowest figure since the 1980s. This may be related to the recent changes in the legal status of cannabis.

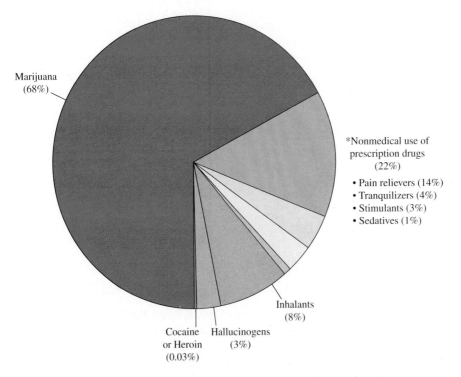

Marijuana
(68%)

*Nonmedical use of
prescription drugs
(22%)

• Pain relievers (14%)
• Tranquilizers (4%)
• Stimulants (3%)
• Sedatives (1%)

Inhalants
(8%)

Cocaine   Hallucinogens
or Heroin   (3%)
(0.03%)

FIGURE 9.1 First drug of use among U.S. residents who started using drugs in 2011. Percentages may not add up to 100 due to rounding or because a few respondents initiated multiple drugs on the same day. In 2011, an estimated 3,083,000 residents initiated drug use in the past year, based on 70,109 completed interviews. *Nonmedical use of prescription drugs is defined as use of pain relievers, tranquilizers, stimulants, and/or sedatives without a prescription belonging to the re-spondent or use that occurred simply for the experience or feeling the drug caused. It does not include the use of over-the-counter drugs. [Adapted by CESAR data from Substance Abuse and Mental Health Services Administration, Results from the 2011 National Survey on Drug Use and Health: Detailed Tables, 2012.]

Did You Know?

Synthetic Marijuana Third Most Reported Substance Used by U.S. High School Students

More high school students report using *synthetic* marijuana than any other substance besides alcohol and marijuana, according to data from a recently released (April 2013) survey of ninth to twelfth graders. Alcohol and marijuana were the most prevalent drugs used, with 57 percent reporting alcohol use and 39 percent reporting marijuana use in the past year in 2012. The third most prevalent substance used was synthetic marijuana (12 percent), often referred to as K2 or Spice. Similar results have been found by other surveys of high school students.

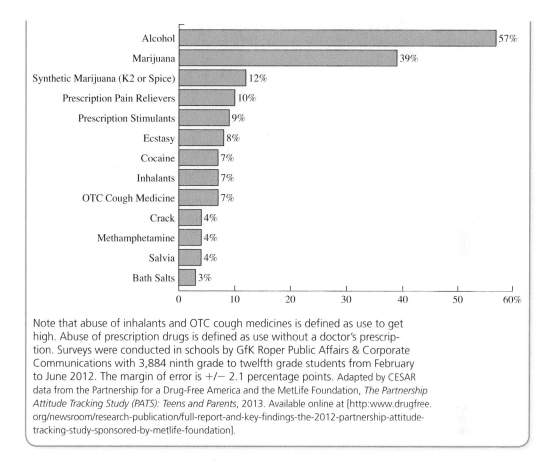

Note that abuse of inhalants and OTC cough medicines is defined as use to get high. Abuse of prescription drugs is defined as use without a doctor's prescription. Surveys were conducted in schools by GfK Roper Public Affairs & Corporate Communications with 3,884 ninth grade to twelfth grade students from February to June 2012. The margin of error is +/− 2.1 percentage points. Adapted by CESAR data from the Partnership for a Drug-Free America and the MetLife Foundation, *The Partnership Attitude Tracking Study (PATS): Teens and Parents*, 2013. Available online at [http:www.drugfree. org/newsroom/research-publication/full-report-and-key-findings-the-2012-partnership-attitude-tracking-study-sponsored-by-metlife-foundation].

History

Cannabis may be the oldest cultivated plant not used for food; the earliest known evidence of cannabis use consists of fibers found in China, from around 4,000 B.C.E. The ancient cultures of China, India, and Tibet treated numerous ailments, including gastrointestinal illness, seizures, malaria, pain of childbirth, and snakebite with the seeds and fruit of the plant. Various religious groups, such as Buddhists and Hindus, incorporated cannabis into their religious ceremonies, and recreational use was also widespread (Seely et al., 2011). Gradually, cannabis use then spread to Asia and the Middle East. The plant had many applications and its primary behavioral effects were well known; it was used for fiber (to make rope, cloth), oil, and medicine, as well as intoxication. For example, the famous Greek physician Galen cautioned that its use might lead to "senseless talk." During the Middle Ages it came to the Muslim world and Africa, where its popularity was perhaps influenced by the Muslim prohibition of alcohol. Over centuries, cannabis was said to have many, sometimes contradictory, properties. It could make you crave sweets, get "high," improve sex and creativity, and also *decrease* the sex drive, produce insanity, and cause an "amotivational" syndrome. The term *assassin* is thought to derive from the word *hashishiyya*, believed to describe common criminals who also used hashish.

Spaniards brought the plant to America in 1545. As a hemp plant, cannabis was very important because it made good rope and rope was important because ships were crucial to the empire and ships needed lots of rope. Because hemp did not grow well in England, American colonists were therefore encouraged to cultivate it. Sir Walter Raleigh was ordered to grow it, which he did in the first season, 1611, next to tobacco. It was a staple crop for over 200 years for rope, clothes, and paper. Even George Washington grew it. It was the major crop before the invention of the cotton gin. It became more popular recreationally in the middle of the nineteenth century, notably after Napoleon's army brought it back from the war in Egypt. Gradually cannabis was again promoted for a variety of illnesses and drug companies marketed cannabis tinctures for medicinal purposes, until the Pure Food and Drug Act of 1906 and the Harrison Narcotic Act of 1914 began to impose some constraints. However, the Harrison Act did not specifically outlaw cannabis, and, when alcohol prohibition was passed the recreational use of cannabis increased greatly, facilitated by the increase in migrant immigration from Mexico. Harry Anslinger, who became the first commissioner of the Federal Narcotics Bureau in 1930, tried to eradicate cannabis when alcohol prohibition failed. He devised dramatic media attacks that led to the Marijuana Tax Act of 1937. This law did not directly outlaw cannabis, but imposed a tax on it, and effectively ended legal medicinal use of cannabis until about 1969, when the Supreme Court declared the law illegal – because imposing a tax on someone who wants to possess an illegal substance is a form of self-incrimination. In 1970 the Comprehensive Drug Abuse Prevention and Control Act (Controlled Substances Act) reduced the federal penalty for possession from a felony to a misdemeanor. Since then, in response to growing evidence for a variety of medicinal properties of cannabis products, a number of states (as of November 2012, 18 states and the District of Columbia) have legalized the medical use of cannabis (Doweicko, 2012; Levinthal, 2012). In fact, on November 6, 2012, the voters of two states, Colorado and Washington, passed a referendum to legalize marijuana for nonmedical purposes. This law violates current federal regulations, and it is unclear how this conflict will be resolved.

What Is Cannabis?

The plant genus for cannabis includes three putative varieties: *Cannabis sativa*, *Cannabis indica*, and *Cannabis ruderalis*. *Cannabis sativa* grows throughout the world and flourishes in most temperate and tropical regions. There are at least 400 different compounds in the plant, of which more than 60 are psychoactive. In 1964 Gaoni and Mechoulam first identified the primary active ingredient *delta-9-tetrahydrocannabinol* (THC) (Figure 9.2A), which renewed interest in the field and led to the discovery of the endogenous endocannabinoids (discussed below).

Names for the numerous products of the cannabis plant include marijuana, hashish, charas, bhang, ganja, and sinsemilla. *Hashish* and *charas*, which consist of the dried resinous exudates of the female flowers, are the most potent preparations, with a THC content averaging between 10 percent and 20 percent. *Ganja* and *sinsemilla* refer to the dried

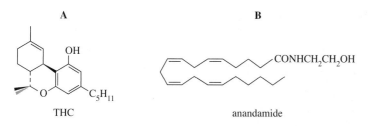

A

B

THC

anandamide

FIGURE 9.2 Structures of delta-9-tetrahydrocannabinol (THC) and anandamide, the endogenous ligand (neurotransmitter) of the cannabinoid receptor.

material found in the tops of the female plants, where the THC content averages about 5 percent to 8 percent. *Bhang* and *marijuana* are lower-grade preparations taken from the dried remainder of the plant, and their THC content varies from 2 percent to 5 percent, although improved growing, harvesting, and processing techniques have boosted this content considerably. A new variation is BHO (butane hash oil), also known as dabs, honey oil, wax, oil, shatter or budder. This is a potent (80 percent THC content) extract, made by using butane, then heated and inhaled as a vapor. Aside from the danger of contaminants, there are reports of explosions caused by accidents during extraction.

Among the other known cannabis constituents with biologic activity, two of the most abundant are cannabinol (CBN) and cannabidiol (CBD). In the plant, CBD is a precursor and CBN a metabolite of THC. As cannabis ages, THC gradually breaks down to CBN. CBN and CBD are not psychoactive themselves, but, as noted below, may modulate the effects of THC. In particular, CBD is thought to have significant analgesic, antipsychotic, and anti-inflammatory activity without the psychoactive effect (the "high") of delta-9-THC (Izzo et al., 2009; Scuderi et al., 2009).

Mechanism of Action: Cannabinoid Receptors

In 1988, the first cannabinoid receptor, designated CB1, was discovered, followed by the discovery of a second, CB2, in the early 1990s. Both of them are in the family of G-protein coupled receptors (GPCRs; see Chapter 3). CB1 receptors are located throughout the body, but they are found in the highest concentration in the central nervous system (CNS). In fact, CB1 receptors are the most common of the GPCRs in the CNS, with concentrations similar to GABA and glutamate (Seely et al., 2011). They are most abundant in the hippocampus, basal ganglia, cerebellum, and frontal cortex, which is very consistent with their well-known effects on memory, motor coordination, perceptual processing, and attention, which are the functions of these brain structures (Figure 9.3 and Figure 9.4) (see Chapter 1). Because there are relatively few cannabis receptors in the brain stem, THC and other agonists have very low toxicity, except at extremely high concentrations.

CB2 receptors are mostly (but not completely) found outside the CNS, primarily in tissues of the immune system, such as the tonsils and thymus. However, in inflammatory conditions, CB2 receptors can be found on the microglia cells that are activated to protect the brain. Acting outside the brain, CB2 receptors may have some protective effects against neurodegeneration. This was shown in a mouse model of Huntington's disease

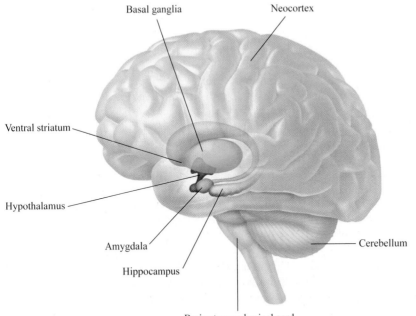

Basal ganglia

Neocortex

Ventral striatum

Hypothalamus

Amygdala

Hippocampus

Cerebellum

Brain stem and spinal cord

FIGURE 9.3 Cannabis produces its psychoactive effects by binding to receptors in several brain sites. These receptors are most concentrated in brain structures that regulate higher-order functions, such as judgment (neocortex), learning and memory (the hippocampus), anxiety (amygdala), drug "high" (ventral striatum), movement (basal ganglia and cerebellum), ingestion (hypothalamus), pain, and the vomiting reflex (brain stem and spinal cord).

(HD). HD mice, given a drug that stimulated CB2 receptors, showed improvement in several measures, such as life span and inflammation, which were blocked by CB2 antagonists. Mice bred without the receptor deteriorated more quickly (Bouchard et al., 2012).

Endocannabinoids

The discovery of the cannabis receptors through which THC produced its effects had significant implications. As stated by Dr. Raphael Mechoulam (in an interview in May, 2010 (http://medicalmarijuana411.com/mmj411_v3/?p=601):

> So now we are sure of two receptors that are present, and THC acts on them and stimulates them. . . . Now receptors are not present in the body because there is a plant outside there. They are present in the body in order to be activated by something the body produces when and where needed. So we went ahead looking for the compounds in the brain

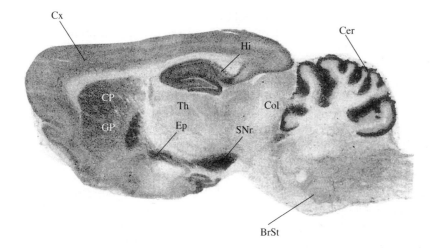

FIGURE 9.4 Autoradiographic binding of potent cannabinoid-to-cannabinoid receptors in the rat brain. BrSt = brain stem; Cer = cerebellum; Col = colliculi; CP = caudate putamen; Cx = cerebral cortex; Ep = entopeduncular nucleus; GP = globus pallidus; Hi = hippocampus; SNr = substantia nigra; Th = thalamus. Autograph [Courtesy of Miles HerKenham, NIMH]

and periphery that would activate these receptors. And in 1992 and 1995, we reported the most important ones. One of them we called anandamide. Ananda comes from the Sanskrit name supreme joy, we were happy after working so hard identifying the compound. Which has, it turns out, to have a different chemical structure from the compound in the plant. It was rather strange, I would say, because the two compounds do exactly the same.

As quoted above, Devane and coworkers (1992) in Dr. Mechoulam's laboratory isolated the first endogenous cannabinoid, *anandamide* (arachidonoylethanolamine, AEA; see Figure 9.2B). Its pharmacology is similar to THC, although its chemical structure is different (Figure 9.5). Anandamide binds to the central (CB1) and, to a lesser extent,

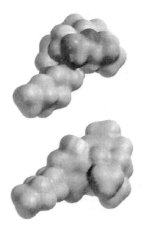

FIGURE 9.5 View of the steric shape and bulk of anandamide (*top*) and THC (*bottom*). [After Thomas et al., 1996, p. 474.]

peripheral (CB2) cannabinoid receptors. It is found in nearly all tissues in a wide range of animals. AEA is a partial agonist at CB1 receptors and a partial agonist, or antagonist, at CB2 receptors (Seely et al., 2011).

Soon after the discovery of AEA, a second endogenous cannabinoid (eCB) was found, *2-arachidonoyl glycerol (2-AG)*. 2-AG binds as a full agonist to both CB1 and CB2 receptors. It is found in even higher concentration in the brain than AEA. Since then, five more substances have been reported to function as endogenous, biologically active cannabinoid substances. Their names and chemical structures are shown in Figure 9.6.

As endogenous neurotransmitters, the eCBs are produced, released, removed, and inactivated by processes similar to those of other neurotransmitters. However, there are some important differences.

First, unlike typical neurotransmitters, AEA and 2-AG are not produced ahead of time and stored in the vesicles of neuronal terminals. Rather, they are synthesized "on demand." What this means is that, only after a postsynaptic endocannabinoid neuron is stimulated (for example, by transmitter released from a presynaptic neuron) does it begin to produce AEA or 2-AG. The transmitter opens calcium channels in the postsynaptic eCB neuron. Calcium entry activates specific enzymes, which then produce either AEA or 2-AG. Once these compounds are synthesized, they immediately diffuse out of the neuron into the synaptic space because they are very lipid soluble.

The second way in which this system differs from classical transmitter function is that once the endocannabinoids are produced and diffuse out of the postsynaptic neuron, *they move back to the presynaptic neuronal terminal, where they bind to CB receptors*. That is, the endocannabinoids move in a *retrograde* direction, and attach to receptors on the *presynaptic neuron*. By binding to presynaptic CB receptors they ultimately inhibit further release of transmitter from the presynaptic terminal. In summary, eCBs are released from depolarized postsynaptic neurons, then travel back to presynaptic neurons, where they activate CB receptors to reduce further transmitter release, such as GABA or glutamate. This represents an important way of modulating neuronal excitability and maintaining equilibrium (Guindon and Hohmann, 2009; Battista et al., 2012).

After the eCBs produce their effects, it is believed that they are taken back up into neurons by an "endocannabinoid membrane transporter" (EMT). Back in the neuron, specific enzymes metabolize them. For AEA the major enzyme is fatty-acid amide hydrolase, or FAAH, which is found in the postsynaptic neuron; for 2-AG the enzyme is monoacylglycerol lipase, or MGL, which is found in the presynaptic neuron. Drugs that inhibit uptake of eCBs have been developed, as well as FAAH inhibitors, which can increase brain levels of anandamide in rodents and produce analgesia and benzodiazepinelike effects in vivo, making FAAH a possible target for pain and anxiety treatment.

It is now known that the eCBs act on other receptor types, beside CB1 and CB2. Whether one of these will turn out to be a third CB receptor remains to be seen. Endocannabinoid neurobiology is complex, and it is not surprising that increasing evidence shows that it is involved in numerous physiological processes, including, but not limited to, memory and learning, neuroprotection, appetite, pain, cancer, and immune function.

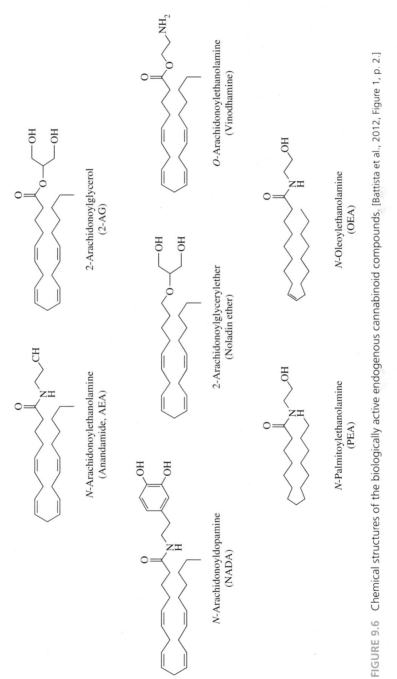

FIGURE 9.6 Chemical structures of the biologically active endogenous cannabinoid compounds. [Battista et al., 2012, Figure 1, p. 2.]

Pharmacokinetics

THC is usually administered in the form of a hand-rolled marijuana cigarette, called a reefer or joint. In general, about one-fourth to one-half of the THC present in a marijuana cigarette is actually available in the smoke. In practice, the amount absorbed into the bloodstream depends on the amount of THC in the cigarette, how deeply the smoker inhales, and how long the smoke is kept in the lungs. Estimates range from 5 percent to 60 percent of the available THC being absorbed into the body (Doweiko, 2012). Whatever the amount, absorption of THC from smoking is rapid and complete. Once absorbed, THC is distributed to the various organs of the body, especially those that have significant concentrations of fatty material, such as the brain and the placenta. The behavioral effects occur almost immediately after smoking begins and correspond with the rapid attainment of peak concentrations in plasma. A "high" is experienced with plasma concentrations of about 5 to 10 nanograms of drug per milliliter of plasma. Within 2 hours, levels fall below 5 nanograms per milliliter and then decline slowly. Unless more is smoked, the effects seldom last longer than 2 to 3 hours.

Marijuana can also be taken orally, and one THC preparation, dronabinol (Marinol), has been available for oral use since the mid-1980s. Taken orally, onset is delayed; acidic degradation, enzyme action, and "first-pass metabolism" may reduce the potency by two-thirds (Grilly and Salamone, 2012). However, the effects will last longer—and there are no associated effects on the lung, or smell of smoke to attract attention.

THC is almost completely metabolized by hepatic cytochrome P450 enzymes to its active metabolite, 11-hydroxy-delta-9-THC, which is subsequently converted to the inactive metabolite carboxy-THC (COOH-THC), which is excreted in the urine (Figure 9.7).

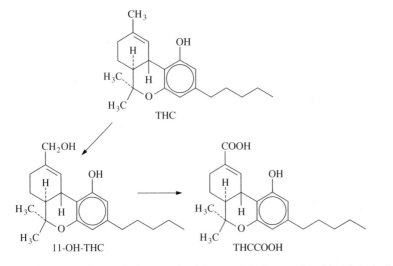

FIGURE 9.7 Major metabolic route for delta-9-tetrahydrocannabinol (THC), including its active metabolite (11-OH-THC) and its primary inactive metabolite (11-nor-9-carboxy-delta-9-tetrahydrocannabinol, or "carboxy-THC").

Much of the THC taken into the body is stored in body fat, from which it is slowly released. Consequently, very low, clinically insignificant amounts in blood may be maintained for a considerable time after drug use ceases, from several days to about 2 weeks and longer in chronic smokers and obese smokers (Huestis, 2005). Such a delay tends to prolong and intensify the activity of subsequently smoked marijuana, forming a type of "reverse tolerance" to the drug, where the persistent low levels are potentiated by subsequently smoked THC cigarettes, which may intensify the psychoactive effects.

As with most psychoactive drugs, only minute quantities of active THC are found in the urine of people who use the drug. Therefore, urine testing for THC focuses on identification of its inactive metabolite, carboxy-THC. Carboxy-THC is only slowly excreted; its half-life in urine varies. In infrequent smokers (less than twice per week), urine samples will generally be positive for 1 to 3 days. In regular smokers (those who smoke several times per week), urine specimens can test positive for 7 to 21 days. In chronic smokers, daily use for prolonged periods of time can yield positive results for 30 days or longer. Thus, a positive urine test does not necessarily mean that a person was under the influence of marijuana at the time the urine specimen was collected; there is little or no correlation between the presence of carboxy-THC in urine and the presence of a pharmacologically significant amount of THC in the blood. This can become quite important in certain legal situations, such as charges of driving while under the influence of marijuana. Exposure to secondhand smoke will usually not result in a positive result for cannabinoid metabolites in urine.

Pharmacological Effects of Cannabis

Acute and Chronic Physiological Effects

Did You Know?

More Kids Exposed to Legal Pot

The decriminalization of medical marijuana in Colorado led to a marked increase in accidental ingestions of the substance among young children, a retrospective, single-center study showed. During the 5 years preceding October 2009, when the Department of Justice determined that medical marijuana users would no longer be prosecuted, there were no cases of marijuana ingestion among the 790 children younger than 12 in a Colorado children's hospital, according to records from the Rocky Mountain Poison and Drug Center in Denver. But between 2009 and 2011, 14 of 588 accidental ingestions were marijuana-related. The children ranged in age from 8 months to 12 years with a median of 2.3 years; two-thirds of the 588 patients were boys. Symptoms of accidental marijuana ingestion among the 14 patients confirmed by urine toxicology included sleepiness and lethargy, ataxia in one case, and respiratory insufficiency in one severe case.

There are currently no requirements for labeling or child-resistant packaging or storing of medical marijuana products, further increasing the need for clinician awareness of the potential hazards.

Cardiovascular System. When someone smokes marijuana there is an initial dose-dependent increase in heart rate; blood pressure might increase, decrease, or remain the same depending on whether the user is standing, sitting, or lying down. Dangerous physical reactions to marijuana are exceedingly rare (Doweicko, 2012), probably because most users are relatively young and healthy. However, a recent study found 59 case reports of cannabis-related stroke in persons with a mean age of 33 years, and a male-to-female ratio of 4.9:1. In many cases the stroke occurred while the drug was being smoked, or within 30 minutes of smoking. This was consistent with a 4.8 times increase in myocardial infarction during the hour after smoking. It seems that cannabis causes brain arteries to constrict, and this may not be easy to see in small blood vessels (Wolff et al., 2013). We know little about the consequences in older persons who might have compromised cardiovascular functions, although middle-aged stroke patients were recently reported 2.3 times more likely to be pot smokers than healthy middle-aged controls (Barber et al., 2013). Perhaps the most well-known cardiovascular effect of smoking marijuana is the bloodshot eyes, due to dilation of the corneal blood vessels.

Respiratory Effects. Marijuana smoking involves repetitive, deep inhalation of unfiltered material, possibly containing contaminants, which is usually smoked as completely as possible, in order not to waste any of the drug. Therefore, it may not be surprising to find that a single marijuana cigarette may be more harmful than a single tobacco cigarette in altering lung tissues and causing bronchial irritation and inflammation (Doweicko, 2012; Grilly and Salamone, 2012; Levinthal, 2012). On the other hand, it is unexpected that, after controlling for tobacco use, there is no definitive evidence that marijuana smokers have an increase in lung cancer. In fact, one 20-year study of pulmonary function found that occasional use (two to three times a month) was not associated with adverse pulmonary effects (Pletcher et al., 2012). However, this conclusion may be premature because, in general, users smoke fewer marijuana cigarettes than nicotine cigarettes, and the cohort of users may only now be reaching the age when such cancers appear.

Effects on the Immune System. Given that CB2 receptors are found primarily in the immune system, it should not be surprising that long-term marijuana use is associated with a degree of immunosuppression, which might be thought to potentially render the smoker susceptible to infections or disease (Hegde et al., 2010). The clinical significance of this occurrence is not known. At this time, little evidence points to cannabinoid-induced immunosuppression as a causative agent in disease, although this action might be relevant to patients with a weakened immune system, such as those with HIV infection.

Effects on the Reproductive System. In Western culture, marijuana is often reported to enhance sexual responsivity, whereas other cultures consider the drug to be a sexual depressant. This difference may be an example of the strong influence of expectation on cannabis's effects. But it is also possible that there is a dose-related mechanism, in that low doses may enhance libido while higher doses depress it (Levinthal, 2012).

Chronic use of marijuana by males can reduce levels of the hormone testosterone and reduce sperm count and viability. Reductions in male fertility and sexual potency, however, have not been reported. On the other hand, there is some evidence that smoking marijuana is associated with an increase in testicular cancer. This is the most common malignancy diagnosed in young men between the ages of 15 and 45. A recent study looking at the relationship between this disease and drug use, revealed that men who reported ever using marijuana had nearly twice the risk of testicular germ cell tumors than those who denied ever using the drug (Lacson et al., 2012).

In females, the levels of follicle-stimulating hormone and luteinizing hormone are reduced by the use of marijuana. Menstrual cycles can be affected and anovulatory cycles have been reported. All these actions reverse when drug use is discontinued. Wang and coworkers (2006) review this complex topic of endocannabinoids in both male and female fertility (one of the few articles to address the endocannabinoid system in the regulation of male fertility).

Marijuana freely crosses the placenta, therefore the developing brain is susceptible to cannabis during gestation. Although cannabis use does not appear to increase the incidence of birth defects, newborns of women who smoked marijuana when pregnant will on average be smaller than normal. One of the greatest risks appears to be the high probability that a pregnant female who smokes marijuana may also use other, more fetotoxic drugs (including nicotine cigarettes). Infants born of marijuana-smoking mothers display mild, transient withdrawal signs, including tremulousness, abnormal responses to stimuli, and neurobehavioral performance deficits (DeMoraes-Barros et al., 2006).

Effects on Pain. In rodents, THC and anandamide are analgesic at spinal, brain stem, and peripheral sites, especially against the pain resulting from persistent inflammation or neuropathic pain, an action similar to but distinct from that of opioids such as morphine (Guindon and Hohmann, 2009; Karst and Wippermann, 2009). This effect is classified as an *opioid-sparing action*, that is, less of the opiate would be needed for pain relief. Such an action might be a result of the presynaptic location of CB receptors, which function to reduce transmitter release, including those responsible for pain. Efforts to develop a cannabis-derived analgesic agent for clinical use, however, have not yet been successful, and there is a great deal of conflicting experimental results. Some people respond very well, others do not. This was illustrated by a study that took brain scans of normal volunteers who were given either 15 milligrams of THC or a placebo, and then rated the intensity of an experimental pain stimulus. With THC, people did not report any change in the pain, but the pain bothered them less. This was matched by a decrease in activity of a brain structure involved in the emotional aspect of pain, not pain sensation (Lee et al., 2013).

Smoking marijuana has long been reported to specifically reduce spasticity-related pain in people diagnosed with multiple sclerosis (MS). This led to the development of an oral medication, Sativex, approved in Canada, New Zealand, and eight European countries for the relief of muscle spasms associated with MS, and in pain associated with end-stage cancer. Sativex contains THC and cannabidiol in a 1:1 mixture, delivered in an oromucosal (mouth) spray. Cannabidiol antagonizes some of the adverse effects of THC, such as dysphoria and sedation (Russo and Guy, 2006) and provides a rational basis for combining the two for clinical efficacy and safety (Pertwee, 2009). Although therapeutic effects are not always observed (Centonze et al., 2009), current research confirms the therapeutic benefit of cannabis for treatment of MS. Cannabis administered either by smoking a marijuana cigarette (Corey-Bloom et al., 2012) or in the form of a capsule containing a cannabis extract (consisting of THC and cannabidiol; Zajicek et al., 2012) decreased spasms, and eased painful muscle stiffness, respectively, in MS patients. These data suggest that the analgesic effect of cannabis may be due to the muscle relaxation as a result of its antispastic action, rather than a direct block of pain.

In spite of the conflicting experimental data, efforts continue to explore the possible direct analgesic effect of cannabis in other illnesses besides MS. In one small study, a group of patients suffering from neuropathic, postsurgical pain, or posttraumatic pain, reported modest pain relief by smoking marijuana cigarettes containing 9.4 percent THC (see Leung, 2011, for a summary; Ware et al., 2010). Among patients diagnosed with fibromyalgia, about 13 percent used cannabinoids, and this behavior was more common in men, in patients also seeking opioids, and in those with a mental illness (Ste-Marie et al., 2012). Because current treatments do not help all pain patients, and because cannabis can produce moderate analgesia in some patients, especially in pain originating in the central nervous system, it may be a useful option (McQuay, 2010). Eloquent and informed arguments "for" and "against" smoking marijuana for medicinal use were recently presented in an editorial in the *New England Journal of Medicine* (Bostwick et al., 2013).

At least one British drug company is so confident of the analgesic potential of cannabis that it is developing a nonsynthetic cannabis mouth spray as a treatment for cancer pain, called nabiximols, currently in phase 3 trials (ClinicalTrials.gov number 01337089). This agent was recently found effective, in low doses, when used as add-on medication for cancer patients with pain that was not responsive to opioids (Portenoy et al., 2012).

Other, more indirect approaches are also being explored. Positive preliminary effects of drugs that block the enzyme FAAH have been reported to be safe for human administration. By blocking the metabolism of AEA, such agents could have a variety of therapeutic effects, especially if they can be formulated not to cross the blood-brain barrier and produce psychoactive effects (Clapper et al., 2010). Research using laboratory models of neuropathic and inflammatory pain conditions demonstrate analgesic effects of AEA (Khasabova et al., 2012) as well as synthetic CB1 and CB2 agonists (You et al., 2011; Ramirez et al., 2012).

Effects on Ingestion. One of the classic effects attributed to marijuana use is appetite stimulation, especially of sweet foods. This ancient association has been confirmed by modern research. THC, AEA, and other CB1 receptor agonists do stimulate appetite especially for sweet and palatable food, even when animals are sated (Seely et al., 2011). In fact, intake of THC can produce significant weight gain (Tibiriça, 2010). This effect has been used to clinical advantage. In 1981, nabilone (Cesamet), a synthetic derivative of THC, and the first licensed cannabis medical product, was approved to treat nausea and vomiting associated with cancer chemotherapy. In 1985 Dronabinol (Marinol), which is synthetic THC, was approved as an antiemetic for similar situations and, in 1992, approval was extended to stimulate appetite in wasting conditions, such as AIDs.

Activation of CB1 receptors in the CNS stimulates appetite, while peripheral stimulation slows metabolism and increases fat deposition. Nevertheless, one study, in a small sample of African American men (30 cannabis users and 30 controls), found that even after long-term use (mean of 12 years) there was little lasting metabolic effect. That is, chronic marijuana smokers had normal glucose tolerance (Muniyappa et al., 2013). Conversely, blockade of the CB1 receptor reduces weight. These experimental findings led to the development of the cannabinoid antagonist *rimonabant* (and other antagonists-inverse agonists, such as taranabant, otenabant, surinabant, and rosonabant). Marketed as the diet drug Acomplia, rimonabant, when combined with a low-calorie diet (Leite et al., 2009) at 20 milligrams per day, significantly reduced body weight and lowered blood glucose levels, cholesterol, and adverse blood lipids in obese patients with type 2 diabetes (Scheen, 2008; Wright et al., 2008). It also reportedly reduced use of (and relapse to) several drugs of abuse, including cigarettes (Gelfand and Cannon, 2006), alcohol (Economidou et al., 2006), opioids and stimulants (Fattore et al., 2007), and other aspects of drug abuse (Beardsley et al., 2009).

Although rimonabant (Acomplia) was approved for clinical use in several European countries in 2006, the U.S. Food and Drug Administration concluded that, despite efficacy, its safety was inadequate. Problems included nausea and potentially serious psychiatric reactions such as anxiety and depression. Because of these side effects rimonabant was removed from the world market and other research programs developing cannabinoid antagonists as antiobesity agents were terminated (Lee et al., 2009).

However, several approaches are being pursued that may reduce the undesirable actions while maintaining the benefits of CB-based medications. Such mechanisms include "partial agonists," "inverse agonists," or "weak antagonists" of the receptor (Fong et al., 2007); receptor modulators that act at a different site from the binding site for AEA; non-brain-penetrating, peripherally acting agents; "neutral antagonists" of the cannabinoid receptor (Janero and Makriyannis, 2009; Lee et al., 2009); blockade of metabolism or reuptake of eCBs (Seely et al., 2011); or development of nonpsychotropic products from *C. sativa.*

Neuroprotection. Cannabinoids and their derivatives have been postulated to possess neuroprotective effects following brain injury. This action is based on the ability of THC to inhibit glutaminergic transmission and reduce reactive oxygen intermediates, which are factors in causing neuronal damage after head injury. One synthetic cannabinoid derivative, dexanabinol, underwent trials as a protective agent after head trauma. Preliminary data were positive, but one double-blind trial found that it was not efficacious in the treatment of traumatic brain injury in humans (Maas et al., 2006).

Acute and Chronic Psychoactive Effects

Subjective Effects. The CNS effects of THC vary with dose, route of administration, experience of the user, vulnerability to psychoactive effects, and the setting in which administration occurs. Users report an increased sense of well-being, mild euphoria, relaxation, and relief from anxiety. Sometimes anxiety is increased in a new user, which may be at least partly due to the perceived increase in heart rate. In general, the senses may be enhanced and the perception of time is usually altered. Often events seem especially funny and laughter is easily elicited. Mundane ideas can seem profound and the loosening of associations and thought intrusions can produce an inflated sense of creativity. Illusions and hallucinations occur infrequently, possibly more at high doses.

It is not really known why marijuana is so rewarding. In humans, there is a range of THC doses that is pleasurable; below that there is no effect, above that, the reaction is unpleasant (Grilly and Salamone, 2012). Nonhuman primates will self-administer THC, AEA, and 2-AG (Justinova et al., 2003, 2011) and these substances activate the mesolimbic dopaminergic reward system (Cooper and Haney, 2009). Filbey and co-workers (2009) demonstrated that in abstinent marijuana users, marijuana cues would activate reward neurocircuitry, and the magnitude of activation was associated with the severity of problems related to marijuana use. On the other hand, the intravenous administration of a synthetic CB1 drug, Org-26828, to healthy male volunteers, produced drowsiness at low doses but caused unpleasant effects of anxiety, paranoia, and hallucinations at higher doses (Zuurman et al., 2010). Moreover, another study found that intravenous injection of THC did not increase dopamine release in the brain of male volunteers, even though it was sufficient to elicit psychotic symptoms in the participants (Barkus et al., 2011).

Huestis and coworkers (2001) demonstrated for the first time in humans that a specific antagonist for cannabinoid receptors would produce a dose-dependent blockade of marijuana-induced intoxication and tachycardia. This demonstration led to speculation that cannabinoid antagonists might be used to reverse cannabinoid intoxication in people who experience unpleasant reactions to marijuana (for example, panic and psychosis), or to treat cannabis addiction, similar to the use of naloxone for opioid overdose or addiction (see Chapter 10). Although cannabis, even when it is the only drug ingested, produces numerous drug-related emergency room visits each year, it is not a lethal substance. Estimates are that a fatal dose would have to be 20,000 to 40,000 times the typically ingested dose (Levinthal, 2012).

Psychomotor Effects. Nevertheless, cannabis use can be dangerous. Impairments of coordination, perception, reaction time, and divided attention that persist for several hours beyond one's perception of the "high" have obvious implications for the operation of a motor vehicle and performance in the workplace or at school. THC blood levels greater than about 2 to 5 nanograms/milliliter may impair driving (Figure 9.8), and blood concentrations greater than 5 to 10 nanograms/milliliter increase accident risk by about three to seven times that seen in nonintoxicated persons (Ramaekers et al., 2006). This increased risk is greatly potentiated by concomitant use of alcohol (Sewell et al., 2009). Interestingly, unlike alcohol, which increases risk-taking, cannabis typically makes drivers more cautious. Drivers under the influence of marijuana apparently try to compensate for its impairment (Grilly and Salamone, 2012). Nevertheless, drivers who use cannabis within 3 hours before driving are nearly twice as likely to cause a vehicle collision as those who have not taken drugs or alcohol (Asbridge et al., 2012).

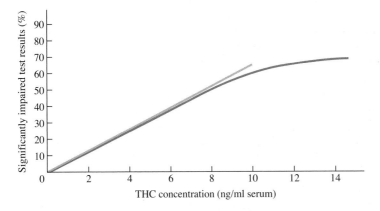

FIGURE 9.8   Percentage of performance decrements observed in the total number of psychomotor tests applied in 87 experimental studies as a function of THC concentration in blood serum (plasma) after eating (blue line) and smoking (red line). [Data from Ramaekers et al., 2004, Figure 1, p. 114.]

Did You Know?

Worker in Philadelphia Demolition Tragedy Allegedly High on Marijuana

In June 2013, during demolition of a four-story building, a wall fell on an adjacent Salvation Army thrift shop, crushing it. Six people died and 13 were injured. The government announced plans to charge construction worker Sean Benschop with 6 counts of involuntary manslaughter, 13 counts of recklessly endangering another person, and 1 count of risking a catastrophe.

Officials allege that Benschop was using an excavator to remove a second-story beam just seconds before the collapse. A toxicology report on blood taken from him about 2 hours after the collapse indicated that Benschop had marijuana and painkillers in his system. Benschop turned himself in to the police. He has a criminal record that includes convictions for drug-related offenses.

In response to this incident, Mayor Michael Nutter is calling for, among other things, random drug testing of operators of heavy equipment.

Cognitive Effects. Perhaps the most well known psychoactive effect of marijuana is the fact that it produces memory impairment. THC impairs all stages of memory, including encoding, consolidation, and retrieval. The ability to focus attention and filter out irrelevant information is disrupted. The marijuana users' speech, and presumably their underlying thought patterns, becomes fragmented. Because of the distracting intrusions of other ideas the user forgets what they, or others, have recently said. This difficulty in concentration impairs performance on many cognitive tasks. And, marijuana may also reduce the motivation to perform well.

The memory-disrupting effects appear to be mediated by CB1 receptors in the hippocampus (Wise et al., 2009). This is consistent with a report that the memory impairment produced by smoking marijuana may depend on the amount of cannabidiol in the product. In this study, users were divided into groups of high (0.75 percent) or low (0.14 percent) *cannabidiol* exposure, with a constant amount of THC. Those who smoked the low cannabidiol cannabis were significantly worse at recalling text material compared to when they were not intoxicated. But, this did not happen in those who smoked cannabis with a high cannabidiol level (Morgan et al., 2010). This result is consistent with other evidence, mentioned below, that cannabidiol has antagonistic actions at cannabis receptors and may mitigate some THC effects.

Cannabis-induced cognitive impairment may have serious implications for efforts to develop therapeutic cannabinoids. At least one study has reported that long-term, heavy cannabis use in MS patients (mean duration, 27 years) may affect cognition beyond what might occur as a result of the disease itself (Honarmand et al., 2011). Although learning and memory were not different between cannabis-using and non-cannabis-using MS patients, other functions, such as executive performance and visuospatial perception were worse, and cannabis users were twice as likely to be globally impaired. Even the medicinal product nabilone has been shown to cause impairments in attention and memory in computerized laboratory tasks in healthy male volunteers (Wesnes et al., 2010).

Research in laboratory animals and simplified neuronal systems suggests possible causes of cannabis-induced memory impairment. Recordings of electrical activity in the brains of rats showed that administration of a CB agonist disrupted the coordination of brain waves between the hippocampus and the frontal cortex (Kucewicz et al., 2011). Because of this "decoupling" of hippocampus and cortex, the rats were unable to correctly navigate around a maze.

The importance of the hippocampal CB1 receptor in cannabis-induced memory impairment was supported by a study that found differential effects of THC on synaptic connections, depending on the location of the CB1 receptors. These experiments used genetically modified mouse strains that specifically lacked CB1 receptors on either hippocampal neurons or on nonneuronal astrocytes, the glial cells associated with the neurons. The results showed that mice lacking CB1 receptors only on the astrocytes were protected from the memory impairment after a dose of THC. Mice that lacked the receptors only on neurons still showed the memory deficit (Han et al., 2012). These data reveal an unexpected effect of nonneuronal glial cells on memory, and further, suggest that cannabis-induced cognitive impairment may be avoided if drugs could be developed that are selective for those CB1 receptors only located on neurons.

The adverse cognitive deficits can persist for at least 1 month following discontinuation of heavy use, and it is generally believed that only minimal effects are likely to persist following a 30-day period of abstinence. However, this conclusion may need to be modified. One study has found that heavy cannabis users have smaller hippocampi and amygdalae than control subjects, and that this was associated with having a certain form of the CB1 gene (Schacht et al., 2012). Given the importance of these two structures for cognition, such long-term changes are concerning, especially considering that the mean age of the men and women in the study was between 27 and 28. These data are consistent with another report by Meier and colleagues (Meier et al., 2012) that people who were persistently diagnosed with cannabis abuse when they were teenagers had statistically significant decreases in IQ by the age of 38. The IQ tests were administered at ages 7 to 13 and again at age 38. Baseline IQ was not different among the groups who subsequently used cannabis and those who did not. But, by age 38 the IQ scores had greatly diverged. If heavy cannabis use began in adulthood, there was no change in IQ. An economist who argues that the IQ changes were confounded by socioeconomic factors, has since questioned the interpretation of this study. He notes that poorer people have less access to good schools, irrespective of cannabis use, and people with low socioeconomic status are on average, likely to show declining IQ as they get older (Røgeberg, 2013).

Psychiatric Effects. For the majority of users, cannabis use does not promote psychiatric problems. A recent longitudinal study in Swedish participants confirms that cannabis use is not associated with an increased risk of depression (Manrique-Garcia et al., 2012). At very high doses, acute depressive reactions, panic reactions, and mild paranoia have been observed, and several surveys indicate that 50 percent to 60 percent of marijuana users have reported at least one anxiety experience. But only at massive doses of THC do delusions, paranoia, hallucinations, confusion, and disorientation, depersonalization, altered sensory perception, and losses of insight occur; these reactions are unusual, however, and generally do not last long.

At the same time, among people with mental illness reporting at least weekly use, the rate of cannabis use was especially high for those with bipolar disorder, personality disorder and, perhaps not surprisingly, other substance use disorders. Specifically, 4.4 percent of persons with a mental illness in the past 12 months reported using cannabis weekly compared to 0.6 percent of persons without mental illness (Lev-Ran et al., 2013). It has long been known that schizophrenia patients have a greater history of cannabis abuse (25 percent) than people in the general population (4 percent). As early as 1958 a study was published that described psychoticlike behavior in healthy volunteers after a single ingestion of cannabis. In the 1970s cannabis-induced psychoses were characterized in the Bahamas and in India. It has also been reported that up to 15 percent of cannabis users experience acute psychotic symptoms. There is compelling epidemiological evidence that cannabis is a risk factor for the onset of psychosis. In 1987 a comprehensive review of over 45,000 Swedish military conscripts found that those who consumed high amounts of cannabis (used more than 50 times) by the age of 18 years, were 6 times more likely to have schizophrenia, even after controlling for contributing variables. In 2002 this result was replicated, showing a 6.7 times increased risk. These, and many other longitudinal studies, indicate some relationship between chronic, perhaps high-dose, cannabis use, and psychotic disorder (Malone et al., 2010). This is not simply due to drug abuse in general; for example, alcohol use does not show this association (Large et al., 2011).

These data raise the question of which comes first, cannabis use or schizophrenia? Perhaps people suffering from psychosis may use the drug to self-medicate and reduce their symptoms. If cannabis actually caused schizophrenia then the incidence of the illness should increase and decrease with the rate of cannabis use. Attempts to determine if that is the case have concluded that that is not what happens. Although there may be a small group of schizophrenic patients who do use cannabis to treat their symptoms, the evidence suggests that cannabis seems to preferentially affect those who had a predisposition to psychosis.

The results of the Swedish conscript study indicated that the age at which cannabis use began was a risk factor for the vulnerability to psychosis. This has prompted numerous efforts to determine whether psychotic symptoms predate the drug or vice versa. One extensive survey was conducted proactively, on a birth cohort of persons in New Zealand, which collected information about psychotic symptoms at age 11 and drug use by age 15. The results showed that early cannabis use increased the risk of psychosis. However, whether this was due to the fact that drug exposure occurred during a time when the brain is still developing, or a result of longer exposure to the drug in early users, is not clear, and both factors may contribute (Lynch et al., 2012).

Subsequent studies have reported the same outcome. Cannabis use by young people increased the risk of a psychotic experience even in those who had no prior psychotic event (Kuepper et al., 2011). In subjects who have a clinically high risk for psychosis, earlier lifetime use is associated with earlier symptomatology (Large et al., 2011; Evins et al., 2012; Nieman et al., 2012; Tosato et al., 2013).

Possible causes for the relationship between early-onset cannabis use and psychosis is currently being investigated. One factor is the increased potency of cannabis. During the last 20 to 30 years the percent of THC in all parts of the marijuana plant has increased, with some reports of up to 18 percent or more, compared to past levels of 3 percent. One study reported that 78 percent of first-episode psychosis patients versus 37 percent of control participants used high-potency cannabis. The first-episode psychosis group was twice as likely to have used cannabis for 5 or more years and six times more likely to be daily smokers.

A second factor involved in cannabis-induced psychosis may be the concentration of cannabidiol (CBD). Leweke and colleagues (2012) report that this component of cannabis reduces psychotic symptoms in patients with acute schizophrenia. (Interestingly, the schizophrenic patients given CBD also had an increase in their blood levels of anandamide.) Similarly, another study found that healthy people had fewer psychotic reactions to intravenous THC if they were pretreated with CBD (Evins et al., 2012). Englund and colleagues (2013) also found that in normal volunteers, CBD inhibited psychotic and paranoid symptoms and even improved the memory impairment produced by THC. Because newer, high-potency cannabis typically has less CBD than in the past, it may be that this natural product has some "antipsychotic" benefit.

Tolerance and Dependence

Experienced users of marijuana often report that they become more sensitive to its psychoactive effects (sensitized), rather than less (tolerant) with continued use. That is, they become "high" more quickly. However, tolerance to cannabis routinely develops in laboratory studies. This difference between experimental and "real world" exposure is believed to be due to several factors. First, novice users have to learn how to get enough of the smoke into the lungs to provide a sufficient THC dose. Second, new users have to learn to be aware of the subjective effects of the drug. Third, because the drug accumulates in fat tissue, regular smokers have some residual amount of THC in their body, which increases the total amount with each cigarette, producing a quicker "high." Nevertheless, tolerance does occur to cannabis. Some degree of tolerance results from learning how to adapt to the drug's disruptive effects. Although rodent studies had shown that CB1 receptors were downregulated after chronic cannabis exposure, which would also mediate tolerance, there was some inconsistency in this regard and it was not known if this occurred in humans. This has now been confirmed. Hirvonen and colleagues (2012) have shown reversible and regionally specific downregulation of CB1 receptors in cortical brain regions of human subjects who chronically smoke cannabis. Downregulation correlated with years of smoking and receptor density returned to normal after about 4 weeks of monitored abstinence.

Originally thought to be a relatively benign and infrequent occurrence, cannabis dependence occurs in about one of every ten persons who start smoking the drug, and is a common reason for admission to a drug treatment program (Benyamina et al., 2008; Cooper and Haney, 2008, 2009; Elkashef et al., 2008; Copeland and Swift, 2009; Vandrey and Haney, 2009). Elkashef and coworkers (2008) report that:

> When cannabis users were asked to rate the effects of their own use as positive, neutral, or negative, they gave overwhelmingly negative ratings of the effects that cannabis had on their social life (70%), their physical health (81%), their cognition (91%), their memory (91%), and their career (79%). (p. 17)

Withdrawal symptoms include irritability, anxiety, marijuana craving, disrupted sleep and strange dreams, anger and aggression, depressed mood, restlessness, decreased appetite, and weight loss. Less common symptoms include chills, headache, physical tension, sweating, stomach pain, and general physical discomfort (Vandrey and Haney, 2009). Reinstituting marijuana use ameliorates withdrawal discomfort (as would be expected). Symptoms begin within 48 hours after drug use stops and last at least 2 days, usually about 7 to 10 days and perhaps longer; EEG changes associated with withdrawal persist for at least 28 days. Although withdrawal from cannabis has been compared to recovering from the flu, or similar to nicotine withdrawal, the intensity, as with other drugs of abuse, depends on the severity of the dependence. The greater the dependence, the more severe the withdrawal syndrome, and the more likely that relapse will occur (Allsop et al., 2012).

Treatment Issues

There are as yet no evidence-based pharmacotherapies available for the management of cannabis withdrawal and craving (Vandrey and Haney, 2009). Psychotherapeutic strategies including cognitive-behavioral therapy, contingency management, family-based interventions, and motivational enhancement interventions have proven effective (Elkashef et al., 2008).

Several pharmacotherapies have been studied. Of these, oral THC and the serotonergic/noradrenergic antidepressant, mirtazapine (Remeron; see Chapter 12) have shown some promise (Benyamina et al., 2008). The antidepressant venlafaxine, given to depressed cannabis-dependent patients, was not effective in reducing the depression and may even increase cannabis use (Levin et al., 2013). The most effective medication so far in reducing cannabis withdrawal is dronabinol, a synthetic formulation of THC intended for oral use (Vandrey and Haney, 2009). Use of dronabinol would be similar to the use of nicotine replacement products to reduce withdrawal during tobacco abstinence. Other investigated medicines include bupropion (Wellbutrin, a dopaminergic antidepressant), buspirone (BuSpar, a serotonergic antidepressant), and the cannabinoid antagonist/inverse agonist, rimonabant. Naltrexone (an opioid antagonist; see Chapter 10) can be modestly effective in specific circumstances, but its effects can be overcome with higher doses of cannabis (Vandrey and Haney, 2009). A recent clinical trial of the drug gabapentin (Neurontin), an anticonvulsant and analgesic (see Chapter 10), showed some effectiveness in a group of 50 chronic, long-term cannabis users. Although 64 percent of the patients dropped out (those who had started earlier, used longer, and had more severe withdrawal), the drug did improve outcomes in conjunction with cognitive behavioral therapy (Mason et al., 2012).

Synthetic Cannabinoid Agonists of Abuse: Herbal Marijuana Alternatives (HMAs)

Classes of Synthetic Cannabinoid Drugs

In 1964, after THC was determined to be the active ingredient of *Cannabis sativa*, efforts were made to develop a synthetic version for possible therapeutic applications. By 1985 this had been accomplished, and dronabinol (Marinol) was approved in the United States as an antiemetic drug. Several other agents that are chemically similar to THC have also been produced, notably, nabilone (Cesamet) and HU-210 (synthesized at the Hebrew University in the 1960s). These are THC analogues, with slight differences in chemical structure. Nabilone is almost as potent as THC, and is the only THC analogue that has ever been approved (also an antiemetic) in the United States. HU-210 has not been approved, mainly because it is 100 to 800 times as potent as THC (Seely et al., 2011).

Additional compounds that differ chemically from THC were also produced. Chemists at the drug company Pfizer developed a group of drugs known as cyclohexylphenols, abbreviated as CP agents. These include substances designated as CP-50, 556-1, and CP-47, 497 and a related form, called (C8)-CP-47, 497, both of which are 30 times more potent than THC.

A third group of related drugs are categorized as aminoalkylindoles (AAIs). These include a drug called pravadoline, and similar compounds such as WIN-55212-2, developed at Sterling Drug Company. These drugs have high affinity for both types of cannabis receptors, produce effects similar to those of THC in laboratory animals, and are blocked by cannabinoid antagonists. Nearly 20 years ago John W. Huffman, a research chemist at Clemson University, created three of these AAIs, designated JWH-018 (1-pentyl-3-(1-naphthoyl)-indole), JWH-073, and JWH-015. These drugs have different binding affinities to the two CB receptors, but generally have similar pharmacological effects as THC, with JWH-018 having the greater relative potency (Seely et al., 2011).

A fourth group of compounds that act at CB receptors, called benzoylindoles include the substances AM-694 and RCS-4 (Fattore and Fratta, 2011). In December 2013, users of even two newer HMAs, ADBICA and ADB-PINACA, became ill at an event in Colorado. These, and several other new derivatives, are described in DOI10.1007/s11419-013-0182-9; http://www.nist.gov/oles/upload/Classes-and-Structures-of-Emerging-Cannabimimetics-and-Cathinones-Berrier.pdf. http://www.nist.gov/oles/upload/NIST-Novel-Hallucinogens-and-Plant-Derived-Highs-Final.pdf

Current Abuse

Several of these compounds became available in the early 2000s, widely sold on the Internet, in "head shops," and convenience stores, and by 2004 they had become globally popular, gaining the attention of American authorities by 2007. Variously called "spice," "mojo" (in Louisiana), "K2," "legal weed," and many other colorful names, the products are routinely labeled and marketed as "incense," not intended for human consumption. They are usually sold as dried leaves, resin, or powder, without age restriction; see Rosenbaum and colleagues (2012) and Seely and colleagues (2011) for a list of the herbs that are used in these products. Typically, about 3 grams of vegetable matter are mixed with one of the synthetic cannabinoids, and smoked, drunk as an infusion, or inhaled. The herbals in these preparations are not psychoactive; it is the synthetic drugs, probably dissolved in a solution and sprayed on the plant product, which produce the psychoactive effects. It is sometimes difficult to determine the active ingredient in spice products because there are natural substances, such as tocopherol (Vitamin E), and some agents, such as nicotine, which might be stated as an ingredient, but not actually present. Forensic assays in Europe and the United States have found that the herbal products are laced with HU-210, JWH-018, JWH-073, CP-47, 49, and (C8)-CP-47, 497, and newer versions (often the methyl derivative) such as JWH-019, JWH-398, JWH-122, JWH-200, JWH-250, and AM-694 (see Fattore and Fratta, 2011, for the specific chemical names) are constantly appearing. Other compounds found in spice products include the synthetic opioid O-desmethyltramadol (see Chapter 10) and a substance called Kratom (*Mitragyna speciosa*), which also has opiate actions, oleamide (a fatty acid derivative that has some sedative property), harmine and harmaline, myristicin (hallucinogens, see Chapter 8), and other substances that might be contaminants.

In summary, these drugs have gained worldwide popularity because they produce psychoactive effects, may still be legal, are easily available, perceived as safe, and are still difficult to detect. Several European countries have banned these compounds. In the United States, starting in February 2011, the Uniform Code of Military Justice (UCM) banned spice and the U.S. Air Force began screening urine for synthetic cannabinoids. In early 2011 the U.S. Drug Enforcement Administration (DEA) placed several of the synthetic cannabinoids on Schedule I. Most states have banned, or are in the process of banning, these products.

Pharmacological, Physiological, Psychoactive Effects and Toxicity

There is currently no definitive description of the absorption, distribution, metabolism, or elimination of HMAs in humans (Rosenbaum et al., 2012). The desired effect of spice is presumably the THC experience of euphoria and well-being. But, there are increasing reports of emergency room cases presenting with the symptoms of nausea, anxiety/agitation/panic attacks, tachycardia, paranoid thoughts, and hallucinations. Anxiety is a common side effect of acute intoxication, which may resolve in 1 to 2 hours after use. One analysis of 1,353 single drug exposures to synthetic cannabinoids, reported to the U.S. National Poison Data System between January and October 2010, provided some general information. The median age of patients was 20 years. Clinical symptoms included tachycardia (40 percent), agitation (23 percent), vomiting (15 percent), lethargy (14 percent), confusion (12 percent) hallucinations or delusions (9 percent), and seizures (4 percent). Treatment generally was supportive and clinical effects usually waned within 24 hours (Simmons et al., 2011; Hoyte et al., 2012). These data were supported by a retrospective study of patients seeking emergency treatment in the German city of Freiburg, between September 2008 and February 2011 (Hermanns-Clausen et al., 2013). The most common acute toxic symptoms of the synthetic cannabinoids were agitation, seizures, hypertension, emesis, and hypokalaemia (low potassium). However, one case reported that a 58-year-old man died as a result of "intentional inhalational abuse" (Hoyte et al., 2012).

Spice blends do not contain cannabidiol, and this may increase the dysphoric effects because, as noted, CBD has antagonistic effects at CB receptors. Tolerance can develop to spice, and cessation of use was reported to elicit a cannabinoid withdrawal syndrome (Zimmermann et al., 2009) in a 20-year-old man who had smoked this product for 8 months as treatment for nervousness. His symptoms were typical of cannabis withdrawal, namely, internal unrest, sweating, drug craving, nightmares, tremor, palpitations, nausea, and vomiting.

Psychotic symptoms have been reported as well as relapse in psychotic patients. Gastrointestinal reactions are common, although some of the most dangerous consequences of spice use are the cardiovascular effects such as increased heart rate and blood pressure. In addition, between March and December 2012, a total of 16 cases of acute kidney injury (AKI) from these agents were reported across the United States (Murphy et al., 2013). Five of the patients needed hemodialysis, four were given corticosteroids and none died. There was no single brand associated with all the cases, but a new, previously unreported fluorinated agent was discovered, methanone, also known as XLR-11, which was a potent CB agonist. Coma and suicide have been reported after use of the substance K2. In the United States, two adolescents died after taking this product, one from a coronary ischemic event and the other from suicide due to extreme anxiety (Fattore and Fratta, 2011).

There is no pharmacologically specific antidote for these substances, especially because the actual contents are usually unknown. In addition to supportive care, benzodiazepines may be helpful for anxiety and agitation. Case reports have not been useful in providing the duration of effects. Selective CB1 antagonists have reversed the psychotropic effects of marijuana in humans, although so far no data are available in regard to HMAs. Interestingly, a congener of HU-210—HU-211 (dexanabinol)—has shown a neuroprotectant effect in animals against soman-induced seizures, perhaps due to an action as a noncompetitive NMDA antagonist (Rosenbaum et al., 2012).

STUDY QUESTIONS

1. Summarize the history of cannabis.

2. What are the endocannabinoids? How do cannabis and the endocannabinoid system work?

3. What are the major acute and chronic physiological effects of cannabis on the body?

4. What are the cognitive effects of cannabis?

5. What are the psychological/psychiatric effects of cannabis?

6. Discuss evidence regarding current and possible future medical uses of marijuana. Should therapeutic uses be pursued?

7. What do you think society's response should be to the continued illicit use of marijuana? Should marijuana be legalized for either medical or recreational use? If so, how should it be regulated or restricted?

8. What are herbal marijuana alternatives? Where did they come from and what are their effects?

REFERENCES

Allsop, D. J., et al. (2012). "Quantifying the Clinical Significance of Cannabis Withdrawal." *PLoS One* 7: e44864.

Asbridge, M., et al. (2012)."Acute Cannabis Consumption and Motor Vehicle Collision Risk: Systematic Review of Observational Studies and Meta-Analysis." *British Medical Journal* 344: e536.

Barber, P. A., et al. (2013). "Cannabis, Ischemic Stroke and Transient Ischemic Attack: A Case Control Study." *International Stroke Conference* Abstract 147.

Barkus, E., et al. (2011). "Does Intravenous Δ9-Tetrahydrocannabinol Increase Dopamine Release? A SPET Study. *Journal of Psychopharmacology* 25: 1462–1468.

Battista, N., et al. (2012). "The Endocannabinoid System: An Overview." *Frontiers in Behavioral Neuroscience* 6: 1–7.

Beardsley, P. M., et al. (2009). "Cannabinoid CB1 Receptor Antagonists as Potential Pharmacotherapies for Drug Abuse Disorders." *International Reviews in Psychiatry* 21: 134–142.

Benyamina, A., et al. (2008). "Pharmacotherapy and Psychotherapy in Cannabis Withdrawal and Dependence." *Expert Reviews in Neurotherapy* 8: 479–491.

Bostwick, J. M., et al. (2013). "Medicinal Use of Marijuana." *New England Journal of Medicine* 368: 866–868.

Bouchard, J., et al. (2012). "Cannabinoid Receptor 2 Signaling in Peripheral Immune Cells Modulates Disease Onset and Severity in Mouse Models of Huntington's Disease." *The Journal of Neuroscience* 32: 18259–18268.

Centonze, D., et al. (2009). "Lack of Effect of Cannabis-Based Treatment on Clinical and Laboratory Measures in Multiple Sclerosis." *Neurological Sciences* 30: 531–534.

Clapper, J. R., et al. (2010). "Anandamide Suppresses Pain Initiation Through a Peripheral Endocannabinoid Mechanism." *Nature Neuroscience* 13: 1265–1270.

Cooper, Z. D., and Haney, M. (2008). "Cannabis Reinforcement and Dependence: Role of the Cannabinoid CB1 Receptor." *Addiction Biology* 13: 188–195.

Cooper, Z. D., and Haney, M. (2009). "Actions of Delta-9-Tetrahydrocannabinol in Cannabis: Relation to Use, Abuse, Dependence." *International Review of Psychiatry* 21: 104–112.

Copeland, J., and Swift, W. (2009). "Cannabis Use Disorder: Epidemiology and Management." *International Review of Psychiatry* 21: 96–103.

Corey-Bloom, J., et al. (2012). "Smoked Cannabis for Spasticity in Multiple Sclerosis: A Randomized, Placebo-Controlled Trial." *Canadian Medical Association Journal* 184: 1143–1150.

Degenhardt, L., and Hall, W. (2012). "Extent of Illicit Drug Use and Dependence, and Their Contribution to the Global Burden of Disease." *Lancet* 379: 55–70.

DeMoraes-Barros, M. C., et al. (2006). "Exposure to Marijuana During Pregnancy Alters Neurobehavior in the Early Neonatal Period." *Journal of Pediatrics* 149: 781–787.

Devane, W. A., et al. (1992). "Isolation and Structure of a Brain Constituent That Binds to the Cannabinoid Receptor." *Science* 258: 1946–1949

Doweiko, H. E. (2012). *Concepts of Chemical Dependency,* 8th ed. Belmont, CA: Brooks/Cole.

Economidou, D., et al. (2006). "Effect of the Endocannabinoid CB1 Receptor Antagonist SR-141716A on Ethanol Self-Administration and Ethanol-Seeking Behaviour in Rats." *Psychopharmacology* 183: 394–403.

Elkashef, A., et al. (2008). "Marijuana Neurobiology and Treatment." *Substance Abuse* 29: 17–29.

Englund, A., et al. (2013). "Cannabidiol Inhibits THC-Elicited Paranoid Symptoms and Hippocampal-Dependent Memory Impairment." *Journal of Psychopharmacology* 27: 19–27.

Evins, A. E., et al. (2012). "The Effect of Marijuana Use on the Risk for Schizophrenia." *Journal of Clinical Psychiatry* 73: 1463–1468.

Fattore, L., et al. (2007). "An Endocannabinoid Mechanism in Relapse to Drug Seeking: A Review of Animal Studies and Clinical Perspectives." *Brain Research Reviews* 53: 1–16.

Fattore, L., and Fratta, W. (2011). "Beyond THC: The New Generation of Cannabinoid Designer Drugs." *Frontiers in Behavioral Neuroscience* 5: 1–12.

Filbey, F. M., et al. (2009). "Marijuana Craving in the Brain." *Proceedings of the National Academy of Sciences USA* 106: 13016–13021.

Fong, T. M., et al. (2007). "Anti-Obesity Efficacy of a Novel Cannabinoid-1 Receptor Inverse Agonist MK-0364 in Rodents." *Journal of Pharmacology and Experimental Therapeutics* 321: 1013–1022.

Gelfand, E. V., and Cannon, C. P. (2006). "Rimonabant: A Selective Blocker of the Cannabinoid CB1 Receptors for the Management of Obesity, Smoking Cessation, and Cardiometabolic Risk Factors." *Expert Opinions on Investigational Drugs* 15: 307–315.

Grilly, D. M., and Salamone, J. D. (2012). *Drugs, Brain and Behavior*, 6th ed. New York: Pearson.

Guindon, J., and Hohmann, A. G. (2009). "The Endocannabinoid System and Pain." *CNS and Neurological Disorders—Drug Targets* 8: 403–421.

Han, J., et al. (2012). "Acute Cannabinoids Impair Working Memory Through Astroglial CB_1 Receptor Modulation of Hippocampal LTD." *Cell* 148: 1039–1050.

Hegde, V. L., et al. (2010). "Cannabinoid Receptor Activation Leads to Massive Mobilization of Myeloid-Derived Suppressor Cells with Potent Immunosuppressive Properties." *European Journal of Immunology* 40: 3358–3371.

Hermanns-Clausen, M., et al. (2013)."Acute Toxicity Due to the Confirmed Consumption of Synthetic Cannabinoids: Clinical and Laboratory Findings." *Addiction* 108: 534–544.

Hirvonen, J., et al. (2012). "Reversible and Regionally Selective Downregulation of Brain Cannabinoid CB_1 Receptors in Chronic Daily Cannabis Smokers." *Molecular Psychiatry* 17: 642–649.

Honarmand, K., et al. (2011). "Effects of Cannabis on Cognitive Function in Patients with Multiple Sclerosis." *Neurology* 76: 1153–1160.

Hoyte, C. O., et al. (2012). "A Characterization of Synthetic Cannabinoid Exposures Reported to the National Poison Data System in 2010." *Annals of Emergency Medicine* 60: 435–438.

Huestis, M. A. (2005). "Pharmacokinetics and Metabolism of the Plant Cannabinoids, Delta9-Tetrahydrocannabinol, Cannabidiol, and Cannabinol." *Handbook of Experimental Pharmacology* 168: 657–690.

Huestis, M. A., et al. (2001). "Blockade of Effects of Smoked Marijuana by the CB1 Selective Cannabinoid Receptor Antagonist SR141716." *Archives of General Psychiatry* 58: 322–328.

Izzo, A. A., et al. (2009). "Non-Psychotropic Plant Cannabinoids: New Therapeutic Opportunities from an Ancient Herb." *Trends in Pharmacological Sciences* 30: 515–527.

Janero, D. R., and Makriyannis, A. (2009). "Cannabinoid Receptor Antagonists: Pharmacological Opportunities, Clinical Experience, and Translational Prognosis." *Expert Opinion on Emerging Drugs* 14: 43–65.

Justinova, Z., et al. (2003). "Self-Administration of Delta(9)-Tetrahydrocannabinol (THC) by Drug Naive Squirrel Monkeys." *Psychopharmacology* 169: 135–140.

Justinova, Z., et al. (2011). " The Endogenous Cannabinoid 2-Arachidonoylglycerol Is Intravenously Self-Administered by Squirrel Monkeys." *Journal of Neuroscience* 31: 7043–7048.

Karst, M., and Wippermann, S. (2009). "Cannabinoids Against Pain. Efficacy and Strategies to Reduce Psychoactivity: A Clinical Perspective." *Expert Opinion on Investigational Drugs* 18: 125–133.

Khasabova, I. A., et al. (2012). "Cannabinoid Type-1 Receptor Reduces Pain and Neurotoxicity Produced by Chemotherapy." *The Journal of Neuroscience* 32: 7091–7101.

Kucewicz, M. T., et al. (2011). "Dysfunctional Prefrontal Cortical Network Activity and Interactions Following Cannabinoid Receptor Activation." *Journal of Neuroscience* 31: 15560–15568.

Kuepper, R., et al. (2011). "Continued Cannabis Use and Risk of Incidence and Persistence of Psychotic Symptoms: 10-year Follow-Up Cohort Study." *British Medical Journal* 342: d738.

Lacson, J. C., et al. (2012). "Population-Based Case-Control Study of Recreational Drug Use and Testis Cancer Risk Confirms an Association Between Marijuana Use and Nonseminoma Risk." *Cancer* 118: 5374–5383.

Large, M., et al. (2011). "Cannabis Use and Earlier Onset of Psychosis." *Archives of General Psychiatry* 68: 555–561.

Lee, M. C., et al. (2013). "Amygdala Activity Contributes to the Dissociative Effect of Cannabis on Pain Perception." *Pain* 154: 124–134.

Lee, H. K., et al. (2009). "The Current Status and Future Prospects of Studies of Cannabinoid Receptor 1 Antagonists as Anti-Obesity Agents." *Current Topics in Medicinal Chemistry* 9: 482–503.

Leite, C. E., et al. (2009). "Rimonabant: An Antagonist Drug of the Endocannabinoid System for the Treatment of Obesity." *Pharmacological Reviews* 61: 217–224.

Leung, L. (2011). "Cannabis and Its Derivatives." *Journal of the American Board of Family Medicine* 24: 452–462.

Levin, F. R., et al. (2013). "A Randomized Double-Blind, Placebo Controlled Trial of Venlafaxine-Extended Release for Co-Occurring Cannabis Dependence and Depressive Disorders." *Addiction* 108: 1084–1094.

Levinthal, C. F. (2012). *Drugs, Behavior and Modern Society,* 7th ed. New York: Allyn & Bacon.

Lev-Ran, S., et al. (2013). "Cannabis Use and Cannabis Use Disorders Among Individuals with Mental Illness." *Comprehensive Psychiatry* 54: 589–598.

Leweke, F. M., et al. (2012). "Cannabidiol Enhances Anandamide Signaling and Alleviates Psychotic Symptoms of Schizophrenia." *Translational Psychiatry* 2: e94.

Lynch, M. -J., et al. (2012). "The Cannabis-Psychosis Link." *Psychiatric Times* 29: 1–5.

Maas, A. I., et al. (2006). "Efficacy and Safety of Dexanabinol in Severe Traumatic Brain Injury: Results of a Phase III Randomized, Placebo-Controlled, Clinical Trial." *Lancet Neurology* 5: 38–45.

Malone, D. T., et al. (2010). "Adolescent Cannabis Use and Psychosis: Epidemiology and Neurodevelopmental Models." *British Journal of Pharmacology* 160: 511–522.

Manrique-Garcia, E., et al. (2012). "Cannabis Use and Depression: A Longitudinal Study of a National Cohort of Swedish Conscripts." *BMC Psychiatry* 12: 112.

Mason, B. J., et al. (2012). "A Proof-of-Concept Randomized Controlled Study of Gabapentin: Effects on Cannabis Use, Withdrawal and Executive Function Deficits in Cannabis-Dependent Adults." *Neuropsychopharmacology* 37: 1689–1698.

McQuay, H. J. (2010). "More Evidence Cannabis Can Help in Neuropathic Pain." *CMAJ* 182: 1494–1495.

Meier, M., et al. (2012). "Persistent Cannabis Users Show Neuropsychological Decline from Childhood to Midlife." *Proceedings of the National Academy of Sciences* 109: E2657–E2664.

Morgan, C. J. A., et al. (2010). "Impact of Cannabidiol on the Acute Memory and Psychotomimetic Effects of Smoked Cannabis: Naturalistic Study." *British Journal of Psychiatry* 197: 285–290.

Muniyappa, R., et al. (2013). "Metabolic Effects of Chronic Cannabis Smoking." *Diabetes Care* 36: 2415–2422.

Murphy, T. D., et al. (2013). "Acute Kidney Injury Associated with Synthetic Cannabinoid Use—Multiple States, 2012." *MMWR* 62: 93–98.

Nieman, D. S., et al. (2012). "Cannabis Use and Age of Onset of Symptoms in Subjects at Clinical High Risk for Psychosis." *Acta Psychiatrica Scandinavia* 125: 45–53.

Pertwee, R. G. (2009). "Emerging Strategies for Exploiting Cannabinoid Receptor Agonists as Medicines." *British Journal of Pharmacology* 156: 397–411.

Pletcher, M. J., et al. (2012). "Association Between Marijuana Exposure and Pulmonary Function Over 20 Years." *Journal of the American Medical Association* 307: 173–181.

Portenoy, R. K., et al. (2012). "Nabiximols for Opioid-Treated Cancer Patients with Poorly-Controlled Chronic Pain: A Randomized, Placebo-Controlled, Graded-Dose Trial." *The Journal of Pain* 13: 438–449.

Ramaekers, J. G., et al. (2004). "Dose Related Risk of Motor Vehicle Crashes After Cannabis Use." *Drug and Alcohol Dependence* 73: 109–119.

Ramaekers, J. G., et al. (2006). "Cognition and Motor Control as a Function of Delta9-THC Concentration in Serum and Oral Fluids: Limits of Impairment." *Drug and Alcohol Dependence* 85: 114–122.

Ramirez, S. H., et al. (2012). "Activation of Cannabinoid Receptor 2 Attenuates Leukocyte-Endothelial Cell Interactions and Blood-Brain Barrier Dysfunction Under Inflammatory Conditions." *The Journal of Neuroscience* 32: 4004–4016.

Røgeberg, O. (2013). *Proceedings of the National Academy of Sciences USA.* http://dx.doi.org/10.1073/pnas. 1215678110.

Rosenbaum, C. D., et al. (2012). "Here Today, Gone Tomorrow . . . and Back Again: A Review of Herbal Marijuana Alternatives (K2, Spice), Synthetic Cathinones (Bath Salts), Kratom, *Salvia divinorum*, Methoxetamine, and Piperazines." *Journal of Medical Toxicology* 8: 15–32.

Russo, E. B., and Guy, G. W. (2006). "The Tale of Two Cannabinoids: The Therapeutic Rationale for Combining Tetrahydrocannabinol and Cannabidiol." *Medical Hypotheses* 66: 234–246.

Schacht, J. P., et al. (2012). "Associations Between Cannabinoid Receptor-1 *(CNR1)* Variation and Hippocampus and Amygdala Volumes in Heavy Cannabis Users." *Neuropsychopharmacology* 37: 2368–2376.

Scheen, A. J. (2008). "CB1 Receptor Blockade and Its Impact on Cardiometabolic Risk Factors: Overview of the RIO Programme with Rimonabant." *Journal of Neuroendocrinology* 20, Supplement 1: 139–146.

Scuderi, C., et al. (2009). "Cannabidiol in Medicine: A Review of Its Therapeutic Potential in CNS Disorders." *Phytotherapeutic Research* 23: 597–602.

Seely, K. A., et al. (2011). "Marijuana-Based Drugs: Innovative Therapeutics or Designer Drugs of Abuse?" *Molecular Interventions* 11: 36–50.

Sewell, R. A., et al. (2009). "The Effect of Cannabis Compared with Alcohol on Driving." *American Journal on Addictions* 18: 185–193.

Simmons, J., et al. (2011). "Three Cases of 'Spice' Exposure." *Clinical Toxicology* 49: 431–433.

Ste-Marie, P. A., et al. (2012). "Association of Herbal Cannabis Use with Negative Psychosocial Parameters in Patients with Fibromyalgia." *Arthritis Care & Research* 64: 1202–1208.

Thomas, B. F., et al. (1996). "Structure-Activity Analysis of Anandamide Analogs: Relationship to a Cannabinoid Pharmacophore." *Journal of Medicinal Chemistry* 39: 471–479.

Tibiriça, E. (2010). "The Multiple Functions of the Endocannabinoid System: A Focus on the Regulation of Food Intake." *Diabetology & Metabolic Syndrome* 2: 5.

Tosato, S., et al. (2013). "The Impact of Cannabis Use on Age of Onset and Clinical Characteristics in First-Episode Psychotic Patients. Data from the Psychosis Incident Cohort Outcome Study (PICOS)." *Journal of Psychiatric Research* 47: 438–444.

Vandrey, R., and Haney, M. (2009). "Pharmacotherapy for Cannabis Dependence: How Close Are We?" *CNS Drugs* 23: 543–553.

Wang, H., et al. (2006). "Jekyll and Hyde: Two Faces of Cannabinoid Signaling in Male and Female Fertility." *Endocrinology Reviews* 27: 427–448.

Ware, M. A., et al. (2010). "Smoked Cannabis for Chronic Neuropathic Pain: A Randomized Controlled Trial." *Canadian Medical Association Journal* 182: E694–E701.

Wesnes, K. A., et al. (2010). "Nabilone Produces Marked Impairments to Cognitive Function and Changes in Subjective State in Healthy Volunteers." *Journal of Psychopharmacology* 24: 1659–1669.

Wise, L. E., et al. (2009). "Hippocampal CB1 Receptors Mediate the Memory Impairing Effects of Delta-9-Tetrahydrocannabinol." *Neuropsychopharmacology* 34: 2072–2080.

Wolff, V., et al. (2013). "Cannabis-Related Stroke: Myth or Reality?" *Stroke* 44: 558–563.

Wright, S. M., et al. (2008). "Rimonabant: New Data and Emerging Experience." *Current Atherosclerosis Reports* 10: 71–78.

You, H., et al. (2011). "Functional Characterization and Analgesic Effects of Mixed Cannabinoid Receptor/T-Type Channel Ligands." *Molecular Pain* 7: 89.

Zajicek, J. P., et al. (2012). "Multiple Sclerosis and Extract of Cannabis: Results of the MUSEC Trial." *Journal of Neurology, Neurosurgery and Psychiatry* 83: 1125–1132.

Zimmermann, U. S., et al. (2009). "Withdrawal Phenomena and Dependence Syndrome After the Consumption of 'Spice Gold'." *Deutsches Ärzteblatt International* 106: 464–467.

Zuurman, L., et al. (2010). "Pharmacodynamic and Pharmacokinetic Effects of the Intravenous CB1 Receptor Agonist Org 26828 in Healthy Male Volunteers." *Journal of Psychopharmacology* 24: 1689–1696.

Chapter 10

Opioid Analgesics

Pain Terminology

Pain is one of the most common of human experiences and one of the most common reasons people seek medical care. Nevertheless, as a sensory phenomenon it is very difficult to measure because it is such a subjective and personal experience. The word itself is thought to be derived from the Latin word *poena* meaning a punishment or penalty (Doweicko, 2012, p. 139), which certainly expresses the concept. The International Association for the Study of Pain defines it as a "highly unpleasant sensory and emotional experience associated with actual or potential tissue damage" (Stone and Molliver, 2009, p. 237).

Acute, short acting, pain is biologically useful because it provides a warning system against real or potential damage to the body, and it resolves once the source of the trauma heals. Chronic pain, however, serves no useful purpose, causes suffering, limits activities of daily living, and increases the costs of health care and disability.

Chronic pain is generally defined as pain lasting more than 3 months. It is classically subdivided into two types, *nociceptive* and *neuropathic* pain. The word *nociception* refers to the physiological processes involved in the transmission of noxious (that is, 'pain producing') stimuli. It represents a neurophysiological phenomenon and does not infer any conscious awareness. A *nociceptor* is a sensory neuron that reacts to a noxious stimulus, such as heat, physical damage, or chemical injury. Processes that increase or decrease nociception are *pronociceptive* or *antinociceptive* (that is, analgesic), respectively.

Nociceptive pain is caused by tissue damage. Neuropathic pain is caused by a lesion or some dysfunction of the nervous system, usually as a result of trauma, neuronal injury or infection. It is characterized by an increased sensitivity (*hyperalgesia*) to pain-producing, or even innocuous (nonpainful), stimuli. Common persistent pain conditions include migraine, back pain, arthritis, neuropathic pain that occurs in diabetes, AIDS, postherpetic neuralgia (PHN), multiple sclerosis and fibromyalgia, among other disorders.

Pain Signaling

Normal pain transmission is triggered when a noxious stimulus activates neurons that innervate a structure in the body, such as the skin, a joint, or an internal organ. These neurons are called primary afferent nociceptive sensory neurons (or just *primary afferents*); their cell bodies are located in ganglia, called *dorsal root ganglia* (DRG)(Figure 10.1), found alongside (parallel to) the spinal cord. Primary afferents send information about noxious stimulation from the body to the spinal cord, specifically to the *dorsal horn* (see Figure 10.1).

The terminals of the primary afferent neurons synapse onto neurons in the dorsal horn of the spinal cord. Those neurons then send the message up to the thalamus, which in turn projects to (makes contact with) the cortex in the forebrain. Here is where the subjective experience of pain occurs. However, as they ascend to the cortex, these fibers also send out branches, which synapse with neurons in the brainstem (*rostral ventral medulla; RVM*) and the midbrain (*periaqueductal gray; PAG*). In addition, the cortex and other structures in the

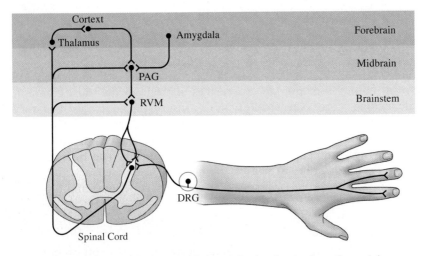

FIGURE 10.1 Overview of pain transmission. Pain signals arise from the periphery (outside of the Central Nervous System), when noxious (painful) stimuli activate sensory endings of nociceptive, primary afferent, neurons. These neurons have their cell bodies in the dorsal root ganglia (DRG) of the spinal cord. The pain signal is transmitted along the axons of the DRG neurons, which synapse on neurons in the dorsal horn of the spinal cord. Spinal cord neurons relay the pain signal to the thalamus and several other structures along the way, in the midbrain (the periaqueductal gray; PAG) and the brainstem (rostral ventral medulla; RVM). The thalamus projects to the higher brain areas where the perception of pain is ultimately experienced. Inhibitory and excitatory pathways descend from the brain back down to the spinal cord, modulating the same PAG and RVM sites that were activated by the ascending pathways. Opiate drugs can affect the pain signal through opiate receptors located at each of these levels, at the periphery, the spinal cord, the limbic system and other supraspinal sites, the midbrain, and the brainstem. In addition, other drugs, such as antidepressants, anticonvulsants, and channel blocking agents, can reduce pain by affecting different mechanisms involved in signal transmission. [Adapted after Stone and Molliver, 2009, Figure 2, p. 237.]

brain, such as the limbic structures, send descending fibers back down to the same mid-brain, brainstem, and spinal centers that transmitted the pain message. In this way various brain structures can either inhibit or facilitate the experience of pain.

As indicated in Figure 10.1, all of these sites may provide a target for analgesic medications. For example, drugs may provide pain relief by reducing the firing of the primary afferent neurons at the periphery, that is, at the site of the injury. This might be accomplished by antagonizing the neurochemical substances that are triggered by pain (the inflammatory reactions) which stimulate the primary afferents. This is essentially how the nonsteroidal anti-inflammatory drugs (NSAIDS) work. Alternatively, drugs such as anticonvulsants may act to reduce the excitation of the primary afferent axons and thereby decrease the signal that is transmitted to the spinal cord. Other drugs may reduce the transmission of the pain signal from within the spinal cord to the brain. Another approach is to activate the descending pathways from the brain to the spinal cord that inhibit ascending pain signals. Some of these descending pathways release the neurotransmitters serotonin and norepinephrine. The reason why some antidepressants can reduce pain (see Chapter 12) is because they increase the amount of these transmitters in the descending pathways (by blocking reuptake). Finally, by acting on higher brain structures, analgesic drugs may also alter the emotional reaction to pain, and reduce the suffering it causes, independently of influencing the sensory phenomenon itself.

Unfortunately, in spite of an expanding knowledge of the underlying pathology and a growing range of therapeutic options, current treatment of chronic pain remains inadequate. One recent review found that across all treatments, only about half of the patients responded to therapy, and the reduction in pain was only about 30 percent (Turk et al, 2011).

History

Morphine, obtained from opium, is still considered the model opioid analgesic, against which all others are compared. Opium is an ancient drug, and there is evidence that the opium poppy, *Papaver somniferum* was cultivated 10,000 years ago, although definite use as an analgesic is dated to about 3500 to 3000 years ago. Extracted from the sap of the seedpod of the poppy (Figure 10.2), opium has been used for thousands of

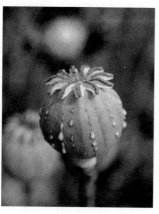

Dr. Jeremy Burgess/Science Source

FIGURE 10.2   Photograph of the opium poppy, showing the sap (resin) released from the scored immature seedpod. The dried powder of the resin is opium.

years to produce euphoria, analgesia, sleep, and relief from diarrhea and cough. The English word *opium* is derived from the Greek word *opion,* which means "poppy juice" (Doweicko, 2012, p. 137). In ancient times, opium was used primarily for its constipating effect and later for its sleep-inducing properties (noted by writers such as Homer, Hippocrates, Dioscorides, Virgil, and Ovid). Although it was used recreationally, not much is known about this aspect before the 18th century (Doweicko, 2012). During the Middle Ages, opium was combined with alcohol and the mixture called *laudanum* (named by Paracelsus in 1520), meaning "something to be praised." Referred to as the "stone of immortality," opium and laudanum were used for practically every known disease.

In 1806, morphine was isolated from opium by the chemist, Sertürner; the chemical formula was determined in 1847. After the invention of the hypodermic needle in 1853 and especially after the Civil War (when opioid addiction was referred to as the "soldier's disease"), clinical and recreational use became widespread. At that time, morphine use was unregulated; it was an unidentified ingredient in patent medicines and elixirs, used liberally in the battlefield and military hospitals, and recreationally by opium smoking (a practice introduced by Chinese immigrants who came to work in the United States during the 19th century).[1] By the year 1900, more than 4 percent of the entire U.S. population was addicted to opium or another opiate (Doweicko, 2012, p. 139). In one survey of 35 Boston drugstores in 1888, 78 percent of the prescriptions that had been refilled three or more times contained opium (Levinthal, 2012, p. 122). This epidemic was one of the factors that led to the passage of the Pure Food and Drug Act of 1906, which required that manufacturers list the ingredients of their products on the labels. Once that happened, people could see that their medicines contained some questionable compounds, and use began to decline. In addition, the Harrison Narcotic Act was passed in 1914, which stated that only a licensed physician or dentist could prescribe opiates (and cocaine) and that they had to register with the Internal Revenue Service if they did prescribe these drugs. Gradually, this law was interpreted by court decisions to mean that opiates could not be prescribed for *nonmedical* reasons, that is, it could only be taken for a medically approved purpose. In other words, it became illegal for opiate addicts to get the drug just to maintain their habit.

Since then, there have been periodic cycles of opiate abuse followed by efforts to reduce the recreational use of opiates, without much success. An important part of this goal has been an ongoing search for drugs that would alleviate pain without the potential for addiction. This search has produced an expanding formulary of natural, semisynthetic and synthetic opiate analgesics, as described below, but so far, the goal to separate the analgesic and addictive (euphoric) properties of opiates has been unsuccessful. Currently, we are in the midst of another ongoing epidemic of prescription opiates, with the epicenter in the United States. As discussed later in this chapter, abuse of prescription

---

[1] The habit of smoking opium was acquired by the Chinese as a result of trade with the West, especially Britain, early in the 19th century. The British needed to balance their large purchases of tea from China. They did this by trading opium, grown in India, for tea. The Chinese government didn't like what the opium trade did to its people, so they outlawed it. But the British did not want to lose this valuable source of income, which led to the Opium Wars of 1839–1842 and 1856–1860 between China and Western countries. The British won the wars because of their naval superiority. Not only did the trade resume, they also gained the island of Hong Kong, until it was returned to China in 1999.

opiates in the United States was recently greater than that of any illicit drug, including cannabis. This prompted development of many new formulations of opiate drugs, pharmacologically designed to prevent recreational misuse. Some evidence now suggests that the epidemic is waning. For the first time since 2006, opioid prescriptions did not increase in 2012, according to the drug market research firm, IMS Health. There were 241 million opioid prescriptions in 2012, compared to 243 million in 2011.

Opioid Terminology

An *opioid* is any exogenous drug (natural, semisynthetic, or synthetic) that binds to an opiate receptor, produces analgesia, and is blocked by an opiate antagonist. Often these drugs are also referred to as *narcotics*. The term *narcotic* is derived from the Greek word *narke*, meaning "numbness," "sleep," or "stupor." Originally referring to any drug that induced sleep, the term later became associated with opioids, such as morphine and heroin. It is an imprecise term, sometimes used in a legal context to refer to a wide variety of abused substances that includes nonopioids, such as cocaine and marijuana. The term is not useful in a pharmacological context, and its use in referring to opioids is discouraged.

There are four naturally occurring alkaloids (plant-derived amines) that can be isolated from the poppy plant: *morphine, codeine, papaverine,* and *thebaine* (Pathan and Williams, 2012). Chemical modification of these opiate alkaloids produced many semisynthetic opiates; totally synthetic opiates then followed. These can be divided into four major groups (which can be further subdivided in terms of chemical structure): morphinan derivatives (levorphanol, butorphanol); diphenylheptane derivatives (methadone, propoxyphene); benzomorphan derivatives (pentazocine, phenazocine); and the phenylpiperidine derivatives (pethidine [a.k.a. meperidine], fentanyl, and similar drugs).

Opioids can also be classified in regard to their action at opiate receptors, as agonists, partial agonists or antagonists. Finally, opiates can be classified according to the type of receptor through which they exert their effects. Some of the most commonly used opiate drugs that are discussed in this chapter, are shown in Table 10.1.

Opioid Receptors

There is general agreement on the existence of at least three types of opioid receptors, all of them G-protein coupled receptors (GPCRs)(see Chapter 1). They are named *mu* (after morphine), *kappa* (after the first agent known to act at this receptor, ketocyclazocine), and *delta* (after vas deferens, the tissue in which it was first isolated) (Pathan and Williams, 2012). In 2000 the nomenclature was changed and the respective receptor types are now also identified as MOP, KOP and DOP. The genes encoding these three families, as well as the receptors themselves, have been cloned and sequenced.

Each receptor type (mu, kappa, delta) arises from its own gene and is expressed through a specific messenger RNA (mRNA). Each receptor is a chain of approximately 400 amino acids, and the amino acid sequences are about 60 percent identical to one another and 40 percent different. Some authorities support the existence of subtypes for the receptors, but this is not universally accepted.

TABLE 10.1 classification of commonly used opiate analgesic agonist and antagonist medications

Opioid (Trade Name)	Origin	Chemical Class	Opioid Receptor Mechanism(s)	Non-Opioid Mechanisms
Morphine	Natural	Morphinan	Full Agonist μ	
Codeine	Natural	Morphinan	Full Agonist μ	
Levorphanol (Levo Dromoran)	Synthetic	Morphinan	Full Agonist μ, κ	NE Reuptake block; NMDA receptor antagonist
Oxycodone (Oxycontin)	Semi-synthetic	Morphinan	Full Agonist μ	
Hydrocodone (Vicodin)	Semi-synthetic	Morphinan	Full Agonist μ	
Hydromorphone (Dilaudid)	Semi-synthetic	Morphinan	Full Agonist μ	
Oxymorphone (Opana)	Semi-synthetic	Morphinan	Full Agonist μ	
Fentanyl (Abstral, Actiq, et al)	Synthetic	Phenylpiperidine	Full Agonist μ	
Meperidine (Demerol)	Semi-synthetic	Phenylpiperidine	Full Agonist μ	
Methadone (Dolophine)	Synthetic	Diphenylheptanes	Full Agonist μ	NE Reuptake block; NMDA receptor antagonist
Buprenorphine (Subutex)	Semi-synthetic	Morphinan	Partial Agonist μ	
Tapentadol (Nucynta)	Synthetic		Agonist μ	NE Reuptake block
Tramadol (Ultram)	Semi-synthetic		Agonist μ	NE Reuptake block; 5-HT Release
Butorphanol (Stadol)	Synthetic	Morphinan	Mixed Ag κ/Antag μ	
Pentazocine (Talwin)	Synthetic	Benzomorphan	Mixed Ag κ/Antag μ	
Naloxone (Narcan)	Semi-synthetic		Agonist μ	
Naltrexone (ReVia; Vivitrol)	Semi-synthetic		Agonist μ	
Nalmefene (Revex)	Semi-synthetic		Partial Ag κ/Antag μ	

TABLE 10.2 Classification of opioid receptors, their precursors and endogenous ligands

Receptor	Precursor	Peptide
DOP	Pro-enkephalin	[Met]-enkephalin
		[Leu]-enkephalin
KOP	Pro-dynorphin	Dynorphin-A
		Dynorphin-B
MOP	POMC	β-Endorphin
	Unknown	Endomorphin-1
		Endomorphin-2
NOP	Pre-pro-nociceptin	N/OFQ

From Pathan, H., and Williams, J. "Basic Opioid Pharmacology: An Update." *British Journal of Pain 6,* 2012:11-16. Copyright © 2012 by British Pain Society. Reprinted by Permission of SAGE Publications Ltd., London, Los Angeles, New Delhi, Singapore, and Washington DC.

The three classical opioid receptors are distributed widely throughout the central nervous system and to a lesser extent, in the periphery (including the vas deferens, knee joint, gastrointestinal tract, and other sites).

The existence of receptors on which the natural substance opium could exert such significant effects, implied that there must be some inherent, endogenous substance(s) within our body that normally acted on those receptors. Presumably the receptors didn't evolve just to respond to an extract of the poppy plant! Soon after the opioid receptors were discovered, these endogenous substances were also determined. Each comes from a precursor compound (Table 10.2). As indicated in the table, the pro-hormone proenkephalin is cleaved to form *met-enkephalin* and *leu-enkephalin*, which have the greatest affinity for the DOP receptor. *Dynorphin A and B* are agonists at the KOP receptor, and are derived from the pro-hormone, prodynorphin.[2] The parent compound of the endogenous agonist for the MOP receptor, β-*endorphin*, is pro-opiomelanocortin (POMC). There are two other MOP agonists, endomorphin 1 and 2, but their precursor has not yet been identified.

As seen in Table 10.2, a fourth type of opiate receptor has also been identified, for which an endogenous ligand and a precursor substance has been determined. However, because this receptor, the nociceptin (NOP) receptor, does not respond to the classical opiate antagonist, naloxone, its categorization has been questioned. It is considered to be a non-opioid 'branch' of the opioid receptor family (Pathan and Williams, 2012).

What is the consequence of the binding of an opioid agonist to a *mu* (MOP) receptor?

Figure 10.3 summarizes this process. As is generally the case with GPCRs, the G-protein (consisting of the α, β and γ subunits) breaks off from the rest of the receptor (dissociates), and separates into two parts, the α component and the βγ components. These components interact with other parts of the neuron: they *activate* potassium channels, *inhibit* calcium channels, and *reduce* the amount of the substance cyclicAMP

---

[2] The hallucinogenic agent salvinorin A (from the psychedelic mint plant *Salvia divinorum*) is a potent agonist of the kappa opioid receptor (discussed in Chapter 8).

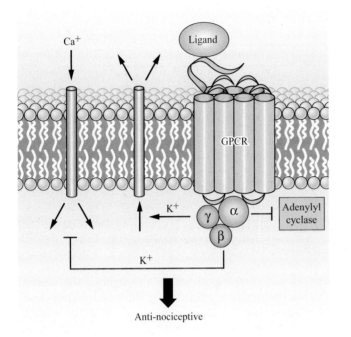

FIGURE 10.3 Schematic of the opiate receptor. The opiate receptor is a G-protein coupled receptor (GPCR). When a molecule of an opiate (ligand), such as morphine, attaches to its binding site on the receptor, it activates the G-protein, causing it to dissociate into its α component and the dual βγ component. The α component inhibits the activity of the enzyme, adenylyl cyclase. The βγ component does two things. First, it opens a channel in the membrane through which potassium ions (K^+) flow out. The movement of positively charged potassium ions *out of the neuron* makes the inside more negative, which means the neuron is inhibited and is less likely to fire. Second, the βγ component *inhibits* channels through which positively charged calcium ions flow *into the neuron*. This reduces neurotransmitter release. All of these processes contribute to reduce the transmission of pain. [Adapted after Stone and Molliver, 2009, Figure 1D, p. 235.]

inside the neuron (by inhibiting the enzyme adenylyl cyclase), as indicated in the figure. These actions hyperpolarize the neuron, that is, the neuron is inhibited. Activating potassium channels will allow more of the positively charged potassium ions to leave the neuron; blocking calcium channels will prevent more of the positively charged calcium ions from entering the neuron. Both of these actions will make the inside of the neuron more negative, relative to the outside. This means the neuron is less likely to fire when stimulated, or, if active, it will release less transmitter.

Exogenous and endogenous opiates exert their effects throughout the body, including the periphery, on neurons in the dorsal horn of the spinal cord, and within various brain sites. In the spinal cord, opioid receptors are located on the presynaptic terminals of the nociceptive primary afferents (see Figure 10.1). When activated by an opioid agonist, the result will be to block the release of pain-producing substances such as glutamate, substance P, and calcitonin gene-related peptide (CGRP). By blocking the release of pain-producing substances, opiates reduce ascending pain signals to higher brain centers.

In the brain, opioid analgesia is believed to be mediated by activation of *mu* (μ, MOP) receptors in the midbrain and brainstem. High densities of opiate receptors are found in midbrain periaqueductal gray (PAG) neurons, and in brainstem nuclei located in the rostral ventral medulla (RVM). Opiate agonists indirectly activate the descending inhibitory input from these sites onto the pain processing neurons of the spinal cord. As noted, these pathways release serotonin, norepinephrine, and enkephalin, which further suppress the transmission of pain signals.

Classification of Opioids

Pure Agonists

All clinically used opioids produce their effects at least partly by acting at the MOP receptor, although some also act at other opiate, and nonopiate receptors. Morphine is the prototype opioid analgesic, but there are many others, as shown in Table 10.1. Of course, morphine also has activity at the other opiate receptors.

Partial Agonists

A partial agonist binds to opioid receptors but has a low intrinsic activity (low efficacy). It therefore exerts an analgesic effect, but the effect has a ceiling at less than the maximal effect produced by a pure agonist. *Buprenorphine* is the prototype partial opioid agonist. When administered to a person who is not opioid dependent, it produces analgesia; when administered to an opioid-dependent person, however, buprenorphine may compete with a full agonist, preventing its full effect, and withdrawal may be precipitated.

Mixed Agonist-Antagonists

A mixed agonist-antagonist drug produces an agonistic effect at one receptor and an antagonistic effect at another. Clinically useful mixed drugs are kappa agonists and weak mu antagonists (they bind to both kappa and mu receptors, but only the kappa receptor is activated). Like a partial agonist, a mixed agonist-antagonist usually displays a ceiling effect for analgesia; in other words, it has decreased efficacy compared to a pure agonist and usually is not so effective in treating severe pain. Also, when a mixed agonist-antagonist is administered to an opioid-dependent person, the antagonistic effect at a mu receptor precipitates an acute withdrawal syndrome. *Pentazocine* (Talwin) is the prototype mixed agonist-antagonist.

Pure Antagonists

Pure antagonists have *affinity* for a receptor (here, the mu receptor), but after attaching they elicit no change in cellular functioning (they lack intrinsic activity). What they do is compete with the mu agonist for the receptor, precipitating withdrawal in an opioid-dependent person and reversing any analgesia caused by the agonist. One example is the clinical use of the opioid antagonist naltrexone in treatment programs for heroin addicts, where heroin taken after the antagonist elicits no analgesic or euphoric effects.

Major Pharmacological Effects of Opiates

Analgesia. Opiates produce analgesia and indifference to pain, reducing the intensity of pain and thus reducing the associated distress by altering the central processing of pain. Analgesia occurs without loss of consciousness and without affecting other sensory modalities. The pain may actually persist as a sensation, but patients feel more comfortable and are able to tolerate it. In other words, the perception of the pain is significantly altered.

Euphoria. Opiates produce a euphoric state, which includes a strong feeling of contentment, well-being, and lack of concern. Regular users of morphine describe the effects of intravenous injection in ecstatic and often sexual terms, but the euphoric effect becomes progressively less intense after repeated use. As with other drugs of abuse, opiates produce their rewarding effects by increasing dopamine release in the limbic reward pathway. It is postulated that opiates act indirectly in the ventral tegmental area by inhibiting GABA neurons via mu opioid receptors. The GABA neurons exert an inhibitory effect on dopamine neurons. Thus opiates are believed to be rewarding at least partly because they *disinhibit dopaminergic neurons and increase dopamine input in the nucleus accumbens and in other areas* (see Chapter 4).

Did You Know?

Risks of Opiate Addiction

The director of the National Institute on Drug Abuse, Dr. Nora Volkow, has personal insight into why people would want to take these drugs. She was badly injured in a car wreck over 15 years ago and was given Demerol. She says, "I was supposed to be in great pain but instead I felt an incredible sense of well-being." Because of her knowledge and sensitiveness about the potential for addiction, after 3 days Dr. Volkow said, "Enough."

Depression of Respiration. Opiates cause a profound depression of respiration by decreasing the brainstem respiratory center's sensitivity to higher levels of carbon dioxide in the blood. Respiratory rate is reduced even at therapeutic doses; at higher doses, the rate slows even further, respiratory volume decreases, breathing patterns become shallow and irregular, and, at sufficiently high levels, breathing ceases.

Respiratory depression is the single most important acute side effect of morphine and is the cause of death from acute opioid overdosage. A respiratory rate of 12 breaths per minute or less, in a patient who is not actually sleeping, strongly suggests acute opioid intoxication, particularly if miosis (pinpoint pupils) or stupor are also present. Treatment, in adults, consists of 0.04 milligrams of the antagonist naloxone, which can be increased up to a maximum of 15 milligrams. If respiratory depression persists after 15 milligrams of naloxone it is unlikely that it is due to opioid overdose. Because naloxone is short-acting, reversal of opioid analgesic toxicity might require continuous infusion (Boyer, 2012). Although the fact that naloxone must be injected is a drawback, other routes, such as a nebulized formulation, may be effective (Weber et al., 2012). The combination of morphine (or other opioid) with alcohol or other sedatives is especially dangerous.

Tolerance of respiratory depression appears to develop at a slower rate than analgesic tolerance. Because of this delay patients with a long history of opioid use are, paradoxically, at increased risk for respiratory depression (Boyer, 2012). Methadone may confer greater risk of overdose toxicity than other opiates, because with this drug respiratory depression may occur *later* than the analgesic effect. A patient may believe that an analgesic dose is too low, and then take more of the drug before it has time to take effect. Moreover, patients tolerant to high doses of other opiates may not be tolerant to methadone (Stachnik, 2011). This may be relevant to recent efforts to understand the current dramatic increase in opiate overdose deaths. Reviews have found that overdose deaths are more likely to occur when patients are 'rotated' from one opioid to another (Webster and Fine, 2012), when higher dosages are prescribed (Bohnert et al., 2011), or when drug addicts either begin or terminate opiate use (Cornish et al., 2010).

Suppression of Cough.   Opiates suppress the cough center in the brain stem and have historically been used as cough suppressants. This is termed an 'antitussive' action. Codeine is particularly popular for this purpose. Today, however, less addicting drugs are used as cough suppressants and opioids have become inappropriate choices for treating persistent cough.

Sedation and Anxiolysis.   Opiates reduce anxiety and produce sedation and drowsiness, but the level of sedation is not so deep as that produced by other CNS depressants. Although people who are taking morphine doze, they can usually be awakened readily. During this state, cognitive slowing is prominent, accompanied by a lack of concentration, apathy, complacency, lethargy, and a sense of tranquility. This effect becomes tolerant with repeated use. Nevertheless, this action may be therapeutically useful, as it has been reported that morphine has helped to reduce the development of Posttraumatic Stress Disorder (PTSD) in soldiers who were injured in combat during the Iraq war (Holbrook et al., 2010).

Nausea and Vomiting.   Opiates stimulate receptors in an area of the medulla called the *chemoreceptor trigger zone*. Stimulation of this area produces nausea and vomiting, which are characteristic and unpleasant side effects of morphine and other opioids, but they are not life threatening. Like drowsiness, this effect becomes tolerant with chronic use.

Gastrointestinal Symptoms.   As a result of their direct actions on the intestine opiates relieve diarrhea, the most important action of opioids outside the CNS. These drugs cause intestinal tone to increase, motility to decrease, feces to dehydrate, and intestinal spasm (and cramping). The combination of decreased propulsion, increased intestinal tone, decreased rate of movement of food, and dehydration hardens the stool and further retards the advance of fecal material. Nothing more effective than the opioids has yet been discovered for treating severe diarrhea. Two opioids have been developed that only very minimally cross the blood-brain barrier into the CNS. One is *diphenoxylate* (the primary active ingredient in Lomotil), and the other is *loperamide* (Imodium). These two drugs are exceedingly effective opioid antidiarrheals.

Unfortunately, as a side effect of chronic opiate treatment, opiate induced constipation (OIC) is often a very undesirable adverse reaction, estimated to occur in 40 to 90 percent of patients (Peppin, 2012). Moreover, there appears to be little tolerance to this side effect. Treatment generally consists of administering an anticonstipatory agent together with the opiate. Although there are numerous options, in the context of this chapter, the opioid antagonists are most relevant. Naloxone, while not officially approved for this indication, is most commonly used. However, because it crosses the blood-brain barrier, naloxone can also reverse the analgesic effect of opiates. Therefore, newer agents have been developed, which have a methyl group added to the opioid antagonist naltrexone. This prevents the antagonist from entering the brain and limits the effects to the periphery. *Methylnatrexone* (Relistor) is currently available as a subcutaneous injection, but an oral formulation is undergoing clinical testing. Methylnaltrexone is intended to restore bowel function in adults with advanced illnesses who are receiving opioids on a continuous basis and suffer from their constipating effects (Thomas et al., 2008). Another injectable opiate antagonist, *alvimopan* (Entereg) is intended to restore normal bowel function in hospitalized patients who have undergone bowel surgery (Webster et al., 2008).

A nonopioid laxative agent, *lubiprostone* (trade name Amitiza), already approved for chronic idiopathic constipation in adults and in adult women with Irritable Bowel Syndrome, was also approved for opioid-induced constipation in chronic pain patients, in April 2013.

Experimental agents, such as TD-1211 (Vickery et al., 2012) and NKTR-118 (Peppin, 2012) are in progress.

Pupillary Constriction.   Opiates cause pupillary constriction (miosis). Indeed, pupillary constriction in the presence of analgesia is characteristic of opioid ingestion. As noted below, one opiate drug that does not elicit this effect is meperidine.

Endocrine Effects.   Opiates exert subtle but important effects on the functioning of the endocrine system (Katz, 2005). Effects include reduced libido in men and menstrual irregularities and infertility in women. These actions occur secondary to drug-induced reductions in sex hormone-releasing agents from the hypothalamus. As a result, testosterone levels in males fall, as do the levels of luteinizing and follicle-stimulating hormones in females. If a person is taking an opioid for chronic pain, both the reduction in sex hormones and the chronic pain may result in loss of sexual desire and impaired performance, alterations in gender role, fatigue, mood alterations, loss of muscle mass and strength, abnormal menses, infertility, and osteoporosis and fractures (Katz, 2005). It may be unclear whether the opioid-induced hypogonadism or the chronic pain was responsible (Brennan, 2013). In addition to changes in sex hormones, patients maintained on opiates for many years may have a variety of hormonal abnormalities (Tennant, 2012).

Other Effects.   Opiates can release histamine from its storage sites in mast cells in the blood, which can result in localized itching or more severe allergic reactions, including bronchoconstriction. Opioids also affect white blood cell function, producing complex alterations in the immune system. It is advisable, perhaps, to avoid the use of morphine in patients with compromised immune function.

Genetic Opioid Metabolic Defects (GOMD)

With the current dramatic increase in opioid prescription abuse and concern about accidental overdose of these medications, the phenomenon of genetic anomalies in opiate metabolism has received greater attention (Pierce and Brahm, 2011;Tennant, 2010, 2011). The primary metabolic opiate pathways are the cytochrome P450 (CYP) 2D6 and 3A4 isoenzymes. These account for over 90 percent of opiate metabolism; the CYP-3A4 alone accounts for 40 to 60 percent. Although the evidence is somewhat indirect, estimates are that 20 to 30 percent of pain patients have a genetic opioid metabolic defect (GOMD) in one of these enzymes (and there are probably more). In some cases the enzyme is too active, the opioid is metabolized, and pain returns, more quickly than usual. These patients require a higher than normal dosage of opiate, which may cause them to be mislabeled as addicts and undertreated. In other cases, the metabolic enzyme is either inactive or absent, which causes the opioid to build up in the blood because it is not being metabolized. These situations may produce life-threatening allergic reactions (due to opioid interactions with the immune system), or respiratory depression.

According to Dr. Tennant, "This mechanism is undoubtedly responsible for some, if not most, of the numerous overdose deaths that have occurred since opioid prescribing for pain became so popular in the last decade," (Tennant, 2010). In his articles, Dr. Tennant discusses simple ways to diagnose and treat these conditions. One very helpful approach is to use opiates that bypass the CYP450 system, and are metabolized by glucuronidation. These include oxymorphone, hydromorphone, and tapentadol.

However, even without a metabolic defect, interactions between opioids and other psychotropic drugs are prevalent and could be dangerous. Many of the metabolic enzymes involved in opiate metabolism are either inhibited or induced by other medications, especially antidepressants, and these effects have important implications for pain prescriptions. Enzyme induction will reduce opioid analgesic efficacy and could even cause withdrawal; enzyme inhibition could cause overdose and respiratory depression. Pierce and Brahm (2011) provide a very useful discussion of these relationships and some of the most relevant specific interactions.

Genetic influences on opiate effects have been found for a variety of responses, in addition to respiratory depression. One study of the reaction to the opiate drug alfentanil in 114 twin pairs, reported that nausea and dislike of the drug had a high degree of heritability (Angst et al., 2012).

Tolerance and Dependence

The development of tolerance and dependence with repeated use is a characteristic feature of all opioid drugs. This reflects a progressive failure of the receptors to initiate a signal after long-term opioid binding, a phenomenon termed receptor desensitization.

The process is thought to involve the uncoupling of the receptors from the G-protein, after which the receptors are taken inside the neuron until they are eventually returned to the membrane and resensitized to opioid binding. It is thought that this cycle limits the degree of tolerance of the mu opioid receptors to their own endogenous opioid ligands. Endogenous opiates are released intermittently and they are metabolized very quickly after being released. As a result, binding of endogenous opiates is short-lived. In contrast, when opioid analgesics are administered for long periods of time they facilitate tolerance because they are constantly attached to the receptors and interfere with receptor recycling and resensitization (Boyer, 2012).

In other words, when morphine or other opioids are used only intermittently, little, if any, tolerance develops, and the opioids retain their initial efficacy. When administration is repeated, tolerance may become so marked that massive doses have to be administered to either maintain a degree of euphoria or prevent withdrawal discomfort. The degree of tolerance is illustrated by the fact that the dose of morphine can be increased from clinical doses (50 to 60 milligrams per day) to 500 milligrams per day over as short a period as 10 days.

Tolerance to one opioid leads to cross-tolerance to all other natural and synthetic opioids, even if they are chemically dissimilar. Cross-tolerance, however, does not develop between the opioids and the sedative hypnotics. In other words, a person who has developed a tolerance for morphine will also have a tolerance for heroin but not for alcohol or benzodiazepines.

Physical dependence is an altered physiological state induced by a drug, whereby withdrawal of a drug elicits biological reactions typical for that class of drugs. Generally, symptoms of withdrawal are the opposite of pharmacological effects (for opiate withdrawal see Table 10.3). The magnitude of these acute withdrawal symptoms depends

TABLE 10.3 Acute effects of opioids and rebound withdrawal symptoms

Acute action	Withdrawal sign
Analgesia	Pain and irritability
Respiratory depression	Hyperventilation
Euphoria	Dysphoria and depression
Relaxation and sleep	Restlessness and insomnia
Tranquilization	Fearfulness and hostility
Decreased blood pressure	Increased blood pressure
Constipation	Diarrhea
Pupillary constriction	Pupillary dilation
Hypothermia	Hyperthermia
Drying of secretions	Lacrimation, runny nose
Reduced sex drive	Spontaneous ejaculation
Peripheral vasodilation; flushed and warm skin	Chilliness and "gooseflesh"

After R. S. Feldman, J. S. Meyer, and L. F. Quenzer, *Principles of Neuropsychopharmacology* (Sunderland, MA: Sinauer, 1997), Table 12.8, p. 533.

on the dose of opioid that had been used, the frequency of previous drug administration, and the duration of drug dependence. Acute opioid withdrawal is not considered to be life threatening.

To help alleviate the symptoms of acute withdrawal, several approaches have been tried (O'Connor, 2005). These approaches include clonidine-assisted detoxification, buprenorphine-assisted detoxification, and rapid anesthesia-aided detoxification. Clonidine is a drug that acts on the sympathetic nervous system to reduce some of the physical manifestations of withdrawal. Buprenorphine will be discussed later in this chapter.

In *rapid anesthesia-aided detoxification* (RAAD), a pure opioid antagonist, such as naloxone or naltrexone, and the sympathetic blocker clonidine are administered intravenously to the opioid-dependent person while he or she is asleep under general anesthesia. The procedure continues for about 72 hours, during which time the withdrawal signs are blunted. The objective is to enable the patient to tolerate high doses of an opioid antagonist and thus undergo complete detoxification while unconscious. After awakening, the patient is maintained on naltrexone and undergoes supportive psychotherapy and group therapies for relapse prevention and to address the underlying causes of addiction. The RAAD technique is controversial, in part because it is expensive, it involves the risks of anesthesia, and it focuses only on short-term dependence rather than on long-term cravings and social adjustments. One study compared the three techniques of detoxification and concluded that RAAD was no less safe or effective than other techniques (Collins et al., 2005).

Regardless of the method, following acute withdrawal there is a protracted opiate *abstinence syndrome,* persisting for up to 6 months. Symptoms include depression, abnormal responses to stressful situations, drug hunger, anxiety, and other psychological disturbances, as well as other psychiatric disorders.

Prescription Opioid Abuse

Opioid tolerance and dependence can develop in anyone who uses the drugs repeatedly, not necessarily people who are abusing them. A patient in the chronic pain of terminal illness should not be denied opioids, despite the inevitable development of tolerance and dependence. Nevertheless, since the previous edition of this book was published, in 2011, the misuse and abuse of prescription medications, particularly opiates, has reached epidemic proportions. The U.S. Centers for Disease Control and Prevention has acknowledged that since 2003 more overdose deaths have involved opioid analgesics than all other illegal drugs (Paulozzi et al., 2011) (Figure 10.4), and that other drugs given for mental disorders are often involved (Paulozzi et al., 2013). Over 10 years there has been a fivefold increase in admissions to substance abuse programs for opioid addiction (Volkow et al., 2011). Between 2000 and 2009 the number of opiate-dependent newborns being treated for neonatal abstinence syndrome (NAS) more than tripled (Hayes and Brown, 2012). The 2011 National Survey on Drug Use and Health (NSDUH) found that nearly one-third of people aged 12 and over, who used drugs for the first time, began by using a prescription drug nonmedically. The same survey found that over 70 percent of people who abused prescription pain relievers got them from friends or relatives. Only 5 percent obtained the drug from dealers.

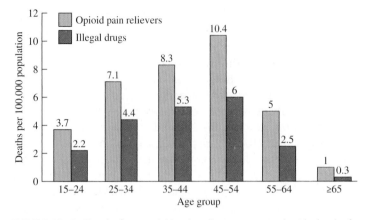

FIGURE 10. 4 Deaths from opioid pain relievers compared with deaths from all other illegal drugs, as a function of age group. (Source: www.nidavic.iqsdev.com Prescription and Over-the-Counter Medications | DrugFacts | National Institute on Drug Abuse.)

The majority of prescriptions and overdose deaths are from methadone, hydroco-done, and oxycodone (Okie, 2010; Volkow et al., 2011), with even the methadone-related deaths linked more to pain management than with opioid addiction treatment programs (Fine et al., 2011). This may be due to its low price and the belief that methadone is less liable to abuse. However, methadone's long half-life makes it difficult to manage and it is especially dangerous when combined with other drugs (Okie, 2010). Disturbingly, evidence suggests that addiction to prescription opiate medications is paralleled by a comparable increase in heroin addiction, which occurs at least partly because heroin is much cheaper. According to the 2011 NSDUH, the number of people ages 18 to 25, who abused prescription drugs fell from 2 million in 2010 to 1.7 million in 2011, but heroin use increased.

These increases in opioid use may be an unintended consequence of well-intentioned efforts to treat chronic pain better, by encouraging physicians to be more proactive in identifying chronic pain conditions. Guidelines intended to improve pain management recommended that pain be treated as a "vital sign," that patients should be asked about their satisfaction with pain control, and that long-term opioid treatment be expanded to include chronic, noncancer-related pain (Lembke, 2012; Perrone and Nelson, 2012). As a result, there has been a 10-fold increase in the medical use of opioids since 1990 and a strong correlation between states in the United States that report high rates of drug-induced poisonings and high rates of opioid use. Unfortunately, according to a 21-state study by the Workers Compensation Research Institute (WCRI), medical management of patients on opiate drugs is not sufficiently meeting the guidelines provided by the American Pain Society and the American Academy of Pain Medicine (Wang et al., 2012). For example, approximately 1 in 12 injured workers were still taking opioid analgesics 7 to 12 months later without receiving recommended follow-up services.

One result of these developments, in which increased medical use has led to overuse, misuse, and abuse of opioid drugs, is the suggestion that the diagnostic term "opioid dependence" be changed to "opioid use disorder" (OUD), and that addiction arising from medical treatment be designated as Prescription Opioid Use Disorder (POUD). Miller and Frankowski (2012) describe this approach and provide terminology and criteria for the diagnosis and treatment of this proposed new medical category.

In addition to these changes in clinical status, the FDA Safety and Innovation Act (FDASIA) and the 2011 Prescription Drug Abuse Prevention Plan from the Office of National Drug Control Policy (ONDCP) called for guidance from the FDA in dealing with the opioid abuse epidemic. The FDA is responding in two ways. First, it is developing protocols for 'abuse-resistant' products, for testing tamper-resistant technology and for evaluating the results of such tests. A draft guidance document released in January 2013 (*Guidance for Industry: Abuse-Deterrent Opioids-Evaluation and Labeling*) is available on the FDA's Web site. This document lists several possible categories of abuse-deterrent formulations:

- Physical and chemical barriers, to prevent chewing, crushing, grinding, and extraction with water or alcohol
- Agonist/antagonist combinations to interfere with the euphoria
- Aversion, to reduce pleasant effects as doses increase
- Delivery systems, such as depot injections and implants
- Prodrugs, which must be transformed in the GI tract to be activated
- Combinations of any of the above.

As yet, the draft does not discuss generic products, which are not manufactured in abuse resistant formulations. The FDA will be seeking public feedback as the recommendations continue to be developed.

The second response from the FDA was a Risk Evaluation and Mitigation Strategy (REMS), approved in July 2012. This announcement called for continuing education programs on the proper use of extended-release and long-acting opioids prescribed for moderate to severe pain. Medical education providers will develop the REMS curriculum under FDA supervision, and drug companies will fund them. The aim is to train clinicians in understanding the risks and benefits of opioid therapy and to recognize signs of misuse, abuse, and addiction. ONDCP and the National Institute on Drug Abuse (NIDA) have already made two online learning modules on opioid analgesics for clinicians, available on the NIDA and Medscape Education Web sites. Information on all drugs included in the REMS program can be found on the FDA Web site.

The pharmaceutical industry has responded to these developments in several ways. First, numerous new formulations of current opioid drugs used to treat pain and opiate addiction have already been produced and marketed (or soon will be). These versions are meant to make misuse and abuse more difficult. Second, there is renewed interest in novel opiate substances that are inherently, biochemically resistant to tampering and abuse. Third, a large number of new compounds, which do not act on the opiate pathway but are designed to block pain transmission by other mechanisms, are being investigated for pain relief.

> ## Did You Know?
>
> **Numerous Well-Known Personalities Have Succumbed to Opiate Addiction.**
>
> Here is just a small sample (most from the list at: http://www.thatspoppycock.com/wp-content/themes/tpc/images/tpc-logo.png
>
> **Marcus Aurelius**—The Roman Emperor initially used the drug for medicinal purposes, but likely became addicted to it at some point during his reign over Rome.
>
> **Charles Dickens**—The author of *A Tale of Two Cities* and *A Christmas Carol* was addicted to opium for many years and used the drug heavily right up to the time of his death (by massive stroke).
>
> **Bela Lugosi**—The star of hundreds of early horror films was a frequenter of several underground opium dens and also used morphine excessively during his life.
>
> **Florence Nightingale**—It was discovered after her death that the most famous nurse who ever lived was a notorious opium user.
>
> 1970: Legendary singer, **Janis Joplin**, is found dead at Hollywood's Landmark Hotel, a victim of an "accidental heroin overdose."
>
> 1982: Comedian **John Belushi** of *Animal House* fame, dies of a heroin-cocaine "speedball" overdose.
>
> 1993: Twenty-three-year-old actor **River Phoenix** dies of a heroin-cocaine overdose, the same "speedball" combination that killed comedian John Belushi.
>
> 1994: **Kurt Cobain**, lead singer of the Seattle-based alternative rock band, Nirvana, dies of heroin-related suicide.
>
> **Robert Downey, Jr.**'s struggle with heroin, and cocaine, addiction has been heavily publicized.
>
> **Matthew Perry** is another example of a talented actor who reached success in his field, but could not stay away from opiates

Common Opiate Drugs

Morphine: A Pure Opioid Agonist

Of the analgesics found in the opium poppy, morphine is the most potent and represents about 10 percent of the crude exudate. Codeine is much less potent and constitutes only 0.5 percent of the crude exudate. Despite decades of research, no other drug has been found that exceeds morphine's effectiveness as an analgesic, and no other drug is clinically superior for treating severe pain.

Morphine can be administered by injection, by inhalation, or taken orally or rectally. An intranasal delivery system (Rylomine) is under development. This product would have a rapid onset of action in situations where oral use is not desired. One spray of Rylomine (7.5 mg) is equivalent to a bolus IV injection of morphine sulfate (5 mg).

Orally, morphine is available in immediate-release formulation and as a long-acting, time-release product (MS-Contin). In general, absorption of morphine from the gastrointestinal tract is slow and incomplete compared to absorption following injection or inhalation. Absorption through the rectum is adequate, and several opioids (morphine, hydromorphone, and oxymorphone) are available in suppository form.[3]

The presence of opioid receptors in the spinal cord means administration of morphine directly onto the spinal cord, an intrathecal route (through small catheters) is effective. This route places the drug right at its site of action and may avoid its effects both on higher CNS centers (maintaining wakefulness and avoiding respiratory depression) and in the periphery (avoiding drug-induced constipation). In medicine, this technique is used to control the pain of obstetric labor and delivery, to treat postoperative pain, and (for long-term use) to relieve otherwise intractable pain associated with terminal cancer and chronic pain. In these situations, an implantable, programmed pump for intraspinal infusion is available.

For millennia, crude opium has been smoked for recreational purposes; the rapidity of onset of drug action rivals that following intravenous injection. Morphine itself is rarely abused in this manner; heroin is the preparation of choice. However, for therapeutic use, a nebulized form of morphine has been found to be effective, for example, in patients who cannot tolerate injections (Thipphawong et al., 2003). Nebulizer preparations of morphine have not yet been marketed.

Morphine crosses the blood-brain barrier fairly slowly, as it is more water soluble than lipid soluble. Other opioids (such as heroin and fentanyl) cross the blood-brain barrier much more rapidly. Only about 20 percent of orally administered morphine reaches the CNS. This may explain why the "flash" or "rush" following intravenous injection of heroin is much more intense than that perceived after injecting morphine.

Opioids reach all body tissues, including the fetus; infants born to addicted mothers are physically dependent on opioids and exhibit withdrawal symptoms. The habitual use of morphine or other opioids during pregnancy does not seem to increase the risk of congenital anomalies; thus, these drugs are not considered to be teratogenic. However, there are increased risks of birth-related problems and fetal growth retardation.

The liver metabolizes morphine, and as much as 40 percent to 60 percent of the drug may not reach the systemic circulation because of first-pass metabolism. One of its metabolites (morphine-6-glucuronide) is actually 10 to 20 times more potent as an analgesic than morphine, and much of its analgesic action is mediated by this active metabolite. The half-lives of morphine and morphine-6-glucuronide are both 3 to 5 hours. Patients with impaired kidney function tend to accumulate the metabolite and thus may be more sensitive to morphine administration.

Urine-screening tests can be used to detect codeine and morphine as well as their metabolites. Because heroin is metabolized to monoacetylmorphine and then to morphine, and because street heroin also contains acetylcodeine, heroin use is suspected when monoacetylmorphine, morphine, and codeine are present in urine. Frequently, urinalysis cannot accurately determine which specific drug (heroin, codeine, or morphine) has been used. However, a specific metabolite of heroin, 6-monoacetylmorphine, is also at times detected and would definitely confirm illicit drug (heroin) use. Furthermore, codeine is widely available in cough syrups and analgesic preparations, and even poppy seeds

---

[3] This kind of preparation might be indicated for patients suffering from muscle-wasting diseases who cannot tolerate other routes of administration.

contain small amounts of morphine. Depending on the drug that was taken, morphine and codeine metabolites may be detected in a patient's urine for 2 to 4 days.

Codeine

Codeine is a commonly prescribed opioid, usually combined with aspirin or acetaminophen for the relief of mild to moderate pain. These combination products are frequently sought drugs of abuse. Because it has been used for so long, codeine never underwent the safety studies required for new drugs. The hepatic drug-metabolizing enzyme CYP-2D6 metabolizes codeine to morphine, and many of codeine's clinical effects (for example, pain relief and euphoria) may, in fact, result from the actions of morphine. The plasma half-life and duration of action is about 3 to 4 hours, but codeine's pharmacokinetics is unpredictable. Moreover, almost 1 in 10 Americans have a genetic variation that causes very rapid metabolism. As a result, abnormally high levels of morphine may accumulate, leading to drowsiness and respiratory depression. And the morphine may also be passed to infants through breast milk. For this reason it has been argued that codeine should be removed from the market, or at least prohibited for infants and young children (MacDonald and McLeod 2010). In February 2013, the FDA warned that products containing codeine should not be used for pain relief in children after tonsillectomy or adenoidectomy because of the risk for adverse effects or death. This was based on medical reports of three deaths and one life-threatening case of respiratory depression in children with sleep apnea given codeine after one of those surgeries. All the children were ultra-rapid metabolizers.

In addition to its inherent pharmacokinetic disadvantages, four of the six selective serotonin reuptake inhibitor (SSRI) antidepressants (fluoxetine, fluvoxamine, sertraline, and paroxetine)(see Chapter 12) can block the pain relief of codeine because they block the conversion of codeine to morphine. For patients taking one of these drugs, an analgesic drug other than codeine may be necessary.

Heroin

Heroin (diacetylmorphine) is three times more potent than morphine and is produced from morphine by a slight modification of chemical structure (Figure 10.5). The increased lipid solubility of heroin leads to faster penetration of the blood-brain barrier, producing an intense rush when the drug is either smoked or injected intravenously. Heroin is metabolized to monoacetylmorphine and morphine; morphine is eventually metabolized and excreted. Although available in Britain (as diacetylmorphine), under restricted clinical guidelines, heroin is not legal in the United States, but is widely used illicitly. When heroin is smoked together with crack cocaine, euphoria is intensified, the anxiety and paranoia associated with cocaine are tempered, and the depression that follows after the effects of cocaine wear off seems to be reduced. Unfortunately, this combination creates a multidrug addiction that is extremely difficult to treat.

Hydrocodone and Oxycodone

Hydrocodone alone is a Schedule II drug, but it is almost always found in combination with acetaminophen in formulations such as Vicodin and Lortab. Those versions are listed under Schedule III, which is less restrictive. This may have been done because

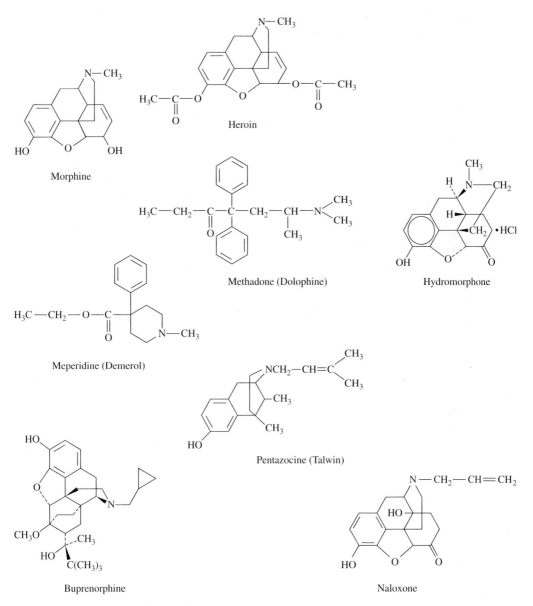

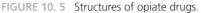

FIGURE 10. 5 Structures of opiate drugs.

originally the products were mainly used as cough medicine and because the risk of liver damage from acetaminophen was believed to be a deterrent for misuse. However, being in Schedule III means that clinicians can call in the prescription, up to a 6-month supply, and don't need to see the patient, whereas Schedule II drugs require office visits (a written prescription) and have only 3-month refills. Consequently, the generic form of

Vicodin is one of the most commonly prescribed, and abused, opiate medications. As long ago as 1999 a citizens Petition was submitted to the Drug Enforcement Agency (DEA), requesting consideration that combination products be moved to Schedule II. In 2004 the DEA conducted an analysis and asked the Department of Health and Human Services to assess the need for rescheduling. Four years later the FDA decided that there was no need to 'up-schedule' hydrocodone combination products and the DEA had to abide by the decision. In 2009 the DEA asked the FDA to reconsider and until the spring of 2012 the FDA had not responded. However, in January 2013 a hearing took place for supporters on both sides to present their arguments, which led to a vote of the FDA advisory committee (19 to 10) to move hydrocodone combinations into the more restrictive schedule II category. (This decision created a great deal of commentary from people on both sides of the issue, which can be accessed online, at *MedPage Today*, for February 3, 2013.)

Concerns about diversion and misuse were obviously involved in the FDA advisory committee vote against recommending approval of a new long-acting hydrocodone formulation (Zohydro ER) in December 2012, because it lacked tamper-resistant technology. Even with the restriction to Schedule II level, and the requirement that Zohydro would require a REMS (that is, a policy for minimizing the risks of using the drug), the committee voted 11 to 2 against approval. The FDA was supposed to make a determination by March 1 2013, but said it needed more time to review the data. If approved, this product would be the first available hydrocodone-only analgesic. (In October 2013 the FDA approved Zohydro ER (extended release) in its current slow-release formulation, meaning that it can be crushed, chewed or mixed with alcohol and still retain full potency.)

An investigational agent, named KP201, is being developed as another new, safer pain treatment. Given the name "benzhydrocodone" it is reported by the company to provide analgesia for moderate to severe pain with both less abuse liability and less opioid-induced constipation. KP201 is composed of hydrocodone chemically bound to a ligand. The company previously reported positive Phase 1 clinical data, which confirmed that KP201 is metabolized in the body as predicted, releasing hydrocodone into the bloodstream. An official application for future approval as a new medication is planned for the first quarter of 2014.

Oxycodone (Percodan, OxyContin) is another semisynthetic opioid similar in action to morphine. The short-acting preparation (Percodan, now generic, as oxycodone and aspirin) is primarily prescribed for the treatment of acute pain. Usual doses are about 5 milligrams every 4 to 6 hours. A combination product is currently under development, which consists of a fixed dose ratio of 3:2 morphine and oxycodone, called MoxDuo CR. This formulation, given once or twice a day, is designed to treat moderate to severe chronic pain. According to the manufacturer, MoxDuo contains proprietary technology that resists tampering or abuse by inhalation or solubilization in water or alcohol.

OxyContin is a long-acting product intended for the treatment of chronic or long-lasting pain. OxyContin goes by many street names: poor man's heroin, hillbilly heroin, oxy, OC, killer, and oxycotton, among others. Abusers crush the pills, destroying the time-release mechanisms, and either snort the powder, smoke the drug, or dilute it in water and inject it. The abuse of OxyContin led to the development of a new formulation approved in April 2010, intended to prevent it from being cut, broken, chewed, crushed, frozen, heated, or dissolved to release more medication. Human pharmacokinetic data demonstrates that dissolving in ethanol and other common drinks or solvents does not cause a rapid release of the drug. One product, called Remoxy is an oral, long-acting oxycodone gelatin capsule that utilizes a controlled-release technology that the FDA has not yet approved for commercial sale, but may decide to in 2013. The second product, Acurox was designed to be both tamper and abuse resistant. It is an immediate release oxycodone tablet with a small amount of niacin as an aversive agent, in addition to the gel-based formulation. The FDA rejected this version in 2010 because of concerns about the niacin. Without the niacin, the drug, called Oxecta was approved in June 2011. According to the manufacturer, this new technology causes the drug to break down into crumbled chunks instead of powder if it is crushed, and turns it "sudsy" if it is mixed with liquid and drawn into a syringe (Bannwarth, 2012). In April 2013, the FDA issued new labeling for OxyContin noting that the product makes abuse difficult. In that statement the agency also stated that it will not approve any generic drug applications that are based on the original formulation. In other words, generic Oxycontin must also be abuse resistant.

The new formulation of oxycodone did successfully reduce abuse liability. A year after the new formula was marketed, it was reported to sell for 28 percent less than the original OxyContin on the black market and abuse fell significantly. However, the use of other opioids, such as fentanyl, heroin and *oxymorphone* (Opana; see below) increased. While 24 percent of drug users said they found a way around the tamper proof mechanism, most (66 percent) said they just switched to another opioid (Cicero et al., 2012).

Hydromorphone and Oxymorphone

Hydromorphone (Dilaudid) and *oxymorphone* (Numorphan, Opana-ER) are both structurally related to morphine and are six to ten times more potent. They produce somewhat less sedation but equal respiratory depression.

Palladone (not to be confused with *paliperidone;* see Chapter 11) and Exalgo are trade names for two new, long-acting formulations of hydromorphone that are taken once daily for treatment of chronic pain in patients who have developed a tolerance to opioids and thus can tolerate the high doses of 10–32 milligrams per day (the dose of short-acting hydromorphone is about 1–2 milligrams). The half-life of both Palladone and Exalgo is about 18 hours. Palladone is formulated as an immediately dissolving capsule containing controlled-release pellets. Exalgo contains hydromorphone in the OROS osmotic delivery system similar to that used for Concerta (see Chapter 15). The FDA first approved Opana ER in 2006. In response to the epidemic of painkiller misuse, the manufacturer developed a crush-resistant formulation (much like Oxycontin did in 2010) that was on the market by the middle of 2012. In January 2013, within a year since the new formulation was marketed in February of 2012, 15 cases of thrombotic thrombocytopenic purpura (TTP) were reported by injection drug users; 14 occurred in addicts who dissolved and injected the reformulated Opana. There were no deaths. TTP is characterized by blood clots in small vessels throughout the body, which can damage organs. The cause is not yet clear; whether the condition was produced by some component of the drug itself, or the methods used to prepare the drug for injection is not yet known (Marder et al, 2013).

At the same time, the company (Endo) filed petitions with the FDA to prevent a generic version of Opana ER from being marketed. The company argued that, because the generic drug was not reformulated to be crush resistant, it was unsafe. The FDA countered that Endo had not recalled the original version of Opana ER, but only stopped marketing it after the crush-resistant version was available. The agency argued that Endos' concerns had less to do with safety than with an effort to delay a generic version from entering the market. Starting in January of 2013 generic versions will be available.

Propoxyphene

Propoxyphene (Darvon; Darvocet, which includes a dose of acetaminophen) is an analgesic compound that is structurally similar to methadone (see Figure 10.5); it is less potent than codeine but more potent than aspirin. Darvon was marketed in 1957 when there were few alternatives for treating pain, except aspirin and strong opioids. In November 2010 the FDA determined that the drug should be banned from commercial sale because of concerns about potentially fatal heart rhythm abnormalities, drug suicide, and overdoses.

Meperidine

Meperidine (Demerol) is a synthetic opioid whose structure differs from that of morphine (see Figure 10.5). Because of this structural difference, meperidine was originally thought to be free of many of the undesirable properties of the opioids. However, meperidine is addictive; it can be substituted for morphine or heroin in addicts. It is one-tenth as potent as morphine, produces a similar type of euphoria, and is equally likely to cause dependence. Meperidine's side effects differ from morphine's and include more excitatory effects, such as tremors, delirium, hyperreflexia, and convulsions. These excitatory actions are produced by a metabolite of meperidine (normeperidine). Unlike other opiates, meperidine does not cause pinpoint pupils but may dilate the pupils because of an anticholinergic action. Meperidine and normeperidine can accumulate in people who have kidney dysfunction or who use only meperidine for their opioid addiction. Following discontinuation, withdrawal symptoms develop more rapidly than with morphine because of meperidine's shorter duration of action.

Fentanyl and Its Derivatives

Fentanyl (Sublimaze) and three related compounds, *sufentanil* (Sufenta), *alfentanil* (Alfenta), and *remifentanyl* (Ultiva), are short-acting, intravenously administered opioid agonists that are structurally related to meperidine. They are meant to be used during and after surgery to relieve surgical pain. Carfentanil, an even more potent compound, is used to immobilize large animals, such as elephants, in veterinary practice.

In addition to its intravenous formulation fentanyl is also available in numerous other forms: a transdermal skin patch (Durapatch); a dissolvable buccal tablet (to be placed above a molar tooth, between the upper cheek and gum, called Fentora (a generic formulation was approved in 2011); a fentanyl buccal soluble film (Onsolis); a sublingual tablet (Abstral); a sublingual spray (Subsys, approved in 2012), and an oral lozenge on a stick (a "lollipop,"Actiq). A pectin nasal spray (available in Europe as PecFent or Instanyl) is under late-stage development for approval in the United States. The transdermal route of drug delivery offers prolonged, rather steady levels of drug in blood; the buccal tablet and lollipop are used for the treatment of unrelieved or breakthrough pain in opioid-dependent chronic pain patients who are intolerant of injections, and for pediatric patients. Reviews of these formulations have been published (Davis, 2011; Paech et al., 2012). Currently, a formulation of sufentanil is under development for acute postoperative pain (ARX-01). This system is designed to allow patients to self-dose a sublingual product called Sufentanil NanoTabs, to manage their post-operative pain. Results of a trial reported in March 2013 showed significant benefit from the drug.

Fentanyl and its three derivatives are 80 to 500 times as potent as morphine as analgesics and profoundly depress respiration. Death from these agents is invariably caused by respiratory failure. Because they are so lipid soluble these drugs may accumulate in fat stores, which means they need an extended period of time to leave the body, that is, to move from the fat cells to the blood and then to the liver. Remifentanil differs from this situation in that, although it is also very lipid soluble, it is metabolized quickly outside of the liver, in the blood and tissues. For this reason, the drug is used for rapid, short-acting analgesia, which can be given for long periods but is cleared quickly (Pathan and Williams, 2012).

In illicit use, fentanyl is known by several nicknames including "china white." Numerous derivatives (such as *methylfentanyl*) have been manufactured illegally; they emerge periodically and have been responsible for many fatalities.

Tramadol

Tramadol (Ultram; Ultram [extended release] ER; generic) became available for use as an analgesic in the United States in 1995. The drug has a unique analgesic profile: (1) it is a partial agonist at mu receptors; (2) it blocks the presynaptic reuptake of norepinephrine; and (3) it releases serotonin. In the United States, tramadol is available only for oral use. Well absorbed orally, the drug undergoes a two-step metabolism, and the first metabolite (monodemethyl tramadol) is as active or more active than the parent compound. As a partial agonist, the drug exhibits a ceiling effect on analgesia, which limits respiratory depression and abuse potential. Side effects include drowsiness and vertigo, nausea, vomiting, constipation, and headache and additive sedation with CNS depressants.

There has been concern about the combination of tramadol and serotonin-type antidepressant drugs: the combination may produce the serotonin syndrome (see Chapter 12).

Tapentadol (Nucynta)

Approved in 2008 for relief of moderate to severe acute pain, tapentadol is structurally similar to *tramadol* (Ultram) and considered to have a potency between tramadol and morphine (Wade and Spruill, 2009). Clinical trials have found it comparable to oxycodone in regard to post-surgical pain relief. Currently, it is FDA scheduled like morphine (Schedule II) rather than tramadol (Schedule III). However, an assessment of the abuse of the immediate release formula concluded that during the first 24 months after it was introduced abuse rates and diversion were very low, similar to those of tramadol and less than the rates for oxycodone and hydrocodone (Dart et al., 2012).

Similar to tramadol, tapentadol has opioid and nonopioid activity, with action as an agonist at the mu opioid receptor and as a norepinephrine reuptake inhibitor. Inhibition of norepinephrine reuptake provides some analgesic efficacy, which should reduce the dose of opioid necessary to relieve pain (an opioid-sparing property). Antidepressants such as *milnacipran* (Savella), *duloxetine* (Cymbalta), and *reboxetine* (Strattera, Edronax) share this norepinephrine reuptake blocking action, and pain relief, but without opioid agonism.

An extended-release formulation of tapentadol was approved in 2011 for treatment of severe chronic pain (such as low back pain and knee pain), and, in 2012, it became the first opioid approved for patients with the neuropathic pain condition of diabetic peripheral neuropathy (DPN).

Mixed Agonist-Antagonist Opioids

Four commercially drugs are classified as mixed agonist-antagonist opioids: pentazocine, butorphanol, nalbuphine, and *dezocine* (Dalgan, discontinued in the United States as of 2011). Each of these drugs binds with varying affinity to the mu and kappa receptors. The drugs are weak mu antagonists; most of their analgesic effectiveness (which is limited) results from their stimulation of kappa receptors (see Table 10.1). Low doses cause moderate analgesia; higher doses produce little additional analgesia. In opioid-dependent people, these drugs precipitate withdrawal. A high incidence of adverse psychotomimetic side effects (dysphoria, anxiety reactions, hallucinations, and so on) is associated with these agents, limiting their therapeutic use.

Pentazocine (Talwin) and *butorphanol* (Stadol) are prototypical mixed agonist-antagonists. Neither has much potential for producing respiratory depression or physical dependence. In 1993 butorphanol, previously available for use by injection, became available as a nasal spray (Stadol NS), the first analgesic so formulated. After it is sprayed into the nostrils, peak plasma levels (and maximal effect) are achieved in 1 hour, with duration of 4 to 5 hours. Use of the nasal spray can result in euphoria, and abuse of butorphanol spray appears to be increasing.

The abuse of pentazocine has also been increasing, particularly in combination with tripelennamine, an antihistamine. This combination of drugs, called "Ts and blues," has caused serious medical complications, including seizures, psychotic episodes, skin ulcerations, abscesses, and muscle wasting. (The latter three effects are caused by the repeated injections rather than by the drugs themselves.)

Nalbuphine (Nubain) is primarily a kappa agonist of limited analgesic effectiveness. Because it is also a mu antagonist, it is not likely to produce either respiratory depression or patterns of abuse.

Methadone

Methadone (Dolophine) is a synthetic mu agonist opioid (see Figure 10.5), very similar to that of morphine. Methadone was first shown to block the effects of heroin withdrawal in 1948. In 1965 it was introduced as a substitute treatment for opioid dependency. The outstanding properties of methadone are its effective analgesic activity, its efficacy by the oral route, its extended duration of action in suppressing withdrawal symptoms in physically dependent people, and its tendency to show persistent effects with repeated administration.

Today, methadone has two primary legitimate uses: (1) as an orally administered substitute for heroin in methadone maintenance treatment programs; and (2) as a long-acting analgesic for the treatment of chronic pain syndromes (Krueger, 2012). This effect is thought to be partly due to an antagonistic activity at the NMDA, glutamatergic receptor (see Table 10.1). Federal prescription regulations clearly separate these two uses. Physicians who do not practice in federally licensed methadone treatment programs may not prescribe the drug for the maintenance of opioid dependency; the drug may be prescribed only through licensed methadone maintenance treatment program centers. However, office-based physicians may prescribe methadone for the treatment of either acute pain or chronic pain.

The main objectives of methadone maintenance treatment programs are rehabilitation of the dependent person and reduction of needle-associated diseases, illicit drug use, and crime. Randomized controlled trials have shown that these aims are generally accomplished. Although there are a number of predictors of the success of a program, the most important is the magnitude of the daily methadone dose. Programs that prescribe average daily doses exceeding 100 milligrams have higher retention rates and lower illicit drug use rates than those in which the average dose is less.

Even where liberal doses are used (sometimes up to 160 milligrams per day or higher), about one-third of the clients regularly experience withdrawal (they are called *nonholders*) and two-thirds (called *holders*) do not experience withdrawal on a once-daily dosing schedule. The generally accepted half-life of methadone is 24 hours.

Multiple CYP hepatic enzymes are required to metabolize methadone. Therefore, methadone is the opioid most susceptible to serious drug interactions resulting from drug-induced enzyme inhibition. For example, some sedatives and antidepressants inhibit methadone's metabolism, resulting in large elevations in blood concentrations, often resulting in unexpected fatalities (Tennant, 2010).

As well as some methadone maintenance programs may work, they reach only 170,000 of the estimated 810,000 opioid-dependent people in the United States. In recent years, diversion of methadone (from methadone clinic programs and from physicians' prescriptions for analgesic effects) has become a major problem. When the large doses prescribed for an opioid-dependent person (40 to 100 milligrams) are taken by a nonopioid-dependent person, severe respiratory depression and death frequently result.

LAAM

Levo-alpha acetylmethadol (LAAM) is related to methadone. It is an oral opioid analgesic that was approved in mid-1993 for the clinical management of opioid dependence in heroin addicts. LAAM has a slow onset and a long duration of action (about 72 hours). Its primary advantage over methadone is its long duration of action; in maintenance therapy it is administered by mouth three times a week.

In general, LAAM and methadone are of equal efficacy, as measured by opioid-free urine samples in heroin-dependent persons. Higher doses of methadone (60 to 100 milligrams) and 75- to 115-milligram doses of LAAM both substantially reduced the use of heroin (Johnson et al., 2000). It is currently not available due to possible serious cardiac complications (Wedam et al., 2007; Wolstein et al., 2009).

Buprenorphine

Although methadone has long been the mainstay of opiate dependence treatment, it is subject to diversion, and the federal government requires patients to receive the drug daily in federally licensed clinics. This makes it difficult for patients with full-time jobs or those who live at a distance, to participate. In 2002 the situation changed dramatically with the approval of *buprenorphine* (Subutex), and then a *buprenorphine/naloxone* combination product (Suboxone) for use in opioid addiction. *Buprenorphine* is a semisynthetic partial mu opioid agonist, which imposes a ceiling to its analgesic effectiveness, respiratory depression and its potential for inducing euphoria. Buprenorphine has a prolonged duration of action (about 24 hours) because it binds very strongly to mu receptors, which limits its reversibility by naloxone should reversal be necessary. It can be given as an intramuscular or intravenous injection, as a sublingual tablet or patch. Because of its high first-pass metabolism, it is not as effective orally.

The most common side effects are flulike symptoms, headache, sweating, sleeping difficulties, nausea, and mood swings.

Although buprenorphine is safe and effective as a maintenance medication in treating heroin addiction, as an agonist, it has also been associated with considerable abuse throughout the world. Use of buprenorphine began to rise rapidly after 2002 and poison control centers throughout the United States reported increases in the number of buprenorphine exposures (Thomas et al., 2012). Buprenorphine may also be used illicitly to avoid withdrawal symptoms (called "bridging") until further use of other illicit substances can resume. Illicit use has already spread beyond the population who started with illicit or prescription opiates; initial exposure has now been described in young adults who were neither heroin users nor dependent on pharmaceutical opiates (Daniulaityte et al., 2012).

Buprenorphine for Treatment of Opiate Abuse. The abuse problem was addressed by the *naloxone/buprenorphine* (Alho et al., 2007) combination of Suboxone, approved as a Schedule III agent for the office-based maintenance treatment of heroin or other opioid dependence under the Federal Drug Addiction Treatment Act of 2000. This means, unlike methadone, a physician in his or her office can prescribe Suboxone for the treatment of opioid dependence. Also, patients can take the drug home instead of appearing at a clinic every day (Barry et al., 2009). The buprenorphine/ naloxone combination (4:1) is less liable to abuse, not only because buprenorphine is a partial agonist, but also because the naloxone causes withdrawal if Suboxone is crushed and injected. When used correctly, however, the naloxone is not well absorbed through the GI tract or mucosa and has a minimal effect. Buprenorphine alone is meant to be used when drug abuse treatment is started, while the combination is administered for maintenance treatment. Recently the federal government removed a requirement that patients had to wait a year to be eligible for buprenorphine therapy, although that rule still applies to methadone treatment. This allows therapists to treat people in early stages of addiction, rather than telling someone who has been addicted for only a few months that they have to come back in a year before they can be treated!

While methadone and buprenorphine are both safe and effective for use in pregnant women, there are some advantages with buprenorphine, particularly in regard to slowing of heart rate in the neonate. Evidence also suggests prenatal buprenorphine reduces the severity of neonatal abstinence syndrome to a clinically significant degree (Jones et al., 2012a, 2012b).

Currently in the United States, more opioid-dependent patients receive buprenorphine than methadone, and most receive this treatment from primary care, office-based physicians. Even adding a cognitive behavioral therapy component does not seem to improve outcomes beyond the benefits of office-based medical management (Fiellin et al., 2013). In 2007, NIDA initiated the Prescription Opioid Addiction Treatment Study (POATS), in which 653 treatment-seeking outpatients, addicted to prescription opiates, received Suboxone in combination with either medical management or addiction counseling. About 49 percent of the participants reduced prescription painkiller abuse during the 12-week Suboxone treatment. But this dropped to 8.6 percent after Suboxone was discontinued. Results were the same for both the addiction counseling and medical supervision only (Weiss et al., 2011).

In 2010 the buprenorphine/naloxone combination became available in a sublingual film, which dissolves faster than the tablet. In 2011 a transdermal form of buprenorphine, the Butrans patch became available. In September 2012 the company that makes Subutex announced that they would withdraw the tablets during the following 6 months, citing evidence that the tablets showed higher rates of accidental overdose by children. (The tablets were packaged in a bottle, but the replacement film formulation comes in individual packets.) At the same time, the company petitioned the FDA not to approve generic Suboxone tablets (the patent expired in 2010) because of safety concerns, unless each tablet was childproofed. The FDA denied this petition.

Although daily Suboxone is effective, adherence and diversion was considered sufficiently concerning that another formulation was recently developed. This version is an implant, called Probuphine, consisting of four solid rods (although a fifth rod can be added), 26 millimeters by 2.5 millimeters, placed subcutaneously in the upper arm, in an office-based surgical procedure. The drug (80 milligrams in each implant) is released slowly by diffusion, for 6 months, after which the implant is removed and replaced at another site.

Clinical trials (Ling et al., 2010) showed efficacy was greater than placebo, with more negative urine samples for illicit opiates (40.4 percent to 28.3 percent, respectively). Overall ratings of craving, withdrawal, and dependence favored the drug; however, only 65.7 percent of the drug-implanted patients completed the study (compared to 30.9 percent of the placebo patients). In January 2013 the FDA granted Priority Review status to Probuphine. On March 21, 2013 the FDA's Psychopharmacologic Drugs Advisory Committee voted 10 to 4 (with one abstention) to recommend approval of Probuphine. However, the panel also had several concerns about the clinical use of this formulation. For example, the product is meant for patients maintained on 12 to 16 milligrams of oral buprenorphine a day, but many patients are maintained on lower doses and there is no information on how to adapt to the lower doses. Other questions concerned diversion, (because the drug can be separated from the implant), and how many times a patient could receive an implant. In May 2013 the FDA denied approval for this indication and requested more information from the company, specifically, the effect of higher doses and training of prescribers on insertion and removal of the implant.

Buprenorphine for Chronic Pain. In the 1980s buprenorphine was introduced under the brand names Temgesic and Buprenex as an analgesic. Currently, transdermal buprenorphine is approved and indicated for the management of moderate to severe chronic pain in patients requiring a continuous, around-the-clock opioid analgesic for an extended period of time. The sublingual buprenorphine formulations have been prescribed off-label for the management of chronic pain since they became available in 2002. Buprenorphine may be especially effective in neuropathic pain, in treating musculoskeletal, visceral, and cancer pain, as well as for chronic headaches. Furthermore, possibly because of kappa antagonism, buprenorphine seems to have antidepressive and antianxiety properties, which also helps in pain management.

According to the FDA, between January 2003 and December 2012, approximately 40 million buprenorphine prescriptions were written.

Pure Opioid Antagonists

Three opioid antagonists are clinically available: naloxone, naltrexone, and nalmefene. Each is a structural derivative of oxymorphone, a pure opioid agonist (see Figure 10.5). All three have an affinity for opioid receptors (especially mu receptors), but after binding they exert no agonistic effects of their own. Therefore, they antagonize the effects of opioid agonists.

Naloxone (Narcan) is the prototype pure opioid antagonist: it has no effect when injected into non-opioid-dependent people, but it rapidly precipitates withdrawal when injected into opioid-dependent people. Naloxone is neither analgesic nor subject to abuse. Because naloxone is neither absorbed from the gastrointestinal tract nor the oral mucosa, it must be given by injection. Its duration of action is very brief, in the range of 15 to 30 minutes. Thus, for continued opioid antagonism, it must be reinjected at short intervals to avoid return of the depressant effects caused by the longer-acting agonist opioid. Naloxone is used to reverse the respiratory depression that follows acute opioid intoxication (overdoses) and to reverse opioid-induced respiratory depression in newborns of opioid-dependent mothers. The limitations of naloxone include its short duration of action and its parenteral route of administration.

Naltrexone (Trexan, ReVia) became clinically available in 1985 as the first orally absorbed, pure opioid antagonist approved for the treatment of heroin dependence. The actions of naltrexone resemble those of naloxone, but naltrexone is well absorbed orally and has a long duration of action, necessitating only a single oral daily dose of about 40 to 100 milligrams. Naltrexone is used clinically in treatment programs when it is desirable to maintain a person on chronic therapy with an opioid antagonist rather than with an agonist such as methadone. In people who take naltrexone daily, injection of an opioid agonist such as heroin is ineffective. Naltrexone can cause nausea (which can be quite severe in some people) and dose-dependent liver toxicity, which can be a problem in patients with preexisting liver disease. One problem with naltrexone is that the drug must be taken in order to be effective. Trite as that sounds, the opioid-dependent person must choose between taking naltrexone or returning to heroin use. Therefore, only highly motivated addicts take the drug.

As discussed in Chapter 5 both oral and long-acting injectable formulations of naltrexone (Vivitrol; in 2006) are approved by the FDA for the treatment of alcoholism to reduce the craving for alcohol during maintenance treatment. The mechanism is believed to be due to antagonism of endorphin action rather than from an as yet unidentified action outside the opioid system. Whether therapy is useful or not is unclear.

In 2010 this drug was also approved for prevention of relapse in opioid-dependent patients. This was based on results of a clinical trial comparing monthly Vivitrol with placebo in 250 patients for 24 weeks. Most were young white men who had been dependent on heroin for about 10 years. (All had to be off opioids for at least 7 days before the experiment.) A total of 47 percent of naltrexone and 62 percent of placebo patients did not complete the trial. But, significantly more patients in the naltrexone group (90 percent), than in the placebo group (35 percent), had urine-screen-confirmed opiate abstinence by the end of the study. Other outcomes, especially less craving, also favored the drug (Krupitsky et al., 2011).

The study was criticized, first, for not obtaining information on safety measures after it ended, because naltrexone can resensitize opioid receptors, which increases the risk of opioid overdose if patients relapse. A second criticism was that the study compared naltrexone with placebo rather than other types of treatment, like methadone or buprenorphine (however, in Russia, where the study took place, opiate agonist treatment is not available for opiate addicts).

Under development and in non-FDA-approved use are implanted naltrexone pellets, or slow-release tablets that are placed under the skin (subcutaneously), and release naltrexone over a period of several months (variable, depending on the preparation). These formulations can reduce opioid use and do not necessitate the dependent person's taking a daily tablet (Kunoe et al., 2009).

Naltrexone has also been reported to have benefits in some other medical conditions. It may have a specific preventive role in reducing self-injurious behaviors (White and Schultz, 2000). It is thought that self-injurious behavior may be used to maintain a high level of endogenous opioids, either to prevent decreases in endorphins or to experience the euphoric effect of opioid stimulation following injury. Jayaram-Lindstrom and coworkers (2008) discuss an anticraving action of naltrexone in amphetamine dependence. For many years, research by Dr. Zagon and colleagues has indicated that low doses of naltrexone may have antitumor and anti-inflammatory actions. These reports, if confirmed, could expand the use of opiate antagonists to other disorders of the immune system, to infections and to neurodegeneration, among others (Zagon et al., 2011a, 2011b).

Nalmefene (Revex), introduced in 1996, is an opioid antagonist at mu and delta receptors and a partial kappa agonist. By injection the drug is useful for the treatment of acute opioid-induced respiratory depression caused by overdosage, because of its long half-life of 8 to 10 hours. Other advantages of nalmefene include greater oral bioavailability and no observed dose-dependent liver toxicity. Nalmefene can precipitate acute withdrawal symptoms in patients who are dependent on opioid drugs, or more rarely when used post-operatively to counteract the effects of strong opioids used in surgery.

Nalmefene is being investigated as a drug treatment for alcoholism, and was studied as a treatment for pathological gambling (Grant et al., 2008). A positive family history of alcoholism was the variable most strongly associated with treatment response.

Agonist/Antagonist Combinations.   In late 2009, the FDA approved a combination of *morphine* and *naltrexone* (Embeda). Here, pellets of an extended-release oral formulation of morphine surround a core of naltrexone. As reported by Katz and coworkers (2010), the naltrexone does not interfere with the analgesic action of the morphine, but abuse potential is considerably reduced. Different dosing regimes were commercially available, all with a morphine-to-naltrexone ratio of 100:4. Embeda was the first FDA-approved long-acting opioid designed to reduce recreational abuse when tampered with by crushing or chewing. In March of 2011 the pharmaceutical firm voluntarily recalled all dosages of Embeda because of unspecified manufacturing problems (Bannwarth, 2012).

A similar combination product using extended-release *oxycodone* (OxyContin) and extended-release naloxone was recently marketed in Europe under the trade name Targin. With this formulation the oxycodone provides analgesic action, but the naloxone remains in the intestine (not being absorbed when taken orally) and blocks the constipating effect of the oxycodone (Lowenstein et al., 2010; Sandner-Kiesling et al., 2010; Hermanns et al., 2012). A combination of oxycodone and ultra-low-dose *naltrexone* (proposed trade name Oxytrex) is under development in the United States (Largent-Milnes et al., 2008). If the dose of naltrexone in the product is sufficient and if the drug is abused by injection, the antagonist would precipitate withdrawal symptoms.

Novel Opioid-Based Compounds Under Development

In addition to the diverse combinations and formulations of classic opioid medications described above, several experimental agents are being investigated as novel options for pain relief, without the side effects and abuse potential of standard drugs. One research group has synthesized a variety of kappa agonists, of which at least one, HS665, was identified as a potential analgesic (Spetea et al., 2012). Another pharmaceutical company is currently testing a kappa receptor agonist (CR845), with an action restricted to the periphery. This drug has already shown efficacy in treating postsurgical pain in women undergoing hysterectomy.

Other companies are modifying the opiate molecule itself to alter its biochemical properties. Nektar Therapeutics has developed an opiate compound, NKTR-181, that is associated with a permanently bound polymer, which slows the rate at which the drug can cross the blood-brain barrier. Because this feature is inherent to the molecule, it cannot be tampered with. The drug is in early clinical trials. The PharmacoFore company has an opiate compound, PF329, that is a pro-drug. When it reaches the small intestine, an amino acid is cleaved off by the digestive enzyme, trypsin, which then activates controlled release of the drug. The molecular bonds cannot be severed by crushing or dissolving. Furthermore, the substance is specifically formulated such that as the amount of drug administered increases, drug release becomes more and more inhibited. In other words, the more you take, the less ability your body has to activate the delivery system. This is an unusual method of limiting abuse and overdose.

Another approach is to deliver the gene that produces the natural opioid enkephalin to patients with intractable cancer pain. This is done by injecting a compound intradermally, that contains the gene for making preproenkephalin. The method is intended to provide increased enkephalin peptides at the local site of the cancer pain.

Yet another novel compound, TRV130 has been developed that is designed to selectively activate the mu opioid receptor. TRV130 stimulates only that part of the receptor mechanism responsible for initiating analgesia; it does not trigger that part of the receptor-linked pathway that initiates other opiate effects. If successful, this type of drug would presumably solve the problem of overdose death from respiratory depression that has been the most problematic side effect of opiate medications for centuries. Of course, even if successful, this mechanism would presumably not influence opiate abuse liability.

Future Pharmacotherapy of Opioid Dependence

Many years ago, Goldstein (1994) reviewed more than 20 years of administering methadone maintenance therapy to heroin addicts in New Mexico. More than half the patients were traced and analyzed. Of these 5001 patients, more than one-third had died from violence, overdosage, or alcoholism. About one-quarter were still enmeshed in the criminal justice system. Another one-quarter had gone on and off methadone maintenance. Data indicated that opioid dependence is a lifelong condition for a considerable fraction of the addict population.

Similarly, Hser and coworkers (2001) reported a remarkable 33-year follow-up of 581 male heroin addicts who were first identified in the early 1960s. At follow-up in 1996–1997, 284 were dead and 242 were interviewed; the mean age at interview was 57 years. Of the 242, 20 percent tested positive for heroin (an additional 9.5 percent refused to provide a urine sample, and 14 percent were incarcerated, so urinalysis was unavailable); 22 percent were daily alcohol drinkers; 67 percent smoked; many reported illicit drug use (heroin, cocaine, marijuana, amphetamines). The group also reported high rates of physical health, mental health, and criminal justice problems. Although long-term heroin abstinence was associated with less criminality, morbidity, and psychological distress, and with higher employment, only a minority of people who were dependent on opioids attained this goal.

Other ways of dealing with opiate addiction continue to be explored. One approach is to try to mitigate the likelihood of overdose death by distributing naloxone to heroin users. Coffin and Sullivan (2013) conducted a simulated analysis that showed that naloxone distribution would prevent over 6 percent of overdose deaths and be very cost effective. This type of program, called the Overdose Education and Nasal Naloxone Distribution initiative (OEND), was implemented in Massachusetts. Between 1996 and 2010, over 10,000 opioid overdose rescues were made with inhaled naloxone. Naloxone was successful in 98 percent of attempts, and even in the failed attempts patients got medical care and survived (Walley et al., 2013).

Another approach, which has also been applied to nicotine and cocaine addiction, is the development of a heroin vaccine (Stowe et al., 2011). This goal is difficult to achieve because heroin is metabolized to other substances that are also psychoactive, such as morphine and its metabolite, 6-acetylmorphine (6AM). The problem was addressed in current vaccine efforts by creating a new type of vaccine "cocktail." Unlike standard vaccines, this type of vaccine slowly degraded in the body and exposed the immune system to the different metabolites of heroin. Using this "dynamic" approach, antibodies were produced to heroin and to 6AM, but not to other opioid drugs or drugs used to treat opiate addiction. So far, research with nonhuman animals is promising.

Other research has, in fact, suggested that the immune system might hold the key to preventing opiate addiction (Hutchinson et al., 2012). Investigators have reported that opiate drugs, in addition to binding classic opiate receptors, also attach to a type of receptor associated with the immune system, called TLR4 (which stands for Toll-Like Receptor 4), which activates a biochemical pathway called MyD88. When the TLR4 receptor was blocked by the "unnatural" isomer of naloxone, (+)-naloxone, in laboratory animals, the rewarding effects of opiate drugs were reduced. The animals no longer made the effort to get opiate injections, and they no longer preferred the location where they used to get the opiate. These results suggest a new direction for development of addiction treatments.

One question raised by these results is whether the mechanism responsible for opiate addiction is the same as that for other drugs of abuse. For example, there is evidence that morphine produces different effects on the brain's reward pathways than cocaine. That is, cocaine and morphine appear to affect neuromodulators involved in the reward system, such as BDNF (Brain-Derived Neurotrophic Factor) in different ways (Koo et al., 2012).

Illicit Opiates of Abuse

In addition to abuse of prescription opiates, current abuse problems with opiate drugs include several substances that are not medications. Desomorphine (*dihydrodesoxymorphine*) is an opiate derived compound, developed in the United States in 1932. It can be synthesized from codeine with other ingredients such as gasoline, paint thinner, hydrochloric acid, iodine, and red phosphorous (from the striking pad of matchboxes), in a manner similar to the production of methamphetamine from pseudoephedrine. This designer drug began to appear in Russia several years ago, after first showing up in Siberia in 2002, perhaps because codeine is commonly sold over-the-counter in Russia. Unfortunately, this homemade mixture has many contaminants, is very toxic, and when injected can produce severe tissue damage, phlebitis and gangrene, sometimes requiring limb amputation. The addict's skin becomes greenish and scaly at the injection site because the blood vessels burst and the tissue dies; this has led to the street name of krokodil (crocodile).

Another agent that has become popular is the herbal drug, Kratom, which comes from the leaves of the medicinal plant *Mitragyna speciosa*, native to Southeast Asia and used for thousands of years. In low doses this substance has a stimulant action, but high doses produce sedation and opiate effects. The major constituent is mitragynine, which acts through the mu opiate receptor. But, in addition to exerting its own opiate effect, Kratom is often combined with another mu agonist, *O*-desmethyltramadol, the active metabolite of tramadol. The combination is referred to as Krypton. *O*-desmethyltramadol is twice as potent as tramadol, and the material is often sold in large quantities. Over a period of less than one year, there were nine cases of poisoning with this agent (Kronstrand et al., 2011). Kratom is usually taken as a tea, but the leaves may also be chewed. Acute side effects include nausea, itching, constipation, and in the worst cases, hallucinations and delusions. Many countries have already banned Kratom, including Thailand, Australia, Finland, Denmark, Poland, Lithuania, Malaysia, and Myanmar. A new urine test just became available for identification of Kratom.

STUDY QUESTIONS

1. How are pain impulses transmitted and modulated within the Central Nervous System?

2. Describe the opioid receptors: What are the endogenous ligands for those receptors? What happens when an opiate agonist activates them?

3. Define an opioid agonist, antagonist, mixed agonist-antagonist, and partial agonist. Give an example of each and how they are therapeutically useful.

4. In addition to analgesia what are the major physiological effects of opioid drugs?

5. How have opiate analgesics been reformulated to reduce undesirable side effects?

6. How have opiate analgesics been reformulated to reduce their abuse potential?

7. Discuss the various options for the pharmacological management of opioid dependence and relapse.

8. What are Krocodil, Kratom, and Krypton?

9. What are some of the new opiate approaches to pain relief?

REFERENCES

Alho, H., et al. (2007). "Abuse Liability of Buprenorphine-Naloxone Tablets in Untreated IV Drug Users." *Drug and Alcohol Dependence* 88: 75–78.

Angst, M. S., et al. (2012). "Aversive and Reinforcing Opioid Effects: A Pharmacogenomic Twin Study." *Anesthesiology* 117: 22–37.

Bannwarth, B. (2012). "Will Abuse-Deterrent Formulations of Opioid Analgesics be Successful in Achieving Their Purpose?" *Drugs* 72: 1713–1723.

Barry, D. T., et al. (2009). "Integrating Buprenorphine Treatment into Office-Based Practice: A Qualitative Study." *Journal of General Internal Medicine* 24: 218–225.

Bohnert, A. S. B., et al. (2011). "Association Between Opioid Prescribing Patterns and Opioid Overdose-Related Deaths." *Journal of the American Medical Association* 305: 1315–1321.

Boyer, E. W. (2012). "Management of Opioid Analgesic Overdose." *New England Journal of Medicine* 367: 146–155.

Brennan, M. J. (2013). "The Effect of Opioid Therapy on Endocrine Function." *The American Journal of Medicine* 126(Suppl. 1): S12–S18.

Cicero, T. J., et al. (2012). "Effect of Abuse-Deterrent Formulation of OxyContin." *New England Journal of Medicine* 367: 187–189.

Coffin, P. O., and Sullivan, S. D. (2013). "Cost-Effectiveness of Distributing Naloxone to Heroin Users for Lay Overdose Reversal." *Annals of Internal Medicine* 158: 1–9.

Collins, E. D., et al. (2005). "Anesthesia-Assisted vs Buprenorphine- or Clonidine-Assisted Heroin Detoxification and Naltrexone Induction: A Randomized Trial." *Journal of the American Medical Association* 294: 903–913.

Cornish, R., et al. (2010). "Risk of Death During and After Opiate Substitution Treatment in Primary Care: Prospective Observational Study in UK General Practice Research Database." *British Medical Journal* 341: c5475.

Daniulaityte, R., et al. (2012)." Illicit Use of Buprenorphine in a Community Sample of Young Adult Non-Medical Users of Pharmaceutical Opioids." *Drug and Alcohol Dependence* 122: 201–207.

Dart, R. C., et al. (2012). "Assessment of the Abuse of Tapentadol Immediate Release: The First 24 Months." *Journal of Opioid Management* 8: 395-402.

Davis, M. P. (2011). "Fentanyl for Breakthrough Pain: A Systematic Review." *Expert Review of Neurotherapeutics* 11: 1197–1216.

Fiellin, D. A., et al. (2013). "A Randomized Trial of Cognitive Behavioral Therapy in Primary Care-based Buprenorphine." *The American Journal of Medicine* 126: e11–e17.

Fine, P. G., et al. (2011). "Deaths Related to Opioids Prescribed for Chronic Pain: Causes and Solutions." *Pain Medicine* 12(Suppl 2): s26–s35.

Goldstein, A. (1994). *Addiction: From Biology to Drug Policy.* New York: Freeman.

Grant, J. E., et al. (2008). "Predicting Response to Opiate Antagonists and Placebo in the Treatment of Pathological Gambling." *Psychopharmacology* 200: 521–527.

Hayes, M. J., and Brown, M. S. (2012). "Epidemic of Prescription Opiate Abuse and Neonatal Abstinence." *Journal of the American Medical Association* 307: 1974–1975.

Hermanns, K., et al. (2012). "Prolonged-Release Oxycodone/Naloxone in the Treatment of Neuropathic Pain – Results from a large Observational Study." *Expert Opinion on Pharmacotherapy* 13: 299–311.

Holbrook, T. L., et al. (2010). "Morphine Use After Combat Injury in Iraq and Post-Traumatic Stress Disorder." *New England Journal of Medicine* 362: 110–117.

Hser, Y. -I., et al. (2001). "A 33-Year Follow-Up of Narcotic Addicts." *Archives of General Psychiatry* 58: 503–508.

Hutchinson, M. R., et al. (2012). "Opioid Activation of Toll-Like Receptor 4 Contributes to Drug Reinforcement." *The Journal of Neuroscience* 32: 11187–11200.

Jayaram-Lindstrom, N., et al. (2008). "Naltrexone for the Treatment of Amphetamine Dependence: A Randomized, Placebo-Controlled Trial." *American Journal of Psychiatry* 165: 1442–1448.

Johnson, R. E., et al. (2000). "A Comparison of Levomethadyl Acetate, Buprenorphine, and Methadone for Opioid Dependence." *New England Journal of Medicine* 343: 1290–1297.

Jones, H. E., et al. (2012a). "Buprenorphine Treatment of Opioid-Dependent Pregnant Women: A Comprehensive Review." *Addiction* 107(Suppl 1); 5–27.

Jones, H. E., et al. (2012b). "Methadone and Buprenorphine for the Management of Opioid Dependence in Pregnancy." *Drugs* 72: 747–757.

Katz, N. (2005). "The Impact of Opioids on the Endocrine System." *Pain Management Rounds* 1 (9): 1–6. Available online at www.painmanagement-rounds.org.

Katz, N., et al. (2010). "ALO-01 (Morphine Sulfate and Naltrexone Hydrochloride) Extended-Release Capsules in the Treatment of Chronic Pain of Osteoarthritis of the Hip or Knee: Pharmacokinetics, Efficacy, and Safety." *Journal of Pain* 11: 303–311.

Koo, J. W., et al. (2012). "BDNF is a Negative Modulator of Morphine Action." *Science* 338: 124–128.

Kronstrand, R., et al. (2011). "Unintentional Fatal Intoxications with Mitragynine and O-Desmethyltramadol From the Herbal Blend Krypton." *Journal of Analytical Toxicology* 35: 242–247.

Krueger, C. (2012). "Methadone for Pain Management." *Practical Pain Management* 12:

Krupitsky, E., et al. (2011)." Injectable Extended-Release Naltrexone for Opioid Dependence: A Double-Blind, Placebo-Controlled, Multicentre Randomized Trial." *Lancet* 377: 1506–1513.

Kunoe, N., et al. (2009). "Naltrexone Implants After In-Patient Treatment for Opioid Dependence: Randomized Controlled Trial." *British Journal of Psychiatry* 194: 541–546.

Largent-Milnes, T. M., et al. (2008). "Oxycodone plus Ultra-Low-Dose Naltrexone Attenuates Neuropathic Pain and Associated Mu-Opioid Receptor-Gs Coupling." *Journal of Pain* 9: 700–713.

Lembke, A. (2012). "Why Doctors Prescribe Opioids to Known Opioid Abusers." *New England Journal of Medicine* 367: 1580–1581.

Levinthal, C. F. (2012). *Drugs, Behavior and Modern Society,* 7ᵗʰ ed. New York: Allyn & Bacon.

Ling, W., et al. (2010)."Buprenorphine Implants for Treatment of Opioid Dependence: A Randomized Controlled Trial." *Journal of the American Medical Association* 304: 1576–1583.

Löwenstein, O., et al. (2010). "Efficacy and Safety of Combined Prolonged-Release Oxycodone and Naloxone in the Management of Moderate/Severe Chronic Non-Malignant Pain: Results of a Prospectively Designed Pooled Analysis of Two Randomised, Double-Blind Clinical Trials." *BMC Clinical Pharmacology* 10:12.

MacDonald, N., and McLeod, S. M. (2010). "Has The Time Come to Phase Out Codeine?" *Canadian Medical Association Journal* 182: 1825.

Miller, S. C., and Frankowski, D. (2012). "Prescription Opioid Use Disorder: A Complex Clinical Challenge." *Current Psychiatry* 11: 15–22.

O'Connor, P. G. (2005). "Methods of Detoxification and Their Role in Treating Patients with Heroin Dependence." *Journal of the American Medical Association* 294: 961–963.

Okie, S. (2010). "A Flood of Opioids, a Rising Tide of Deaths." *New England Journal of Medicine* 363: 1981–1985.

Paech, M. J., et al. (2012). "New Formulations of Fentanyl for Acute Pain Management." *Drugs Today* 48: 119–132.

Pathan, H., and Williams, J. (2012)."Basic Opioid Pharmacology: An Update." *British Journal of Pain* 6:11–16.

Paulozzi, L. B., et al. (2011). "A National Epidemic of Unintentional Prescription Opioid Overdose Deaths: How Physicians Can Help Control It." *Journal of Clinical Psychiatry* 72: 589–592.

Paulozzi, L. B., et al. (2013). "Pharmaceutical Overdose Deaths, United States, 2010." *Journal of the American Medical Association* 309: 657–659.

Peppin, J. F. (2012). "Opioid-Induced Constipation." *Practical Pain Management* 12: 59–66.

Perrone, J., and Nelson, L. S. (2012). "Medication Reconciliation for Controlled Substances-An "Ideal" Prescription-Drug Monitoring Program." *New England Journal of Medicine* 366: 2341– 2343.

Pierce, A. M., and Brahm, N. C. (2011). "Opiates and Psychotropics: Pharmacokinetics for Practitioners." *Current Psychiatry* 10: 83–86.

Sandner-Kiesling, A., et al. (2010). "Long-Term Efficacy and Safety of Combined Prolonged-Release Oxycodone and Naloxone in the Management of Non-Cancer Chronic Pain." *International Journal of Clinical Practice* 64: 763–774.

Spetea, M., et al. (2012). "Discovery and Biological Evaluation of a Diphenethylamine Derivative (HS665), a Highly Potent and Selective κ Opioid Receptor Agonist." *BMC Pharmacology and Toxicology* 13(Suppl 1): A43.

Stachnik, J. M. (2011). "Medications for Chronic Pain – Opioid Analgesics." *Practical Pain Management* 11:110–119.

Stone, L. S., and Molliver, D. C. (2009). "In Search of Analgesia." *Molecular Interventions* 9: 234–251.

Stowe, G. N., et al. (2011). "A Vaccine Strategy That Induces Protective Immunity Against Heroin." *Journal of Medicinal Chemistry* 54: 5195–5204.

Tennant, F. (2010). "Making Practical Sense of Cytochrome P450." *Practical Pain Management* 10: 12–18.

Tennant, F. (2011). "Genetic Screening for Defects in Opioid Metabolism: Historical Characteristics and Blood Levels." *Practical Pain Management* 11:26–30.

Tennant, F. (2012). "Endocrine Abnormalities After 20 Years of Opioid Therapy." Presented at the 2012 American Association of Pain Medicine Annual Meeting, Poster 248.

Thipphawong, J. B., et al. (2003). "Analgesic Efficacy of Inhaled Morphine in Patients After Bunionectomy Surgery." *Anesthesiology* 99: 693–700.

Thomas, J., et al. (2008). "Methylnaltrexone for Opioid-Induced Constipation in Advanced Illness." *New England Journal of Medicine* 358: 2332–2343.

Turk, D., et al. (2011). "Treatment of Chronic Non-Cancer Pain." *Lancet* 377: 2226–2235.

Vickery, R., et al. (2012). "TD-1211 Demonstrates Improvement in Bowel Movement Frequency and Bristol Stool Scores in a Phase IIb Study of Patients With Opioid-Induced Constipation (OIC)." *American College of Gastroenterology* Abstract 36.

Volkow, N. D., et al. (2011). "Characteristics of Opioid Prescriptions in 2009." *Journal of the American Medical Association* 305: 1299–1301.

Wade, W. E., and Spruill, W. J. (2009). "Tapentadol Hydrochloride: A Centrally Acting Oral Analgesic." *Clinical Therapeutics* 31: 2804–2818.

Wang, D., et al. (2012). "Longer-Term Use of Opioids." Vol WC-12-39. Cambridge, MA: Workers Compensation Research Institute.

Weber, J. M., et al. (2012). "Can Nebulized Naloxone be Used Safely and Effectively by Emergency Medical Services for Suspected Opioid Overdose?" *Prehospital Emergency Care* 16: 289–292.

Webster, L. R., and Fine, P. G. (2012). "Review and Critique of Opioid Rotation Practices and Associated Risks of Toxicity." *Pain Medicine* 13: 562–570.

Webster, L., et al. (2008). "Alvimopan, a Peripherally Acting Mu-Opioid Receptor (PAM-OR) Antagonist for the Treatment of Opioid-Induced Bowel Dysfunction: Results from a Randomized, Double-Blind, Placebo-Controlled, Dose-Finding Study in Subjects Taking Opioids for Chronic Non-Cancer Pain." *Pain* 137: 428–440.

Wedam, E. F., et al. (2007). "QT-Interval Effects of Methadone, Levomethadyl, and Buprenorphine in a Randomized Trial." *Archives of Internal Medicine* 167: 2469–2475.

Weiss, R. D., et al. (2011). "Adjunctive Counseling During Brief and Extended Buprenorphine-Naloxone Treatment for Prescription Opioid Dependence." *Archives of General Psychiatry* 68: 1238–1246.

White, T., and Schultz, S. K. (2000). "Naltrexone Treatment for a 3-Year-Old Boy with Self-Injurious Behavior." *American Journal of Psychiatry* 157: 1574–1580.

Wolstein, J., et al. (2009). "A Randomized, Open-Label Trial Comparing Methadone and Levo-Alpha-Acetylmethadol (LAAM) in Maintenance Treatment of Opioid Addiction." *Pharmacopsychiatry* 42: 1–8.

Zagon, I. S., et al. (2011a). "B Lymphocyte Proliferation is Suppressed by the Opioid Growth Factor-Opioid Growth Factor Axis: Implication for the Treatment of Autoimmune Diseases." *Immunobiology* 216: 173–183.

Zagon, I. S. et al. (2011b). " T Lymphocyte Proliferation is Suppressed by the Opioid Growth Factor ([Met^5] – Enkephalin) – Opioid Growth Factor Receptor Axis: Implication for the Treatment of Autoimmune Diseases." *Immunobiology* 216: 579–590.

PART 3

Psychotherapeutic Drugs

The chapters in this part introduce the drugs that are used to treat psychological disorders. These medications include the traditional and "atypical" antipsychotics (Chapter 11), the antidepressants (Chapter 12), the medications used classically to treat anxiety and insomnia (Chapter 13), and the "mood stabilizers" for treating bipolar disorder (Chapter 14).

Important advances have been made in the pharmacological treatment of psychological disorders, allowing affected people to lead much more "normal" lives than they have ever been able to before in human history. Nevertheless, progress has been slow and modest. The goals of these next four chapters are to impart a sense of the historical development of therapeutics of each disorder, to cover the pharmacology of drugs currently being used to treat these disorders, and to convey a sense of excitement about the promise of even better therapies. The drugs are compartmentalized in these chapters under descriptive headings (antidepressants, mood stabilizers, antipsychotics, and so forth), but the headings do not adequately describe or define the drugs. For example, besides being used to relieve major depression, antidepressants are used as antianxiety drugs and analgesics. Many of the mood stabilizers, besides being used to treat bipolar disorder, are used to treat chronic pain syndromes, psychological disorders associated with agitation and aggression, and even substance abuse. Antipsychotic drugs, besides being used to treat schizophrenia, are being used to treat bipolar disorder, explosive and aggressive disorders, autism, and other pervasive developmental disorders. Newer antipsychotic agents are being used to treat depression and dysthymia. Nevertheless, the artificial distinctions are maintained to present the pharmacology of the drugs in a logical manner.

Chapter 11

Antipsychotic Drugs

Schizophrenia

Schizophrenia is a debilitating neuropsychiatric illness that typically strikes young people just when they are maturing into adulthood (Freedman, 2003). Affecting approximately 1 percent of the population, the disorder is associated with marked social and/or occupational dysfunction, and its course and outcome vary greatly. In the premorbid phase of the illness subtle motor, cognitive, or social impairments are often observed but are not severe enough to place affected people outside the normal range of functioning (Miyamoto et al., 2003). In the prodromal phase mood symptoms, cognitive symptoms, social withdrawal, or obsessive behaviors may develop. The onset of the full syndrome leads to substantial functional deterioration in self-care, work, and interpersonal relationships, especially during the first 5 years, after which clinical deterioration reaches a plateau and, in some situations, function may actually improve. Jobe and Harrow (2010) followed a group of individuals diagnosed with schizophrenia for 26 years. In studying their course of illness and comparing their data with data from other long-term longitudinal studies, a common set of findings emerged: the course and outcome for schizophrenic patients are poorer than those of other psychotic and nonpsychotic disorders, even 10 years after the diagnosis.

Despite apparent gains in treatment during the early phase of illness, there is no overall agreement on whether the long-term outcome for schizophrenia has been improved.

Approximately 10 to 15 percent of people with this disorder take their own lives, usually within the first 10 years of developing the illness (Keltner and Folks, 2005; Sadock and Sadock, 2007).

In general, individuals with schizophrenia have a lifespan that is up to 25 years shorter than individuals in the general population without the disorder with the most common cause of death being cardiovascular and cerebrovascular disease (Colton and Manderscheid, 2006). With regard to violent offenses, however, there is only a minimal link between violent crime and schizophrenia in the absence of substance abuse (Fazel etal., 2009).

Schizophrenia is thought to be a neurodevelopmental disease, associated with significant abnormalities in brain structure and function. Because these abnormalities can be observed in patients who have never been treated with antipsychotic medications, they are considered to be inherent in the disease, not medication related (Torrey, 2002). Based on an analysis of twin studies, schizophrenia is thought to be a highly heritable disorder (Sullivan et al., 2003). Genetic testing suggests that if a person carries a certain gene combination, they may be less susceptible to the effects of antipsychotic medication (Zhang et al., 2010). However, the field of genomics for the study of mental illness is still in the development phase and at present, genetic testing cannot be used to determine diagnosis, to select treatment medications, or to predict response to treatment (Zhang and Malhotra, 2013). The illness is currently viewed as a misconnection syndrome, reflecting a basic disorder in neural circuits, caused by many factors that affect brain development (Miyamoto et al., 2003; Javitt and Coyle, 2004).

The symptoms of schizophrenia have classically been divided into positive and negative clusters. The positive symptoms are the symptoms typical of psychosis and include abnormalities in perception (hallucinations) and inferential thinking (delusions) as well as disorganized, incoherent, and illogical speech (thought disorder). The negative symptoms reflect the absence of some normal human quality and include blunting of emotional expression (constricted range and decreased intensity of affect), impoverishment of speech and mental creativity (alogia), loss of motivation and interest (avolition), the loss of the ability to experience pleasure (anhedonia), and social withdrawal. This differentiation of symptomatology is important because current agents affect primarily the positive symptoms, while there is less benefit for negative symptoms. Patients with schizophrenia also have impairments in many different cognitive systems, such as memory, attention, and executive function. Therefore, treatment is now aimed at more than reducing abnormal perceptions and thought processes; efforts are also being directed to improving cognitive functioning and quality of life so that patients with severe and persistent mental illness can successfully reintegrate into the community (Weickert et al., 2003; American Psychiatric Association, 2004; Janicak et al., 2011).

Dopamine Involvement

Early scientific evidence supported a specific *dopamine theory* of schizophrenia, which proposed that the disorder developed from dysregulation of dopaminergic brain pathways, resulting in overactivity of dopaminergic function (McGowan et al., 2004). This conclusion was derived from two known facts: (1) Abuse of stimulant drugs that are known to increase synaptic dopamine concentration, such as amphetamine, produce a syndrome indistinguishable from the paranoid type of schizophrenia; and (2) Antipsychotic drugs are *dopamine receptor antagonists* that block dopamine receptors in the brain. Dopamine receptors can be classified as either D_1 (of which there are two subtypes, D_1 and D_5) or D_2 (which has three subtypes, D_2, D_3, and D_4). It is now appreciated not only that all antipsychotic drugs have an affinity for the D_2 receptor but that this affinity remains the single best predictor of the effective clinical dose of an antipsychotic (Figure 11.1).

Unfortunately, dopamine, released by neurons in the basal ganglia of the brain, is crucial for maintaining normal coordination of movement. In fact, the loss of these neurons is responsible for the neurological disorder Parkinson's disease. Similarly, by

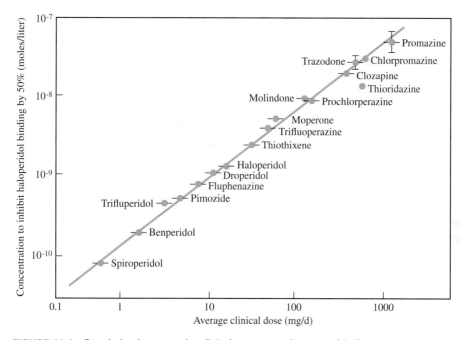

FIGURE 11.1 Correlation between the clinical potency and receptor-binding activities of neuroleptic drugs. Clinical potency is expressed as the daily dose used in treating schizophrenia, and binding activity is expressed as the concentration needed to produce 50 percent inhibition of haloperidol binding. Haloperidol binds to dopamine-2 receptors; other antipsychotic drugs compete for the same receptors. Thus, measuring the competitive inhibition of haloperidol binding correlates with potency of an antipsychotic drug.

blocking dopamine receptors, antipsychotic drugs produce the neurological side effect of parkinsonian symptoms (also known as extrapyramidal symptoms—EPS). Long-term, chronic antipsychotic administration may also elicit other syndromes of abnormal motor function such as tardive dyskinesia (TD), which may be irreversible.

It has been generally assumed that the risk of these neurological symptoms was an unavoidable consequence of antipsychotic drug therapy. However, the discovery of the second-generation antipsychotics (SGAs) has shown that this assumption is incorrect and that antipsychotic efficacy can be obtained with little or no EPS or TD (Correll et al., 2004; Janicak et al., 2011). This is the primary advantage of the newer agents relative to the first-generation drugs.

Serotonin Involvement

As with dopamine, early investigations into the possible role of serotonin (5-HT) in schizophrenia followed from observations of the actions of psychoactive drugs. Because the psychedelic drug LSD produces hallucinations, it was initially proposed to be involved in the clinical syndrome seen in schizophrenia. LSD is one of a group of hallucinogenic drugs that are thought to exert their psychedelic effect as agonists at 5-HT$_{2A}$ receptors. For this reason, it was hypothesized that *5-HT$_2$ receptor antagonism* might be responsible for some of the beneficial actions of antipsychotics. Although it has since been concluded that serotonin does not play an important role in the etiology of schizophrenia, antagonism of this transmitter at 5-HT$_2$ receptors may be involved in the improved neurological side effect profile of the newer antipsychotic medications. Meltzer (2002) discusses the history of this concept.

Glutamate Involvement

In addition to amphetamine and LSD, the two psychedelic drugs *phencyclidine* (PCP) and *ketamine* (see Chapter 8) have also provided insight into the neurochemistry of schizophrenia. These drugs also produce some schizophrenia-like symptoms, such as hallucinations, out-of-body experiences, negative symptomatology, and cognitive deficits. The mechanism responsible for these effects is a potent blockade of NMDA-type glutamate receptors. This relationship suggests that there may be a glutamatergic dysfunction in the etiology of schizophrenia, which has prompted a glutamate-NMDA hypothesis of schizophrenia. This theory proposes that NMDA hypofunction results in excessive release of the excitatory neurotransmitters glutamate and acetylcholine in the frontal cortex, damaging cortical neurons and triggering the deterioration seen in patients with schizophrenia (Farber, 2003; Laruelle et al., 2003; Moghaddam, 2003; Rujescu et al., 2006).

However, none of these models completely explains nor exactly mimics the phenotypic presentation of behaviors associated with schizophrenia. And that should not be expected since schizophrenia is understood to be multiple types of disorders, perhaps having multiple gene involvement. Serotonin agonists like LSD produce positive symptoms of illusions/hallucinations, but serotonin antagonists alone are not effective in the treatment of schizophrenia; NMDA/glutamatergic drugs like PCP and ketamine produce more negative symptoms, but GABA or glutamate antagonists are not effective antipsychotics; and dopamine agonists like stimulants and cannabinoid agonists like THC produce more paranoid ideation. But the one consistent finding is that any drug shown to be effective in the treatment of schizophrenia has to block dopamine receptors, primarily the D$_2$ receptor (Paparelli et al., 2011).

HISTORICAL BACKGROUND AND CLASSIFICATION OF ANTIPSYCHOTIC DRUGS

Prior to 1950, there were no effective drugs for treating psychotic patients; these patients were usually permanently or chronically hospitalized. By 1955, more than half a million psychotic patients in the United States were residing in mental hospitals. A dramatic and steady reversal in this trend began in 1956, and by 1983 fewer than 220,000 patients were institutionalized despite a doubling in the number of admissions to state hospitals. By the early 1990s, people with schizophrenia were routinely stabilized on medication and rapidly discharged from institutions. What accounted for this dramatic shift was a class of drugs called phenothiazines, the first category of antipsychotic agents.

Phenothiazines were initially developed as antihistamines and were first studied for their mildly sedating action. The sedative properties led the French anesthesiologist and surgeon Henri Laborit to use *promethazine,* the first phenothiazine, to deepen anesthesia. This drug was administered in a "lytic cocktail" to patients the night before surgery to allay their fears and anxieties. Promethazine was soon followed by a second phenothiazine, *chlorpromazine* (Thorazine), which was found to reduce the amount of anesthetic drugs a patient needed without making the patient unconscious; rather, this treatment produced a state characterized by calmness, conscious sedation, and lack of interest in and detachment from external stimuli. This condition was termed a *neuroleptic state,* and chlorpromazine was the first neuroleptic drug.

Laborit persuaded many clinicians to try chlorpromazine, and later the same year the French research psychiatrists Delay and Deniker studied its effect in schizophrenic patients. Although it did not provide a permanent cure, chlorpromazine was found to be remarkably effective in alleviating the clinical manifestations of psychosis (López-Muñoz et al., 2005). In conjunction with supportive therapy, its use allowed thousands of patients who otherwise would have been permanently hospitalized to return to their communities, albeit in a less than satisfactory state.

In the continuing search for more effective drugs with fewer side effects, alternatives to the phenothiazines have been developed. The second class of neuroleptics was the *butyrophenones,* developed in Belgium in the mid-1960s. Two butyrophenones are currently available, *haloperidol* (Haldol) and *droperidol* (Inapsine). Haloperidol is used in the treatment of schizophrenia, droperidol in the treatment of nausea and vomiting associated with surgery.

These first-generation antipsychotics (FGAs) are most effective against the positive symptoms of schizophrenia, and, as noted, the doses required for clinical improvement were significantly correlated with their ability to block D_2 dopamine receptors.

Unfortunately, D_2 antagonism as noted above also produced EPS and TD. Therefore, for the FGAs, binding to D_2 receptors not only resulted in clinical efficacy but also increased the likelihood of EPS. Indeed, the antipsychotic and EPS effects of neuroleptics were generally thought to be linked and inseparable. This idea led to a *neuroleptic threshold concept* of treatment, which held that the neuroleptic dose should be gradually increased until EPS was produced. Thus, the "right" dose was the one that caused some degree of motor side effects.

Beginning in the late 1980s, breakthroughs occurred that seemed to offer improvements in regard to such side effects. These developments began with the discovery of the first second-generation antipsychotic, clozapine (Clozaril). Clozapine was a major advance because it was effective for many patients (about 30 percent) who did not respond to standard treatment and because it produced little or no symptoms of movement disorders such as EPS or TD (and, in fact, may even reduce TD caused by other antipsychotics).

Unfortunately, clozapine itself had some serious side effects, which limited its use to patients who had not responded to conventional treatment. However, it prompted the development of other SGAs, collectively referred to as "atypical" antipsychotics. In addition to *clozapine* (Clozaril), they include *risperidone* (Risperdal), *olanzapine* (Zyprexa), *quetiapine* (Seroquel), *ziprasidone* (Geodon), *aripiprazole* (Abilify), *paliperidone* (Invega), *iloperidone* (Fanapt), *asenapine* (Saphris), and *lurasidone* (Latuda). Aripiprazole may actually be the first of a new, third generation of antipsychotics (TGAs) because of its unique mechanism of action.

All the SGAs differ pharmacologically from the FGAs by having relatively less affinity for D_2 receptors (Grunder et al., 2003) and greater affinity for 5-HT (serotonergic) receptors. For some reason, this allows a separation between antipsychotic efficacy and induction of EPS or other movement disorders (with the exception of risperidone at higher doses) (Kapur and Remington, 2001; Kapur and Seeman, 2001; Horacek et al., 2006). Although none of the others share clozapine's superior efficacy for treatment of schizophrenic patients who are refractory to treatment, these drugs have shown that it is possible to separate therapeutic benefit from parkinsonian side effects (Advokat, 2005).[1]

Initially, the SGAs also appeared to be more effective than FGAs against negative symptoms. However, it is now appreciated that an apparent improvement in negative symptoms may be secondary to the absence of EPS or to other indirect causes, such as improvement in socialization and cognition, rather than a direct therapeutic effect (Rosenheck et al., 2003). Negative symptoms, especially social and emotional withdrawal, poor rapport, and blunted affect are still prominent, even in patients treated in routine clinical practice. Their presence was associated with being male, older, and single/unmarried; having greater illness severity and fewer positive symptoms; and receiving a high antipsychotic dose (Bobes et al., 2010). Unfortunately, efforts to alleviate negative symptoms with drugs like the wakefulness/antifatigue drug modafinil have not proven successful (Freudenreich et al., 2009).

Criticisms of the comparative efficacy, safety, and cost-benefit ratio of the SGAs have been discussed in several meta-analyses and comparative studies of the first- and second-generation agents (Davis et al., 2003; Davis and Chen, 2004). The largest meta-analysis combined results from 124 clinical trials, including some unpublished data from the U.S. Food and Drug Administration (FDA; Davis et al., 2003). There were two conclusions. The first, not surprising, was that clozapine was superior to FGAs. The second was that, among the other SGAs, only olanzapine and risperidone appeared to be better than FGAs. But there were two major criticisms of this conclusion. First, it was suggested that some SGAs didn't separate from FGAs because the doses may have been too low. Second, it was argued that patient recruitment might now be more difficult. With more patients experiencing some improvement, perhaps the population of participants is less responsive to standard treatment. A smaller meta-analysis, appearing around the same time (Leucht et al., 2003), concluded that there were no meaningful differences among the SGAs, while a subsequent comparison found small differences favoring olanzapine, followed by risperidone (Leucht et al., 2009a). Nevertheless, even before some of these literature reviews, the National Institute of Mental Health (NIMH)

[1] Several possible mechanisms might account for this property. First, 5-HT is known to inhibit dopamine release in the nigrostriatal but not the mesolimbic dopamine pathway. By blocking this action (either through 5-HT$_2$ receptor antagonism at the dopamine terminal or by 5-HT$_{1A}$ antagonism at the cell body), SGAs selectively enhance dopamine release in the striatum, which mitigates neuroleptic-induced EPS. Second, clozapine and quetiapine have a low affinity for the D_2 receptor and do not attach very tightly to these binding sites. Because the natural amount of dopamine in the nigrostriatal pathway is greater than that in the mesolimbic pathway, clozapine and quetiapine may be more easily displaced from the striatal dopamine receptors by the higher concentration of the endogenous transmitter. This occurrence would normalize dopaminergic activity in the nigrostriatal system and reduce pseudoparkinsonian side effects.

conducted a large, double-blind, active control clinical trial, designed to directly compare the relative effectiveness of SGAs with the effectiveness of the FGA perphenazine. This was the largest, longest, and most comprehensive independent trial ever done to examine existing therapies for schizophrenia.

CATIE and CUtLASS Studies

The Clinical Antipsychotic Trials of Intervention Effectiveness (CATIE) study was conducted in the United States between January 2001 and December 2004 at 57 clinical sites for up to 18 months or until treatment was discontinued for any reason. In the first of three phases, 1493 patients were randomly assigned to receive either one of three SGAs (olanzapine, risperidone, or quetiapine) or perphenazine under double-blind conditions. Ziprasidone was added later following its FDA approval. Results showed that patients discontinued antipsychotic medications at a high rate, 64 to 82 percent across all the drugs, primarily because of lack of efficacy or intolerable side effects (EPS in the case of perphenazine and weight gain or metabolic changes from olanzapine). There was no overall difference in the rate of discontinuation between the SGAs and the FGA, perphenazine (Lieberman et al., 2005).

Of the 1493 patients enrolled in the study, 1052 were eligible for phase 2. This part of the study provided two treatment pathways. Patients who had not shown optimal improvement on one of the SGAs in the first phase or who had stopped treatment for any other reason were offered the option of random assignment to clozapine or to an SGA other than the one they had received in phase 1. A total of 99 patients entered this "efficacy" pathway. Patients who discontinued treatment for intolerability were offered the opportunity to receive treatment with an SGA other than the one they had previously received—excluding clozapine. A total of 444 patients entered this "tolerability" pathway. The remaining 509 patients (48 percent) did not enter phase 2.

In the "efficacy" pathway, clozapine treatment was found to be more effective than the other SGAs; patients receiving clozapine were less likely to discontinue therapy because of lack of therapeutic response than patients receiving any of the other newer agents. In the "tolerability" pathway, olanzapine and risperidone were more effective than quetiapine or ziprasidone in "time until discontinuation" for any reason. Neither of the phase 2 pathways included either aripiprazole or any first-generation antipsychotic (McEvoy et al., 2006; Stroup et al., 2006).

A British comparison between SGAs and FGAs—Cost Utility of the Latest Antipsychotic Drugs in Schizophrenia Studies (CUtLASS 1)—was reported in October 2006 (Jones et al., 2006). It evaluated 227 people with a diagnosis of schizophrenia who had an inadequate response or adverse reaction to their previous medication. Prescriptions for either an FGA or an SGA (excluding clozapine) were monitored for one year, with blind assessments at 12, 26, and 56 weeks. The primary outcomes were a measure of quality of life, symptoms, adverse effects, participant satisfaction, and costs of care. Like the CATIE trial, the results of this study showed that patients with schizophrenia did just as well on antipsychotic drugs from either category, with patients taking FGAs actually showing a trend toward greater improvement on the quality-of-life scale and symptom scores. Participants expressed no clear preference, and the costs were similar.

Although antipsychotic drugs remain the "cornerstone of treatment for schizophrenia" (Lieberman et. al., 2005), the results of the CATIE and CUtLASS 1 trials have prompted a reassessment of the perceived advantages of the second-generation antipsychotics. The initial optimism generated by these new, "atypical" neuroleptics has been tempered by evidence that they do not improve clinical outcome as much as anticipated and are much more expensive than the older drugs.

This perspective was supported by the most recent meta-analysis of SGAs versus FGAs (Leucht et al., 2009b), which included 150 studies and more than 21,500 patients. In 95 of the 150 studies, haloperidol was the comparator. In this case, amisulpride, clozapine, olanzapine, and risperidone were significantly more effective at reducing overall symptoms than the FGAs, whereas aripiprazole, quetiapine, sertindole, ziprasidone, and zotepine (not available in the United States) were not more effective than FGAs. All SGAs produced significantly fewer EPS than haloperidol. Even though some differences were statistically significant, they were not absolutely very large. Essentially, it is now understood that not all SGAs are the same (Komossa et al., 2009a, 2009b); they don't all produce better outcomes than FGAs, even in cases of acute toxic ingestion (Ciranni et al., 2009); and the merits of each drug have to be determined independently, taking into account side effects and cost benefits (Rosenheck and Sernyak, 2009). In situations where EPS may preclude the use of FGAs, such as autism, bipolar disorder, borderline personality disorder, and aggressive disorders, SGAs may be the first choice. The transition to generic status of the SGAs (reducing their cost) will most likely affect such considerations as well.

Kane and Correll (2010) provide a comprehensive summary of the history of the role of drug treatments for schizophrenia; the evolution from the FGAs to the SGAs; successes and lack of success for novel interventions; and future directions for research.

First-Generation Antipsychotic Drugs: FGAs

Antipsychotics (Figure 11.2 and Table 11.1) are not only the most widely used drugs for treating schizophrenia, they are also used for other purposes, such as to treat nausea and vomiting, to sedate patients before anesthesia, to delay ejaculation, to relieve severe itching, to cure hiccups, and to manage psychosis regardless of cause (such as acute manic attacks, alcoholic hallucinosis, and psychedelic agents). Today, treatment of most of these conditions now involves the use of newer drugs.

Did You Know?

Now We Know Why Old Schizophrenia Medicine Works On Antibiotic-Resistant Bacteria

In 2008 researchers from the University of Southern Denmark showed that the drug thioridazine, which has previously been used to treat schizophrenia, is also a powerful weapon against antibiotic-resistant bacteria such as staphylococci (*Staphylococcus aureus*). Antibiotic-resistant bacteria are a huge problem all over the world: For example, 25—50 percent of the inhabitants in southern Europe are resistant to *staphylococci*. So any effective anti-inflammatory candidate is important to investigate, even if the candidate is an antipsychotic that was originally developed to alleviate one of the hardest mental illnesses, schizophrenia.

Until now, scientists could only see that thioridazine works effectively and can kill *staphylococcus* bacteria in a flask in the laboratory, but now a new study reveals that thioridazine works by weakening the bacterial cell wall: thioridazine weakens the bacterial cell wall by removing glycine (an amino acid) from it. In the absence of glycine, the antibiotics can attack the weakened cell wall and kill *staphylococcus* bacteria. And now that researchers know that thioridazine works they can concentrate on improving this ability. They can remove or inactivate the parts of thioridazine that treats schizophrenia, and develop a nonpsychopharmacological drug that can save people from potentially fatal infections that do not respond to antibiotics.

Pharmacokinetics

First generation antipsychotics are lipid soluble, and highly bound to protein and tissue, with large volumes of distribution. Oral absorption is unpredictable, and several undergo first-pass metabolism in the liver, which means that oral bioavailability is low or variable. However, most have long half-lives, of 20 to 40 hours, which allows doses to be given only once or twice a day after stabilization. All FGAs are extensively metabolized and some have

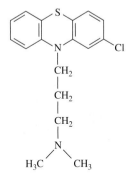

Chlorpromazine (Thorazine)

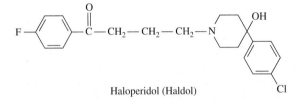

Haloperidol (Haldol)

FIGURE 11.2 Structural formulas of a phenothiazine (chlorpromazine) and a butyrophenone (haloperidol). Both are traditional antipsychotic drugs.

TABLE 11.1 Antipsychotic drugs

Chemical classification	Drug name: Generic (Trade)	Dose equivalent (mg)	Sedation	Autonomic side effects[a]	Involuntary movement
Phenothiazine	Chlorpromazine (Thorazine)	100	High	High	Moderate
	Prochlorperazine (Compazine)	15	Moderate	Low	High
	Fluphenazine (Prolixin)	2	Low	Low	High
	Trifluoperazine (Stelazine)	5	Moderate	Low	High
	Perphenazine (Trilafon)	8	Low	Low	High
	Acetophenazine (Tindal)	20	Moderate	Low	High
	Carphenazine (Proketazine)	25	Moderate	Low	High
	Triflupromazine (Vesprin)	25	High	Moderate	Moderate
	Mesoridazine (Serentil)	50	High	Moderate	Low
	Thioridazine (Mellaril)	100	High	Moderate	Low
Thioxanthene	Thiothixene (Navane)	4	Low	Low	High
	Chlorprothixene (Taractan)	100	High	High	Moderate
Butyrophenone	Haloperidol (Haldol)	2	Low	Low	Very high
Miscellaneous	Loxapine (Loxitane)	10	Moderate	Low	Moderate
	Molindone (Moban)	10	Moderate	Moderate	Moderate
	Pimozide (Orap)	2	Low	Low	Moderate
New generation	Clozapine (Clozaril)	50	Moderate	Moderate	Low
	Risperidone (Risperdal)	1	Low	Low	Low-Moderate
	Olanzapine (Zyprexa)	1.5	Moderate	Low	Low
	Quetiapine (Seroquel)	40	Low	Low	Low
	Ziprasidone (Geodon)	15	Low	Low	Low
	Aripiprazole (Abilify)	3	Low	Low	Low
	Amisulpride (Solian)	NA	Low	Low	Low
	Paliperidone (Invega)	NA	Low	Low	Low
	Iloperidone (Fanapt)	NA	Moderate	Moderate	Low
	Asenapine (Saphris)	NA	Moderate	Low	Low
	Lurasidone (Latuda)	NA	Moderate	Low	Moderate

[a]Autonomic side effects include dry mouth, blurred vision, constipation, urinary retention, and reduced blood pressure.

active metabolites. Metabolites of some of the phenothiazines can be detected for several months after the drug has been discontinued. Slow elimination may also contribute to the slow rate of recurrence of psychotic episodes following cessation of drug therapy.

Pharmacological Effects

In addition to blocking D_2 receptors, most FGAs also block acetylcholine (muscarinic), histamine, and norepinephrine receptors. Cholinergic blockade produces dry mouth, dilated pupils, blurred vision, cognitive impairments, constipation, urinary retention, and tachycardia. Noradrenergic blockade can result in hypotension and sedation. Histaminergic blockade has sedating as well as antiemetic effects. Through actions on the brain stem, antipsychotics suppress the centers involved in behavioral arousal (the ascending reticular activating center) and vomiting (the chemoreceptor trigger zone).

Dopaminergic pathways extend from the hypothalamus to the pituitary gland. The pituitary gland is responsible for regulating the secretion of sex hormones; therefore, dopaminergic blockade increases the release of the hormone prolactin, which can produce breast enlargement in males and lactation in females. In men, ejaculation may be blocked; in women, libido may be decreased, ovulation may be blocked, and normal menstrual cycles may be suppressed, resulting in infertility.

Basal Ganglia. By blocking dopamine receptors in the basal ganglia, FGAs produce two main kinds of motor (neurologic) disturbances, which comprise the most bothersome and potentially serious side effects associated with the use of these agents. The two syndromes are (1) acute extrapyramidal reactions, which develop early in treatment in up to 90 percent of patients, and (2) tardive ("tardy," or late) dyskinesia, which occurs much later, during and even after cessation of chronic neuroleptic treatment. *Acute extrapyramidal (EPS)* side effects include the following:

- Akathisia, a syndrome characterized by the subjective feeling of anxiety, manifested by restlessness, pacing, constant rocking back and forth, and other repetitive, purposeless, actions. Because it can be extremely upsetting to the patient, akathisia is a common cause of nonadherence to psychotropic treatment and may lead to an increased risk for suicide. Although its cause is not well established, a decrease in dopaminergic activity appears to be an important etiological factor. In addition to reducing the dose, the most effective treatment of akathisia includes either a beta-adrenergic antagonist (for example, propranolol) or a serotonergic, 5-HT$_2$, receptor antagonist (for example, ritanserin). Emerging evidence suggests that the likelihood of eliciting akathisia may be increased when antipsychotic drugs (particularly the second generation antipsychotic *aripiprazole* (Abilify) and antidepressant drugs, especially the serotonergic agents) are combined, such as in the treatment of bipolar disorder (Advokat, 2010).
- Dystonia, which presents as involuntary muscle contractions and sustained abnormal, bizarre postures of the limbs, trunk, head, and tongue.
- Neuroleptic-induced parkinsonism, which resembles idiopathic (of unknown etiology) Parkinson's disease. Neuroleptic-induced parkinsonism is characterized by tremor at rest, "cogwheel type" rigidity of the limbs, and slowing of movement, with a reduction in spontaneous activity. In idiopathic parkinsonism, these symptoms occur when the concentration of dopamine in the nuclei of the basal ganglia (caudate nucleus, putamen, and globus pallidus) decreases to about 20 percent of normal. The same symptoms are produced when neuroleptic drug-induced blockade of dopamine receptors reaches 80 percent or greater. If necessary, antiparkinsonian agents can be administered to control these symptoms, although tolerance may eventually develop to neuroleptic-induced parkinsonism.

Tardive dyskinesia (TD) is a much more puzzling and serious form of movement disorder. Victims exhibit involuntary hyperkinetic movements, often of the face and tongue but also of the trunk and limbs, which can be severely disabling. More characteristic are sucking and smacking of the lips; lateral jaw movements; and darting, pushing, or twisting of the tongue. Choreiform (dancelike) movements of the extremities are frequent. The syndrome appears a few months to several years after the beginning of neuroleptic treatment and is sometimes (about 20 percent of the time) irreversible. The incidence of tardive dyskinesia has been estimated at about 20 percent of patients who are treated with FGAs, increasing about 4 percent annually for the first 5 years, but this side effect depends greatly on the particular drug, the dosage, presence of any organic brain disorder, presence of affective symptoms, and the age of the patient (it is most common in patients older than 50, with approximately 50 percent of the elderly affected after 5 years). Although the incidence of TD is much less with the SGAs, it is not zero. One recent study found an incidence of 0.74 percent (Tenback et al., 2010). Unfortunately, there is no adequate treatment for this condition, except perhaps clozapine or another SGA, although it is not clear if some SGAs are more effective than others or what mediates this phenomenon (Peritogiannis and Tsouli, 2010). Although dyskinesia may be controlled by restarting or increasing the dose of neuroleptic, in the short run parkinsonian side effects may be elicited, and eventually the intensity of the abnormal movements may increase.

A novel approach to treating movement disorders, whether in schizophrenia or other neurological conditions, is being developed by Neurocrine Biosciences, Inc. This company is developing a drug (NBI-98854) that selectively blocks the transporter for the storage vesicles in dopamine neurons, called the vesicular monoamine transporter 2 (VMAT2). By blocking the transporter, the drug would prevent dopamine from being repackaged. The aim is to provide sustained, low levels of dopamine to minimize side effects associated with excessive dopamine depletion. The company is currently in Phase IIb clinical trial testing. Results thus far suggest some reduction in Abnormal Involuntary Movement Scale (AIMS) scores (a clinical measure of TD) in schizophrenia patients with TD.

Limbic System. Dopaminergic neurons of the central midbrain portion of the brain stem project to limbic structures, which regulate emotional expression, as well as to forebrain areas, where emotion and cognition are integrated. Increased sensitivity of dopamine receptors in these areas may be responsible for the positive symptoms of schizophrenia. Thus, antipsychotics reduce the intensity of schizophrenic delusions and hallucinations, which are particularly sensitive to treatment. They decrease paranoia, fear, hostility, and agitation, and may dramatically relieve the restlessness and hyperactivity associated with an acute schizophrenic episode.

Side Effects and Toxicity

Much of the art of treating schizophrenic patients with antipsychotics lies in diagnosing and managing side effects. In general, the high-potency agents—agents that block dopamine receptors most strongly and require lower doses—produce more extrapyramidal side effects but less sedation, fewer anticholinergic actions, and less postural hypotension than the low-potency neuroleptics (Table 11.2). The choice of drug depends on the specific situation. When sedation is desired, a low-potency agent may be sufficient or

TABLE 11.2 Major adverse effects of receptor blockade by neuroleptics	
Receptor	Effects
D_2 dopamine	Extrapyramidal symptoms; prolactin increase
α_1 norepinephrine	Postural hypotension
H_1 histamine	Sedation/drowsiness; weight gain
M_1 muscarinic acetylcholine	Memory deficits; constipation/urinary retention; tachycardia; blurred vision; dry mouth
5 HT (1B; 2C) serotonin	Weight gain

a high-potency drug may be combined with a benzodiazepine. If anticholinergic side effects limit adherence, a high-potency drug may be more appropriate, and drug-induced movement disorders, if elicited, may be controlled with antiparkinsonian agents.

It has long been recognized that cognitive disturbances are evident in 40 to 60 percent of patients with schizophrenia. Neuropsychological tests show deficits in numerous "executive" functions which appear in the very first episode. These include deficits in: attention, memory, problem solving, judgment, concept formation, planning, and language. Measured IQ and other cognitive abilities decline the most just before symptoms appear and the first episode occurs but then stabilize (Mesholam-Gately, 2009).

Although it is generally agreed that antipsychotic drugs improve schizophrenic symptomatology, anticholinergic and antihistaminergic actions of the antipsychotics produce memory impairment and sedation, respectively. If these effects are responsible for producing or worsening cognitive dysfunction, then agents without these side effects, such as some SGAs, may improve cognition (Carpenter and Gold, 2002; Weiss et al., 2002).

The NIMH has recently sponsored two initiatives to develop assessments for cognition in schizophrenia and evaluate new medicines: Measurement and Treatment Research to Improve Cognition in Schizophrenia (MATRICS) and Treatment Units for Research on Neurocognition and Schizophrenia (TURNS). Studies are currently being published using the MATRICS assessment battery. But, there are no major reviews of outcomes at this time. TURNS is recruiting for participants in the project and no studies have been reported thus far.

Other potentially serious but less common side effects of antipsychotics include altered pigmentation of the skin, pigment deposits in the retina, permanently impaired vision, allergic (hypersensitivity) reactions (including liver dysfunction and blood disorders), as well as the previously noted hormonal impairments. Although rare, one potentially lethal reaction is the neuroleptic malignant syndrome (NMS). The NMS is an acute reaction that may occur in response to a variety of agents that increase dopaminergic tone. Its incidence in FGA-treated patients is 0.02 to 2.4 percent, and it has been reported to occur in response to the SGAs clozapine, risperidone, and olanzapine. The most common symptoms include fever, severe muscle rigidity of the "lead pipe" type, autonomic changes (such as fluctuating blood pressure), and altered consciousness that may progress to stupor or coma. The most important aspect of effective treatment is early recognition, immediate withdrawal of the responsible agent, and initiation of supportive measures.

Tolerance and Dependence

One of the positive attributes of antipsychotics is that they are not prone to compulsive abuse. They do not produce tolerance or physical or psychological dependence. Psychotic patients may take them for years without increasing their dose because of tolerance; if a dose is increased, it is usually to increase control of psychotic episodes.

Individual First-Generation Antipsychotics

Following the introduction of chlorpromazine and the other phenothiazines during the late 1950s and early 1960s, the limitations of these agents soon became apparent. Pharmaceutical manufacturers therefore attempted to find drugs with novel chemical structures that might exert antipsychotic efficacy without the accompanying side effects, especially the movement disorders. Although this goal was not realized until the mid-1990s, a few nonphenothiazine antipsychotic agents were developed in the 1960s and early 1970s.

Haloperidol

In 1967, *haloperidol* (Haldol), shown in Figure 11.2, was introduced as the first therapeutic alternative to the phenothiazines. A related compound, *droperidol* (Inapsine), was subsequently introduced into anesthesia for the treatment of postoperative nausea and vomiting. Although haloperidol is structurally different, its pharmacological efficacy and side effects are comparable to that of the phenothiazines. It is well absorbed orally and has a moderately slow rate of metabolism and excretion; stable blood levels can be seen for up to 3 days after the drug is discontinued. It takes approximately 5 days for 40 percent of a single dose to be excreted by the kidneys.

Haloperidol's mechanism of antipsychotic action is the same as that of the phenothiazines—it competitively blocks D_2 receptors. It does not produce some of the serious side effects occasionally seen in patients taking phenothiazines (such as jaundice and blood abnormalities). But because it is a high-potency D_2 antagonist, it causes parkinsonism and other motor disorders comparable to those induced by high-potency phenothiazines, and it may require adjunctive prophylactic antiparkinsonian medication. In general, however, haloperidol is effective for treating acutely psychotic patients, as it has a rapid onset, especially when given by injection.

Molindone

The two alternative medications *molindone* (Moban) and *loxapine* (Loxitane) were introduced in the early 1970s. Molindone is a structurally unique molecule resembling the neurotransmitter serotonin. Whether this similarity is relevant to its antipsychotic action is unknown. Molindone is comparable to the traditional antipsychotic drugs in dopamine receptor occupancy, therapeutic efficacy, and side effects, except that it has been shown to produce weight loss. It produces moderate sedation, although it has also been reported to increase motor activity and possibly induce a euphoric effect in rare cases. Both effects may be related to its reported block of the enzyme monoamine oxidase. Molindone may also produce parkinsonian movements similar to those seen in patients taking phenothiazines.

Loxapine

Loxapine (Loxitane) structurally resembles the atypical antipsychotic clozapine, and like the newer SGAs, it binds strongly to both dopaminergic and serotonergic receptors. Nevertheless, its actions differ little from those of the traditional antipsychotic drugs. It has antipsychotic, antiemetic, and sedative properties, and causes abnormal motor movements. It lowers convulsive thresholds somewhat more than the phenothiazines. Taken orally, loxapine is well absorbed, and it is metabolized and excreted within about 24 hours.

Alexza Pharmaceuticals, Inc. has developed an inhalation formulation of *loxapine* (Adasuve) which was FDA approved in December 2012 to treat acute agitation in patients with schizophrenia or bipolar disorder. Previously, the available treatments were either intramuscular injection, which sometimes requires restraint, or rapidly dissolving or standard tablets, which are slower in onset than the inhalation product. The inhaled drug is quickly absorbed through the lungs into the bloodstream, which is as therapeutically rapid as intravenous administration.

Pimozide

Although *pimozide* (Orap) is an antipsychotic drug, it is currently marketed in the United States for the treatment of motor and phonic tics in patients with Tourette's disorder who are unresponsive to other medications. In Europe and South America it is more widely used as a neuroleptic antipsychotic drug. Besides the usual movement disorders of EPS and TD, the side effects that most limit the use of pimozide are electrocardiographic abnormalities (called QT prolongation) that are potentially dangerous. QT prolongation is discussed later in this chapter.

The discovery and development of the first-generation antipsychotics was a major advance in the treatment of schizophrenia. Nevertheless, it is recognized that there are three types of unsatisfactory outcomes for schizophrenic patients treated with phenothiazines and other FGAs. The first category includes patients who are treatment-resistant and refractory to medication, despite an adequate trial of an antipsychotic. The second consists of patients who have persistent negative symptoms, despite successful control of positive symptoms. The third consists of patients who are unable to tolerate the side effects of the antipsychotics. Current evidence suggests that, at the very least, SGAs may provide better options for patients in the third category.

Second-Generation (Atypical) Antipsychotic Agents

From 1975 to 1989, not a single new antipsychotic was marketed in the United States. Since then, clozapine (1989), risperidone (1994), olanzapine (1996), sertindole (1997), quetiapine (1997), ziprasidone (2001), aripiprazole (2002), paliperidone (2006), iloperidone (2009), asenapine (2009), and lurasidone (2010) have been introduced. *Amisulpride* (Solian) is available in Europe and Australia but not yet in the United States.

Clozapine

Clozapine (Clozaril), shown in Figure 11.3, the first atypical antipsychotic, has been demonstrated to be clinically superior to traditional antipsychotics, first, because it is effective in about one-third of patients who are resistant to conventional medications, and second, because it lacks the extrapyramidal side effects associated with the traditional neuroleptics (Volavka et al., 2002). In fact, for patients with primary parkinsonism who demonstrate psychotic symptoms (such as hallucinations and delusions), clozapine can effectively treat their psychosis without exacerbating the movement disorder (Parkinson Study Group, 1999; Comaty and Advokat, 2001). Third, the FIN11 study found that clozapine compared to either FGAs or other SGAs reduced all cause mortality rates in schizophrenics over an 11 year period and reduced suicide rates in the same population (Tiihonen et al., 2009). Clozapine is indicated for treatment-resistant schizophrenia and the treatment of suicidal behavior in schizophrenia.

Background. Synthesized in 1959, clozapine was introduced into clinical practice in Europe in the early 1970s. Its lack of extrapyramidal effects was immediately appreciated. However, in 1975 several schizophrenic patients in Finland died of severe infectious diseases after developing agranulocytosis (loss of white blood cells in the blood) while taking clozapine. As a result, clinical testing ceased and the drug was withdrawn from unrestricted use in Europe. Later, clozapine was re-examined for two major reasons: (1) the agranulocytosis was found to be reversible when the drug was discontinued, and (2) the drug was found to be therapeutically beneficial in patients who had failed to respond to the traditional antipsychotic medications.

In 1986 a large, multicenter trial of the drug in the United States found improvement in 30 percent of severely psychotic patients who were unresponsive to other drugs; only 1 to 2 percent developed agranulocytosis. More recent studies show that the rate of improvement may approach 60 percent with longer therapy. In some patients the improvements are striking; they are able to be discharged from hospitals or to participate meaningfully in rehabilitation. Other clozapine responders do not improve substantially in their positive symptoms but report that their mood and sense of well-being are improved and their quality of life is better. These clinical data are confirmed by real-world improvements (Wheeler et al., 2009).

Evidence that clozapine reduced the risk of suicide in schizophrenia relative to other antipsychotics led to the International Suicide Prevention Trial (InterSePT) study, which compared clozapine with another SGA, olanzapine, in patients with schizophrenia or schizoaffective disorder at risk for suicide (Meltzer et al., 2003). Clozapine was better at reducing suicidal behaviors and has been approved by the FDA for reduction of suicide risk in patients with schizophrenia or schizoaffective disorder.

Pharmacokinetics. Clozapine is well absorbed orally, and plasma levels of the drug peak in about 1 to 4 hours. The drug has two major metabolites, both of which are pharmacologically inactive. Its metabolic half-life varies from 9 to 30 hours. A reasonable daily dose of clozapine is about 300 to 450 milligrams, although dosage must be individualized and may be as high as 900 milligrams per day (maximum daily

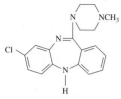

Clozapine (Clozaril)

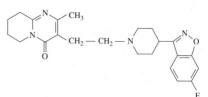

Risperidone (Risperdal)

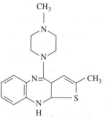

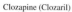

Olanzapine (Zyprexa)

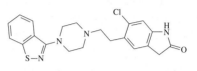

Ziprasidone (Geodon)

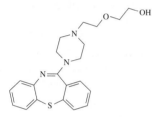

Quetiapine (Seroquel)

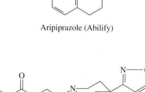

Aripiprazole (Abilify)

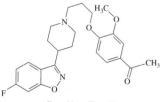

Iloperidone (Fanapt)

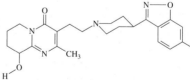

Paliperidone (Invega)

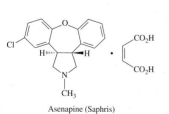

Asenapine (Saphris)

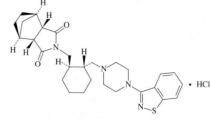

Lurasidone (Latuda)

FIGURE 11.3 Structural formulas of some second-generation, atypical, antipsychotic drugs.

dose), if clinically warranted. Monitoring plasma levels may be useful in optimizing treatment to determine whether nonadherence or abrupt discontinuation of the drug might be at fault when psychotic symptoms recur (Tollefson et al., 1999). Studies have shown that plasma levels of at least 350 ng/ml are necessary to constitute an adequate trial of clozapine.

Pharmacodynamics. As noted, clozapine has a receptor profile that differs from that of the FGAs. It antagonizes D_2 receptors less strongly than D_1 receptors and substantially less than $5\text{-}HT_2$ receptors. Other receptor types antagonized by clozapine include D_3 and D_4 receptors and $5\text{-}HT_{1A}$, histaminergic, cholinergic (muscarinic), and adrenergic receptors.

Side Effects and Toxicity. Although clozapine's efficacy is well documented, its use is severely limited by its side effects and potential for serious toxicity. Common side effects include sedation, extreme weight gain, decrease in seizure threshold, sialorrhea (hypersalivation), and constipation, with rare instances of agranulocytosis.

Sedation, most likely an antihistaminergic action, occurs in about 40 percent of patients taking clozapine; it may be dose limiting and have a negative impact on adherence. Taking the drug at bedtime may help improve adherence. Weight gain is a problem for up to 80 percent of patients; it can be severe, with gains of 20 pounds or more not unusual. Seizures occur at a greater rate with clozapine than with other antipsychotics, especially at high doses (600 to 900 milligrams per day), and it has a specific warning for this adverse event.

Sialorrhea (increased saliva production) occurs in one-third to one-half of patients, not only during the day but often much more extensively at night, with patients complaining of waking up with a wet pillow. The mechanism is believed to be due to an impaired ability to swallow, which causes saliva to accumulate. It may be severe and difficult to treat, although it can disappear over time. Constipation occurs in about 30 percent of patients and can be quite bothersome.

The greatest concern with clozapine is the risk of developing severe, life-threatening (although reversible) agranulocytosis, with an incidence of about 1 to 2 percent (Tschen et al., 1999). White blood cell counts and absolute neutrophil counts must be monitored weekly for the first 6 months of therapy, then every 2 weeks for the next 6 months, then monthly thereafter, with more frequent monitoring if the white blood cell count decreases. Other drugs that can reduce white blood cell count (most notably carbamazepine; see Chapter 14) should not be taken concomitantly. The etiology of clozapine-induced agranulocytosis appears to involve an unusual cellular-toxic mechanism. Eutrecht (1992) demonstrated that clozapine could be metabolized not only in the liver but also by the white blood cells themselves (an extremely unusual situation). An intermediate compound in this metabolic process is reactive and toxic to the cell, possibly destroying the white cells that produced the metabolite.

Clozapine is also associated with the risk for metabolic syndrome that includes abnormalities of blood pressure, lipids, glucose utilization, and Body Mass Index (BMI). These abnormalities contribute to an increased risk for cardiovascular disease and therefore require monitoring in those individuals who are prescribed clozapine.

Clozapine is the least prescribed of all the SGAs due to the need for frequent blood tests and its array of potentially serious side effects. However, it is also one of the most effective antipsychotic medications, especially for those individuals who have not responded to one or more trials of other FGA or SGA drugs. There is increasing interest in supporting the use of clozapine earlier rather than later in the course of treatment. Due to restrictions clozapine cannot be used as a first-line agent, but some clinicians argue that it should not be the treatment of 'last resort' either (Remington et al., 2013). Clozapine has been shown particularly effective in reducing mortality as noted above, specifically reducing both aggressive behavior and suicide risk (Citrome, 2009; Meltzer, 2012). It may also be beneficial in reducing smoking and use of other drugs of abuse in schizophrenic patients who have those comorbidities.

Risperidone

Risperidone (Risperdal), shown in Figure 11.3, the second atypical antipsychotic drug, was introduced in 1994. It is a potent antagonist at both D_2 and $5\text{-}HT_2$ receptors, resulting in improved control of psychotic symptoms with a minimum of neuroleptic-induced EPS at low doses, less than 6 milligrams per day. However, the incidence of parkinsonism and other effects of dopaminergic blockade (such as prolactin release) increases at higher doses. In 2008, the FDA approved the first generic versions of risperidone tablets, again lowering the cost.

Risperidone is indicated for the treatment of schizophrenia, bipolar disorder, and irritability in individuals with autism.

Pharmacokinetics. Risperidone is well absorbed when taken orally, is highly bound to plasma proteins, and is metabolized to an active intermediate, 9-hydroxy-risperidone. A long-acting injectable form of *risperidone* (Risperdal Consta) is available. Using novel technology, the drug in this formulation is encapsulated in biodegradable polymer microspheres suspended in a water-based solution. A single intramuscular injection can last up to 2 weeks (Fleishhacker et al., 2003; Kane et al., 2003).

In 2009, Risperdal Consta (risperidone) long-acting injection was approved for a new indication, as either a monotherapy or as adjunctive therapy to lithium or valproate in the maintenance treatment of bipolar I disorder. One clinical trial showed that, over the course of 2 years, it was better than placebo, or monotherapy, at delaying time to relapse for any mood episode (depression, mania, hypomania, or mixed). A second study showed that over the course of 52 weeks, for patients already on lithium or valproate, it delayed the time to relapse compared with a combination of current treatment plus placebo.

The metabolic half-life of risperidone is about 3 hours; that of the metabolite, which accounts for much of risperidone's action, is about 23 hours. In fact, recognition of this characteristic led to the approval in 2006 of the active metabolite 9-hydroxy-risperidone (paliperidone), under the trade name Invega (see Figure 11.3). This metabolite is a once-daily oral medication, available in 3-, 6-, or 9-milligram doses, that delivers the drug through the OROS[2] extended-release formulation, with a recommended dose of

---

[2] OROS is a trademarked delivery system. It is a capsule-shaped tablet consisting of a multilayer core surrounded by a semipermeable membrane that allows slow release of the drug from the tablet. Concerta (methylphenidate; see Chapter 15) is formulated in this **OROS** formulation.

6 milligrams and a range of 3 to 12 milligrams. Invega is not metabolized in the liver, so patients with liver failure can take it. Nussbaum and Stroup (2008) analyzed five studies comparing paliperidone with placebo, olanzapine, or Risperidal. Paliperidone was more effective than placebo, with a side effect profile similar to that of risperidone. But unlike risperidone, paliperidone cannot be crushed and administered in food.

An injectable, long-lasting form (1 month) of paliperidone was recently compared with placebo for maintenance. The average time to first recurrence on placebo was 163 days (after being stable on a fixed dose of medication for 12 weeks). So few paliperidone patients had relapsed that the corresponding number could not be calculated. In mid-2009, the FDA approved Invega Sustenna (*paliperidone palmitate*), an extended-release injectable suspension, for the acute and maintenance treatment of schizophrenia in adults. It is the first once-monthly, long-acting, injectable atypical antipsychotic approved in the United States for this use (Sedky et al., 2010). Unfortunately, its expense may limit its use. In fact more recent studies have not shown any outcome benefit for Invega Sustenna compared to oral medications and therefore its potential benefits would not outweigh the costs (Rosenheck et al., 2011; Barnett et al., 2012).

Risperidone is also supplied as a rapidly dissolving tablet (Risperidal M-Tab).

Pharmacodynamics. Risperidone is as effective as haloperidol in reducing the positive symptomatology of schizophrenia at doses that do not produce a high incidence of EPS. Although this drug might not be quite as effective as clozapine, its safety profile can make it a first-line agent for treating schizophrenia.

Side Effects. Common side effects of risperidone include somnolence, agitation, anxiety, insomnia, headache, elevation of prolactin levels, EPS at higher doses, and nausea. Weight gain is about 50 percent of that seen with either clozapine or olanzapine. Extrapyramidal symptoms are minimal at low doses (6 milligrams or less), although even low doses may elicit EPS in newly diagnosed patients with no previous exposure to antipsychotic drugs (Rosebush and Mazurek, 1999). Risperidone is considered to be safe in breast-fed infants; infant levels are only about 4 percent of the mother's (Ilett et al., 2004).

In 2004 the manufacturer reported an increased incidence of strokes and CNS ischemic attacks in elderly patients taking risperidone (see Chapter 16 for a more complete discussion).

Olanzapine

Introduced in 1996, *olanzapine* (Zyprexa) (see Figure 11.3) structurally and pharmacologically resembles clozapine, without clozapine's toxicity on white blood cells. It is indicated for the treatment of schizophrenia, bipolar disorder acute mixed or manic states, bipolar disorder maintenance, and agitation associated with schizophrenia or bipolar disorder.

Pharmacokinetics. Olanzapine is well absorbed orally. Peak plasma levels occur in about 5 to 8 hours. Metabolized in the liver, olanzapine has an elimination half-life in the range of 27 to 38 hours in both adults and children (Grothe et al., 2000). Gardiner and coworkers (2003) and Ambresin and coworkers (2004) studied olanzapine levels in infants of breast-feeding mothers who were taking the drug. They reported that infants received doses of only about 1 to 4 percent of that given to the mother, resulting in plasma levels of about 38 percent of those in the mother with no adverse effects.

Pharmacodynamics. Olanzapine is at least comparable to haloperidol in efficacy (Rosenheck et al., 2003), with minimal EPS, although it is more expensive and produces much more weight gain. There is a complete block of 5-HT$_2$ receptors at low doses (5 milligrams/day), with increasing D$_2$ blockade as doses increase from 5 to 20 milligrams/day. Olanzapine has not been reported to cause agranulocytosis, which eliminates the need for white blood cell counts and may improve adherence. Olanzapine is also provided in an orally disintegrating tablet (Zydis) that is designed to rapidly dissolve on the tongue, which aids those who have trouble swallowing pills and reduces opportunities for 'cheeking' medications.

Zyprexa IntraMuscular was as or more effective than either lorazepam or haloperidol in treating aggressive and agitated behaviors, usually in an emergency room scenario. In December 2009, a long-acting depot formulation of olanzapine was approved by the FDA, which had rejected it the previous year. Called Zyprexa Relprevv, it is given IM every 2 to 4 weeks, depending on the dose approved for treatment of schizophrenia in adults. Previous concerns were raised about a side effect called post-injection delirium/sedation syndrome (PDSS), which occurs in about 2 percent of patients. Patients have fallen asleep in public places or walked into walls. Labeling now includes a requirement that patients stay under observation at a health care facility for at least 3 hours after each injection and have an escort when leaving the facility. Dispensers must also register in a patient care education program to learn about the risks.

Sertindole

Sertindole (Serlect) was released in 1997 as the fourth atypical antipsychotic. It is primarily a 5-HT$_2$-receptor antagonist with lesser blockade of D$_2$ receptors. It therefore provides the requisite dual action of blocking 5-HT$_2$ and D$_2$ receptors thought to define SGAs. This dual action predicted therapeutic efficacy in treating schizophrenia, with a low incidence of EPS. Unlike risperidone and clozapine, sertindole has no affinity for histamine receptors and therefore is less sedative.

The drug can adversely affect the heart, an action that can lead to severe cardiac arrhythmias. For this reason, sertindole was removed from the market in 1998. Although clinical trials are ongoing, sertindole has not been approved by the FDA for a return to the U.S. market.

Quetiapine

Quetiapine (Seroquel) (see Figure 11.3) is the fifth SGA with 5-HT$_2$/D$_2$ receptor-blocking action (Arvanitis and Miller, 1997). It is comparable to haloperidol in reducing positive symptoms, with little EPS. Quetiapine is currently approved for the acute and maintenance treatment of schizophrenia, bipolar disorder (manic phase), and as an adjunctive treatment for major depressive disorder and bipolar disorder maintenance. The initial formulation has a relatively short biological half-life (about 6 hours);

a long-acting version, quetiapine XR, was approved in June 2007 in 200-, 300-, and 400-milligram doses. In December 2008, tentative approval was given to market the generic tablet version. Consequently, efforts are under way to show that the drug is useful for a number of other disorders (Adityanjee, 2002). Seroquel is used a great deal to treat adolescent mania (see Chapter 15). Unfortunately, its potent sedative/anxiolytic action has led to abuse, especially in prisons, where it is used to promote sleep and reduce anxiety and drug cravings. However, this sedative property contributes to its off-label use as a sleep aide in individuals with a variety of mental disorders. Although rare, one side effect of this drug is a prolongation of the QTc interval that can in the extreme lead to a fatal cardiac arrthymia. Therefore, it should not be combined with other drugs that can also prolong the QTc interval or it should be used cautiously or not at all in individuals with pre-existing cardiac rhythm disturbances.

Ziprasidone

Ziprasidone (Geodon) (see Figure 11.3), approved in 2001, shows efficacy for treating schizophrenia with low liability for causing EPS (Goodnik, 2001; Arato et al., 2002; Gunasekara et al., 2002). It is also approved for the treatment of bipolar disorder, acute manic or mixed episodes, or as an adjunctive treatment of bipolar disorder combined with either lithium or valproic acid. Its half-life appears to be short, in the range of 6 hours. Perhaps its major clinical advantage is that it causes negligible weight gain. Ziprasidone has some unique receptor actions. In addition to blocking 5-HT$_2$ and D$_2$ receptors, it is a partial agonist at 5-HT$_{1A}$ receptors and a moderate inhibitor of serotonin and norepinephrine uptake. These receptor actions confer antidepressant and anxiolytic effects to the drug. It reduced both depressive and psychotic symptoms in people with schizoaffective disorder (Keck et al., 2001; Swainston and Scott, 2006). It has not demonstrated clear efficacy in the treatment of unipolar or bipolar depression although sufficient carefully controlled trials have not been completed (Andrade, 2013). Ziprasidone was the first SGA to be approved for intramuscular use. An injectable formulation was approved in 2003 for rapid control of agitated behavior and psychotic symptoms. The limiting factor to the wide use of ziprasidone is its effect on the heart. The drug prolongs the QT interval, causing concern, but as yet no fatal reactions have occurred. However, QT prolongation may be a more serious problem in children and adolescents (Blair et al., 2005) or those with pre-existing rhythm disturbances.

Aripiprazole

Aripiprazole (Abilify), shown in Figure 11.3, was approved in 2002 as perhaps the first of a new "third generation" antipsychotic (Potkin et al., 2003) because it has a different mechanism of action from those of the FGAs and SGAs. Aripiprazole is a partial agonist at D$_2$ and 5-HT$_{1A}$ receptors as well as an antagonist at 5-HT$_2$ receptors (Jordan et al., 2002). This "dopaminergic partial agonism" is meant to "stabilize" the system because, although the drug binds with high affinity to D$_2$ receptors, it has lower intrinsic activity (less efficacy). This means that under conditions of high dopamine levels, aripiprazole may replace dopamine at the receptor, but it will not produce as strong an effect as the natural transmitter. Conversely, when dopamine concentration is low, aripiprazole can produce a net increase in dopaminergic action (Stahl, 2002; Tamminga and Carlsson, 2002; Lieberman, 2004). Partial agonism at 5-HT_{1A} receptors confers anxiolytic or antidepressant actions, and this drug has been reported to augment the effect of SSRIs in patients with depression and anxiety disorders who were partial responders to the antidepressants (Schwartz et al., 2007). In 2007, the FDA approved aripiprazole as an adjunctive, or add-on, treatment to antidepressant therapy in adults with major depressive disorder. This was the first medication approved by the FDA as an add-on treatment for major depressive disorder. In addition, Abilify was approved in 2008 as an adjunct in patients whose manic episodes have not responded to lithium or valproate. This approval was based on a trial in 384 patients, with most receiving 15 milligrams during a 6-week period. The reduction in the Young Mania Rating Scale scores for aripiprazole was -13.3 versus -10.7 for placebo, with 19 percent of aripiprazole patients reporting akathisia (Vieta et al., 2008).

In late November 2009, the FDA approved an expanded indication for aripiprazole for the treatment of irritability associated with autism spectrum disorder in children aged 6 to 17 years. Oral aripiprazole had previously been approved for acute and maintenance treatment (with or without lithium or valproate) of manic and mixed episodes of bipolar disorder in patients aged 10 years and older as well as for acute and maintenance treatment of schizophrenia in patients aged 13 years and older (see Chapter 15).

To date, aripiprazole appears to be as effective as conventional and other second-generation agents. It does not cause QT prolongation or prolactin elevation, and it is not associated with weight gain or other glucose or lipid abnormalities. However, although rare, some cases of neuroleptic malignant syndrome have been reported after treatment with this drug, and some evidence for the development of movement disorders, like akathisia, has been noted.

Aripiprazole is provided in tablets, IM acute injection, oral solution, and a rapidly dissolving tablet (DiscMelt). In February 2013, the FDA approved a new extended release injectable formulation of *aripiprazole* (Abilify Maintena) that allows for once a month IM injections of the drug.

Iloperidone

In 2009 the FDA approved *iloperidone* (Fanapt), shown in Figure 11.3, for the acute treatment of schizophrenia in adults. Two placebo and active control short-term trials (of 4 weeks and 6 weeks) showed efficacy, and safety data have been obtained from more than 2000 patients. Final doses are usually 12 to 24 mg/day, and titration to 12 mg should be gradually achieved over 4 days, because of the potent alpha antagonism. Like older SGAs, iloperidone is a $D_2/5\text{-HT}_{2A}$ antagonist. It also has high affinity for the D_3 receptor. It is a 5-HT_{2C} and 5-HT_6 antagonist as well as a partial agonist at 5-HT_{1A} receptors (suggesting antidepressant benefit; see Chapter 12), with relatively high alpha-1 blockade, which produces orthostatic hypotension. This risk requires gradual titration initially producing a delay in onset of clinical effectiveness compared to other SGAs without strong alpha-1 blockade. But low histamine blockade produces less sedation and weight gain, and little muscarinic antagonism indicates low anticholinergic side effects. This drug has had a long history of development, and early trials did not always show an impressive degree of efficacy relative to the comparator drug. It produced dose-dependent increases in QT interval, mild weight gain similar to risperidone, with mild glucose elevation. However, it elicited less akathisia than other compounds. For a clinical review of iloperidone, see Weiden (2012).

Iloperidone is indicated for the treatment of schizophrenia and is provided as oral tablets.

Asenapine

Asenapine (Saphris), shown in Figure 11.3, was approved in 2009 for the treatment of schizophrenia (5 mg, two times a day) and manic or mixed episodes of bipolar disorder (10 mg, two times a day). It received an additional indication in 2010 for the acute treatment of bipolar disorder manic or mixed episodes as an adjunct to either lithium or valproic acid. Asenapine has a chemical structure related to the antidepressant mirtazepine. It is unique in that it must be dissolved under the tongue, with no eating or drinking for 10 minutes afterward; otherwise, it will not be adequately absorbed into the bloodstream. Bioavailability is less than 2 percent orally but 35 percent sublingually. It binds to more receptors than most other antipsychotics, with strong antagonism of D_1 through D_4, 5-HT_{2A} and 5-HT_{2C}, 5-HT_{1A}, alpha-1 and H_1 receptors (Lincoln and Preskorn, 2009). A six-week comparison of asenapine with risperidone and placebo in 174 schizophrenic patients, in which patients who had failed other drug treatments were excluded, showed that both drugs separated from placebo. A three-week trial that assigned 488 patients with acute mania to Saphris, Zyprexa, or placebo reported adverse events in 60.8 percent of the Saphris treated patients, 52 percent of the Zyprexa treated patients, and 36.2 percent of those who received placebo. Additional studies have shown asenapine to be equivalent to other SGAs with fewer risks for EPS (other than akathisia), dyslipidemia, or cardiotoxicity in the treatment of schizophrenia or bipolar disorder (McIntyre and Wong, 2012; Stoner and Pace, 2012; Fagiolini et al., 2013). For a review of asenapine's efficacy in the acute and maintenance treatment of schizophrenia, see Cortese, et al. (2013). The most prominent side effects included weight gain, sleepiness, akathisia, dizziness, oral numbness, and, in some patients, a chalky taste sensation. A long-term extension study (26 weeks, after 26 weeks of "acute" treatment) showed a favorable comparison with olanzapine. However, treatment-emergent adverse events were 85.1 percent for asenapine and 74.1 percent for olanzapine. In September 2011, the FDA issued a warning about asenapine's risk of producing severe allergic reactions in sensitive individuals, even after a single dose.

Lurasidone

Lurasidone (Latuda), shown in Figure 11.3, was approved for the treatment of schizophrenia by the FDA in 2010. Data have been obtained from 40 clinical studies and approximately 2,500 patients. Lurasidone is also in late-stage clinical testing for the treatment of bipolar mania as monotherapy and adjunctive treatment of bipolar depression. It is a potent antagonist of 5-HT_{2A}, D_2, 5-HT_7, and 5-HT_{1A} receptors, with little affinity for most other receptors. Its efficacy was demonstrated in four controlled trials showing it superior to placebo or not inferior to olanzapine; most common side effects were akathisia, sedation, nausea, parkinsonism, and agitation. It is considered weight neutral and does not have any significant effects on lipid or glucose metabolism. It may cause increased prolactin levels in females, but has no significant effect on QTc intervals (Citrome, 2011; Lincoln and Tripathi, 2011; Citrome, 2012). Steady state is reached within 7 days. It is metabolized primarily by the CYP 3A4 enzyme family in the liver. The dose range is 40 mg/day or 80 mg/day administered once daily with food. Some authors have suggested that lurasidone may improve cognitive status based on animal studies, but there is no evidence that it produces any cognitive enhancement in patients (Sewell, 2011).

Prominent Side Effects of Second-Generation Antipsychotics

Although the use of SGAs is generally associated with fewer parkinsonian-like symptoms than the use of FGAs, the SGAs are not without side effects, the most prominent of which are weight gain, a propensity to produce glucose intolerance (diabetes) along with elevation in blood lipids, and specific cardiac electrographic abnormalities that can be serious and even fatal. Collectively, these side effects have been termed the *metabolic syndrome*.

Weight Gain

As a group, SGAs have a propensity to induce weight gain, with clozapine and olanzapine inducing the most, ziprasidone, aripiprazole, and lurasidone the least (Allison and Casey, 2001; Citrome, 2012) (Figure 11.4). Weight gain occurs in 20 to 30 percent of people taking risperidone, olanzapine, and quetiapine, although the gain with risperidone is about half that brought on by the other two drugs. Weight gain in adolescents may be even greater than in adults (Ratzoni et al., 2002; Correll, 2007). This side effect may contribute to patient nonadherence with treatment and may adversely affect clinical outcome (Poyurovsky et al., 2003). Weight gain may also be related to an individual's BMI at the time the drug was first prescribed. Studies suggest that those individuals with higher BMI's tend to lose weight on SGAs while those with normal or low BMI's tend to gain weight (Bushe et al., 2013).

The mechanism responsible for this weight gain is still being elucidated (Newcomer, 2005); however, data suggest that this phenomenon is associated with the antihistaminergic aspects of the second-generation antipsychotics. Snyder and colleagues (discussed by Hampton, 2007) found a relationship between the SGAs that are most associated with this side effect and the stimulation of a hypothalamic AMP-activated protein kinase (AMPK). This enzyme, AMPK, is important for maintaining energy balance and has been linked to the regulation of food intake. The investigators found that histaminergic antagonism stimulated AMPK, and histamine decreased this stimulation. In mice given clozapine, AMPK activity quadrupled. This discovery may lead to the development of antipsychotics that retain their therapeutic benefit but do not produce weight gain and other metabolic problems.

Did You Know?

There May be a Way to Determine Which Patients Will Gain Weight When Taking Antipsychotic Medications.

It is well known that one of the side effects of many antipsychotic medications is weight gain, which can be substantial. But clinicians do not currently have any reliable method of predicting in advance, who would be susceptible to this common side effect. If clinicians had such a predictor, then they could tailor their drug selection to agents that are least likely to produce weight gain and they could also counsel patients on proper nutrition, exercise, and weight loss strategies. Recently, researchers studied a group of individuals who had never taken antipsychotic medication previously and followed them closely for 12 weeks to make sure they took their medication as prescribed and to monitor their metabolic status. They also carried out genetic studies to identify any gene variants that might be related to those individuals within the group who gained significant weight. Their results identified markers in a gene called the melanocortin 4 receptor (MC4R) that were associated with severe weight gain in people taking second-generation antipsychotics. The MC4R region overlaps somewhat with another region previously identified as being associated with obesity in the general population. In addition, the results were replicated in three independent cohorts. Although particular gene variants were implicated, the study's sample size was small. Further research with larger samples is needed to extend the findings.

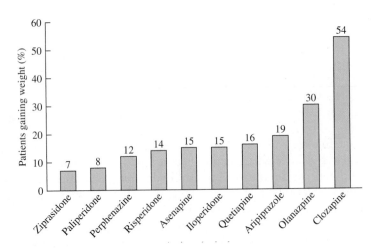

FIGURE 11.4 Percentage of patients who gained 7 percent or more of their baseline body weight while being treated with the indicated antipsychotic drugs. The 7 percent threshold is the accepted measure for determining a significant effect. [Data from Ellinger et al., (2010), 44:668-679.]

Diabetes and Hyperglycemia

Patients who receive certain atypical antipsychotics are 9 to 14 percent more likely to develop adult-onset (type 2) diabetes than patients who receive traditional first-generation antipsychotic drugs (Sernyak et al., 2002; Lindenmayer et al., 2003; Newcomer, 2005). Increases in diabetes rates are seen in patients over 40 years of age who were taking clozapine, olanzapine, and quetiapine, but not risperidone (Gianfrancesco et al., 2003). There is little evidence to suggest that the four newest SGAs (paliperidone, iloperidone, asenapine, and lurasidone) have a significant impact on glucose metabolism at this time. In patients under the age of 40, all agents have been found to increase the incidence of diabetes. These changes are independent of the weight gain induced by these drugs and seem to reflect a more rapid onset of diabetes. The American Diabetes Association and American Psychiatric Association have published suggested monitoring schedules for insulin resistance, recommending that blood levels be taken at 6 months and 1 year and then every 5 years thereafter. The long-term consequences of small elevations in blood glucose are unknown at this time but may include increased risk of cardiovascular disease (Wirshing et al., 2002). In one meta-analytic review, it was determined that the antidiabetic drug metformin significantly reduced body weight in nondiabetic patients who had gained weight on their antipsychotic medications. But there was a great deal of variability among the studies, and metformin is not approved for this indication (Björkhem-Bergman et al., 2010). Metformin is not universally helpful in weight reduction and should not be used as a preventative agent. Lifestyle changes, diet, and exercise are better approaches to weight management and metabolic control (Hasnain et al., 2011).

Electrocardiographic Abnormalities (Sudden Cardiac Death)

The "pacemaker" of the heart is the sinoatrial node, located in the right atrium of the heart. An electrical signal from the pacemaker flows over the atria and into the ventricles through the atrioventricular node. The ventricles then contract, propelling blood forward into the aorta and the arteries. Following depolarization and mechanical contraction, the ventricles repolarize to be ready for the next depolarization. Figure 11.5 illustrates the electrocardiogram (ECG) for one electrical cycle. The QT interval is the time from the start of spread of electricity to the ventricles to the end of ventricular repolarization. In essence, if this period is prolonged to about 500 milliseconds (0.5 second), the patient is at significant risk of developing the arrhythmia *torsades de pointes* (Figure 11.6), which can result in sudden death. The normal range for the QT interval for men below the age of 55 years is 350 to 430 milliseconds; for women, it is 350 to 450 milliseconds. Concern should arise when the QT interval is between 450 and 500 milliseconds; that is, the risk increases with a prolongation of 20 milliseconds or more. Besides drug-induced QT interval prolongation, *torsades de pointes* arrhythmias may at least partly be involved in sudden death in athletes and in infants (SIDS).

Many psychotropic medications, including neuroleptics, antidepressants, stimulants, and anxiolytics, may cause *torsades de pointes* (Glassman and Bigger, 2001; Khatib et al., 2003; Witchel et al., 2003). Even nonpsychotropic drugs have caused this side effect. Some drugs, such as the antihistamine Seldane and the gastric stimulant Propulsid, have been removed from the market for this reason. Among the FGAs, thioridazine is

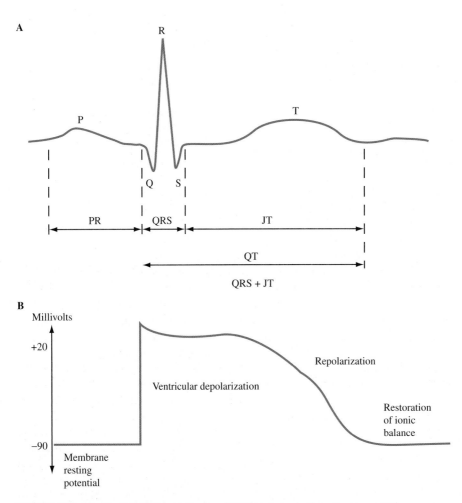

FIGURE 11.5 **A.** Normal electrocardiogram (ECG) in sinus rhythm. P wave - atrial electrical depolarization and leads to muscular contraction of the right and left ventricles. QRS complex - ventricular electrical depolarization and leads to muscular contraction of the right and left ventricles. JT - the time from the end of ventricular depolarization (QRS) to the end of ventricular repolarization. The QT interval includes both ventricular depolarization (QRS) and ventricular repolarization. **B.** Rapid ventricular depolarization and slower repolarization. Most of the QT interval represents ventricular repolarization.

most associated with this side effect and is rarely prescribed. Among the SGAs, this was one reason sertindole was removed from the market. In 2009 an FDA review found that patients taking sertindole had a significantly higher risk of sudden cardiac death (SCD) compared with those taking risperidone (13 versus 3). Approval of ziprasidone was delayed until additional safety data could be examined: it prolongs the interval by about 10 or 15 milliseconds. In a large retrospective cohort of adults, current users of the atypicals had a dose-dependent increase in the risk of sudden cardiac death that was

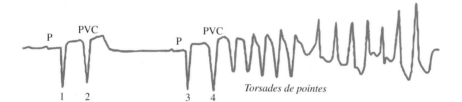

Torsades de pointes

FIGURE 11.6 Characteristic development of *torsades de pointes* ventricular arrhythmia. Sinus beat with normal ventricular complex (1) followed by a premature ventricular contraction (PVC; 2) closely coupled to the sinus beat. After a long pause (2–3), this paired complex is repeated (3–4). The second PVC initiates a bizarre ventricular arrhythmia consistent with *torsades de pointes*. This ventricular arrhythmia is accompanied by poor contraction of ventricular muscle and therefore loss of contractility and output of blood from the heart, leading to a cardiac arrest.

essentially identical to that among users of the typical agents. With regard to this side effect, the SGAs are no safer than the older drugs (Karlsson et al., 2009; Ray et al., 2009).

New Agents and Updated Recommendations for the Treatment of Schizophrenia

Cariprazine is a drug in clinical testing for schizophrenia, acute bipolar mania, bipolar depression, and treatment-resistant depression. It "prefers" D_3 over D_2, with both effects being partial agonism rather than antagonism. This selectivity would theoretically predict higher doses for mania and schizophrenia, for greater antagonist action, and lower doses for depression, for greater agonistic effect. Little weight gain or other metabolic problems have been reported so far. This agent has two long-acting active metabolites, which might offer the option of weekly to monthly depot administration. Four phase II and III studies have been completed examining the acute treatment of schizophrenia showing efficacy and a longer-term study examining the efficacy for prevention of relapse is ongoing. Cariprazine does not appear to adversely impact metabolic variables, prolactin, or the electrocardiogram (ECG) QT interval (Citrome, 2013b). Similar efficacy for the treatment of bipolar disorder is being found in manufacturer sponsored clinical trials (Citrome, 2013a).

GABAergic agents are currently in clinical trials. One such drug, BL-1020 is a dopamine/serotonin blocking agent combined with $GABA_A$ receptor agonist activity with antihistaminic properties. In clinical trials it has shown some efficacy in the treatment of schizophrenia and it is hypothesized to produce little EPS and based on the GABA agonist activity, to either prevent cognitive side effects or improve cognition in those treated with other agents (Geffen et al., 2012).

Blonanserine (Lonasen) has been used in Japan and Korea and is in clinical trials here in the United States. It is a SGA with the usual dopamine/serotonin antagonist profile with some D_3 and alpha-receptor blocking activity. It has no muscarinic or histamine-blocking effects. It is said to have the highest D_2 receptor occupancy and lowest 5-HT receptor blocking potential of all SGAs (Kishi et al., 2013).

The schizophrenia Patient Outcomes Research Team (PORT) recommendation summary has been updated. The review groups identified 41 treatment areas for review and conducted literature searches to identify all clinical studies published since the last review in 2002. Studies in areas not covered in 2002 were also reviewed. A total of 16 psychopharmacologic and 8 psychosocial treatments were recommended; another 13 psychopharmacologic and 4 psychosocial treatments had insufficient evidence for a recommendation (Buchanan et al., 2010; Kreyenbuhl et al., 2010).

Additional Applications for Second-Generation Antipsychotics

The use of SGAs in nonpsychotic disorders has rapidly increased in the last few years Table 11.3 [Trémeau and Citrome, 2006] and Table 11.4 [Maher and Theodore, 2012]). With the exception of bipolar disorder, most of these applications have been "off-label," that is, they have not received FDA approval (Crystal et al., 2009). Although the FGAs were also known to be efficacious in some of these disorders, the improved neurological profile of the new agents and the inadequate response of many patients to the approved FGA medications for their respective illnesses have expanded the use of SGAs. While most information has been obtained from studies of risperidone and olanzapine, there are numerous case reports and open-label studies describing benefits of all the SGAs in a variety of conditions. At present, it should be kept in mind that most of the available evidence comes from evaluations of SGAs as adjuncts to other psychotropics, that few direct comparisons between FGAs and SGAs have been published, and that there is not yet a great deal of information on the long-term safety of the newer agents. Current reports suggest that FDA-required warnings about risks concerning the use of atypical antipsychotics are not receiving sufficient attention (Kuehn, 2010).

As we will now see, atypical antipsychotic drugs are being used both on-label and off-label for multiple disorders, such as bipolar disorder, resistant depression, dysthymia, as well as behavioral problems associated with dementia, autism spectrum disorders, severe resistant anxiety disorders, and borderline personality disorder. These drugs are also being used to aid in controlling anger, aggression, and tantrums in various behavioral dyscontrol disorders. In these treatments the term "antipsychotic" seems inappropriate. Therefore, we introduce the term *thymic stabilizer* to encompass a variety of uses—comparable to use of the terms *mood stabilizer* or *neuromodulator* to refer to antiepileptic drugs used in nonepileptic disorders.

Bipolar Disorder

Except for clozapine, paliperidone, and iloperidone, all the newer antipsychotics are approved by the FDA for treatment of some aspect of bipolar disorder. Olanzapine (in 2000), risperidone (in 2004), quetiapine (in 2004), ziprasidone (in 2004; Keck et al., 2003b), aripiprazole (in 2004; Keck et al., 2003a), and asenapine (2009) are approved for monotherapy of acute bipolar mania and (with the exception of quetiapine) for mixed episodes. Olanzapine, risperidone, quetiapine, and asenapine (2010) are also approved as add-ons for treating bipolar mania in patients with a poor response to monotherapy.

TABLE 11.3 Nonpsychotic indications in adults for second-generation antipsychotic agents

SGA[a]	Bipolar mania	Bipolar depression	Bipolar maintenance	Other
Aripiprazole	Acute mania or mixed episodes	Bipolar I disorder, most recent episode manic or mixed	Maintenance therapy	Resistant depression, irritability in autism
Asenapine	Acute mania or mixed episodes			
Clozapine				Risk of recurrent suicidal behavior in schizophrenia or schizoaffective disorders
Olanzapine	Acute mania or mixed episodes; monotherapy or with lithium or valproate for manic episodes		Bipolar disorder maintenance monotherapy	
Olanzapine/fluoxetine combination		Bipolar depressive episodes		Resistant depression
Quetiapine	Acute manic episodes; monotherapy or with lithium or valproate	Bipolar depressive episodes	Maintenance therapy	Resistant depression (XR formulation)
Risperidone	Acute mania or mixed episodes; monotherapy or with lithium or valproate			Irritability in autism
Ziprasidone	Acute mania or mixed episodes		Maintenance therapy	

[a]SGA - second-generation antipsychotic (oral form)

Safety issues. SGAs' safety profiles warrant caution. SGAs are less likely than first-generation antipsychotics (FGAs) to cause extrapyramidal symptoms (EPS) and tardive dyskinesia (TD) at therapeutic dosages, but they increase the risks of weight gain, diabetes, glucose intolerance, dyslipidemia, and hyperprolactinemia. Akathisia and hypotension also may occur.

Prescribing decisions. SGAs' potential adverse effects complicate clinical decision making. First it must be decided whether to use an SGA for the patient with a nonpsychotic disorder.

Adapted from Trémeau and Citrome (2006), p. 39.

TABLE 11.4 Efficacy of atypical antipsychotics by condition and strength of evidence.

	Aripiprazole	Olanzapine	Quetiapine	Risperidone	Ziprasidone
Anxiety					
Generalized anxiety disorder	o	−	++	−	−
Social phobia	o	+	−	o	o
Attention-deficit hyperactivity disorder					
No co-occurring disorders	o	o	o	+	o
				o	o
Bipolar children	−	o	o		
Mentally retarded children	o	o	o	+	o
Dementia					
Overall	++	+	+	++	o
Psychosis	+	+−	+−	++	o
Agitation	+	++	+−	++	o
Depression					
MDD augmentation of SSRI/SNRI	++[a]	+[a]	++[a]	++	+
MDD monotherapy	o	−	++	o	o
Eating disorders	o	−−	−	o	o
Insomnia	o	o	−	o	o
Obsessive-compulsive disorder					
Augmentation of SSRI	o	+	−−	++	−
Augmentation of citalopram	o	o	+	+	o
Personality disorder					
Borderline	+	+−	+	o	−
Schizotypal	o	o	o	+−	o
Post-traumatic stress disorder	o	+−	+	++	o
Substance abuse					
Alcohol	−−	−	−	o	o
Cocaine	o	−	o	−	o
Methamphetamine	−	o	o	o	o
Methadone clients	o	o	o	−	o
Tourette's syndrome	o	o	o	+	−

Symbol legend: For strength of evidence; ++ = moderate or high evidence of efficacy; + = low or very low evidence of efficacy; +− = mixed results; − = low or very low evidence of inefficacy; −− = moderate or high evidence of inefficacy; o = no trials.
Source: Maglione M, Ruelaz Maher A, Hu J, et al. Off-label use of atypical antipsychotics: an update. AHRQ comparative effectiveness review no. 43 September 2011.
[a]FDA approval for this indication.
FDA = U.S. Food and Drug Administration; MDD = major depressive disorder; SNRI = serotonin norepinephrine reuptake inhibitor; SSRI = selective serotonin reuptake inhibitor.
From Maher, A.R. and Theodore, G. "Summary of the Comparative Effectiveness Review on Off-Label Use of Atypical Antipsychotics" *Journal of Managed Care Pharmacy Supplement* June 2012, Vol. 18, No. 5B p. S7. Reprinted by permission of Rockwater, Inc. and Academy of Managed Care Pharmacy.

A combination product containing *olanzapine* and *fluoxetine* (Symbyax) was approved in 2003 for treating acute bipolar depression. However, in August 2009, the label for Symbyax was updated, and in October of the same year, labels were revised for olanzapine to warn of the possible development of leukopenia/neutropenia and agranulocytosis, that is, low white blood cells or neutrophils; in 2010 warnings were added for risk of hypoglycemia, dyslipidemia, weight gain, and increases in prolactin levels; and in 2013, warnings were added for combining Symbyax with MAOIs and risk of serotonin syndrome.

Quetiapine is also approved for treating bipolar depressive episodes. For a review of the use of SGAs in bipolar disorder, see Fountoulakis et al. (2012).

Unipolar Depression

Only about one-third of patients with major depressive disorder (MDD) receiving initial antidepressant treatment achieve remission (see STAR*D study in Chapter 12). Among the many agents used for augmentation, the traditional antipsychotic drugs were known to be effective, but the risk of TD and EPS discouraged their use. The first report of an SGA for augmentation in MDD appeared in 1999, when eight patients with lack of response to selective serotonin reuptake inhibitors (SSRIs) showed rapid improvement with risperidone. This was followed by the first placebo-controlled study of the olanzapine-fluoxetine combination in fluoxetine-resistant depression (Shelton et al., 2005). Currently, the evidence for SGAs is greater than that for any other strategy, and they are becoming widely used for this purpose (Papakostas et al., 2004, 2005; Yargic et al., 2004; Simon and Nemeroff, 2005; Rapaport et al., 2006). As noted, in 2008 aripiprazole was the first atypical agent and first pharmacologic treatment of any type to be approved by the FDA for use as an augmentation agent in MDD. In December of 2009, quetiapine (extended release) was the second SGA approved for this indication.[3] One possible reason for quetiapine's antidepressant effects is the metabolite norquetiapine's potent inhibition of the NE transporter.

Nelson and Papakostas (2009) reviewed this area and reported no significant differences in efficacy among the different atypical agents. Efficacy did not appear to be affected by the duration of the trial or how treatment resistance was determined. However, the discontinuation rate due to adverse events was significantly higher for the atypicals: 9.1 percent compared to 2.3 percent for placebo. While rates of discontinuation did not differ among the SGAs, rates of specific side effects may be very different.

Research to date indicates support for use of quetiapine, risperidone, and aripiprazole as augmenting agents, and quetiapine as monotherapy in major depressive disorder (Maglione et al., 2011; Maher and Theodore, 2012).

Dementia

Although not approved for this indication, antipsychotic drugs are widely used to treat delusions, aggression, and agitation in elderly patients (Jeste et al., 2005; Carson et al., 2006).

---

[3] Perhaps because the immediate-release formulation lost its patent in 2011, the manufacturer of quetiapine applied for approval of the drug as monotherapy for MDD and general anxiety disorder (GAD). The FDA advisory committee concluded that quetiapine was effective as an adjunctive therapy for MDD and monotherapy for MDD and GAD, but there was concern about safety. In the end, the panel voted that quetiapine was not safe to use as *monotherapy* for MDD or GAD. Increases in glucose and lipids were greater for quetiapine.

Because FGAs may cause EPS, lower blood pressure, and increase the risk of falls, the use of SGAs for this population has become more common. The National Institute of Mental Health sponsored the CATIE-AD study to compare olanzapine, risperidone, and quetiapine with placebo in outpatients with symptoms of psychosis, agitation, and aggressiveness. Results showed no significant differences in effectiveness, measured as discontinuation for any cause, among the medications (Schneider et al., 2006). Other data suggest that olanzapine and quetiapine, perhaps because of their anticholinergic potency, may worsen cognition in older patients with dementia (Ballard et al., 2005).

However, an increased risk of stroke was noted in manufacturer-sponsored trials of risperidone and olanzapine (Wang et al., 2005), and in 2005 the FDA released an advisory stating that treatment with SGA medications of behavioral disorders in elderly patients with dementia is associated with a slight increase in mortality. This was extended to FGAs in 2008. Most of the deaths were due to heart-related events or infections (primarily pneumonia). Because the four SGAs that were studied belong to three different chemical classes, the FDA concluded that the effect was probably common across all atypical antipsychotics. The agency announced that it would require a "black box" warning describing this risk on the labels of the drugs and that it would also so designate the olanzapine-fluoxetine combination of Symbyax. To assess the impact of the warning, Dorsey and colleagues (2010) evaluated antipsychotic use in patients 65 and older with dementia, from 2003 to 2008. In the first year after the advisory, atypical antipsychotic prescriptions decreased by 2% overall, and by 19% for patients with dementia.

Autism Spectrum Disorders, Pervasive Developmental Disorder, Agitation, and Aggression

Antipsychotics represent one-third of all filled psychotropic prescriptions for patients with pervasive developmental disorders (PDD). Conventional antipsychotics are known to be effective in treating agitation, hyperactivity, aggression, stereotypic behaviors, tics, and affective lability in PDD (Lott et al., 2004) and autism spectrum disorders (McDougle et al., 1998, 2005; McCracken et al., 2002). Impairments of communication and social interaction are less affected. The undesirable neurologic side effects of FGAs, especially when used on a long-term basis, have shifted the focus toward SGAs. Indeed, in 2007 risperidone received FDA approval for the treatment of irritability associated with autistic behavior in children. The majority of the studies with SGAs in children with PDD have been conducted with risperidone and a few with olanzapine or aripiprazole. In an analysis of these studies, risperidone and to a lesser extent aripiprazole, have shown some benefit for the disruptive behaviors associated with PDD but not for the core behaviors of the disorder itself and these drugs seemed to work best in those patients with the more severe symptoms (Zuddas et al., 2011). Nevertheless, even in short-term studies, as many as 30 percent of children may fail to respond to risperidone, and after 6 months 33 percent of initial responders may fail to maintain their improvement. Concerns have also been raised about the long-term safety of this agent in children, particularly because of the increased release of prolactin. Chronic prolactin elevation may exert variable effects on puberty; may reduce bone mass; and is a risk factor in infertility, breast cancer, heart disease, and prostate abnormalities (Gagliano et al., 2004). Like other SGAs, risperidone, even in low doses, has been associated with weight gain and symptoms of the metabolic syndrome; in higher doses, it has been associated with EPS, tardive dyskinesia, and the neuroleptic malignant syndrome. As with risperidone, olanzapine has improved symptoms associated with PDD in children and adults, but has high risk for weight gain and metabolic disorder. The use of antipsychotics in the management of agitation and aggression in youth has been reviewed and is covered in more detail in Chapter 15, where the use of antipsychotic drugs for aggression is compared with other agents.

Posttraumatic Stress Disorder

There is evidence for the effectiveness of SGAs in treating psychotic symptoms of posttraumatic stress disorder (PTSD). Most of the data come from studies of combat-related PTSD in patients either unresponsive or partially responsive to antidepressants. Clinical case reports support the use of risperidone (Bartzokis et al., 2005), olanzapine (Stein et al., 2002), quetiapine (Adityanjee, 2002), ziprasidone (Siddiqui et al., 2005), and aripiprazole (Lambert, 2006) in war veterans for reducing such symptoms as hyperarousal, reexperiencing, avoidance, nightmares, and flashbacks. Similarly, risperidone monotherapy was found useful for women with a current diagnosis of PTSD as a result of domestic violence or sexual abuse. A mean final risperidone dose of 2.6 milligrams per day significantly reduced avoidant and hyperarousal PTSD symptoms compared with the response of the placebo group, although there were no differences between the two groups on the Hamilton Rating Scales for Anxiety or Depression (Padala et al., 2006). Several small-scale studies have suggested that risperidone in particular may have benefit for reducing reexperiencing symptoms in PTSD, but the results are based on small samples and lack of control for other interventions being received at the same time. A large scale, long-term study conducted by the VA did not find any benefit of risperidone in reducing any of the core symptoms of PTSD (Spaulding, 2012). At present, it is still an open question whether SGAs have any benefit for the core symptoms of PTSD. Certainly, if a patient is not responsive to other pharmacological treatments for PTSD like the use of antidepressants, then a trial of a SGA may be warranted. It has been indicated that symptoms associated with the co-occurring disorders are more responsive to treatment with SGAs than are the primary symptoms of PTSD.

Obsessive-Compulsive Disorder

Risperidone (McDougle et al., 2000), olanzapine (Bystritsky et al., 2004), quetiapine (Atmaca et al., 2002; Mohr et al., 2002; Denys et al., 2004), and aripiprazole (Storch et al., 2008) have been reported to be effective in augmenting the clinical response of patients with obsessive-compulsive disorder who were treatment-refractory to antidepressants. Other anxiety disorders that have been responsive to SGAs, as either monotherapy or add-on, include social anxiety (Barnett et al., 2002), generalized anxiety (Brawman-Mintzer et al., 2005), and panic disorder (Khaldi et al., 2003). Gao and coworkers (2006) reviewed the use of SGAs in the management of anxiety disorders. At present the SSRIs remain the mainstay for the treatment of OCD and there is not enough research to determine if adjunctive SGAs are of routine benefit apart from the earlier studies mentioned here (Fineberg; et al., 2012).

Borderline Personality Disorder

Borderline personality disorder (BPD) affects about 2 percent of the population; about 75 percent of patients with the diagnosis are female. The condition is characterized by brief, intense episodes of impulsiveness, hostility, and anger (including self-injurious behavior), as well as anxiety and depression.

Several reports had shown positive results with SGAs, including risperidone (Rocca et al., 2002), clozapine (Grootens and Verkes, 2005), quetiapine (Villeneuve and Lemelin, 2005), olanzapine (Bogenschutz and Nurnberg, 2004), and aripiprazole (Nickel et al., 2006). However, in two meta-analyses of pharmacotherapy for severe personality disorders, antipsychotics were found to have a very small effect (with aripiprazole being more effective than other antipsychotics; Mercer et al., 2009), whereas mood stabilizers were more efficacious (Mercer et al., 2009; Ingenhoven et al., 2010). Mood stabilizers were also found to be more effective for specific symptoms of BPD than antidepressants in a review by Lieb and colleagues (2010), although these authors concluded that aripiprazole and olanzapine were also beneficial. A Cochrane Library review found some evidence for olanzapine, ziprasidone, and aripiprazole but more data is needed (Stoffers et al., 2010).

Parkinson's Disease

It has long been appreciated that clozapine can reduce psychotic reactions in patients with Parkinson's disease who are receiving dopaminergic agents. Because of clozapine's undesirable side effect profile, quetiapine has become the preferred treatment (Comaty and Advokat, 2001; Reddy et al., 2002). The efficacy of these drugs may be due to their low affinity for the dopamine receptor, which prevents interference with the treatment of Parkinson's disease. This is supported by a report that aripiprazole was not very effective for medication-induced psychosis in "probable" parkinsonian patients (Fernandez et al., 2004).

Experimental Agents and Future Developmental Efforts

To determine whether *omega-3 polyunsaturated fatty acids* (omega-3-PUFA) reduce the rate of progression to first-episode psychotic disorder in adolescents and young adults aged 13 to 25 years with subthreshold psychosis, a randomized, double-blind, placebo-controlled trial was conducted between 2004 and 2007 in the "psychosis detection" unit of a large public hospital in Vienna, Austria. It included 81 patients at high risk of psychotic disorder. A 12-week intervention period of 1.2 grams/day of omega-3-PUFA or placebo was followed by a 40-week monitoring period, for a total study period of 12 months. Of the 81 participants, 76 completed the protocol (93.8%). At the end, 2 of 41 patients in the omega group and 11 of 40 in the placebo group had transitioned to psychotic disorder. Omega-3-PUFA may offer a safe and efficacious preventive strategy for young people with subthreshold psychotic states (Amminger et al., 2010).

The NIMH is launching a large-scale research project to explore whether using early and aggressive treatment, individually targeted and integrating a variety of different therapeutic approaches, will reduce the symptoms and prevent the gradual deterioration of functioning that is characteristic of chronic schizophrenia. The Recovery After an Initial Schizophrenia Episode (RAISE) project is being funded by the NIMH, with additional support from the American Recovery and Reinvestment Act (ARRA). Other early intervention studies have been completed and results to date are considered inconclusive and there are questions about whether any positive effects are sustained over time (Marshall and Rathbone, 2011).

Efforts have been especially directed toward novel pharmacological approaches to treat cognitive deficits and negative symptoms. These efforts have focused on the cholinergic and glutamatergic systems, both of which may be involved in cognitive function. The two cholinergic receptor types are nicotinic and muscarinic. In 2008, a trial of one compound, a partial agonist of the alpha-7 nicotinic receptor subtype named anabaseine (DMXB-A), was conducted in 31 schizophrenic patients. DMXB-A was added to the patients' antipsychotic medications, mostly nonclozapine SGAs. Unfortunately, neither of the two DMXB-A doses differentiated from placebo on the battery of cognitive tests, although there was some evidence for effectiveness against negative symptoms. In the same year, a pilot clinical trial was conducted of the muscarinic agonist xanomeline in 20 schizophrenic patients. The xanomeline group showed significantly greater improvement in symptomatology and in some cognitive measures. But one drawback of this drug is that it also activates M_2, M_3, and M_5 receptors, which produces undesirable side effects. For this reason, the Eli Lilly Company and collaborators at several institutions developed a drug, LY2033298, that is an allosteric modulator of M_4 receptors. That is, it acts on a site that is different from the one at which acetylcholine binds, and it potentiates the action of the neurotransmitter. Preclinical laboratory studies were promising and research is ongoing (Leach et al., 2009). *Atomoxetine* (Strattera), a selective norepinephrine (NE) uptake blocker, was also found to be ineffective for improving cognitive function in schizophrenia (Kelly et al., 2009).

Several observations implicate glutamate in the etiology of schizophrenia, although it is not clear what the most relevant mechanism might be. Antagonists of the ionotropic NMDA receptor, like PCP and ketamine, increase cortical excitability, which suggests that drugs that reduce such *hyperexcitation* might be antipsychotic.

Presynaptic metabotropic glutamate receptors, of the 2/3 subtype, modulate glutamate release. Agonists at this receptor decrease glutamate release, reducing neuronal excitation and possibly the pathological substrate of schizophrenia. In fact, mGlu2/3 receptor agonists block the effects of PCP and ketamine, as well as those of other neurotransmitter stimulants, on some behaviors and are under development as a new category of antipsychotic.

At the same time, PCP itself elicits some characteristic symptoms of schizophrenia. This led to the hypothesis that schizophrenia involves *hypofunction* of the NMDA receptor. The neuromodulator glycine is a required coagonist of the NMDA receptor, and administration of glycine has been shown to produce some modest improvement in schizophrenic patients. This suggests that increasing glycine levels and *enhancing* NMDA function might be therapeutic. For this reason, there is interest in the development of drugs that inhibit the transport system for glycine, specifically, the GlyT1 type, which has a similar distribution in the brain as the NMDA receptor. By blocking the glycine transporter, such drugs would increase NMDA activity and reverse the hypothesized deficit (Conn et al., 2008).

At present, research and development is focusing on agents that affect a wide variety of receptors thought to be involved in the phenotypic symptoms of schizophrenia, if not the underlying disorder. A list of these targets includes: metabotropic glutamate agonists; alpha nicotinic receptor agonists; muscarinic agonists; histamine-3 receptor antagonists; glycine transporter inhibitors; ampakines; phosphodiesterase-10 inhibitors; D_1 agonists; D_3 antagonists; $5-HT_{2A}$ antagonists; and partial dopamine agonists (Kane and Correll, 2010). Research is shifting focus from treatment of positive symptoms which are affected by all antipsychotics to negative symptoms and the cognitive effects of schizophrenia for which we do not currently have effective treatments. This shift in focus is based on the understanding that it is the negative symptoms of schizophrenia and in particular the cognitive impairments associated with the disorder that are responsible for the morbidity and more importantly, the barrier to recovery seen in individuals with schizophrenia (Minzenberg and Carter, 2012).

Finally, based on advances in genetic technology, research is ongoing to identify genotypic targets for schizophrenia. Although some studies have been published that suggest discovery of genetic variations that may be associated with some schizophrenic behaviors, this area of research is still too new to have produced any reliable information that could inform drug development or clinical use.

STUDY QUESTIONS

1. What are the positive and negative symptoms of schizophrenia? Why are these symptoms important in drug therapy?

2. Which neurotransmitters are most involved in the pathogenesis of schizophrenia?

3. What are the primary clinical differences between traditional and atypical antipsychotic drugs?

4. Discuss the mechanisms of action of traditional antipsychotics and atypical antipsychotics.

5. Discuss the side effects of first- and second-generation antipsychotics.

6. Name the currently available atypical antipsychotic drugs. How are they alike? How do they differ? What appears unique about ziprasidone, aripiprazole, and amisulpride?

7. Why might antipsychotic drugs induce weight gain and/or diabetes?

8. Compare and contrast the newer atypical antipsychotics in terms of their efficacy, diabetes potential, effect on weight gain, QT effects, and other side effects.

REFERENCES

Adityanjee, S. C. (2002). "Clinical Use of Quetiapine in Disease States Other Than Schizophrenia." *Journal of Clinical Psychiatry* 63, Supplement 13: 32–38.

Advokat, C. (2005). "Differential Effects of Clozapine, Compared with Other Antipsychotics, on Clinical Outcome and Dopamine Release in the Brain." *Essential Psychopharmacology* 6: 73–90.

Advokat, C. (2010). "A Brief Overview of Iatrogenic Akathisia." *Clinical Schizophrenia & Related Psychoses* 3: 226–236.

Allison, D. B., and Casey, D. E. (2001). "Antipsychotic-Induced Weight Gain: A Review of the Literature." *Journal of Clinical Psychiatry* 62, Supplement 7: 22–31.

Ambresin, G., et al. (2004). "Olanzapine Excretion into Breast Milk: A Case Report." *Journal of Clinical Psychopharmacology* 24: 93–95.

American Psychiatric Association. (2004). "Practice Guideline for the Treatment of Patients with Schizophrenia," 2nd ed. *American Journal of Psychiatry* 161 (February Supplement).

Amminger, G. P., et al., (2010). "Long-Chain Omega-3 Fatty Acids for Indicated Prevention of Psychotic Disorders: A Randomized Placebo-Controlled Trial." *Archives of General Psychiatry* 67: 146–154.

Andrade, C. (2013). "Antidepressant Action of Atypical Antipsychotics: Focus on Ziprasidone Monotherapy, With a Few Twists in the Tale." *Journal of Clinical Psychiatry* 74: e193–e196.

Arato, M., et al. (2002). "A 1-Year, Double-Blind, Placebo-Controlled Trial of Ziprasidone 40, 80 and 160 mg/day in Chronic Schizophrenia: The Ziprasidone Extended Use in Schizophrenia (ZEUS) Study." *International Clinical Psychopharmacology* 17: 207–215.

Arvanitis, L. A., and Miller, B. G. (1997). "Multiple Fixed Doses of 'Seroquel' (Quetiapine) in Patients with Acute Exacerbation of Schizophrenia: A Comparison with Haloperidol and Placebo. The Seroquel Trial 13 Study Group." *Biological Psychiatry* 42: 233–246.

Atmaca, M., et al. (2002). "Quetiapine Augmentation in Patients with Treatment Resistant Obsessive-Compulsive Disorder: A Single-Blind, Placebo-Controlled Study." *International Clinical Psychopharmacology* 17: 115–119.

Ballard, C., et al. (2005). "Quetiapine and Rivastigmine and Cognitive Decline in Alzheimer's Disease: Randomized Double Blind Placebo Controlled Trial." *British Medical Journal* 330: 874.

Barnett, P. G., et al. (2012). "Cost and Cost-effectiveness in a Randomized Trial of Long-acting Risperidone for Schizophrenia." *Journal of Clinical Psychiatry* 73: 696-702.

Barnett, S. D., et al. (2002). "Efficacy of Olanzapine in Social Anxiety Disorder: A Pilot Study." *Journal of Psychopharmacology* 16: 365–368.

Bartzokis, G., et al. (2005). "Adjunctive Risperidone in the Treatment of Combat-Related Posttraumatic Stress Disorder." *Biological Psychiatry* 57: 474–479.

Björkhem-Bergman, L., et al. (2011). "Metformin for Weight Reduction in Non-Diabetic Patients on Antipsychotic Drugs: A Systematic Review and Meta-Analysis." *Journal of Psychopharmacology* 25: 299–305.

Blair, J., et al. (2005). "Electrocardiographic Changes in Children and Adolescents Treated with Ziprasidone: A Prospective Study." *Journal of the American Academy of Child and Adolescent Psychiatry* 44: 73–79.

Bobes, J., et al. (2010). "Prevalence of Negative Symptoms in Outpatients with Schizophrenia Spectrum Disorders Treated with Antipsychotics in Routine Clinical Practice: Findings from the CLAMORS Study." *Journal of Clinical Psychiatry* 71; 280–286.

Bogenschutz, M. P., and Nurnberg, G. (2004). "Olanzapine versus Placebo in the Treatment of Borderline Personality Disorder." *Journal of Clinical Psychiatry* 65: 104–109.

Brawman-Mintzer, O., et al. (2005). "Adjunctive Risperidone in Generalized Anxiety Disorder: A Double-Blind, Placebo-Controlled Study." *Journal of Clinical Psychiatry* 66: 1321–1325.

Bressan, R. A., et al. (2003). "Is Regionally Selective D_2/D_3 Dopamine Occupancy Sufficient for Atypical Antipsychotic Effect? An In Vivo Quantitative [^{123}I] Epidepride SPET Study of Amisulpride-Treated Patients." *American Journal of Psychiatry* 160: 1413–1420.

Buchanan, R. W., et al. (2010). "The 2009 Schizophrenia PORT Psychopharmacological Treatment Recommendations and Summary Statements." *Schizophrenia Bulletin* 36: 71–93.

Bushe, C. J., et al. (2013). "Weight Change by Baseline BMI from Three-year Observational Data: Findings from the Worldwide Schizophrenia Outpatient Health Outcomes Database." *Journal of Psychopharmacology* 27: 358–365.

Bystritsky, A., et al. (2004). "Augmentation of Serotonin Reuptake Inhibitors in Refractory Obsessive-Compulsive Disorder Using Adjunctive Olanzapine: A Placebo-Controlled Trial." *Journal of Clinical Psychiatry* 65: 565–568.

Carpenter, W. T., Jr., and Gold, J. M. (2002). "Another View of Therapy for Cognition in Schizophrenia." *Biological Psychiatry* 52: 969–971.

Carson, S., et al. (2006). "A Systematic Review of the Efficacy and Safety of Atypical Antipsychotics in Patients with Psychological and Behavioral Symptoms of Dementia." *Journal of the American Geriatric Society* 54: 354–361.

Ciranni, M. A., et al. (2009). "Comparing Acute Toxicity of First- and Second-Generation Antipsychotic Drugs: A 10-year, Retrospective Cohort Study." *Journal of Clinical Psychiatry* 70: 122–129.

Citrome, L. (2009). "Clozapine for Schizophrenia: Life-threatening or Life-saving Treatment?" *Current Psychiatry* 8: 57–63.

Citrome, L. (2011). "Lurasidone for Schizophrenia: A Brief Review of a New Second-generation Antipsychotic." *Clinical Schizophrenia & Related Psychoses* 4: 251–257.

Citrome, L. (2012). "Lurasidone for the Acute Treatment of Adults with Schizophrenia: What is the Number Needed to Treat, Number Needed to Harm, and Likelihood to be Helped or Harmed?" *Clinical Schizophrenia & Related Psychoses* 6: 1–10.

Citrome, L. (2013a). "Cariprazine in Bipolar Disorder: Clinical Efficacy, Tolerability, and Place in Therapy." *Advances in Therapy* 30: 102–113.

Citrome, L. (2013b). "Cariprazine in Schizophrenia: Clinical Efficacy, Tolerability, and Place in Therapy." *Advances in Therapy* 30: 114–126.

Colton, C. W., and Manderscheid, R. W. (2006). "Congruencies in Increased Mortality Rates, Years of Potential Life Lost, and Causes of Death Among Public Mental Health Clients in Eight States." Preventing Chronic Disease 3: 1–14.

Comaty, J. E., and Advokat, C. (2001). "Indications for the Use of Atypical Antipsychotics in the Elderly." *Journal of Clinical Geropsychology* 7: 285–309.

Conn, P. J., et al. (2008). "Schizophrenia: Moving Beyond Monoamine Antagonists." *Molecular Interventions* 8: 99–107.

Correll, C. U. (2007). "Weight Gain and Metabolic Effects of Mood Stabilizers and Antipsychotics in Pediatric Bipolar Disorder: A Systematic Review and Pooled Analysis of Short-Term Trials." *Journal of the American Academy of Child and Adolescent Psychiatry* 46: 687–700.

Correll, C. U., et al. (2004). "Lower Risk for Tardive Dyskinesia Associated with Second-Generation Antipsychotics: A Systematic Review of 1-Year Studies." *American Journal of Psychiatry* 161: 414–425.

Cortese, L., et al. (2013). "Management of Schizophrenia: Clinical Experience with Asenapine." *Journal of Psychopharmacology* March: 1-9: doi: 10.1177/1359786813482533.

Crystal, S., et al. (2009). "Broadened Use of Atypical Antipsychotics: Safety, Effectiveness, and Policy Challenges." *Health Affairs* 28: W770–W781.

Davis, J. M., and Chen, N. (2004). "Dose Response and Dose Equivalence of Antipsychotics." *Journal of Clinical Psychopharmacology* 24: 192–208.

Davis, J. M., et al. (2003). "A Meta-Analysis of the Efficacy of Second-Generation Antipsychotics." *Archives of General Psychiatry* 60: 553–564.

Denys, D., et al. (2004). "A Double-Blind, Randomized, Placebo-Controlled Trial of Quetiapine Addition in Patients with Obsessive-Compulsive Disorder Refractory to Serotonin Reuptake Inhibitors." *Journal of Clinical Psychiatry* 65: 1040–1048.

Dorsey, E. R., et al. (2010). "Impact of FDA Black Box Advisory on Antipsychotic Medication Use." *Archives of Internal Medicine* 170: 96–103.

Ellinger, L. K., et al. (2010). "Efficacy of Metformin and Topiramate in Prevention and Treatment of Second-generation Antipsychotic-induced Weight Gain." *The Annals of Pharmacotherapy* 44: 668–679.

Eutrecht, J. P. (1992). "Metabolism of Clozapine by Neutrophils: Possible Implications for Clozapine-Induced Agranulocytosis." *Drug Safety* 7, Supplement 1: 51–56.

Fagiolini, A., et al. (2013). "Asenapine for the Treatment of Manic and Mixed Episodes Associated with Bipolar I Disorder: From Clinical Research to Clinical Practice." *Expert Opinion on Pharmacotherapy* 14:489–504.

Farber, N. B. (2003). "The NMDA Receptor Hypofunction Model of Psychosis." *Annals of the New York Academy of Sciences* 1003: 119–130.

Fazel, S., et al. (2009). "Schizophrenia, Substance Abuse and Violent Crime." *Journal of the American Medical Association* 301: 2016–2023.

Fernandez, H. H., et al. (2004). "Aripiprazole for Drug-Induced Psychosis in Parkinson Disease: Preliminary Experience." *Clinical Neuropharmacology* 27: 4–5.

Fineberg, N. A., et al. (2012). "Evidence-based Pharmacotherapy of Obsessive-compulsive Disorder." *International Journal of Neuropsychopharmacology* 15: 1173–1191.

Fleishhacker, W. W., et al. (2003). "Treatment of Schizophrenia with Long-Acting Injectable Risperidone: A 12-Month Open-Label Trial of the First Long-Acting, Second-Generation Antipsychotic." *Journal of Clinical Psychiatry* 64: 1250–1257.

Freedman, R. (2003). "Schizophrenia." *New England Journal of Medicine* 349: 1738–1749.

Fountoulakis, K. N., et al. (2012). "Efficacy of Pharmacotherapy in Bipolar Disorder: A Report by the WPA Section on Pharmacopsychiatry." *European Archives of Psychiatry and Clinical Neuroscience* 262 (Suppl 1): S1–S48.

Freudenreich, O., et al. (2009). "Modafinil for Clozapine-Treated Schizophrenia Patients: A Double-Blind, Placebo-Controlled Pilot Trial." *Journal of Clinical Psychiatry* 70: 1674–1680.

Gagliano, A., et al. (2004). "Risperidone Treatment of Children with Autistic Disorder: Effectiveness, Tolerability, and Pharmacokinetic Implications." *Journal of Child and Adolescent Psychopharmacology* 14: 39–47.

Gao, K., et al. (2006). "Efficacy of Typical and Atypical Antipsychotics for Primary and Comorbid Anxiety Symptoms or Disorders: A Review." *Journal of Clinical Psychiatry* 67: 1327–1340.

Gardiner, S. J., et al. (2003). "Transfer of Olanzapine into Breast Milk, Calculation of Infant Drug Dose, and Effect on Breast-Fed Infants." *American Journal of Psychiatry* 160: 1428–1431.

Geffen, Y., et al. (2012). "BL-1020, a New Y-aminobutyric Acid-enhanced Antipsychotic: Results of 6-week, Randomized, Double-blind, Controlled, Efficacy and Safety Study." *Journal of Clinical Psychiatry* 73: e1168–e1174.

Gianfrancesco, F., et al. (2003). "Antipsychotic-Induced Type 2 Diabetes: Evidence from a Large Health Plan Database." *Journal of Clinical Psychopharmacology* 23: 328–335.

Glassman, A. H., and Bigger, J. T. (2001). "Antipsychotic Drugs: Prolonged QTc Interval, Torsade de Pointes, and Sudden Death." *American Journal of Psychiatry* 158: 1774–1782.

Goodnik, P. J. (2001). "Ziprasidone: Profile on Safety." *Expert Opinions in Pharmacotherapy* 2: 1655–1662.

Grootens, K. P., and Verkes, R. J. (2005). "Emerging Evidence for the Use of Atypical Antipsychotics in Borderline Personality Disorder." *Pharmacopsychiatry* 38: 20–23.

Grothe, D. R., et al. (2000). "Olanzapine Pharmacokinetics in Pediatric and Adolescent Inpatients with Schizophrenia." *Journal of Clinical Psychopharmacology* 20: 220–225.

Grunder, G., et al. (2003). "Mechanism of New Antipsychotic Medications: Occupancy Is Not Just Antagonism." *Archives of General Psychiatry* 60: 974–977.

Gunasekara, N. S., et al. (2002). "Ziprasidone: A Review of Its Use in Schizophrenia and Schizoaffective Disorder." *Drugs* 62: 1217–1251.

Hampton, T. (2007). "Antipsychotic's Link to Weight Gain Found." *Journal of the American Medical Association* 297: 1305–1306.

Hasnain, M., et al. (2011). "Metformin for Obesity and Glucose Dysregulation in Patients with Schizophrenia Receiving Antipsychotic Drugs." *Journal of Psychopharmacology* 25: 715–721.

Hirschfeld, R. M. A. (2005). "Introduction: The Role of Atypical Antipsychotics in the Treatment of Bipolar Disorder." *Journal of Clinical Psychiatry* 66, Supplement 3: 3–4.

Horacek, J., et al. (2006). "Mechanism of Action of Atypical Antipsychotic Drugs and the Neurobiology of Schizophrenia." *CNS Drugs* 20: 389–409.

Ilett, K., et al. (2004). "Transfer of Risperidone and 9-Hydroxyrisperidone into Human Milk." *Annals of Pharmacotherapy* 38: 273–276.

Ingenhoven, T., et al. (2010). "Effectiveness of Pharmacotherapy for Severe Personality Disorders: Meta-Analyses of Randomized Controlled Trials." *Journal of Clinical Psychiatry* 71: 14–25.

Janicak, P. G., et al. (2011). *Principles and Practice of Psychopharmacotherapy (5th Ed.)*. Philadelphia: Lippincott Williams & Wilkins.

Javitt, D. C., and Coyle, J. T. (2004). "Decoding Schizophrenia: A Fuller Understanding of Signaling in the Brain of People with This Disorder Offers a New Hope for Improved Therapy." *Scientific American* 290: 48–56.

Jeste, D. V., et al. (2005). "Atypical Antipsychotics in Elderly Patients with Dementia or Schizophrenia: Review of Recent Literature." *Harvard Review of Psychiatry* 13: 340–351.

Jobe, T. H., and Harrow, M. (2010). "Schizophrenia Course, Long-term Outcome, Recovery, and Prognosis." *Current Directions in Psychological Science* 19: 220–225.

Jones, P. B., et al. (2006). "Randomized Controlled Trial of the Effect on Quality of Life of Second- vs First-Generation Antipsychotic Drugs in Schizophrenia: Cost Utility of the Latest Antipsychotic Drugs in Schizophrenia Study (CUtLASS 1)." *Archives of General Psychiatry* 63: 1079–1087.

Jordan, S., et al. (2002). "The Antipsychotic Aripiprazole Is a Potent, Partial Agonist at the Human 5-HT1A Receptor." *European Journal of Pharmacology* 441: 137–140.

Kane, J. M., et al. (2003). "Long-Acting Injectable Risperidone: Efficacy and Safety of the First Long-Acting Atypical Antipsychotic." *American Journal of Psychiatry* 160: 1125–1132.

Kane, J. M., and Correll, C. U. (2010). "Past and Present Progress in the Pharmacologic Treatment of Schizophrenia." *Journal of Clinical Psychiatry* 71: 1115–1124.

Kapur, S., and Remington, G. (2001). "Atypical Antipsychotics: New Directions and New Challenges in the Treatment of Schizophrenia." *Annual Reviews of Medicine* 52: 503–517.

Kapur, S., and Seeman, P. (2001). "Does Fast Dissociation from the Dopamine D_2 Receptor Explain the Action of Atypical Antipsychotics? A New Hypothesis." *American Journal of Psychiatry* 158: 360–369.

Karlsson, J., et al. (2009). "Sudden Cardiac Death in Users of Second-generation Antipsychotics." *Journal of Clinical Psychiatry* 70: 1725–1726.

Keck, P. E., et al. (2001). "Ziprasidone in the Short-Term Treatment of Patients with Schizoaffective Disorder: Results from Two Double-Blind, Placebo-Controlled, Multicenter Studies." *Journal of Clinical Psychopharmacology* 21: 27–35.

Keck, P. E., et al. (2003a). "A Placebo-Controlled, Double-Blind Study of the Efficacy and Safety of Aripiprazole in Patients with Acute Bipolar Disorder." *American Journal of Psychiatry* 160: 1651–1658.

Keck, P. E., et al. (2003b). "Ziprasidone in the Treatment of Acute Bipolar Mania: A Three-Week, Placebo-Controlled, Double-Blind, Randomized Trial." *American Journal of Psychiatry* 160: 741–748.

Kelly, D. L., et al. (2009). "Randomized Double-Blind Trial of Atomoxetine for Cognitive Impairments in 32 People with Schizophrenia." *Journal of Clinical Psychiatry* 70: 518–525.

Keltner, N. L., and Folks, D. G. (2005). *Psychotropic Drugs*, 4th ed. Philadelphia: Mosby.

Khaldi, S., et al. (2003). "Usefulness of Olanzapine in Refractory Panic Attacks." *Journal of Clinical Psychopharmacology* 23: 100–101.

Khatib, S. M. al-, et al. (2003). "What Clinicians Should Know About the QT Interval." *Journal of the American Medical Association* 289: 2120–2127.

Kishi, T., et al. (2013). "Blonanserin for Schizophrenia: Systematic Review and Meta-analysis of Double-blind, Randomized, Controlled Trials." *Journal of Psychiatric Research* 47: 149–154.

Komossa, K., et al. (2009a). "Sertindole versus Other Atypical Antipsychotics for Schizophrenia." *Cochrane Database System Review*. Issue 4. Art. No. CD006752.

Komossa, K., et al. (2009b). "Ziprasidone versus Other Atypical Antipsychotics for Schizophrenia." *Cochrane Database System Review*. Issue 4. Art. No. CD006627.

Kreyenbuhl, J., et al. (2010). "The Schizophrenia Patient Outcomes Research Team (PORT): Updated Treatment Recommendations." *Schizophrenia Bulletin* 36: 94–103.

Kuehn, B. M. (2010). "Questionable Antipsychotic Prescribing Remains Common, Despite Serious Risks." *Journal of the American Medical Association* 303:1582–1584.

Lambert, M. T. (2006). "Aripiprazole in the Management of Post-Traumatic Stress Disorder Symptoms in Returning Global War on Terrorism Veterans." *International Clinical Psychopharmacology* 21: 185–187.

Laruelle, M., et al. (2003). "Glutamate, Dopamine and Schizophrenia from Pathophysiology to Treatment." *Annals of the New York Academy of Sciences* 1003: 138–158.

Leach, K., et al. (2009). "Molecular Mechanisms of Action and *In Vivo* Validation of an M_4 Muscarinic Acetylcholine Receptor Allosteric Modulator with Potential Antipsychotic Properties." *Neuropsychopharmacology* 35: 855–869.

Leucht, S., et al. (2003). "New Generation Antipsychotics versus Low-Potency Conventional Antipsychotics: A Systematic Review and Meta-Analysis." *Lancet* 361: 1581–1589.

Leucht, S., et al. (2009a). "A Meta-Analysis of Head-to-Head Comparisons of Second-Generation Antipsychotics in the Treatment of Schizophrenia." *American Journal of Psychiatry* 166: 152–163.

Leucht, S., et al. (2009b). "Second-Generation versus First-Generation Antipsychotic Drugs for Schizophrenia: A Meta-Analysis." *Lancet* 373: 31–41.

Lewis, R., et al. (2005). "Sertindole for Schizophrenia." *Cochrane Database System Review.* Issue 3. Art. No. CD001715.

Lieb, K., et al. (2010). "Pharmacotherapy for Borderline Personality Disorder: Cochrane Systematic Review of Randomised Trials." *British Journal of Psychiatry* 196: 4–12.

Lieberman, J. A. (2004). "Dopamine Partial Agonists: A New Class of Antipsychotic." *CNS Drugs* 18: 251–267.

Lieberman, J., A., et al. (2005). "Effectiveness of Antipsychotic Drugs in Patients with Chronic Schizophrenia." *New England Journal of Medicine* 353: 1209–1223.

Lincoln, J., and Preskorn, S. (2009). "Asenapine for Schizophrenia and Bipolar I Disorder." *Current Psychiatry* 8: 75–85.

Lincoln, J., and Tripathi, A. (2011). "Lurasidone for Schizophrenia." *Current Psychiatry* 10: 67–70.

Lindenmayer, J.-P., et al. (2003). "Changes in Glucose and Cholesterol in Patients with Schizophrenia Treated with Typical or Atypical Antipsychotics." *American Journal of Psychiatry* 160: 290–296.

López-Muñoz, F., et al. (2005). "History of the Discovery and Clinical Introduction of Chlorpromazine." *Annals of Clinical Psychiatry* 17: 113–135.

Lott, I. T., et al. (2004). "Longitudinal Prescribing Patterns for Psychoactive Medications in Community-Based Individuals with Developmental Disabilities: Utilization of Pharmacy Records." *Journal of Intellectual Disabilities Research* 48, Part 6: 563–571.

Maglione, M., et al. (2011). "Off-Label Use of Atypical Antipsychotics: An Update." Comparative Effectiveness Review No. 43. (Prepared by the Southern California Evidence-based Practice Center under Contract No. HHSA290-2007-10062-1.) Rockville, MD: Agency for Healthcare Research and Quality. September 2011. Available at: www.effectivehealthcare.ahrq.gov/reports/final.cfm.

Maher, A. R., and Theodore, G. (2012). "Summary of the Comparative Effectiveness Review on Off-Label Use of Atypical Antipsychotics." *Journal of Managed Care Pharmacy* 18 (Suppl 5): S1–S20.

Marshall, M., and Rathbone, J. (2011). "Early Intervention for Psychosis." *Cochrane Database of Systematic Reviews*, Issue 6. Art. No.: CD004718. DOI: 10.1002/14651858.CD004718.pub3.

McCracken, J. T., et al. (2002). "Risperidone in Children with Autism and Serious Behavioral Problems." *New England Journal of Medicine* 347: 314–321.

McDougle, C. J. (1998). "A Double-Blind, Placebo-Controlled Study of Risperidone in Adults with Autistic Disorder and Other Pervasive Developmental Disorders." *Archives of General Psychiatry* 55: 633–641.

McDougle, C. J., et al. (2000). "A Double-Blind, Placebo-Controlled Study of Risperidone Addition in Serotonin Reuptake Inhibitor-Refractory Obsessive-Compulsive Disorder." *Archives of General Psychiatry* 57: 794–801.

McDougle, C. J., et al. (2005). "Risperidone for the Core Symptom Domains of Autism: Results from the Study by the Autism Network of the Research Units on Pediatric Psychopharmacology." *American Journal of Psychiatry* 162: 1142–1148.

McEvoy, J. P., et al. (2006). "Effectiveness of Clozapine versus Olanzapine, Quetiapine and Risperidone in Patients with Chronic Schizophrenia Who Did Not Respond to Prior Atypical Antipsychotic Treatment." *American Journal of Psychiatry* 163: 600–610.

McGowan, S., et al. (2004). "Presynaptic Dopaminergic Dysfunction in Schizophrenia: A Positron Emission Tomographic [18F] Fluorodopa Study." *Archives of General Psychiatry* 61: 134–142.

McIntyre, R. S., and Wong, R. (2012). "Asenapine: A Synthesis of Efficacy Data in Bipolar Mania and Schizophrenia." *Clinical Schizophrenia & Related Psychoses* 5: 217–220.

McKeage, K., and Plosker, G. L. (2004). "Amisulpride: A Review of Its Use in the Management of Schizophrenia." *CNS Drugs* 18: 933–956.

Meltzer, H. Y., (2002). "Commentary on 'Clinical Studies on the Mechanism of Action of Clozapine: The Dopamine–Serotonin Hypothesis of Schizophrenia.'" *Psychopharmacology* 163: 1–3.

Meltzer, H. Y., (2012). "Clozapine: Balancing Safety with Superior Antipsychotic Efficacy." *Clinical Schizophrenia & Related Psychoses* 6: 134–144.

Meltzer, H. Y., et al. (2003). "Clozapine Treatment for Suicidality in Schizophrenia: International Suicide Prevention Trial (InterSePT)." *Archives of General Psychiatry* 60: 82–91.

Mercer, D., et al. (2009). "Meta-Analyses of Mood Stabilizers, Antidepressants and Antipsychotics in the Treatment of Borderline Personality Disorder: Effectiveness for Depression and Anger Symptoms." *Journal of Personality Disorders* 23: 156–174.

Mesholam-Gately, R. I. (2009). "Neurocognition in First-Episode Schizophrenia: A Meta-Analytic Review." *Neuropsychology* 23: 315–336.

Minzenberg, M. J., and Carter, C. S. (2012). "Developing Treatments for Impaired Cognition in Schizophrenia." *Trends in Cognitive Sciences* 16: 35–42.

Miyamoto, S., et al. (2003). "Recent Advances in the Neurobiology of Schizophrenia." *Molecular Interventions* 3: 27–39.

Moghaddam, B. (2003). "Bringing Order to the Glutamate Chaos in Schizophrenia." *Neuron* 40: 881–884.

Mohr, N., et al. (2002). "Quetiapine Augmentation of Serotonin Reuptake Inhibitors in Obsessive-Compulsive Disorder." *International Clinical Psychopharmacology* 17: 37–40.

Nelson, J. C., and Papakostas, G. I. (2009). "Atypical Antipsychotic Augmentation in Major Depressive Disorder: A Meta-Analysis of Placebo-Controlled Randomized Trials." *American Journal of Psychiatry* 166: 980–991.

Newcomer, J. W. (2005). "Second-Generation (Atypical) Antipsychotics and Metabolic Effects: A Comprehensive Literature Review." *CNS Drugs* 19, Supplement 1: 1–93.

Nickel, M. K., et al. (2006). "Aripiprazole in the Treatment of Patients with Borderline Personality Disorder: A Double-Blind, Placebo-Controlled Study." *American Journal of Psychiatry* 163: 833–838.

Nussbaum, A., and Stroup, S. (2008). "Paliperidone for Treatment of Schizophrenia." *Schizophrenia Bulletin* 34: 419–422.

Padala, P. R., et al. (2006). "Risperidone Monotherapy for Post-Traumatic Stress Disorder Related to Sexual Assault and Domestic Abuse in Women." *International Clinical Psychopharmacology* 21: 275–280.

Papakostas, G. I., et al. (2004). "Ziprasidone Augmentation of Selective Serotonin Reuptake Inhibitors (SSRIs) for SSRI-Resistant Major Depressive Disorder." *Journal of Clinical Psychiatry* 65: 217–221.

Papakostas, G. I., et al. (2005). "Aripiprazole Augmentation of Selective Serotonin Reuptake Inhibitors for Treatment-Resistant Major Depressive Disorder." *Journal of Clinical Psychiatry* 66: 1326–1330.

Paparelli, A., et al. (2011). "Drug-induced Psychosis: How to Avoid Star Gazing in Schizophrenia Research by Looking at More Obvious Sources of Light." *Frontiers in Behavioral Neuroscience* 5: 1–9.

Parkinson Study Group (1999). "Low-Dose Clozapine for the Treatment of Drug-Induced Psychosis in Parkinson's Disease." *New England Journal of Medicine* 340: 757–763.

Peritogiannis, V., and Tsouli, S. (2009). "Can Atypical Antipsychotics Improve Tardive Dyskinesia Associated with Other Atypical Antipsychotics? Case Report and Brief Review of the Literature." *Journal of Psychopharmacology* 24: 1121–1125.

Potkin, S. G., et al. (2003). "Aripiprazole, an Antipsychotic with a Novel Mechanism of Action, and Risperidone vs. Placebo in Patients with Schizophrenia and Schizoaffective Disorder." *Archives of General Psychiatry* 60: 681–690.

Poyurovsky, M., et al. (2003). "Attenuation of Olanzapine-Induced Weight Gain with Reboxetine in Patients with Schizophrenia: A Double-Blind, Placebo-Controlled Study." *American Journal of Psychiatry* 160: 297–302.

Rapaport, M. H., et al. (2006). "Effects of Risperidone Augmentation in Patients with Treatment-Resistant Depression: Results of Open-Label Treatment Followed by Double-Blind Continuation." *Neuropsychopharmacology* 31: 2501–2513.

Ratzoni, G., et al. (2002). "Weight Gain Associated with Olanzapine and Risperidone in Adolescent Patients: A Comparative Prospective Study." *Journal of the American Academy of Child and Adolescent Psychiatry* 41: 337–343.

Ray, W. A., et al. (2009). "Atypical Antipsychotic Drugs and the Risk of Sudden Cardiac Death." *New England Journal of Medicine* 360: 225–235.

Reddy, S., et al. (2002). "The Effect of Quetiapine on Psychosis and Motor Function in Parkinsonian Patients with and Without Dementia." *Movement Disorders* 17: 676–681.

Remington, G., et al. (2013). "Clozapine's Role in the Treatment of First-Episode Schizophrenia." *American Journal of Psychiatry* 170:146–151.

Rocca, P., et al. (2002). "Treatment of Borderline Personality Disorder with Risperidone." *Journal of Clinical Psychiatry* 63: 241–244.

Rosebush, P. I., and Mazurek, M. F. (1999). "Neurologic Side Effects in Neuroleptic-Naive Patients Treated with Haloperidol or Risperidone." *Neurology* 52: 782–785.

Rosenheck, R., et al. (2003). "Effectiveness and Cost of Olanzapine and Haloperidol in the Treatment of Schizophrenia: A Randomized Controlled Trial." *Journal of the American Medical Association* 290: 2693–2702.

Rosenheck, R. A., et al. (2011). "Long-acting Risperidone and Oral Antipsychotics in Unstable Schizophrenia." *New England Journal of Medicine* 364: 842–851.

Rosenheck, R., and Sernyak, M. J. (2009). "Developing a Policy for Second-Generation Antipsychotic Drugs." *Health Affairs* 28: 782–793.

Rujescu, D., et al. (2006). "A Pharmacological Model for Psychosis Based On N-Methyl-D-Aspartate Receptor Hypofunction: Molecular, Cellular, Functional and Behavioral Abnormalities." *Biological Psychiatry* 59: 721–729.

Sadock, B. J., and Sadock, V. A. (2007). *Kaplan and Sadock's Synopsis of Psychiatry.* New York: Lippincott Williams & Wilkins.

Schneider, L. S., et al. (2006). "Effectiveness of Atypical Antipsychotic Drugs in Patients with Alzheimer's Disease." *New England Journal of Medicine* 355: 1525–1538.

Schwartz, T. L., et al. (2007). "Aripiprazole Augmentation of Selective Serotonin or Serotonin Norepinephrine Reuptake Inhibitors in the Treatment of Major Depressive Disorder." *Primary Psychiatry* 14: 67–69.

Sedky, K., et al. (2010). "Paliperidone Palmitate: Once-Monthly Treatment Option for Schizophrenia." *Current Psychiatry* 9: 48–50.

Sernyak, M. J., et al. (2002). "Association of Diabetes Mellitus with Use of Atypical Neuroleptics in the Treatment of Schizophrenia." *American Journal of Psychiatry* 159: 561–566.

Sewell, R. A. (2011). "Latuda: "Procognitive" or Pro-Profit?" *The Carlat Report Psychiatry* 9: 1–3.

Shelton, R. C., et al. (2005). "Olanzapine/Fluoxetine Combination for Treatment-Resistant Depression: A Controlled Study of SSRI and Nortriptyline Resistance." *Journal of Clinical Psychiatry* 66: 1289–1297.

Siddiqui, Z., et al. (2005). "Ziprasidone Therapy for Post-Traumatic Stress Disorder." *Journal of Psychiatry & Neuroscience* 30: 430–431.

Simon, J. S., and Nemeroff, C. B. (2005). "Aripiprazole Augmentation of Antidepressants for the Treatment of Partially Responding and Nonresponding Patients with Major Depressive Disorder." *Journal of Clinical Psychiatry* 66: 1216–1220.

Spaulding, A. M. (2012). "A Pharmacotherapeutic Approach to the Management of Chronic Posttraumatic Stress Disorder." *Journal of Pharmacy Practice* 25: 541–551.

Stahl, S. M. (2002). "Dopamine System Stabilizers, Aripiprazole, and the Next Generation of Antipsychotics. Part 1: Goldilocks Actions at Dopamine Receptors; Part 2: Illustrating Their Mechanism of Action." *Journal of Clinical Psychiatry* 62: 841–842, 923–924.

Stein, M. B., et al. (2002). "Adjunctive Olanzapine for SSRI-Resistant Combat-Related PTSD: A Double-Blind, Placebo-Controlled Study." *American Journal of Psychiatry* 159: 1777–1779.

Stoner, S. C., and Pace, H. A. (2012). "Asenapine: A Clinical Review of a Second-Generation Antipsychotic." *Clinical Therapeutics* 34: 1023–1040.

Stoffers, J., et al. (2010). "Pharmacological Interventions for Borderline Personality Disorder." Cochrane Database of Systematic Reviews 2010, Issue 6. Art. No.: CD005653. DOI: 10.1002/14651858.CD005653.pub2.

Storch, E. A., et al. (2008). "Aripiprazole Augmentation of Incomplete Treatment Response in an Adolescent Male with Obsessive-Compulsive Disorder." *Depression and Anxiety* 25: 172–174.

Stroup, T. S., et al. (2006). "Effectiveness of Olanzapine, Quetiapine, Risperidone, and Ziprasidone in Patients with Chronic Schizophrenia Following Discontinuation of a Previous Atypical Antipsychotic." *American Journal of Psychiatry* 163: 611–622.

Sullivan, P. F., et al. (2003). "Schizophrenia as a Complex Trait." *Archives of General Psychiatry* 60: 1187–1192.

Swainston, H. T., and Scott, L. J. (2006). "Ziprasidone: A Review of Its Use in Schizophrenia and Schizoaffective Disorder." *CNS Drugs* 20: 1027–1052.

Tamminga, C. A., and Carlsson, A. (2002). "Partial Dopamine Agonists and Dopaminergic Stabilizers, in the Treatment of Psychosis." *Current Drug Targets—CNS & Neurological Disorders* 1: 141–147.

Tenback, D. E., et al. (2009). "Incidence and Persistence of Tardive Dyskinesia and Extrapyramidal Symptoms in Schizophrenia." *Journal of Psychopharmacology* 24: 1031–1035.

Tiihonen, J., et al. (2009). "11-Year Follow-up of Mortality in Patients with Schizophrenia: A Population-based Cohort Study (FIN11 study)." *Lancet* 374: 620-627.

Tollefson, G. D., et al. (1999). "Controlled, Double-Blind Investigation of the Clozapine Discontinuation Symptoms with Conversion to Either Olanzapine or Placebo." *Journal of Clinical Psychopharmacology* 19: 435–443.

Torrey, E. F. (2002). "Studies of Individuals with Schizophrenia Never Treated with Antipsychotic Medications: A Review." *Schizophrenia Research* 58: 101–115.

Trémeau, F., and Citrome, L. (2006). "Antipsychotics for Patients Without Psychoses?" *Current Psychiatry* 5: 33–44.

Tschen, A. C., et al. (1999). "The Cytotoxicity of Clozapine Metabolites: Implications for Predicting Clozapine-Induced Agranulocytosis." *Clinical Pharmacology and Therapeutics* 65: 526–532.

Vieta, E., et al. (2008). "Efficacy of Adjunctive Aripiprazole to Either Valproate or Lithium in Bipolar Mania Patients Partially Nonresponsive to Valproate/Lithium Monotherapy: A Placebo-Controlled Study." *American Journal of Psychiatry* 165: 1316–1325.

Villeneuve, E., and Lemelin, S. (2005). "Open-Label Study of Atypical Neuroleptic Quetiapine for Treatment of Borderline Personality Disorder: Impulsivity as Main Target." *Journal of Clinical Psychiatry* 66: 1298–1303.

Volavka, J., et al. (2002). "Clozapine, Olanzapine, Risperidone, and Haloperidol in the Treatment of Patients with Chronic Schizophrenia and Schizoaffective Disorder." *American Journal of Psychiatry* 159: 255–262.

Wang, P. S., et al. (2005). "Risk of Death in Elderly Users of Conventional vs. Atypical Antipsychotic Medications." *New England Journal of Medicine* 353: 2335–2341.

Weickert, T., et al. (2003). "Comparison of Cognitive Performance During a Placebo Period and an Atypical Antipsychotic Treatment Period in Schizophrenia: Critical Examination of Confounds." *Neuropsychopharmacology* 28: 1491–1500.

Weiden, P. J. (2012). "Iloperidone for the Treatment of Schizophrenia: An Updated Clinical Review." *Clinical Schizophrenia & Related Psychoses* 6: 34–44.

Weiss, E. M., et al. (2002). "The Effects of Second-Generation Atypical Antipsychotics on Cognitive Functioning and Psychosocial Outcomes in Schizophrenia." *Psychopharmacology* 162: 11–17.

Wheeler, A., et al. (2009). "Outcomes for Schizophrenia Patients with Clozapine Treatment: How Good Does It Get?" *Journal of Psychopharmacology* 23: 957–965.

Wirshing, D. A., et al. (2002). "The Effects of Novel Antipsychotics on Glucose and Lipid Levels." *Journal of Clinical Psychiatry* 63: 856–865.

Witchel, H. J., et al. (2003). "Psychotropic Drugs, Cardiac Arrhythmia, and Sudden Death." *Journal of Clinical Psychopharmacology* 23: 58–77.

Yargic, L. I., et al. (2004). "A Prospective Randomized Single-Blind, Multicenter Trial Comparing the Efficacy and Safety of Paroxetine with and Without Quetiapine Therapy in Depression Associated with Anxiety." *International Journal of Psychiatry in Clinical Practice* 8: 205–211.

Zhang, J-P., et al. (2010). "D_2 Receptor Genetic Variation and Clinical Response to Antipsychotic Drug Treatment: A Meta-Analysis." *American Journal of Psychiatry* 167: 763–772.

Zhang, J-P., and Malhotra, A. K. (2013). "Genetics of Schizophrenia: What Do We Know?" *Current Psychiatry* 12: 25–33.

Zuddas, A., et al. (2011). "Second Generation Antipsychotics (SGAs) for Non-psychotic Disorders in Children and Adolescents: A Review of the Randomized Controlled Studies." *European Neuropsychopharmacology* 21: 600–620.

Chapter 12

Antidepressant Drugs

In the 55 years since antidepressant medications were first introduced into medicine, these drugs have been heavily promoted (by the pharmaceutical industry) and prescribed (by physicians) in the hope that they may:

- Alleviate the signs, symptoms, and distress associated with clinical depression
- Relieve anxiety either as a single diagnosis or as part of comorbid anxiety/depression
- Improve the lives of persons with debilitating depression
- Repair the neuronal damage associated with depression

To what extent has this been accomplished?

- Depression is only modestly improved. This implies only limited efficacy.
- Side effects can be very bothersome and clinically limiting.

Fifty years ago we asked whether or not antidepressants work at all. Today, this same question is still being asked (Holtzheimer and Mayberg, 2011; Nierenberg, 2011) (Figure 12.1). Today, as stated by Fournier and coworkers (2010, p. 47):

> The magnitude and benefit of antidepressant medication compared with placebo increases with severity of depression symptoms and may be minimal or non-existent, on average, in patients with mild to moderate symptoms. For patients with very severe depression, the benefit of medications over placebo is substantial.

Unfortunately, in patients with mild to moderate depression, antidepressants remain frequently prescribed, with little efficacy and with bothersome side effects, including sexual dysfunction, weight gain, possible adverse cognitive effects, and even suicidal ideation. This lack of response is frequently termed "treatment-resistant depression" and

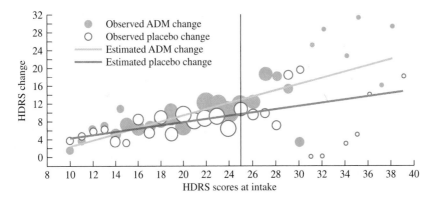

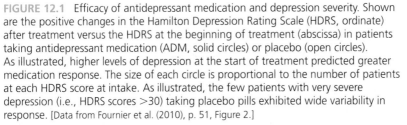

FIGURE 12.1 Efficacy of antidepressant medication and depression severity. Shown are the positive changes in the Hamilton Depression Rating Scale (HDRS, ordinate) after treatment versus the HDRS at the beginning of treatment (abscissa) in patients taking antidepressant medication (ADM, solid circles) or placebo (open circles). As illustrated, higher levels of depression at the start of treatment predicted greater medication response. The size of each circle is proportional to the number of patients at each HDRS score at intake. As illustrated, the few patients with very severe depression (i.e., HDRS scores >30) taking placebo pills exhibited wide variability in response. [Data from Fournier et al. (2010), p. 51, Figure 2.]

additional medications are added, usually with little improvement and additional side effects. There is little consensus on how to improve treatment outcomes. Combinations of antidepressants and psychotherapy differ only slightly from either alone and alternative therapies have minimal efficacy. Perhaps "the type of treatment offered is less important than getting depressed patients involved in an active therapeutic program" (Khan, et al., 2012).

Depression

Depression, or major depressive disorder (MDD), is a chronic, recurring, and potentially life-threatening illness. MDD is currently the third most disabling disease worldwide, and by the year 2020, it will be the second leading cause of disability across the globe. Depression accounts for 4.5 percent of the total worldwide burden of disease in terms of disability-adjusted life years. Depression worsens the health of people with other chronic illnesses, has a tendency to recur, and is associated with increasing disability over time. About 10 percent of men and up to 25 percent of women experience depression in their lifetime, and each year about 9 to 10 percent of the U.S. population, or approximately 30 million Americans, suffer with this illness. Depression is responsible for up to 70 percent of psychiatric hospitalizations and about 40 percent of suicides. Unfortunately, it has been estimated that only about 21 percent of persons with depression are adequately treated. Holtzheimer and Mayberg (2011) call for a rethinking of depression and its treatment.

Depression is an *affective disorder*, characterized by (sometimes profound) alterations of emotion or mood. Beside mood alterations, there may be decreased interest in pleasurable activities and in the ability to experience pleasure, sleep difficulties, fatigue or loss of energy, feelings of worthlessness or excessive guilt, and possible thoughts of death or suicide. Symptoms may be mild, moderate, or severe, depending on the extent of impairment in daily social and occupational functioning. Severe depression may be associated with symptoms of psychosis or loss of touch with reality. People with relatively mild but prolonged symptoms that persist for at least 2 years are considered to have "dysthymia."

Symptoms of anxiety are also seen in many people with depression. Although many of the anxiety disorders have historically been treated with benzodiazepine anxiolytics (see Chapter 13), today antidepressant treatment is also indicated for most anxiety disorders. Not only are the antidepressant drugs efficacious for treating anxiety, they are less prone to compulsive use and less likely to impair learning, memory, and concentration than the benzodiazepines.[1]

Pathophysiology of Depression

Classically, depression was conceptualized as a deficiency involving neurotransmitters, particularly the "monoamines" serotonin, norepinephrine, and dopamine. Restoring these neurotransmitters, usually by prolonging their presence in the synaptic cleft, was responsible for recovering a normal mood state. One weakness of this model was that the neurotransmitter changes occurred soon after drug administration—but the clinical antidepressant effect develops more slowly, often during several weeks of continuous treatment. This delay was hypothesized to be due to changes in receptor sensitivity caused by the chronic increase in synaptic levels of neurotransmitter. However, in the last few years, this view has broadened, and attention has shifted to the study of the long-term actions of antidepressant treatments on intracellular processes, such as second messengers, and their functions in the neuron.

Two of these second-messenger functions are (1) to protect neurons from damage due to injury or trauma and (2) to promote and maintain the health and stability of newly formed neurons. Research into these processes has led to a new way of thinking about depression (and the effect of antidepressant treatment) called the *neurogenic theory of depression*.

The neurogenic theory is a result of the relatively recent discovery that, contrary to what we once believed, (1) existing neurons are able to "repair" or "remodel" themselves and (2) the brain is capable of making new neurons (Andrade and Rao, 2010). In particular, it is now known that new neurons are produced throughout life in the hippocampus and the frontal cortex of several species, including humans. The birth of new neurons is called *neurogenesis*. This finding is especially relevant to understanding depressive disorders because the hippocampus influences many functions that are impaired in a depressed person, such as attention, concentration, and memory. At the same time, we know that the hippocampus is also very vulnerable to the effects of trauma, such as hypoglycemia, lack of oxygen, toxins, infections, and especially stress,

---

[1] According to current diagnostic criteria, anxiety disorders include panic disorder (PD), obsessive-compulsive disorder (OCD), posttraumatic stress disorder (PTSD), social phobia, and generalized anxiety disorder (GAD).

and to the hormones that are activated by stressful situations (such as corticosterone). In fact, stressful situations are known both to reduce hippocampal and frontal cortical neurogenesis and to damage existing neurons.

Among the stressful conditions that can damage the hippocampus is a state of depression—not surprising, as stress is believed to be one of the most significant causes of depression; about 50 percent of depressed patients have some abnormality in their physiological responses to stress. Moreover, hippocampal nerve cells are among the most sensitive to stress-induced damage. For example, depressed women with a history of child abuse have an 18 percent smaller left hippocampal volume than nonabused women (Grande et al., 2010). Remarkably this hippocampal shrinkage is reversible with antide-pressant treatment, consistent with a role of neurotropic factors in neuronal plasticity in the hippocampus (Neto et al., 2011; Autry and Monteggia, 2012). Consequently, depres-sion is now viewed as a neurodegenerative disorder (Andrade and Rao, 2010; Lucassen et al., 2010; Tripp et al., 2012).

Just as a variety of stimuli can damage neurons and decrease neurogenesis, several factors are known to repair neurons and increase neurogenesis—among them, antide-pressant drugs.[2] It has been proposed that the therapeutic delay in the clinical effect of antidepressants occurs because of the time required for new neurons to develop, mature, and become functional. This hypothesis is supported by the observation that the increase in neurogenesis requires chronic antidepressant administration, which is consistent with the time course for the therapeutic action of these medications. A major focus of cur-rent research is to identify the cellular processes in the hippocampus and frontal cortex that are responsible for the protective effects of antidepressants. Most current studies are directed toward the second-messenger systems, which are activated by the synaptic action of neurotransmitters. This action in turn stimulates production of intracellular proteins that control the expression of certain genes.

One of the intracellular targets of second-messenger systems is called *cAMP response-element-binding protein* (CREB). The fact that the amount of CREB protein increases in the hippocampus during chronic antidepressant treatment provides additional evidence for the neurogenic hypothesis. In turn, it is known that CREB activates genes that con-trol the production of a protein called *brain-derived neurotrophic factor* (BDNF). BDNF is one of a group of substances called *neurotrophins*, produced by many brain structures, which are important for the normal development and health of the nervous system. For example, when injected into the brain of rats, BDNF not only prevents the spontane-ous death of some neurons but also helps to protect neurons that have been poisoned with various toxins. Conversely, in animals, chronic stress decreases the production and amount of BDNF (and other neurotrophic substances) in the brain and increases cell death. As predicted by the neurogenic hypothesis, levels of BDNF (and some other neu-rotrophic substances) increase in the hippocampus of rats chronically exposed to a wide range of antidepressants. Of particular significance, blood levels of BDNF are decreased in depressed patients, and some studies have found that antidepressant treatment can reverse this effect (Neto et al., 2011). (Figure 12.2).

---

[2] Other stimuli include electroconvulsive therapy, exercise, light therapy, and so on.

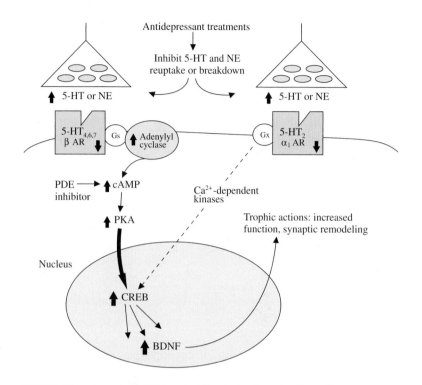

FIGURE 12.2 A model for the molecular mechanism of action of long-term antidepressant treatments. Antidepressants induce short-term increases in 5-HT and NE. Longer-term use decreases the function and expression of their receptors, but the cAMP signal transduction pathway is increased, including increased levels of adenylyl cyclase and cAMP-dependent protein kinase (PKA), as well as translocation of PKA to the cell nucleus. Antidepressants increase expression and function of the transcription factor cAMP response element-binding protein (CREB), suggesting that CREB is a common postreceptor target for antidepressants. Brain-derived neurotrophic factor is also increased by antidepressant treatment; up regulation of CREB and BDNF could influence the function of hippocampal neurons or neurons innervating this brain region, increasing neuronal survival, function, and remodeling of synaptic or cellular architecture. [After Duman et al. (1997), p. 600.]

Launay and coworkers (2011) discuss the link between fluoxetine (Prozac), serotonin reuptake blockade, and secretion of *neurotropic factors* in the hippocampus. This mechanism may explain the synaptic action of fluoxetine and how its effect leads to the relief of depression. As stated, this appears to be the "missing link" between fluoxetine treatment and hippocampal neurogenesis; an intracellular protein (microRNA, or miR-16) sustains the hippocampal response to fluoxetine and other serotonergic agents.

If BDNF is deficient in depression and if this deficiency leads to depressive symptomatology, might there be genetic influences that predispose a person to depression and perhaps offer new insights into therapy? Much has been done to elucidate candidate genes associated with major depression. Kupfer and coworkers (2012), Mitjans and

Arias (2012), Schosser and coworkers (2012), Narasimhan and Lohoff (2012), and Saveanu and Nemeroff (2012) all offer recent reviews of genetic factors in depression. Certainly, genetic variability in BDNF as well as serotonin transporter genes appears to increase the risk of developing depressive disorders, including suicide (Sher, 2011). To date, these studies have not translated into new therapeutic drugs or into better choices of medicating depressive disorder, especially in treatment-resistant patients (Masi and Brovedani, 2011).

In summary, several lines of evidence suggest that depression is a consequence of stress, which, like any injury, disease, or other type of physical trauma, damages the brain and weakens its ability to recover. Antidepressants relieve depressed mood by acting at the cellular level to promote neuronal survival and reverse stress-induced neuronal damage (Figure 12.3). Although the immediate effect of antidepressants is to modulate

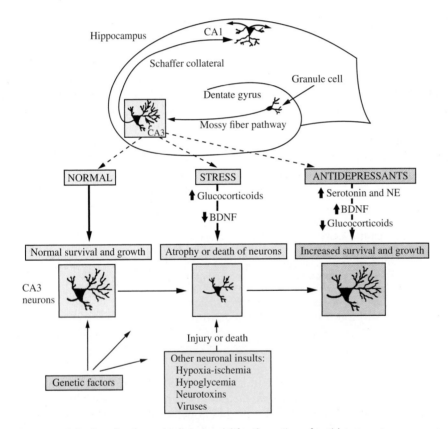

FIGURE 12.3 A molecular and cellular model for the action of antidepressants and the pathophysiology of stress-related disorders. Chronic stress decreases the expression of BDNF in the hippocampus, contributing to atrophy or death of neurons in the hippocampus. Elevated levels of glucocorticoids also decrease survival of these neurons, as do many other insults. Antidepressants increase the expression of BDNF and prevent the down regulation of BDNF elicited by stress, increasing neuronal survival or helping repair or protect neurons from further damage. [After Duman et al. (1997), p. 603.]

synaptic levels of neurotransmitters, their ultimate targets are the intracellular molecules responsible for maintaining neuronal health and plasticity. This reconceptualization of depressive disorder has broadened the search for new drug treatments; including agents that block the effect of stress hormones or that directly stimulate neurotrophic processes (Cazorla et al., 2011).

Evolution of Antidepressant Drug Development

Fifty-five years ago, the antidepressant properties of the drug *imipramine* were discovered accidentally. Since then, it has been learned that imipramine and similar drugs, called *tricyclic antidepressants* (TCAs; Table 12.1), block the presynaptic transporter protein receptors for the neurotransmitters norepinephrine and serotonin. Note that the term *tricyclic antidepressant* refers to a commonality in chemical *structure,* in contrast to newer antidepressants, which are defined by their mechanism of action. That is because, when the antidepressant effect of imipramine was discovered, its mechanism of action was unknown; thus, a structural classification had to suffice and persists today.

At about the same time the TCAs were discovered, another class of early antidepressant drugs, called the *monoamine oxidase inhibitors* (MAOIs), was identified. The MAOIs bind to and block the enzyme monoamine oxidase. This enzyme normally metabolizes and regulates the amount of the biogenic amine transmitters in the presynaptic nerve terminal. Thus, the levels of these neurotransmitters increase and more transmitter is available for release when stimulated by an action potential reaching the nerve terminal. Both the TCAs and the MAOIs are effective in the treatment of major depression, but both possess adverse side effects, discussed later in this chapter. Together, we refer to these two classes of drugs as *first-generation antidepressants.*

Many problems with the first-generation agents prompted the search for new antidepressants that were equally effective and better tolerated, but less toxic. First was the development of several drugs that were slight modifications of the basic tricyclic structure but that still exhibited antidepressant efficacy. These drugs were termed *second-generation,* or *atypical, antidepressants* (see Table 12.1).

During the late 1980s and continuing through the 1990s, the *selective serotonin reuptake inhibitors* (SSRIs) were developed, the first of which was fluoxetine (Prozac) (see Table 12.1). Six more were eventually marketed. Today, because of the limitations and side effects of the SSRIs, antidepressant drug research is progressing to identify compounds that act by different mechanisms. These drugs are not necessarily more clinically efficacious than the older TCAs, but they may have a more favorable profile of toxicity or side effects. The availability of the newer drugs has not yet reduced the number of treatment-resistant patients with major depression; the new drugs have only altered the profile of side effects. Three main therapeutic improvements still must be met: (1) superior efficacy, especially in the treatment of therapy-resistant depression; (2) faster onset of action; and (3) improved side effect profile. The following discussion of specific antidepressant drugs is subdivided into categories according to the chronology of their introduction into medicine and the neurotransmitters on which each group is thought to act.

TABLE 12.1 Drugs used to treat depression

Drug name: Generic (trade)	Sedative activity	Anticholinergic activity[a]	Elimination half-life (h)	Reuptake inhibition		
				Norepinephrine	Serotonin	Dopamine
TRICYCLIC COMPOUNDS						
Imipramine (Tofranil)	Moderate	Moderate	10–20	++	++	0
Desipramine (Norpramin)	Low	Low	12–75	+++	+	0
Trimipramine (Surmontil)	High	Moderate	8–20	+	+	0
Protriptyline (Vivactil)	Low	Moderate	55–125	+++	+	0
Nortriptyline (Pamelor, Aventil)	Low	Low	15–35	++	++	0
Amitriptyline (Elavil)	High	High	20–35	++	++	0
Doxepin (Adapin, Sinequan)	High	High	8–24	++	++	0
Clomipramine (Anafranil)	Low	Low	19–37	++	++++	0
SECOND-GENERATION (ATYPICAL) COMPOUNDS						
Amoxapine (Asendin)[b]	Moderate	Moderate	8–10	++	+	0
Maprotiline (Ludiomil)	Moderate	Moderate	27–58	+++	0	0
Trazodone (Desyrel, Oleptro)	High	Low	6–13	0	++	0
Bupropion (Wellbutrin)	Low	Low	8–14	0/+	0/+	++
Venlafaxine (Effexor)	Moderate	None	3–11	++	++++	0
Desvenlafaxine (Pristiq)	Moderate	None	3–11	++	++++	0
SELECTIVE SEROTONIN REUPTAKE INHIBITORS						
Fluoxetine (Prozac)	Moderate	None	24–96	0	++++	0
Sertraline (Zoloft)	Moderate	None	26	0	++++	0
Paroxetine (Paxil)	Moderate	None	24	+	++++	0
Citalopram (Celexa)	Moderate	None	33	0	++++	0
Fluvoxamine (Luvox)	Moderate	None	15	0	++++	0

Escitalopram (Lexapro)	Low	None	2–5	0	++++	0
Vilazodone (Viibryd)	Low	None	20–24	0	++++	0
DUAL-ACTION ANTIDEPRESSANTS						
Nefazodone (Serzone)	High	None	3–4	0	++++	0
Mirtazapine (Remeron)	High	Low	20–40	++	++++	0
Duloxetine (Cymbalta)	Moderate	Low	11–16	+++	+++	0
MAO INHIBITORS: IRREVERSIBLE						
Phenelzine (Nardil)	Moderate	None	2–4[c]	0	0	0
Isocarboxazid (Marplan, Enerzer)	Low	None	1–3[c]	0	0	0
Tranylcypromine (Parnate)	Moderate	None	1–3[c]	0	0	0
Selegiline (Emsam)						
SELECTIVE NOREPINEPHRINE REUPTAKE INHIBITORS						
Atomoxetine (Strattera)	None	Low	5	++++	0	0

[a]Anticholinergic side effects include dry mouth, blurred vision, tachycardia, urinary retention, and constipation.
[b]Also has antipsychotic effects due to blockage of dopamine receptors (Chapter 4).
[c]Half-life does not correlate with clinical effect (see text).
0 = no effect; + = mild effect; ++ = moderate effect; +++ = strong effect; ++++ = maximal effect.
Several generic products have been marketed under new brand names, here, only classic trade names are given.

> ## Did You Know?
>
> ### Mystery Biography
>
> I was born on September 2, 1948, in Shreveport, Louisiana. By the time I reached high school, I was well known for my athletic abilities—I set a national record for the javelin throw at 245 feet, and was featured in *Sports Illustrated's Faces in the Crowd.* I purposely failed my entrance exam to LSU, choosing to attend Louisiana Tech University. I was a big frat boy, pledging with Tau Kappa Epsilon. By the time 1970 rolled around, I was the first-round draft pick in the NFL, having amassed quite a record during my college years in the sport of football. In 1996, I was voted into the College Football Hall of Fame. During my time in the NFL, I started out a bit erratic, but quickly settled into my role as a team leader to four Super Bowl titles over the course of my career. I am even a key player in one of the most well-known football plays of all time. I had a 13-year football career, eventually retiring due to elbow, neck, and shoulder injuries. I was admitted into the Hall of Fame in 1989. I recently divulged to the media my corticosteroid use in the '70's, and have been known to abuse alcohol. Specifically, following each of my divorces, I would often sink into a deep depression and have severe anxiety attacks. I attempted to self-medicate with alcohol, and experienced weight loss, sleeplessness, and frequent crying episodes. I finally hit rock bottom and got myself to a psychiatrist, where I was diagnosed with clinical depression. I am currently taking Paxil CR, and feel that my depression has been well-managed, though I have been living with this illness for more than 5 years. In 2001, I received a star on the Hollywood Walk of Fame, the only NFL player to achieve this accomplishment. I've written several best-selling books as well. I am living proof that one can live a successful life without being hindered by depression, as long as it is successfully treated. It took me taking that first step to ask for help in order to get myself where I am today; I am currently a spokesman for depression education programs.
>
> Who am I?...Terry Bradshaw

First-Generation Antidepressants

The first two classes of antidepressants (TCAs and MAOIs) were introduced into medicine in the late 1950s and early 1960s. Drugs of both classes increased the levels of norepinephrine and serotonin in the brain, leading to the concept that depression resulted from a relative deficiency of these neurotransmitters. Conversely, excesses in the amounts of these transmitters were thought to lead to a state of mania. This was called the *monoamine (receptor) hypothesis of mania and depression.* Although this interpretation is much too simplistic, until recently the concept has been extremely useful for guiding the development of new antidepressants.

Tricyclic Antidepressants

The term *tricyclic antidepressant* describes a class of drugs that all have a characteristic three-ring molecular core (Figure 12.4). TCAs not only effectively relieve symptoms of depression; they also possess significant anxiolytic and analgesic actions. Historically, the

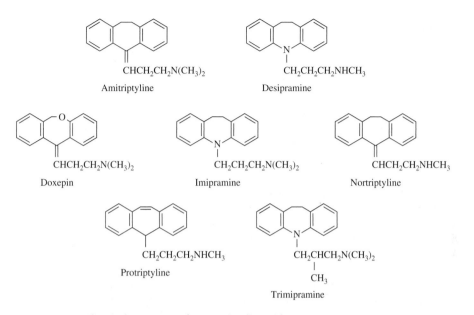

FIGURE 12.4   Chemical structures of seven tricyclic antidepressants.

TCAs were drugs of first choice for the treatment of major depression. The SSRIs, which today are widely prescribed, are no more effective and may be considerably more expensive; they are, however, less toxic, and their use is associated with a higher rate of patient comfort and compliance.

Imipramine (Tofranil) is the prototype TCA, but another clinically available TCA, *desipramine* (Norpramin), is the pharmacologically active intermediate metabolite of imipramine. Likewise, *amitriptyline* (Elavil) has an active intermediate metabolite, *nortriptyline* (Pamelor, Aventil). In fact, these two active intermediates may actually be responsible for much of the antidepressant effect of both imipramine and amitriptyline.

Mechanism of Action.   TCAs exert two significant pharmacologic actions that are presumed to account for both the therapeutic effects and most side effects of these drugs:

1. They block the *presynaptic reuptake transporter* for norepinephrine and serotonin. They were therefore the first "dual action" antidepressants, decades before venlafaxine (Effexor) and duloxetine (Cymbalta).
2. They block *postsynaptic receptors* for histamine and acetylcholine. Such blockade accounts for most of the side effects of this class of drugs.

The therapeutic effects of the TCAs result from blockade of presynaptic serotonin and norepinephrine reuptake transporters. Blockade of histamine receptors results in drowsiness and sedation, an effect similar to the sedation seen after administration of the classic antihistamine *diphenhydramine* (Benadryl). Blockade of acetylcholine receptors results in confusion, memory and cognitive impairments, dry mouth, blurred vision, increased heart rate, and urinary retention. In general, nortriptyline and desipramine are reasonable choices for initial treatment of depression when therapy with a TCA is chosen. These two TCAs cause less sedation and exert fewer anticholinergic side effects, such as cognitive impairment, than most other TCAs. Moreover, nortriptyline is known to have a therapeutic range, or window: the maximum response is most likely at blood drug concentrations between 0.05 and 0.15 micrograms per milliliter, although such measurement is uncommon in clinical practice.

Pharmacokinetics. The TCAs are well absorbed when administered orally. Because most of them have relatively long half-lives (see Table 12.1), taking them at bedtime can reduce the impact of unwanted side effects, especially persistent sedation. These drugs are metabolized in the liver. As discussed earlier, two TCAs (imipramine and amitriptyline) are converted into pharmacologically active intermediates (desmethylimitramine and nortriptyline, respectively) that are detoxified later. This combination of a pharmacologically active drug and active metabolite results in a clinical effect lasting up to 4 days, even longer in elderly patients (who can be adversely affected by the detrimental cognitive effects of these drugs).

TCAs readily cross the placental barrier. However, in utero exposure does not affect global IQ, language development, or behavioral development in preschool children. No fetal abnormalities from these drugs have yet been reported.

Pharmacological Effects. All the TCAs attach to and inhibit (to varying degrees) the presynaptic transporter proteins for both norepinephrine and serotonin, which is thought to account for their therapeutic efficacy. The TCAs, however, have three clinical limitations. First, they are claimed to have a slow onset of action, although overall, TCAs seem to start acting as fast as any other antidepressant drug, provided that comparable dosage strategies can be tolerated. Second, the TCAs exert a wide variety of effects on the CNS, causing numerous adverse side effects that the SSRIs do not cause. Third, in overdosage (as in suicide attempts), TCAs are cardiotoxic and potentially fatal because they can cause cardiac arrhythmias.

Because TCAs do not produce euphoria, they have no recreational or addictive liability. Therefore, abuse and psychological dependence are not concerns. The clinical choice of TCA is determined by effectiveness, tolerance of side effects, prior good response, family history of good response, and duration of action of the particular agent.

In depressed patients, TCAs elevate mood, increase physical activity, improve appetite and sleep patterns, and reduce morbid preoccupation. They are useful in treating acute episodes of major depression as well as in preventing relapses. Some patients resistant to other antidepressants respond favorably to a TCA. In addition, TCAs are clinically effective in the long-term therapy of dysthymia and in treating bipolar depression (as an adjunct to a mood stabilizer), although the SSRIs are equally efficacious and better tolerated.

TCAs are effective analgesics in a variety of clinical pain syndromes; they are consistently superior to placebo in the treatment of chronic pain. Uses include diabetes-associated peripheral neuropathies, post-herpetic neuralgia, migraine headache, fibromyalgia, chronic back pain, myofascial pain, and chronic fatigue. The antidepressant action may not only provide analgesic relief, but also promote well-being and improve affect as it reduces physical discomfort. One review compared the analgesic effect of three types of antidepressants, and it concluded that the TCAs were slightly more efficacious than the selective norepinephrine reuptake inhibitors (SNRIs), which were more analgesic than the selective serotonin reuptake inhibitors (Sindrup et al., 2005).

Side Effects. Side effects follow from the anticholinergic, antihistaminic, and antiadrenergic actions. In the patient on long-term TCA therapy, tolerance may develop to many of these side effects, but some will persist. Often, choosing a particular TCA with an awareness of its side effects can turn a disadvantage into a therapeutic advantage. For example, amitriptyline and doxepin are the most sedating of the TCAs, making them useful in treating people with comorbid depression and insomnia. Administering one of these drugs at bedtime would provide both the antidepressant effect and the needed sedation. Recently, *doxepin* was formulated in a very low dose and marketed as Silenor. This formulation (3 or 6 mg of doxepin) is about 50-times the price of 10 mg preparations of generic doxepin (Patel and Goldman-Levine, 2011). It has been shown effective in older adults with insomnia, less so in younger adults.

The effects of TCAs on memory and cognitive function are significant. The direct adverse effects on cognition are related to the anticholinergic and antihistaminic properties of the drugs, which may be partly compensated for by the improvement in mood. Relatively nonsedating compounds with minimal anticholinergic side effects cause less impairment of psychomotor or memory functions. Therefore, because the young and the elderly may be more susceptible to the anticholinergic-induced impairment of memory, patients at the extremes of age, if treated with TCAs, should probably receive a drug with low potency at blocking histaminic and cholinergic receptors.

As already noted, cardiac effects can be life threatening when an overdose is taken, as in suicide attempts. The patient commonly exhibits excitement, delirium, and convulsions, followed by respiratory depression and coma, which can persist for several days. Cardiac arrhythmias can lead to ventricular fibrillation, cardiac arrest, and death. Thus, all TCAs can be lethal in doses that are commonly available to depressed patients. For this reason, it is unwise to dispense more than a week's supply of an antidepressant to an acutely depressed patient.

There have been reports of about 12 cases of sudden death in children receiving desipramine for the treatment of attention deficit/hyperactivity disorder (ADHD) or depression. These deaths are cause for concern when using TCAs to treat depression in children, and the therapeutic efficacy of TCAs in treating major depression in children is questionable anyway (see Chapter 15). In cases where efficacy is more demonstrable—enuresis (bed-wetting), obsessive-compulsive disorder (OCD), and ADHD—use may be appropriate, but caution is warranted.

Monoamine Oxidase Inhibitors

Monoamine oxidase (MAO) is an enzyme that regulates the amount of monoamine neurotransmitters (norepinephrine, dopamine, and serotonin) in the body and the brain. Drug-induced inhibition of MAO (by *MAO-inhibitors*, or MAOI) allows monoamine transmitters to accumulate within the end-terminals of neurons. Such blockade of monamine metabolism causes transmitter molecules to build up in the terminal, which means that more transmitter than usual is released into the synaptic cleft upon activation. Such accumulation results in robust antidepressant action, resulting in the most *efficacious* antidepressants ever developed. Such efficacy, however, has been limited by potentially serious, even fatal, side effects. Multiple fatalities have limited the widespread clinical utility of these drugs.

Three monoamine oxidase inhibitors were developed in the mid-1950s for treating major depressive illnesses (see Table 12.1). Because of toxicity, none of the three have been in much use for several years. However, one of these, *isocarboxazid* (Marplan, marketed in 1959), which disappeared in 1994 when the FDA required additional data to maintain commercial availability, has recently reappeared under a new trade name (Enerzer). It likely will have limited use, although recent trials are unavailable.

The use of the three traditional MAOIs is limited by potentially fatal interactions when taken with certain foods and medicines. Medicines include adrenalinelike drugs found in nasal sprays, antiasthma medications, and cold medicines. Foods include those that contain tyramine, a by-product of fermentation, such as in many cheeses, wines, beers, liver, and some beans. Tyramine induces release of monoamine neurotransmitter, both elevating mood[3], but also increasing blood pressure. Too much tyramine release can elevate blood pressure to extreme levels, resulting in a heart attack or rupture of an aneurism or vascular malformation, either possibly resulting in death. Because MAO is also found in the gastrointestinal tract, inhibition of the enzyme blocks the metabolism of dietary tyramine, with increased absorption of the compound. In the absence of MAO, tyramine may modestly elevate blood pressure; in patients on MAOIs, such elevation may be extreme. Nevertheless, although they are potentially dangerous, MAOIs can be used safely with strict dietary restrictions.[4]

Interest in MAOIs has remained strong because: (1) they can be as safe as SSRIs; (2) they can work in many patients who respond poorly to both TCAs and SSRIs; and (3) they are particularly effective drugs for the treatment of atypical depression, masked depression (such as hypochondriasis), anorexia nervosa, bulimia, bipolar depression, dysthymia, depression in the elderly, panic disorder, and phobias. They just must be used with caution.

The three classic MAOIs are irreversible in their effect, since they form a chemical bond with the MAO enzyme that cannot be broken; enzyme function returns only as new enzyme is slowly biosynthesized. For this reason, patients who need to switch from an MAOI to another type of antidepressant must still observe the dietary restrictions and other precautions for approximately 10 to 14 days, until new enzyme is produced.

A few years ago, a specific MAO-A inhibitor (moclobemide) was developed that was reversible in action; it did not bond as tightly to the enzyme as the classic MAOIs. When detachment occurred, MAO was again able to metabolize the tyramine and the cardiotoxic risk was minimized. Unfortunately, although this was a logical approach for developing a better MAOI, moclobemide was not a very efficacious antidepressant.

Interest in the MAOIs has undergone recent resurgence because of the availability of a new selective, irreversible MAO-B inhibitor (*selegiline*, Eldapril), which increases dopamine neurotransmission in the brain. Initially, selegiline was used in the treatment

---

[3] Do we "feel better" after drinking red wine and eating tyramine-containing meats and cheeses?

[4] Multiple sites on the Web detail tyramine-free diets for use when MAOIs are prescribed.

of Parkinson disease (Fabbrini et al., 2012). Selegiline then became commercially available as a transdermal patch that allows for slow, continuous absorption (in this form, it was marketed under the new trade name Emsam). At the low doses absorbed across the skin, food and drug interactions were not a concern because transdermal administration bypasses the gastrointestinal tract and did not achieve blood concentrations sufficient to seriously elevate blood pressure.[5] As initially reported by Amsterdam (2003), selegiline (as a 6-milligram patch applied daily) was robustly effective in reducing moderate to severe depression, with onset of effect in only a few days. Sexual functioning was not impaired, and compliance was excellent. These initial positive results were confirmed in a long-term study in which patients with MDD who responded to selegiline during acute treatment (10 weeks) were either maintained on the drug or switched to placebo. After 52 weeks, significantly fewer patients taking selegiline relapsed (16.8 percent) compared with the placebo group (30.7 percent), and they did so after a significantly longer time on the drug than those given the placebo (Amsterdam and Bodkin, 2006). Pae and coworkers (2012) recently stated in their analysis of selegiline that "Very few patients reported a hypertensive effect, and there were no objectively confirmed reports of hypertensive crisis with food at any selegiline dose" (page 662). Therefore, for refractory patients with severe depression, transdermal selegiline may be unique in its efficacy.[6]

Atypical Antidepressants

Efforts from the late 1970s to the mid-1980s to find structurally different agents that might overcome some of the disadvantages of the TCAs (slow onset of action, limited efficacy, and significant side effects) and the MAOIs (hypertensive crises) produced the so-called heterocyclic, or *atypical*, antidepressants (Figure 12.5; see Table 12.1).

Maprotiline (Ludiomil), developed in the early 1980s, was one of the first clinically available antidepressants (other than the MAOIs) that modified the basic tricyclic structure (see Figure 12.5). It has a long half-life, blocks norepinephrine reuptake, and is as efficacious as imipramine (the gold standard of TCAs). However, it offers few, if any, therapeutic advantages. A major limitation of maprotiline is that it can cause seizures (although it rarely does), presumably because of the accumulation of active metabolites that excite the CNS. It is generally not an antidepressant of first choice.

Amoxapine (Ascendin) (see Figure 12.5), also introduced in the early 1980s, is the second atypical antidepressant, structurally different from the TCAs. It is primarily a norepinephrine reuptake inhibitor, clinically as effective as imipramine, although it may be slightly better at relieving accompanying anxiety and agitation. Amoxapine may produce parkinsonianlike side effects as a result of postsynaptic dopamine receptor blockade. The drug is metabolized to an active intermediate, 8-hydroxy-amoxapine, which may be responsible for the dopamine receptor blockade. As with TCAs, overdosage can result in fatality. Amoxapine is not generally an antidepressant of first choice.

---

[5] There is some evidence, however, that with the 9- and 12-milligram patches, the effect may be no different than with any other oral MAOI and dietary restrictions may again be needed.

[6] See also: Nandagopal and DelBello (2009).

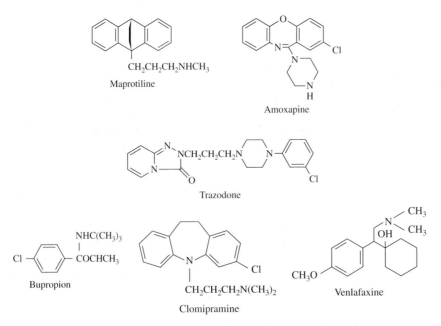

FIGURE 12.5 Chemical structures of six second-generation "atypical" antidepressants.

Trazodone (Desyrel), FDA-approved in 1981, is the third atypical antidepressant (see Figure 12.5), therapeutically as efficacious as the TCAs. However, it is not a potent reuptake blocker of either norepinephrine or serotonin, although its active metabolite, m-chlorophenyl-piperazine, is a serotonin agonist. Drowsiness is the most common side effect, and, until recently, the drug's main use was as an antidepressant sleeping pill. Taken at bedtime, in the 25–100-mg range, trazodone essentially blocks all $5HT_{2A}$ receptors (at 10 milligrams), and about half of the alpha-1 adrenergic receptors and histamine receptors, producing a good night's sleep. While about 50 percent of the serotonin transporters are also blocked at these doses that is not enough for an antidepressant action. Therefore, traditional trazodone, available as a short-acting immediate-release (IR) formulation, has often been used as a hypnotic (even though the FDA has not approved it for this indication). Its peak effect is reached and then declines relatively rapidly, and this "pulsatile" action is less likely to produce tolerance.

A new formulation of trazodone—an extended-release, once-daily preparation with the trade name Oleptro—was approved in 2010 for the treatment of MDD in adults. This formulation, in a dose of 300 milligrams, apparently provides sufficient constant blood levels for an antidepressant effect; tolerance gradually develops to the sedation over several days. With this pharmacokinetic modification, it may be possible to regain the antidepressant benefit of trazodone. Certainly, daytime sedation may be a continuing problem with this extended-release formulation of trazodone.

Trazodone's main side effect can be serious: in rare instances, priapism (prolonged and painful penile erection) occurs. This side effect requires prompt attention because it can lead to permanent impotence and infertility. Any detrimental effects of an overdose of trazodone on cognitive functioning appear modest.

Clomipramine (Anafranil) (see Figure 12.5) is structurally a TCA (see Figure 12.4), but it has a greater effect on serotonin reuptake than the classic TCAs. It is an effective antidepressant and anxiolytic. In addition, it and its active metabolite, desmethylclomipramine, also inhibit norepinephrine reuptake. Thus, it is classified as a *mixed serotonin-norepinephrine reuptake inhibitor,* similar to venlafaxine (discussed below). Clomipramine is approximately equal to the TCAs in both its efficacy and its profile of side effects.

Clomipramine has long been used to treat obsessive-compulsive disorder (OCD); about 40 to 75 percent of patients with OCD respond favorably. The drug has also been used in the treatment of panic disorder and phobic disorders. Historically, it was the first antidepressant medication to be appreciated as having efficacy in the treatment of anxiety disorders, an observation later applied to the SSRI-type antidepressants.

Psychostimulants, such as the *amphetamines* and *methylphenidates* release the neurotransmitters dopamine and norepinephrine from nerve terminals in the brain. They are occasionally examined for antidepressant efficacy (Howland, 2012). Widely used for over 60 years to treat attention-deficit hyperactivity disorder (ADHD), they promote alertness and reduce fatigue, both important features of depression. In low doses, their action is of rapid onset, and they are well tolerated with only modest side effects (see Chapter 15). However, they have to be prescribed carefully because of the potential for abuse and dependence. Despite this, psychostimulants are being reexamined for short-term use in treatment-resistant depression and perhaps in depression associated with palliative care and in the elderly (Candy et al., 2008; Parker and Brotchie, 2010; Abbasowa et al, 2013).

Bupropion (Wellbutrin, Zyban)(see Figure 12.5) is a reuptake inhibitor of the neurotransmitters dopamine and norepinephrine, potentiating the synaptic effects of these transmitters. Therefore, clinically they have effects similar to those exerted by the psychostimulants, but with a lower potential for abuse. Bupropion is without effect on serotonin neurons, and therefore it does not have the side effects associated with the use of SSRIs (discussed below).

Bupropion has several uses in medicine. It has been used to treat children with ADHD, although efficacy is not very robust. Under the trade name "Zyban", it is FDA-approved for use in smoking-cessation programs. Bupropion is also useful and quite widely used for the treatment of depression. Here, it has been used as mono-therapy, as an add-on (augmenting) therapy in patients only partially responsive or nonresponsive to SSRIs, and in patients with difficult-to-treat bipolar depression. It may also reduce the fatigue associated with depression (like the psychostimulants). Its therapeutic efficacy is comparable to that of the SSRIs, discussed next, but with a different profile of side effects (Gartiehner et al., 2011).

On the positive side, bupropion is devoid of the sexual side effects associated with use of the SSRIs, including loss of libido. In fact, the drug may actually enhance sexual functioning in both male and female patients. Unfortunately, used in combination with an SSRI (as augmentation therapy), this effect is less robust. Short-term treatment with long-acting *bupropion* (Wellbutrin SR) may result in weight loss; an advantage in patients for whom weight gain is a problem, although tolerance to this action appears to develop.

Perhaps the most bothersome side effects of bupropion include anxiety, restlessness, tremor, and insomnia. The dopaminergic actions can result in more serious anxiety disorders including the induction of psychosis *de novo*, similar to that seen in abusers of cocaine and methamphetamine. Seizures have been reported at higher doses. Bupropion is not effective in the treatment of panic disorder, and it may even exacerbate or precipitate panic in susceptible people.

Because bupropion and cocaine share similar mechanisms of action (blockade of dopamine reuptake), it's possible that bupropion exerts a reinforcing or dependency-inducing action. Although there are a few reports of snorting this drug, it does not seem to have a high abuse potential in humans, perhaps because of the occurrence of seizures (Kim and Steinhart, 2010). Because bupropion reinforces dopaminergic neurotransmission, it can exert a reinforcing action and has been tried in the treatment of abuse of other reinforcing drugs such as cocaine, methamphetamine, and especially nicotine.

Selective Serotonin Reuptake Inhibitors (SSRIs)

Six SSRIs have been available for 12 or more years, a seventh (*vilazodone*) was released in 2011, and the eighth (vortioxetine) was released in late 2013. Older SSRIs (Figure 12.6) include *fluoxetine* (Prozac), *paroxetine* (Paxil), *sertraline* (Zoloft), *fluvoxamine* (Luvox), *citalopram* (Celexa), and escitalopram (structure not shown because it is the optical isomer of citalopram).

These six drugs are all potent blockers of the presynaptic transporter for serotonin reuptake. The degree to which they block reuptake of other neurotransmitters, primarily norepinephrine, varies greatly, with more than a twelvefold difference between citalopram (the most selective for serotonin) and fluoxetine (the least selective for serotonin). More selectivity implies a more severe discontinuation syndrome and greater potential for inducing serotonin syndrome (both discussed below).

These SSRIs do not block postsynaptic serotonin receptors. Therefore, the primary acute neuronal effect of SSRIs is to make more serotonin available in the synaptic cleft, which activates all of the many postsynaptic receptors for serotonin. The action of serotonin at all its postsynaptic receptors is responsible for both their therapeutic actions and their serotonergic side effects.

Vilazodone (Viibryd) (see Figure 12.6) is claimed to have a "dual serotonin action" by inhibiting serotonin reuptake (SSRI) and by being a partial agonist (weak stimulant action) at the serotonin-1A (5-HT_{1A}) receptor. To date, despite theoretical advantages and additional expense, no therapeutic advantages over preexisting older agents (which, as generics, are much less expensive) have been demonstrated (Guay, 2012).

Vortioxetine (Brintellix) is claimed to be a "multi-modal" antidepressant. It inhibits serotonin reuptake, is an agonist of the serotonin-1A (5-HT_{1A}) receptor, a partial agonist of the serotonin-1B (5-HT_{1B}) receptor, and an antagonist of 5-HT_3, 5-HT_{1D}, and 5-HT_7 receptors. How each action translates into antidepressant action is unknown (Stahl et al., 2013). However, it is the first antidepressant to exhibit this combination of pharmacodynamics actions. Comparative studies with other antidepressants have not been published.

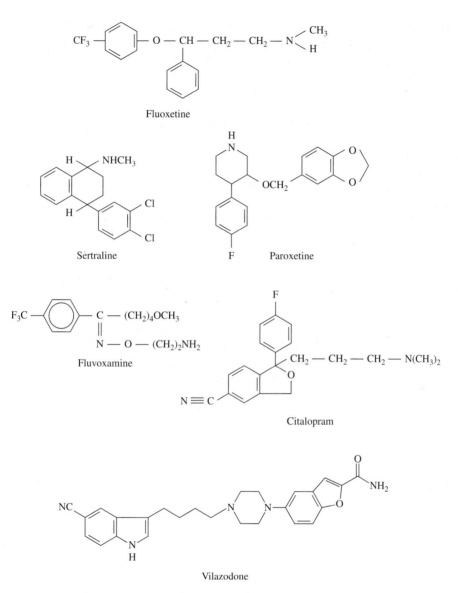

FIGURE 12.6 Chemical structures of six selective serotonin reuptake inhibitor (SSRI) antidepressants. Escitalopram is the active isomer of citalopram and is therefore not shown.

The current view is that increased serotonin availability at 5-HT$_{1A}$-type receptors is associated with antidepressant and anxiolytic effects, whereas increased serotonin availability at 5-HT$_2$-type and 5-HT$_3$-type receptors produces adverse effects. Increased 5-HT$_2$ receptor activity is associated with insomnia, anxiety, agitation, sexual dysfunction, and the production of a *serotonin syndrome* at higher doses (see below). Increased 5-HT$_3$

receptor activity is responsible for the nausea that these drugs can cause. Because of their receptor selectivity, SSRIs exert few anticholinergic or antihistaminic side effects. Most important, these drugs are not fatal in overdose because they are devoid of the cardiac toxicity produced by TCAs.

As a general statement, the clinical differences among individual SSRIs are minimal; all are equally effective and about as effective as older antidepressants (Undurraga and Baldessarini, 2012). As noted above, TCAs can be fatal in overdose and MAOIs are associated with hypertensive crises. SSRIs are not fatal in overdose. As a class, they have an efficacy of about 17 percent over placebo in clinical trials. This is not a huge improvement, but their popularity appears to be due to their perceived safety (despite side effects), ease of use, and broad clinical utility (anxiety and depression), rather than to well-demonstrated superior efficacy.

It has long been recognized that if a patients fails to respond to one SSRI, another might be tried, sometimes with improved response. This suggests some differences between drugs; the seven SSRIs are not necessarily interchangeable. Differences lie in individual pharmacokinetics (half-lives), receptor selectivity, and in effects that inhibit cytochrome P450 (CYP) drug-metabolizing enzymes in the liver (Table 12.2). Different SSRIs inhibit hepatic drug-metabolizing enzymes differently, and thereby differentially affect the metabolism of other drugs the patient may be taking. For example, fluoxetine, sertraline, and paroxetine are potent inhibitors of CPY2D6 while fluvoxamine markedly inhibits CYP1A2 and 2C19. Citalopram and escitalopram are very weak inhibitors of drug-metabolizing enzymes and may be safer to use when a patient is on multiple medications (Spina et al., 2008).

Approved therapeutic indications for SSRI therapy include major depression, dysthymia, and all the anxiety disorders (panic disorder, OCD, GAD, PTSD, phobias), although SSRIs also have benefit in other clinical situations. The conditions for which each of the newer drugs is currently FDA-approved are summarized in Table 12.3.

Before discussing individual SSRIs, we address several concerns associated with SSRI therapy:

- The treatment-resistant patient
- Serotonin syndrome

TABLE 12.2 Ability of SSRIs to inhibit various subtypes of CYP liver enzymes

Drug	CYP-450 1A2	CYP-450 2C9	CYP-450 2C19	CYP-450 2D6	CYP-450 3A4
Citalopram (Celexa)	0	0	0	+	0
Escitalopram (Lexapro)	0	0	0	+	0
Fluoxetine (Prozac)	+	+ +	+/+ +	+ + +	+/+ +
Paroxetine (Paxil)	+	+	+	+ + +	+
Sertraline (Zoloft)	+	+	+	+/+ +	+
Fluvoxamine (Luvox)	+	+ +	+ +	+ + +	+ +
Vilazodone (Viibryd)			+ +	+ +	

TABLE 12.3 FDA-approved indications for antidepressant medications

	ADHD	MDD	GAD	OCD	Panic	PTSD	Social anxiety	Bulimia	Premenstrual dysphoria	Smoking cessation	Diabetic neuropathy	Fibromyalgia
SSRI												
Fluoxetine		✓		✓	✓			✓	✓			
Sertraline		✓		✓	✓	✓	✓		✓			
Fluvoxamine				✓			✓(CR)					
Paroxetine		✓	✓	✓	✓	✓	✓		✓(CR)			
Citalopram		✓										
Escitalopram		✓	✓									
Vilazodone		✓										
SSNRI												
Duloxetine		✓	✓								✓	
Venlafaxine		✓	✓(XR)		✓(XR)		✓(XR)					
Mirtazepine		✓										
Desvenlafaxine		✓										
Milnacepran												✓
SNRI												
Atomoxetine	✓											
NDRI												
Bupropion		✓								✓		

SSRI = selective serotonin reuptake inhibitor
SSNRI = selective serotonin norepinephrine reuptake inhibitor
SNRI = selective norepinephrine reuptake inhibitor
NDRI = norepinephrine dopamine reuptake inhibitor
CR = controlled-release formulation
XR = extended-release formulation

- The SSRI discontinuation syndrome
- SSRI-induced sexual dysfunction

A fifth issue, the possible fetal effects if the mother takes the SSRI during pregnancy or while breast-feeding, is discussed in Chapter 15.

The Treatment-Resistant Patient

Many, if not most, patients either fail to respond or only partially respond to a trial of SSRI medication. This can be due to several reasons including inadequate dose or inadequate length of treatment. It might also be the result of administration to a "rapid metabolizer" such that therapeutic blood concentrations are not achieved. Guidelines to improve partial- or non-responders include the following: increase the dose of antidepressant, switch to a different antidepressant, augment with a non-antidepressant (such as a mood stabilizer or atypical antipsychotic drug), or add a second antidepressant to the original drug (Garcia-Toro et al., 2012).

Serotonin Syndrome

High doses of an SSRI or the combination of an SSRI plus another serotonergic drug can induce the disturbing reaction termed the *serotonin syndrome*. Accumulation of serotonin leads to a cluster of responses, characterized by cognitive disturbances (disorientation, confusion, hypomania), behavioral agitation and restlessness, autonomic nervous system dysfunctions (fever, shivering, chills, sweating, diarrhea, hypertension, tachycardia), and neuromuscular impairment (ataxia, increased reflexes, myoclonus). Visual hallucinations have even been reported. Some of these symptoms might result from excess serotonin at 5-HT$_2$ receptors, the site of action of the psychedelic drug LSD. There is a positive relationship between the specificity of the SSRI for blocking the 5-HT transporter and the likelihood of producing the syndrome. For example, *paroxetine* (Paxil) is one of the most specific SSRIs, and it is perhaps the SSRI most implicated in causing the serotonin syndrome.

In theory, any drug that has the net effect of increasing serotonin function can produce the syndrome; usually, however, it results from the combination of an SSRI and other serotonergic drugs, especially since these drugs can inhibit each other's metabolic detoxification and potentiate each other's effects. The syndrome can even occur when SSRIs are combined with herbal substances such as St. John's wort or valerian. Once the drugs are discontinued, the syndrome usually resolves within 24 to 48 hours; during this time, support is the primary treatment.

SSRI Discontinuation Syndrome

A discontinuation syndrome occurs in perhaps 60 percent of SSRI-treated patients following abrupt cessation of drug intake. This SSRI discontinuation syndrome was originally associated with abrupt cessation of paroxetine, but it can occur following discontinuation of any SSRI, although it is least likely with fluoxetine because of the drug's long half-life. Onset of the syndrome is usually within a few days and persists perhaps

3 to 4 weeks. There are six core sets of somatic signs and symptoms represented by the mnemonic "FINISH" (Muzina, 2010):

1. **F**lulike symptoms (fatigue, lethargy, myalgias, chills, headache)
2. **I**nsomnia (sleep disturbances, vivid dreams)
3. **N**ausea (gastrointestinal symptoms, vomiting, diarrhea)
4. **I**mbalance (dizziness, vertigo, ataxia)
5. **S**ensory disturbances (sensation of electric shocks in the arms, legs, or head)
6. **H**yperarousal (anxiety, agitation)

Other, less frequently reported symptoms of SSRI discontinuation syndrome include hyperactivity, depersonalization, depressed mood, and memory problems (confusion, decreased concentration, and slowed thinking). The dual-action antidepressants (discussed later), venlafaxine (Effexor), and duloxetine (Cymbalta), because of their serotoninergic action, can also produce this discontinuation syndrome.

Risk factors for antidepressant discontinuation symptoms include abrupt termination of the antidepressant (or noncompliance or drug holidays), short half-life of the drug, long treatment duration, female gender, pregnancy, younger age, newborn infants of mothers who have been on antidepressants (see Chapter 15), and vulnerability to depressive relapse.

All the somatic and psychological phenomena abate over time and obviously disappear when the SSRI is restarted. It is believed that the syndrome results from a relative deficiency of serotonin when the SSRI is stopped; however, the exact mechanism may be more complex. Therefore, tapering of all antidepressants that are being discontinued is recommended.

SSRI-Induced Sexual Dysfunction

Sexual dysfunction is often associated with major depressive disorder, and SSRI medications can further compound it (Schweitzer et al., 2009). Up to 80 percent of depressed patients treated with SSRIs exhibit sexual dysfunction, including problems with orgasm, erection, sexual interest, desire, and psychological arousal. In males, ejaculatory dysfunction seems most prominent. Loss of desire and sexual dysfunction can affect medication compliance and impair interpersonal relationships. Treatment of sexual dysfunction may involve discontinuation of the SSRI and switching to an antidepressant in another class (for example bupropion). *Sildenafil* (Viagra) has been found useful for some patients, including females (Nurnberg et al., 2008).

Additional Side Effects of SSRIs

In addition to the specific issues described above, there are several other notable consequences of long-term antidepressant use:

- *Suicidality*. A review of FDA trials in pediatric and adolescent patients indicated that antidepressants increased the risk of suicidal ideation/behavior. In 2005, the FDA required that manufacturers include a warning in product labeling, recommending

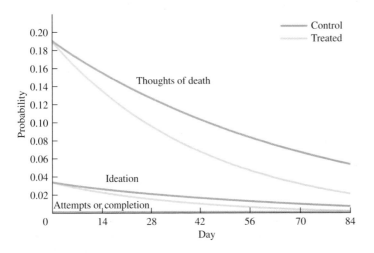

FIGURE 12.7   Probabilities of suicide risk in adult and geriatric fluoxetine and venlafaxine studies. Dark blue lines indicate estimated probabilities for control patients receiving placebo; light blue lines, estimated probabilities for treated patients; thoughts of death curves, "wishes he or she were dead or any thoughts of possible death to self" or worse; ideation curves, "suicide ideas or gestures" or worse; and attempts or completion curves, "suicide attempts or suicides." [Data from Gibbons et al., 2012, Figure 1, page 583.]

that young patients be monitored for the occurrence of suicidality. After that, the number of prescriptions for youth fell dramatically, followed by an *increase* in adolescent suicide. In 2007, the FDA extended the suicidality warning to young adults aged 18 to 24, with the emphasis that depression itself may lead to suicide and that anyone started on antidepressants should be monitored for worsening symptoms. The use of antidepressants in children and adolescents is discussed further in Chapter 15. In adults as well as geriatric patients, suicidal risk lessens as depression severity decreases, the antidepressant reducing suicide risk as well as depression severity (Figure 12.7).

- *Sleep Disturbance.* SSRIs interfere with sleep function, although these difficulties vary among the agents. They may produce insomnia with sleep fragmentation (episodes of awakening).

- *Apathy.* Although uncommon, lack of motivation and apathy have been reported in children and adults treated with SSRIs.

- *Physiological Symptoms.* A variety of physiological symptoms have been reported with SSRIs. *Hyponatremia* (serum sodium concentration below 130 mEq/L) may occur within the first few weeks of treatment but will resolve after discontinuation. Symptoms include nausea, headache, lethargy, muscle cramps, seizures, coma, and possibly respiratory arrest. In adults over 50 years of age, SSRI use may slightly increase the risk of sustaining *fractures* in a fall and of osteoporosis (Eom et al., 2012). SSRIs increase the risk of *gastrointestinal bleeding and easy bruising*, although this is magnified by the use of certain nonsteroidal anti-inflammatory agents, such as aspirin. Both agents inhibit platelet aggregation (Bismuth-Evenzal et al., 2012). Rare cases of *cardiovascular problems*, such as arrhythmias, prolonged QTc intervals, and cardiovascular depressant effects, have been reported (Cooke and Waring, 2013). Indeed, the FDA has warned that citalopram should not be used in doses exceeding 40 mg daily; Vieweg and coworkers (2012) have refuted this statement.

Specific SSRIs

Fluoxetine.   *Fluoxetine* (Prozac) (see Figure 12.6) became clinically available in the United States in 1988 as the first SSRI-type antidepressant and the first non-TCA that could be considered a first-line antidepressant. Fluoxetine's efficacy is comparable to that of the TCAs, with few or no anticholinergic or antihistaminic side effects.

Besides major depression, fluoxetine has been used in the treatment of dysthymia, bulimia (an eating disorder), alcohol withdrawal, and virtually all the various subtypes of anxiety disorders. Specific formulations of fluoxetine, sertraline, and paroxetine have been shown to be effective in relieving the symptoms of a controversial syndrome termed *premenstrual dysphoric disorder.* For this use, the manufacturer of Prozac marketed fluoxetine under the trade name Sarafem.

Fluoxetine has a half-life of about 2 to 3 days, but its active metabolite (*norfluoxetine,* which is an even stronger reuptake inhibitor than fluoxetine) has a half-life of about 6 to 10 days. This prolonged action distinguishes fluoxetine from other SSRIs, which have half-lives of about 1 day and no active intermediates. Also because of its long half-life, fluoxetine need not be administered every day; it can be taken as infrequently as once a week, and a once-weekly oral formulation of fluoxetine is commercially available under the trade name *Prozac Weekly*.

As with all SSRIs, fluoxetine's antidepressant action is of slow onset (about 4 to 6 weeks), and the drug and its metabolite thus tend to accumulate with repeated doses over about 2 months, presumably because levels of both compounds continue to increase. This action can explain not only the slow onset of peak therapeutic effect but also the late onset of side effects and the prolonged duration of action following drug discontinuation. Therapeutic trials with fluoxetine should continue for at least 8 weeks before the drug is determined to be ineffective. Significant and important side effects of fluoxetine include anxiety, agitation, and insomnia, and the serotonin syndrome. As discussed, sexual dysfunction is common.

Fluoxetine, sertraline, paroxetine, and fluvoxamine inhibit certain of the drug-metabolizing enzymes in the liver (see Table 12.2). Therefore, coadministration of any of these four drugs can increase the level of other drugs that the patient might be taking.

In 2004, the FDA-approved a novel combination of fluoxetine and olanzapine (an atypical antipsychotic) for the treatment of depressive episodes associated with bipolar disorder. The trade name of the combination product is Symbyax. One review supports the benefit of this combination in treatment-resistant depression (Bobo and Shelton, 2009), although it produced greater increases in body weight, prolactin, and total cholesterol than either of the two agents independently or a combination of fluoxetine plus an atypical antipsychotic (e.g., aripiprazole) with less potential for weight gain.

Sertraline. *Sertraline* (Zoloft) (see Figure 12.6) was the second SSRI approved for clinical use in the United States. Clinically, like all SSRIs, it is as effective as TCAs in the treatment of major depression and dysthymia, and it has fewer side effects and improved patient compliance (Ravindran et al., 2000).

Sertraline is four to five times more potent than fluoxetine in blocking serotonin reuptake and is more selective. Because of increased selectivity, serotonin-associated side effects (serotonin syndrome and serotonin discontinuation syndrome) may be more intense than with fluoxetine. Steady-state levels of the drug in plasma are achieved within 4 to 7 days, and its metabolites are much less pharmacologically active. Like all SSRIs, sertraline has few anticholinergic, antihistaminic, and adverse cardiovascular effects, as well as a low risk of toxicity in overdose.

Paroxetine. *Paroxetine* (Paxil) (see Figure 12.6) was the third SSRI to become available in the United States for clinical use in treating major depression, dysthymia, various anxiety disorders, and premenstrual dysphoric disorder. The FDA has also approved paroxetine for treating generalized anxiety disorder (GAD), although this capability is probably shared by all SSRIs. Like sertraline, paroxetine is more selective than fluoxetine in blocking serotonin reuptake. The drug's metabolic half-life is about 24 hours, and steady state is achieved in about 7 days; its metabolites are relatively inactive.

Paroxetine is perhaps the SSRI most associated with serotonin syndrome, serotonin discontinuation syndrome, new onset or precipitation of psychosis, paranoid ideations, temper dyscontrol, delusions, and even visual hallucinations. In 2006, it was reported that the use of paroxetine was associated with a small but statistically significant increase in the risk of cleft lip/palate deformities in newborns of women who took the drug during their pregnancy. In December 2006, the American College of Obstetricians and Gynecologists published a position statement that paroxetine probably should not be used during pregnancy (see Chapter 15).

Fluvoxamine. *Fluvoxamine* (Luvox) is a structural derivative of fluoxetine (see Figure 12.6). Like all SSRIs, fluvoxamine has well-described antidepressant properties, comparable in efficacy to the TCA imipramine, but fewer serious side effects and superior patient compliance. It has been shown effective in the treatment of all anxiety disorders. The FDA approved an extended-release formulation of this drug (Luvox CR) in 2008 for the treatment of social anxiety disorder and OCD in adult patients.

Citalopram. *Citalopram* (Celexa) (see Figure 12.6) is an SSRI available in Europe since 1989 and introduced into the United States in 1998 as the fifth SSRI. Citalopram was claimed to have a more rapid onset of action than fluoxetine, but this observation is probably overstated. Efficacy was also likely overstated, with the drug being only modestly more effective than placebo-treatment (Apler, 2011). As discussed above, high doses of citalopram have been associated with ECG irregularities and rare fatalities. It has a lower incidence of inhibition of drug-metabolizing hepatic enzymes, so it might be better for patients who are taking multiple medications.

Citalopram is well absorbed orally; peak plasma levels are reached in about 4 hours. Steady state is achieved in about 1 week, and maximal effects are seen in about 5 to 6 weeks. The elimination half-life is about 33 hours, enabling once-per-day dosing. The elderly have a reduced ability to metabolize citalopram; for older people, a 33 to 50 percent reduction in dose is necessary.

Citalopram has been reported to moderately reduce alcohol consumption in problem alcoholics. Citalopram might be expected to exert anxiolytic effects similar to those exerted by other SSRIs. Adverse effects of citalopram resemble those of other SSRIs.

Escitalopram. *Escitalopram* (Lexapro) was released in the United States in 2002 for the treatment of major depression. It is also approved for the treatment of GAD. The drug is the therapeutically active isomer (mirror-image molecule) of citalopram. As an active isomer, the major difference is potency: escitalopram is twice as potent as citalopram, so the prescribed dose is 50 percent of the dose of citalopram. In other words, 10 milligrams of escitalopram is equivalent to 20 milligrams of citalopram. Wade and coworkers (2011) noted that while a dose of 20 mg (comparable to 40 mg of citalopram) was marginally effective in treating depression, doses to 50 mg were very effective in achieving remission, with 40 to 50 percent of patients eventually reaching remission over a 12 week study period (Figure 12.8). No cardiac complications were observed, even though doses were increased to as much as 50 mg daily.

Vilazodone. As discussed above, *vilazodone* (Viibryd) (see Figure 12.6) is an SSRI that is also a weak stimulant at 5-HT$_{1A}$ receptors. Modest SSRI-like efficacy has been demonstrated, but comparative studies with any active antidepressant (e.g., another SSRI) have not been reported (Reinhold, et al., 2012; Singh and Schwartz, 2012). Claims of more rapid onset of action and less sexual side effects have not been verified.

Vortioxetine. *Vortioxetine* (Brintellix) is a multi-modal SSRI that exerts several different actions at various serotonin receptor subtypes. Short-term, non-comparative tri-

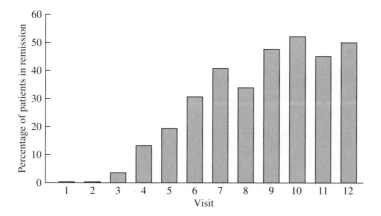

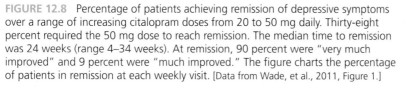

FIGURE 12.8 Percentage of patients achieving remission of depressive symptoms over a range of increasing citalopram doses from 20 to 50 mg daily. Thirty-eight percent required the 50 mg dose to reach remission. The median time to remission was 24 weeks (range 4–34 weeks). At remission, 90 percent were "very much improved" and 9 percent were "much improved." The figure charts the percentage of patients in remission at each weekly visit. [Data from Wade, et al., 2011, Figure 1.]

als have been reported with low doses (2.5–5.0 mg daily) being ineffective (Jain et al., 2013) and higher doses (10–20 mg daily) likely effective. Like other SSRIs, vortioxetine was effective in the treatment of generalized anxiety disorder (Rothschild et al., 2012).

Dual-Action Antidepressants

Historically, the TCAs were the first dual-action antidepressants: they block the presynaptic reuptake of both norepinephrine and serotonin, but side effects limited their widespread use. The unitary action of the SSRIs, while associated with efficacy against a wide variety of anxiety and depressive disorders, is limited by side effects common to serotonin overactivity. Vilazodone does not overcome these SSRI-related problems. Therefore, attempts have been made to expand on the concept that actions at two different synaptic sites may improve or maintain efficacy while limiting side effects. Most attempts to develop a dual-action antidepressant have resulted in medicines that inhibit the active presynaptic reuptake of both serotonin and norepinephrine. *Venlafaxine* and its active metabolite *desvenlafaxine* followed the TCAs and are protypes of this action.

Nefazodone

Nefazodone (Serzone) (see Figure 12.9) is a dual-action antidepressant chemically related to trazodone (see Figure 12.5) but with some important pharmacological distinctions. Nefazodone's strongest pharmacological action is 5-HT$_2$ receptor blockade, which distinguishes it from the SSRIs; however, it also inhibits both serotonin and norepinephrine reuptake at its therapeutic dose. Nefazodone, however, can produce liver failure at a rate about three to four times greater than that in the general population, resulting in death or necessitating liver transplantation. The drug was removed from the market in Canada in 2004, and although it is still available in generic formulations in the United States, it is little used.

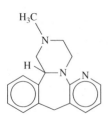
Mirtazepine (Remeron)

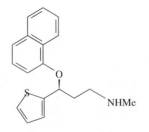
Duloxetine (Cymbalta)

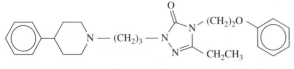
Nefazodone (Serzone)

FIGURE 12.9 Chemical structures of three dual-action antidepressants.

Milnacipran

Milnacipran (Savella) is another drug that blocks norepinephrine and serotonin reuptake It is FDA-approved for the treatment of fibromyalgia. Perhaps uniquely, milnacepram blocks NMDA-type glutamate receptors in the spinal cord, contributing to analgesic action (Kohno et al., 2012). Used in many countries as an antidepressant, such use has not been FDA-approved in this country. The approval of milnacepram for fibromyalgia in 2009 was the third such approval for a drug for this disorder (following pregabalin and duloxetine). Milnacipran reduces the chronic pain associated with fibromyalgia with concomitant improvements in global well-being, fatigue, and other domains of the disorder.

Venlafaxine

Venlafaxine (Effexor) (see Figure 12.5) is classified as a mixed *serotonin-norepinephrine reuptake inhibitor*. The serotonin blockade occurs at lower doses than does the norepinephrine blockade, and at higher doses venlafaxine also inhibits the reuptake of dopamine. Venlafaxine lacks anticholinergic or antihistaminic effects, a distinct advantage. On the other hand, it was reported that, while the response and remission rates to venlafaxine XR were the same as to bupropion XL, venlafaxine produced significantly more sexual side effects (Thase et al., 2006). Some evidence also suggests that venlafaxine may be more likely than other antidepressants to trigger a manic state in people who are taking the drug as treatment for bipolar depression. This suggests a possibility that venlafaxine might precipitate agitated or aggressive behavior in some patients.

Concern was raised about venlafaxine's known association with blood pressure elevation in some 3 to 4 percent of patients using the sustained-release formulation and 2 to 13 percent of those taking the immediate-release preparation. Essentially, higher overdose fatality rates were seen according to studies using population datasets. In December 2006, the U.S. manufacturer issued a warning stating that prescriptions for venlafaxine should be written for the smallest quantity of capsules consistent with good patient management, in order to reduce the risk of overdose. However, in 2010, a large population study from the United Kingdom looked at the sudden cardiac death, or near death, rate of new users (18 to 89 years old) of several antidepressants. The results found no association of venlafaxine, used for either depression or anxiety, with increased cardiac risk over a period of 3.3 years (Martinez et al., 2010).

In an extended-release formulation *venlafaxine* (Effexor XR) is FDA-approved for the treatment of GAD as well as panic and social anxiety. Venlafaxine appears to have only minimal effects on drug-metabolizing enzymes, and drug interactions are few. Venlafaxine's primary metabolite, desvenlafaxine, is pharmacologically active; the half-lives of the parent compound and the primary metabolite are 5 hours and 11 hours, respectively.

Desvenlafaxine

In 2008, desvenlafaxine was approved for the treatment of MDD under the brand name Pristiq (Pae et al., 2009). As stated above, desvenlafaxine is the active metabolite of venlafaxine. Therefore, it has the antidepressant efficacy, safety, and tolerability, of venlafaxine (Ferguson et al., 2012). With an 11-hour half-life, it requires only once-daily dosing. Desvenlafaxine has also been shown to reduce the frequency and severity of hot flashes in postmenopausal women; but in 2011 the FDA refused approval for this use.

Duloxetine

Duloxetine (Cymbalta) (see Figure 12.9) is another dual-action antidepressant that binds to and blocks the reuptake transporters for norepinephrine and serotonin. The blockade seems to be more complete than that of *venlafaxine* (Bymaster et al., 2005). Duloxetine seems to be mildly effective in the treatment of both depression and anxiety. Cipriani and coworkers (2012), however, found evidence of superiority over other antidepressants to be underwhelming. Hellerstein and coworkers (2012) recently reported duloxetine useful in the acute treatment (10-week) of chronic nonmajor depression, including dysthymic disorder.

Duloxetine has been reported to significantly reduce physical symptoms of pain (such as backaches, headache, muscle and joint pain, and back and shoulder pain), to reduce interference with daily activities, and to reduce time in pain while awake. This drug has been approved for the management of neuropathic pain associated with diabetic peripheral neuropathy and fibromyalgia. There is also evidence that this agent may induce a manic or hypomanic episode in patients with bipolar disorder (Peritogiannis et al., 2009). Duloxetine is also FDA-approved for the treatment of generalized anxiety disorder.

The half-life of duloxetine is about 12 hours, allowing once-daily dosing. Nausea is the most common side effect. Weight gain and sexual dysfunction have not yet been problems with the drug (Clayton et al., 2012). Elevations in blood pressure (hypertension), theorized to be possible with duloxetine, has not yet been a major problem in clinical studies.

Mirtazepine

Mirtazepine (Remeron) (see Figure 12.9) was introduced into clinical use in the United States in 1997. The drug is clinically effective, and its antidepressant action may be more rapid than that achieved with other antidepressants (Watanabe et al., 2011). Overall, mirtazepine is a dual-action antidepressant that increases the presynaptic release of both norepinephrine and serotonin through several actions:

- It blocks central alpha$_2$ autoreceptors. By blocking adrenergic autoreceptors, it causes an increase in the release of norepinephrine.

- It blocks adrenergic heteroceptors located on the terminals of serotonin-releasing neurons, where they normally inhibit the release of serotonin. When these adrenergic heteroceptors are blocked, 5-HT neurons release more serotonin.

- The increased release of serotonin stimulates only 5-HT$_1$ receptors because 5-HT$_2$- and 5-HT$_3$-type receptors are specifically blocked by mirtazepine.

Although complicated, this mechanism explains how mirtazepine enhances both norepinephrine and serotonin neurotransmission. Because mirtazepine is a potent antagonist of postsynaptic 5-HT$_2$ and 5-HT$_3$ receptors, it does not produce the side effects of SSRIs (especially anxiety, insomnia, agitation, nausea, and sexual dysfunction).

Mirtazepine is also a potent blocker of histamine receptors, and drowsiness is a prominent and often therapeutically limiting side effect. Sedation may be advantageous in depressed patients with symptoms of anxiety and insomnia, a common occurrence. Because of the drowsiness, the drug is best taken at bedtime and probably should not be combined with alcohol or other CNS depressants.

Other side effects of mirtazepine include increased appetite and weight gain. The drug may therefore be advantageous in certain situations, such as in the treatment of patients with anorexia, in patients with wasting diseases (for example, cancers and AIDS), and in the elderly where bedtime sedation and maintenance of body weight are a goal.

Mirtazepine is rapidly absorbed orally; peak blood levels occur 2 hours after administration. The elimination half-life is 20 to 40 hours, allowing once-a-day administration, usually at bedtime to maximize sleep and minimize daytime sedation.

Selective Norepinephrine Reuptake Inhibitors

Until recently, no antidepressant exhibited specific norepinephrine reuptake blockade in the absence of dopamine (bupropion) or serotonin (venlafaxine, duloxetine) reuptake blockade. Then two agents, *reboxetine* (Vestra) and *atomoxetine* (Strattera), were developed as selective norepinephrine reuptake inhibitors (NRIs). Unfortunately, in two separate clinical trials, reboxetine was not found to have any greater effect than placebo, and it was found to be ineffective as an antidepressant (Eyding et al., 2010). *Atomoxetine* became commercially available in 2003 as the first nonstimulant drug to be approved by the FDA for the treatment of ADHD in children, adolescents, and adults. It is claimed to be as effective as methylphenidate, probably without abuse potential. The use of atomoxetine in children and adolescents is discussed in Chapter 15.

Atomoxetine has also been examined as an antidepressant. In persons with ADHD, the drug was efficacious and improved quality of life and executive functioning (Durell et al., 2013). This implies potential use in patients with comorbid ADHD and depressive symptoms.

STAR*D Study

While basic research continues to improve our understanding of the pathophysiology of depressive disorders and the mechanisms of action of antidepressants, progress has been much slower in the clinical management of depression. A nationwide clinical trial, the Sequenced Treatment Alternatives to Relieve Depression (STAR*D) study, was conducted at a cost of $35M over a six-year period ending in 2006. The aim was to identify specific treatment strategies that would improve the long-term outcome of people with depressive disorder. The study started with almost 3,000 patients at 41 clinical sites. Patients were started on citalopram at standard doses. The primary outcome was remission; patients not responding were offered a medication switch, combination, or augmentation strategies. No placebo group was included and augmentation strategies did not include the atypical antipsychotics that are today FDA-approved for the treatment of resistant depression (quetiapine and aripiprazole). Switch options included sertraline, bupropion-SR, or venlafaxine-XR; add-on options included either bupropion-SR or buspirone. An option for cognitive treatment was also offered. Participants who became symptom-free continued with the treatment in a follow-up period; participants who did not or who experienced intolerable side effects could continue on to other options, including mirtazepine or nortriptyline (a TCA) for up to 14 weeks.

Finally, participants who had not become symptom-free were taken off all other medications and randomly switched to one of two treatments, the MAOI tranylcypromine or the combination of extended-release venlafaxine with mirtazepine.

Results

Only about 30 percent of patients placed on citalopram reached "remission," and about 10 to 15 percent more were "responders," who did not achieve remission but whose symptoms decreased to at least half of what they had been at the start of the trial. On average, it took nearly 6 weeks for a participant to respond and nearly 7 weeks to achieve remission. With a historical response to placebo usually around 20 to 25 percent, these results were very discouraging because they documented the poor efficacy of the chosen SSRI to achieve significant therapeutic benefits.

Of the nonresponders, 51 percent agreed to switch their medication, 39 percent agreed to receive "medication augmentation"; the rest received cognitive behavioral therapy (CBT). About 25 percent of the participants who switched became symptom-free. This result was the same for each of the three medication groups: no one drug was best, none worked more quickly than another, and there was no difference in side effects or serious problems. About one-third of the participants in the augmentation group achieved remission. Among patients who did not respond adequately to citalopram, CBT produced outcomes comparable to those of medications; antidepressant therapy was more rapidly effective than CBT, but CBT was better tolerated than were the antidepressants.

Conclusions

Over the course of all four treatment levels (a total of 48 weeks), about two-thirds of participants were able to achieve remission if they did not withdraw from the study. However, dropout rates were high: 21 percent after Level 1, 30 percent after Level 2, and 42 percent after Level 3. The data show that, overall, many patients with treatment-resistant depression can get better, but the odds of remission diminish with every additional treatment strategy needed. This study illustrated for the first time what to expect with treatment changes in attempts to bring treatment-resistant patients to remission (Preskorn, 2009; Sinyor et al., 2010). Overall, there appeared to be no antidepressant that was superior to all the others, and clinical decisions currently need to be based not only on effectiveness but also on side effects, cost, and patient preference.

Where Do We Go From Here in Antidepressant Treatment?

The STAR*D study was essentially a "shotgun" approach to treating depression: start with an SSRI and then make multiple switches or medication combinations in hopes of achieving treatment success. Overall, despite the strategy, efficacy of treatment was moderate at best and the side effect burden was high. New approaches are needed for the next decade. Needed are the following:

• Development of genetic predictability to help guide therapy, and
• More effective medications, hopefully with a reduced side effect burden

Genetic Influences

As discussed already, cost-effective genetic testing is available to identify genetic deficits in drug metabolism (CYP enzymes) that predict drug interactions with many antidepressants. These interactions are important with many antidepressants as they inhibit the action of these enzymes and increase the blood concentrations of other drugs. However, recent interest has centered on how genetic alterations may influence the clinical response (or lack of response) to these medications.

Recently, Hall-Flavin and coworkers (2012) studied polymorphisms on five genes: (1) cytochrome P4502D6 gene, (*CYP2D6*); (2) cytochrome P450 2C19, (*CYP2C19*); (3) cytochrome P450 1A2 gene, (*CYP1A2*); (4) the serotonin transporter gene (*SLC6A4*); and (5) the serotonin 2A receptor gene (*HTR2A*). Using therapy guided by these results, remission of depression was significantly improved. While currently expensive for routine clinical practice, as genetic testing costs continue to fall, this may become a more common clinical practice.

Other genetic testing protocols also seem initially hopeful. Ellsworth and coworkers (2013) studied genetic variation of a glucocorticoid receptor protein (FKBP51) with a genotype-phenotype association between rs352428 being associated with positive responses in the STAR*D study. Adkins and coworkers (2012) studied similar genomic variations possibly involved in the side effects of citalopram, again from the STAR*D study. Singh and coworkers (2012) did much the same for dosing strategies with escitalopram. Certainly, over the coming decade more about genetic influences involved in depression and antidepressant response will become more commonplace with likely entry into clinical practice.

Antidepressants of the Future: More Effective? Fewer Side Effects?

The history of antidepressant drugs now encompasses almost 60 years. As is apparent in the descriptions of current drugs, we are still seeking the "perfect" antidepressant, one that is widely effective in bringing about the remission of acute episodes and preventing future relapses in the absence of significant side effects. In this section, we discuss:

- Agents currently used to augment the therapeutic action of standard antidepressants. These include modafinil, lamotrigine, quetiapine, aripiprazole, and ziprasidone.
- Serotonin receptor agonists.
- Non-pharmaceutical, natural substances that may have antidepressant properties: Omega-3 polyunsaturated fatty acids, folate, St. John's wort, SAM-e (Table 12.4).
- Ketamine and other glutaminergic agonists.
- Miscellaneous agents with potential antidepressant actions.

Augmenting Agents

Modafinil (Provigil) is a nonstimulant wakefulness-promoting drug used to combat daytime fatigue in patients with narcolepsy. It does not produce typical psychostimulant-induced side effects, and, in narcoleptic patients, modafinil may also improve subjective

TABLE 12.4 Summary of complementary and alternative medicine therapies for MDD

Intervention	Body of evidence
St. John's wort	Reduction in Ham-D scores in meta-analysis of 29 RCTs as monotherapy
Folate	Small reduction in Ham-D scores in 2 of 3 RCTs as adjunct therapy; folate deficiency related to refractory and severe MDD; other benefits of treating folate deficiency
SAM-e	Reduction of Ham-D scores in 4 of 5 RCTs as oral monotherapy
Acupuncture	No reduction in Ham-D scores in 1 meta-analysis (30 RCTs) and 5 other RCTs as monotherapy or adjunct therapy
Exercise	Reduction in Ham-D scores in 3 meta-analysis (25, 5, and 12 RCTs) as monotherapy or adjunct therapy; other benefits
Omega-3 fatty acids	Small reduction in Ham-D scores in meta-analysis of 16 RCTs as monotherapy; other benefits

Ham-D – Hamilton Rating Scale for Depression, MDD – major depressive disorder, RCT – randomized controlled trial
SAM-e – S-Adenosylmethionine
From Nahas, R. and Sheikh, O. "Complementary and alternative medicine for the treatment of major depressive disorder" *Canadian Family Physician*, Vol. 57, June 2011. Originally published in and reprinted with permission from Canadian Family Physician.

well-being, reduce fatigue, and enhance cognition and concentration. Abolfazli and coworkers (2011) demonstrated augmentation of the antidepressant action of fluoxetine by the addition of modafinil. Ferraro and coworkers (2012) discuss the mechanism of action of modafinil to achieve this effect.

Modafinil has two isomers, each of which is active. One is eliminated from the body much more quickly than the other, so essentially the activity really comes from one isomer. *Aromodafinil* (marketed as Nuvigil) is the longer-acting isomer formulation of modafinil for the treatment of narcolepsy and shift-work sleep disorders. Niemegeers and coworkers (2012) reviewed the pharmacology of armodafinil and its potential use as an augmenting agent in bipolar depression.

Lamotrigine (Lamictal) is an effective anticonvulsant and mood stabilizer. Lamotrigine is unique as an anticonvulsant in that it has clearly stated antidepressant properties. Therefore, it has become a staple in the treatment of bipolar depression. Lamotrigine has also been reported to be useful as an augmenting agent in treatment-refractory unipolar depression (Barbee et al., 2011), in treatment-resistant obsessive-compulsive disorder (Bruno et al., 2012), and in severe cases of premenstrual dysphoric disorder (Sepede et al., 2013).

Certain *atypical antipsychotics*, including *aripiprazole* and *quetiapine* have demonstrated antidepressant activity and are now approved by the FDA for the treatment of treatment-resistant depression. In addition, the combination product containing a combination of *olanzapine* and *fluoxetine* (Symbyax) is also FDA-approved for the same indication. Casey and coworkers (2012) included review of three studies in patients with inadequate response to an SSRI; aripiprazole accelerated early response and this predicted maintenance of response through the endpoint (Figure 12.10). Richardson and coworkers (2011) noted that aripiprazole potentiated inadequate SSRI-response in treating comorbid military-related PTSD and depression. Han and coworkers (2013) noted that aripiprazole potentiated escitalopram in improving both antidepressant response

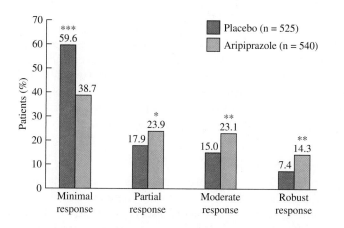

FIGURE 12.10 Percentage of 1,065 patients exhibiting minimal to maximal response to aripiprazole (blue bars) or placebo (red bars) as measured by the Massachusetts General Hospital Antidepressant Treatment Response Questionnaire. Patients were classified as nonresponders to standard medication treatment and aripiprazole or placebo was added for a six-week trial of combination therapy. Asterisks indicate a statistical difference between the two treatments. [Data from Casey et al., 2012, Figure 1.]

and reducing alcohol dependence. Similarly, *quetiapine* (Seroquel) was an effective antidepressant as a sole-agent (Maneeton et al., 2012), and also improving both depression and poor sleep quality (Sheehan et al., 2012; Frey et al., 2013). Finally, although not yet approved by the FDA for this use, Ziprasidone (Geodon) has been shown effective for the treatment of depression (Patkar et al., 2012; Papakostas et al., 2012a) (Figure 12.11). The complete pharmacology of atypical antipsychotics was presented in Chapter 11.

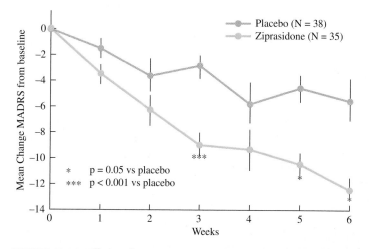

FIGURE 12.11 Efficacy of Ziprasidone versus placebo on the Montgomery Asberg Depression Rating Scale (MADRS) over a six-week period where Ziprasidone dosing began at 40 mg/day and increased by 20–40 mg/day to a target dose of 80–160 mg/day. Baseline psychotropic drugs were left unchanged throughout the study. Patients had diagnoses of acute depressive mixed states. [Data from Patkar et al., 2012, Figure 2.]

Serotonin Receptor Partial Agonists

Buspirone (BuSpar) is an anxiolytic agent (see Chapter 13) that exerts its effects secondary to weak stimulation of serotonin 5-HT$_{1A}$ receptors. This drug also exerts modest antidepressant properties likely by either antagonizing presynaptic 5-HT$_{1A}$ autoreceptors (which would increase serotonin release) or by directly stimulating postsynaptic 5-HT$_{1A}$ receptors. The combination of melatonin and buspirone was shown to be clinically effective (Fava et al., 2012). A related serotonin 5-HT$_1$ partial agonist, *gepirone*, is not yet available in this country.

Natural Substances That May have Antidepressant Properties

Omega-3 Fatty Acids.   Two types of omega-3 fatty acids are found in fatty fish like salmon, sardines, and mackerel: eicosapentaenoic acid, or EPA, and docosahexaenoic acid, or DHA. The American Heart Association recommends eating at least two servings of fatty fish each week, indicating that the omega-3 fats found in the fish help protect against cardiovascular disease. Omega-3 oils are also essential during pregnancy for normal brain maturation in the neonate. Much speculation has developed about the potential efficacy of omega-3 oils in the treatment of depression, Here, efficacy is weak, although certainly side effects are minimal and the oils (especially EPA) are neuroprotective (Hegarty and Parker, 2013). While Omega-3s may indeed "improve mood" (Lin et al., 2012), recent studies indicate that as treatments for major depressive disorder, they appear to be of minimal significant benefit with only "trends toward efficacy"(Lesperance et al., 2011; Sublette et al., 2011; Bloch and Hannestad, 2012). However, considering the minimal expense, lack of side effects, and neuroprotective actions, there is little harm in a personal trial of fish oils high in DHA.

Folate.   Folate is a "B" vitamin that occurs naturally in food and in nutritional supplements. The possible significance of *folate* in depressive disorder is a topic of wide discussion. Indeed, there seems to be a relationship between low folate levels in blood and depressive disorder. Thus, replacement might be a treatment for depression. The relationship between folate and antidepressants is that folate enhances the production of all three monoamines, dopamine, norepinephrine, and serotonin. Since deficiencies in these neurotransmitters are linked to depressive disorder, this might underlie the etiology of some cases of depression. It has been postulated that some people have a genetic defect in folate metabolism that might increase the risk of depression (Jamerson et al., 2013). There is ongoing controversy whether, in depressed patients with folate deficiency who have not responded to antidepressants, augmentation with a new, expensive folate metabolite (L-methylfolate, Deplin) might be more effective than dietary folate.

Folate in blood is converted into dihydrofolate and then into L-methylfolate that is perhaps the major form of folate capable of crossing the blood-brain-barrier (BBB). There, L-methylfolate helps form tetrahydrobiopterin (BH4), a cofactor in neurotransmitter production. BH4 is not entirely dependent on L-methylfolate and some folate also crosses the BBB. Balt (2012) questions whether any of this is important; folate may help some persons with dietary deficiencies and depression, but whether the expense of Deplin is justified is quite unclear. A few individuals (e.g., 22 percent of Hispanics and those of Mediterranean descent) may have a genetic mutation (called MTHFR C677T) that may reduce the folate to L-methylfolate conversion. This may or may not have clinical significance. Papakostas and coworkers (2012b) reported on two trials of L-methylfolate in depression. The substance was ineffective in one trial but was effective in the second. They concluded that L-methylfolate "may be effective." Both trials compared L-methylfolate with placebo but not with folate.

Much of what can be said of folate can be said of *Vitamin D* where low vitamin D levels can be associated with depression (Hoang et al., 2011) and dietary replacement may be therapeutically effective as an adjunct to SSRI therapy (Khoraminya et al., 2013).

S-Adenosylmethionine.   *S-Adenosylmethionine (SAM-e)* is a naturally occurring molecule present in all body cells. It catalyzes "methylating reactions, including L-methylfolate. There is some evidence for deficiency in depression with supplementation perhaps assisting to relieve mild depression; evidence does not support use in severely depressed persons (Carpenter, 2011 following L-methylfolate.). Part of this difficulty may be due to the fact that oral absorption of SAM-e is poor, and less than 1 percent of the ingested drug reaches the bloodstream. Papakostas and coworkers (2012c) reviewed SAM-e for depression and claimed that efficacy was similar to the efficacy of tricyclic antidepressants. Use is limited primarily by expense.

St. John's wort.   *St. John's wort* is an extract of *Hypericum perforatum*, a perennial herb. It has been used to treat depression since initial German reports of efficacy. In most studies, the compound was superior to placebo and equivalent to standard drugs (Nahas and Skeikh, 2011; Sarris et al., 2012).). Mechanistically, St. John's wort mimics the neurotropic effect of BDNF in the hippocampus (Leuner et al., 2013). Most studies had significant bias. St. John's wort likely should not be combined with most other antidepressants because of a potential to induce serotonin syndrome. The drug also induces drug-metabolizing enzymes, so multiple other drugs may become more toxic at usual doses (Rahimi and Abdollahi, 2012). Other side effects may further reduce its utility.

Did You Know?

You Are—and Your Mood Is—What You Eat

In one study 10,094 initially healthy participants were followed for a median of 4.4 years. To better understand the association between diet and mood, participants were assigned a Mediterranean dietary pattern score, which positively weighted the consumption of vegetables, fruit, nuts, cereal, legumes, and fish. The researchers found an inverse relationship between adherence to the Mediterranean diet and risk for depression, suggesting this diet has a protective role against the development of mood disorders.

Similarly, a study comparing a diet high "whole" foods (e.g., high in vegetables, fruits and fish) with a diet high in processed foods, found that those who most closely followed the whole foods diet had lower odds of depression as measured by the Center for Epidemiologic Studies–Depression scale while those who had ate diets high in processed foods had increased odds of developing depression.

In a study of 7,114 adolescents aged 10–14 years, participants completed dietary questionnaires, which were then used to determine healthy and unhealthy diet quality scores. The Short Mood and Feelings Questionnaire was used to measure depression. Once again, this study found an inverse relationship between good, healthy eating and the development of depression. Adolescents with higher unhealthy diet scores had a 79 percent increased risk of depression.

Ketamine and Other Glutaminergic Agonists

Ketamine, for the past 50 years, has been an anesthetic drug characterized by amnesia, analgesia and out-of-body experiences. It was used for anesthesia because it was one of the only anesthetics that could produce amnesia and analgesia without perilous drops in blood pressure. Its psychedelic properties were tolerated. However, because of psychedelic side effects, it and its precursor (phencyclidine, PCP) were considered drugs of abuse. In recent years, however, remarkably, low dose intravenous infusions of ketamine have been demonstrated to produce rapid, although transient, relief from depression in the majority of patients to whom it was administered. Indeed, administered in a dose of 0.5 mg/kg body weight three times weekly over a 12-day period, response rates in treatment-resistant depression were about 70 percent, sustained for an average of 18 days posttreatment (Murrough et al., 2013). The response is often seen within hours and is accompanied by increases in synaptogenesis, including increased density and function of spine synapses in the prefrontal cortex. This has led to a reversal of the deficits in synaptic number and function resulting from chronic stress exposure (Duman et al., 2012). This remarkable, albeit short-lived, antidepressant response is one of the more remarkable advances in recent years in the area of depression research.

Currently, administration of ketamine is limited by its abuse potential, by the need for intravenous administration, and by the need for a supervising anesthesiologist for administration. It does point out, however, that glutaminergic antagonists (like ketamine) may reverse both the synaptic and behavioral symptoms of depression. Much remains to be learned in this area, but the results with ketamine are remarkable. Other drugs that may ultimately antagonize NMDA-glutamate receptors, possibly with the psychedelic properties of ketamine are under study; one such agent is termed *GLYX-13* (Burgdorf et al., 2013). Regardless, this is further evidence of the link between deficits in BDNF and a predisposition to depressive symptomatology (Liu et al., 2012). The next several years should add considerable information to this most interesting area of research.

Miscellaneous Agents with Potential Antidepressant Actions

At this point in time, because of economic potential, many other experimental compounds are being evaluated for use in the clinical treatment of depression.

Tianeptine. *Tianeptine* (Stablon) increases the presynaptic neuronal uptake of serotonin in the brain and thus decreases serotonin neurotransmission. However, tianeptine appears to reduce stress-induced atrophy of neuronal dendrites, exerting a neuronal protective effect against stress and restoring intracellular mechanisms adversely affected by stress and other insults. Its efficacy against major depression is well documented. It does not appear to produce adverse cognitive, psychomotor, sleep, cardiovascular, body weight, or sexual side effects. Tianeptine is also effective in bipolar depression, dysthymia, and anxiety. It seems quite useful in the elderly and in patients with chronic alcoholism. This unusual compound offers both an alternative medication to standard antidepressants and new insights into the patho-physiology of depression and anxiety. Because its patent has expired, the drug has not been marketed in the United States.

Agomelatine. Chapter 13 discusses agomelatine as an anxiolytic agent that acts as a melatonergic agonist and a serotonin 5-HT_{2C} receptor antagonist. Potential adverse effects on the liver limit its use. Agomelatine also possesses antidepres-sant properties (Kasper et al., 2013), again with the same limitation (Carney and Shelton, 2011). The drug has also been demonstrated to effectively treat anhedonia, an effect that was superior to that produced by venlafaxine (Di Giannantonio and Martinotti, 2012).

In addition to the substances discussed in this chapter, because of widespread need for more effective medications with fewer side effects, the pharmaceutical industry is and will continue to investigate new agents. Among those under trial, serdaxin is a serotonin- and norepinephrine-releasing agent; and GSK372475 releases serotonin, norepinephrine, and dopamine. To help keep abreast of new agents, as they are encoun-tered we suggest performing a "PubMed" search. Here, we suggest a trial search using the drug listed above as *GLYX-13*. Go to www.pubmed.gov and, in the search bar at the top, type "GLYX-13" and "depression". All medical literature references with those two terms will be displayed. If the number is too large, add the term "review" to the search. Note that several articles are available as full text, an excellent way to learn about a given topic.

STUDY QUESTIONS

1. What is the relationship between depression and the biological amine transmitters in the brain?

2. Describe the probable mechanism of both acute and ultimate effects of antidepressant drugs. What might account for the delay in clinical effect?

3. List and differentiate the major classes of antidepressants.

4. Compare and contrast imipramine and fluoxetine.

5. Discuss what happens when a patient overdoses on a tricyclic antidepressant.

6. Discuss the side effects of SSRIs. What is the serotonin syndrome? What is the SSRI withdrawal syndrome? Discuss the effects of these drugs on sexual function.

7. Which drug or class of drugs do you think is the "best" antidepressant? Why?

8. Which antidepressants are used in the treatment of anxiety disorders? Why? How do these drugs differ from the benzodiazepine-type anxiolytics?

9. Discuss the strategies being used to discover the next generation of antidepressant drugs and the types of drugs that are being developed from those approaches.

10. Discuss the role of neutraceuticals and vitamins in the treatment of depression.

REFERENCES

Abbasowa, L., et al. (2013). "Psychostimulants in Moderate to Severe Affective Disorder: A Systematic Review of Randomized Controlled Trials." *Nordic Journal of Psychiatry*. 67: 369–382.

Abolfazli, R., et al. (2011). "Double-Blind, Randomized, Parallel-Group Clinical Trial of Efficacy of the Combination Fluoxetine plus Modafinil versus Fluoxetine plus Placebo in the Treatment of Major Depression." *Depression and Anxiety* 28: 297–302.

Adkins, D. E., et al. (2012). "Genone-Wide Pharmacogenomic Study of Citalopram-Induced Side Effects in STAR*D." *Translational Psychiatry* July 3; 2: e129.

American College of Obstetricians and Gynecologists. (2006). "Position Statement on Paroxetine." *Obstetrics and Gynecology* 108: 1601–1603.

Amsterdam, J. D. (2003). "A Double-Blind, Placebo-Controlled Trial of the Safety and Efficacy of Selegiline Transdermal System Without Dietary Restrictions in Patients with Major Depressive Disorder." *Journal of Clinical Psychiatry* 64: 208–214.

Amsterdam, J. D., and Bodkin, A. (2006). "Selegiline Transdermal System in the Prevention of Relapse of Major Depressive Disorder: A 52-Week, Double-Blind, Placebo-Substitution, Parallel-Group C Clinical Trial." *Journal of Clinical Psychopharmacology* 26: 579–586.

Andrade, C., and Rao, N. S. K. (2010). "How Antidepressant Drugs Act: A Primer on Neuroplasticity as the Eventual Mediator of Antidepressant Efficacy." *Indian Journal of Psychiatry* 52: 378–386.

Apler, A. (2011). "Citalopram for Major Depressive Disorder in Adults: A Systematic Review and Meta-Analysis of Published Placebo-Controlled Trials." *BMJ Open* 2:e000106.

Autry, A. E., and Monteggia, L. M. (2012). "Brain-Derived Neurotropic Factor and Neuropsychiatric Disorders." *Pharmacological Reviews* 64: 238–258.

Balt, J. (2012). "Deplin: Is it Just Folate by Another Name?" *The Carlat Psychiatry Report* 10(1): 1–8.

Barbee, J. G., et al. (2011). "A Double-Blind Placebo-Controlled Trial of Lamotrigine as an Antidepressant Augmentation Agent in Treatment-Refractory Unipolar Depression." *Journal of Clinical Psychiatry* 72: 1405–1412.

Bismuth-Evenzal, Y., et al. (2012). "Decreased Serotonin Content and Reduced Agonist-Induced Aggregation in Platelets of 58 Patients Chronically Medicated with SSRI Drugs." *Journal of Affective Disorders* 136: 99–103.

Bloch, M. H., and Hannestad J. (2012). "Omega-3 Fatty Acids for the Treatment of Depression: Systematic Review and Meta-Analysis." *Molecular Psychiatry* 17: 1272–1282.

Bobo, W. V., and Shelton, R. C. (2009). "Fluoxetine and Olanzapine Combination Therapy in Treatment-Resistant Major Depression: Review of Efficacy and Safety Data." *Expert Opinion in Pharmacotherapy* 10: 2145–2159.

Bruno, A., et al. (2012). "Lamotrigine Augmentation of Serotonin Reuptake Inhibitors in Treatment-Resistant Obsessive-Compulsive Disorder: A Double-Blind, Placebo-Controlled Study." *Journal of Psychopharmacology* 26: 1456–1462.

Burgdorf, J., et al. (2013). "GLYX-13, An NMDA Receptor Glycine-Site Functional Partial Agonist, Induces Antidepressant-Like Effects Without Ketamine-Like Side Effects." *Neuropsychopharmacology* 385: 729–742.

Bymaster, F. P., et al. (2005). "The Dual Transporter Inhibitor Duloxetine: A Review of Its Preclinical Pharmacology, Pharmacokinetic Profile, and Clinical Results in Depression." *Current Pharmaceutical Design* 11: 1475–1493.

Candy, M., et al. (2008). "Psychostimulants for Depression." *Cochrane Database of Systematic Reviews* April 16;(2): CD006722.

Carney, R. M., and Shelton, R. C. (2011). "Agomelatine for the Treatment of Major Depressive Disorder." *Expert Opinion on Pharmacotherapy* 12: 2411–2419.

Carpenter, D. J., (2011). "St. John's wort and S-adenosyl methionine as "Natural" Alternatives to Conventional Antidepressants in the Era of the Suicidality Boxed Warning: What is the Evidence for Clinically Relevant Benefit." *Alternative Medicine Reviews* 16: 17–39.

Casey, D. E., et al. (2012). "Efficacy of Adjunctive Aripiprazole in Major Depressive Disorder: A Pooled Response Quartile Analysis and the Predictive Value of Week 2 Early Response." *Primary Care Companion CNS Disorders* 14(3). Pii: PCC. 11m01251.

Cazorla, M., et al. (2011). "Identification of a Low-Molecular Weight TrkB Antagonist with Anxiolytic and Antidepressant Activity in Mice." *Journal of Clinical Investigation* 121: 1846–1857.

Ciprianai, A., et al. (2012). "Duloxetine versus Other Anti-Depressive Agents for Depression." *Cochrane Database of Systematic Reviews* October 17; 10: CD006533.

Clayton, A. H., et al. (2013). "An Evaluation of Sexual Functioning in Employed Outpatients with Major Depressive Disorder Treated with Desvenlafaxine 50 mg or Placebo." *Journal of Sex Medicine* 10: 768–778.

Cooke, M. J., and Waring, W. S. (2013). "Citalopram and Cardiac Toxicity." *European Journal of Clinical Pharmacology*. 69: 755–760.

Di Giannantonio, M. and Martinotti, G. (2012). "Anhedonia and Major Depression: The Role of Agomelatine." *European Neuropsychopharmacology* 22, Supplement 3: S505–S510.

Duman, R. S., et al. (1997), "A Molecular and Cellular Theory of Depression." *Archives of General Psychiatry* 54: 597–606.

Duman, R. S., et al. (2012). "Signaling Pathways Underlying the Rapid Antidepressant Actions of Ketamine." *Neuropharmacology* 62: 35–41.

Durell, T. M., et al. (2013). "Atomoxetine Treatment of Attention-Deficit/Hyperactivity Disorder in Young Adults with Assessment of Functional Outcomes: A Randomized, Double-Blind, Placebo-Controlled Clinical Trial." *Journal of Clinical Psychopharmacology* 33: 45–54.

Ellsworth, K. A., et al. (2013). "FKBP5 Genetic Variation: Association with Selective Serotonin Reuptake Inhibitor Treatment Outcomes in Major Depressive Disorder." *Pharmacogenetic Genomics* 23: 156–166.

Eom, C. S., et al. (2012). "Use of Selective Serotonin Reuptake Inhibitors and Risk of Fracture: A Systematic Review and Meta-Analysis." *Journal of Bone Mineralization Research* 27: 1186–1195.

Eyding, D., et al. (2010). "Reboxetine for Acute Treatment of Major Depression: Systematic Review and Meta-Analysis of Published and Unpublished Placebo and Selective Serotonin Reuptake Inhibitor Controlled Trials." *British Medical Journal (BMJ)* October 12; 341: c4737.

Fabbrini, G., et al. (2012). "Selegiline: A Reappraisal of its Role in Parkinson Disease." *Clinical Neuropharmacology* 35: 134–140.

Fava, M., et al. (2012). "An Exploratory Study of Combination Buspirone and Melatonin SR in Major Depressive Disorder (MDD): A Possible Role for Neurogenesis in Drug Discovery." *Journal of Psychiatric Research* 46: 1553–1563.

Ferguson, J. M., et al. (2012). "High-Dose Desvenlafaxine in Outpatients with Major Depressive Disorder." *CNS Spectrums* 17: 121–130.

Ferraro, L., et al. (2013). "The Vigilance Promoting Drug Modafinil Modulates Serotonin Transmission in the Rat Prefrontal Cortex and Dorsal Raphe Nucleus. Possible Relevance for its Postulated Antidepressant Activity." *Mini-Reviews in Medicinal Chemistry* 13: 478–492.

Fournier, J. C., et al. (2010). "Antidepressant Drug Effects and Depression Severity: A Patient-Level Meta-analysis." *Journal of the American Medical Association* 303: 47–53.

Frey, B. N., et al. (2013). "Effects of Quetiapine Extended Release on Sleep and Quality of Life in Midlife Women with Major Depressive Disorder." *Archives of Women's Mental Health* 16: 83–85.

Garcia-Toro, M., et al (2012). "Treatment Patterns in Major Depressive Disorder after an Inadequate Response to First-Line Antidepressant Treatment." *BMC Psychiatry* 12:143.

Gartliehner, G., et al. (2011). "Comparative Benefits and Harms of Second-Generation Antidepressants for Treating Major Depressive Disorder: An Updated Meta-Analysis." *Annals of Internal Medicine* 155: 772–785.

Gibbons, R. D., et al. (2012). "Suicidal Thoughts and Behavior with Antidepressant Treatment." *Archives of General Psychiatry* 69:580–587.

Grande, I., et al. (2010). "The Role of BDNF as a Mediator of Neuroplasticity in Bipolar Disorder." *Psychiatry Investigations* 7: 243–250.

Guay, D. R., (2012). "Vilazodone Hydrochloride: A Combined SSRI and 5-HT1A Receptor Agonist for Major Depressive Disorder." *The Consulting Pharmacist* 27: 857–867.

Guilloux, J. P., et al. (2012). "Molecular Evidence for BDNF- and GABA-Related Dysfunctions in the Amygdala of Female Subjects with Major Depression." *Molecular Psychiatry* 17: 1130–1142.

Hall-Flavin, D. K., et al. (2012). "Using a Pharmacogenomic Algorithm to Guide the Treatment of Depression." *Translational Psychiatry* 2: e172.

Han, D. H., et al. (2013). "Adjunctive Aripiprazole Therapy with Escitalopram in Patients with Co-Morbid Major Depressive Disorder and Alcohol Dependence: Clinical and Neuroimaging Evidence." *Journal of Psychopharmacology* 27: 282–291.

Hegarty, B., and Parker G. (2013). "Fish Oil as a Management Component for Mood Disorders – An Evolving Signal." *Current Opinions in Psychiatry* 26: 33–40.

Hellerstein, D. J., et al. (2012). "A Randomized Controlled Trial of Duloxetine versus Placebo in the Treatment of Nonmajor Chronic Depression." *Journal of Clinical Psychology* 73: 984–991.

Hoang, M. T., et al. (2011). "Association Between Low Serum 25-Hydroxyvitamin D and Depression in a Large Sample of Healthy Adults: The Cooper Center Longitudinal Study." *Mayo Clinic Proceedings* 86: 1050–1055.

Holtzheimer, P. E., and Mayberg, H. S. (2010). "Stuck in a Rut: Rethinking Depression and its Treatment." *Trends in Neurosciences* 34: 1–9.

Howland, R. H., (2012). "The use of Dopaminergic and Stimulant Drugs for the Treatment of Depression." *Journal of Psychosocial Nursing and Mental Health Services* 50: 11–14.

Jain, R., et al. (2013). "A Randomized, Double-Blind, Placebo-Controlled 6-wk Trial of the Efficacy and Tolerability of 5 mg Vortioxetine in Adults with Major Depressive Disorder." *International Journal of Neuropsychopharmacology* 16: 313–321.

Jamerson, B. D., et al. (2013). "Folate Metabolism Genes, Dietary Folate and Response to Antidepressant Medications in Late-Life Depression." *International Journal of Geriatric Psychiatry* 28: 925–932.

Kasper, S., et al. (2013). "Antidepressant Efficacy of Agomelatine versus SSRI/SNRI: Results from a Pooled Analysis of Head-to-Head Studies Without a Placebo Control." *International Clinical Psychopharmacology* 28: 12–19.

Khan, A. (2012). "A Systematic Review of Comparative Efficacy of Treatments and Controls for Depression." *Plos One* 7: e41778.

Khoraminya, N., et al. (2013). "Therapeutic Effects of Vitamin D as Adjunctive Therapy to Fluoxetine in Patients with Major Depressive Disorder." *Australian & New Zealand Journal of Psychiatry* 47: 271–275.

Kim, D., and Steinhart, B. (2010). "Seizures Induced by Recreational Abuse of Bupropion Tablets via Nasal Insufflation." *Canadian Journal of Emergency Medicine* 12: 158–161.

Kohno, T., et al. (2012). "Milnacipram Inhibits Glutamatergic n-methyl-D-Aspartate Receptor Activity in Spinal Dorsal Horn Neurons." *Molecular Pain* 8: 45.

Kupfer, D. J., et al. (2012). "Major Depressive Disorder: New Clinical, Neurobiological, and Treatment Perspectives." *Lancet* 379: 1045–1055.

Launay, J. M., et al. (2011). "Raphe-Mediated Signals Control the Hippocampal Response to SRI Antidepressants via miR-16." *Translational Psychiatry* 1, e56.

Lesperance, F., et al. (2011). "The Efficacy of Omega-3 Supplementation for Major Depression." *Journal of Clinical Psychiatry* 72: 1054–1062.

Leuner, K., et al. (2013). "Hyperforin Modulates Dendritic Spine Morphology in Hippocampal Pyramidal Neurons by Activating Ca(2+) –Permeable TRPC6 Channels." *Hippocampus* 23: 40–52.

Lin, Pao-Yen, et al. (2012). "Are Omega-3 Fatty Acids Anti-Depressants or Just Mood-Improving Agents." *Molecular Psychiatry* 17: 1161–1163.

Liu, C. Y., et al. (2012). "Metabotropic Glutamate Receptor 5 Antagonist 2-methyl-6-(phenethyl) pyridine Produces Antidepressant Effects in Rats: Role of Brain-Derived Neurotropic Factor." *Neuroscience* 223C: 219–224.

Lucassen, P. J., et al. (2010). "Regulation of Adult Neurogenesis by Stress, Sleep Disruption, Exercise and Inflammation: Implications for Depression and Antidepressant Action." *European Neuropsychopharmacology* 20: 1–17.

Maneeton, N., et al. (2012). "Quetiapine Monotherapy in Acute Phase for Major Depressive Disorder: A Meta-Analysis of Randomized, Placebo-Controlled Trials." *BMC Psychiatry* 12(1): 160.

Martinez, C., et al. (2010). "Use of venlafaxine Compared with other Antidepressants and the Risk of Sudden Cardiac Death or Near Death: A Nested Case-Control Study." *British Medical Journal* February 5; 340: c249.

Masi, G., and Brovedani, P. (2011). "The Hippocampus, Neurotropic Factors and Depression: Possible Implications for the Pharmacotherapy of Depression." *CNS Drugs* 25: 913–931.

Mitjans, M., and Arias, B. (2012). "The Genetics of Depression: What Information can New Methodologic Approaches Provide?" *Actas Espanolas de Psiquitria* 40: 70–83.

Murrough, J. W., et al. (2013). "Rapid and Longer-Term Antidepressant Effects of Repeated Ketamine Infusions in Treatment-Resistant Major Depression." *Biological Psychiatry* 15: 250–256.

Muzina, D. J. (2010). "Discontinuing an Antidepressant? Tapering Tips to Ease Distressing Symptoms." *Current Psychiatry* 9: 51–61.

Nahas, R., and Sheikh, O. (2011). "Complimentary and Alternative Medicine for the Treatment of Major Depressive Disorder." *Canadian Family Physician* 57: 659–663.

Nandagopal, J. J., and DelBello, M. P. (2009). "Selegiline Transdermal System: A Novel Treatment Option for Major Depressive Disorder." *Expert Opinions in Pharmacotherapy* 10: 1665–1673.

Narasimhan, S., and Lohoff, F. W. (2012). "Pharmacogenetics of Antidepressant Drugs: Current Clinical Practice and Future Directions." *Pharmacogenomics* 13: 441–464.

Niemegeers, P., et al. (2012). "Pharmacokinetic Evaluation of Armodafinil for the Treatment of Bipolar Depression." *Expert Opinion in Drug Metabolism and Toxicology* 8: 1189–1197.

Neto, F. L. et al. (2011). "Neurotropins Role in Depression Neurobiology: A Review of Basic and Clinical Evidence." *Current Neuropharmacology* 9: 530–552.

Nierenberg, A. A. (2011). "The Current Crisis of Confidence in Antidepressants." *Journal of Clinical Psychiatry* 72: 27–33.

Nurnberg, H. G., et al. (2008). "Sildenafil Treatment of Women with Antidepressant-Associated Sexual Dysfunction: A Randomized Controlled Trial." *Journal of the American Medical Association* 300: 395–404.

Pae, C. U., et al. (2009). "Desvenlafaxine: A New Antidepressant or Just Another One?" *Expert Opinion on Pharmacotherapy* 10: 875–887.

Pae, C. U., et al. (2012). "Safety of Selegiline Transdermal System in Clinical Practice: Analysis of Adverse Events from Postmarketing Exposures." *Journal of Clinical Psychiatry* 73: 661–668.

Papakostas, G. I., et al. (2012a). "A 12-Week, Randomized, Double-Blind, Placebo-Controlled, Sequential Parallel Comparison Trial of Ziprasidone as Monotherapy for Major Depressive Disorder." *Journal of Clinical Psychiatry* 73: 1541–1547.

Papakostas, G. I., et al. (2012b). "L-Methylfolate as Adjunctive Therapy for SSRI-Resistant Major Depression: Results of Two Randomized, Double-Blind, Parallel-Sequential Trials." *American Journal of Psychiatry* 169: 1267–1274.

Papakostas, G. I., et al. (2012c). "Folates and S-Adenosylmethionine for Major Depressive Disorder." *Canadian Journal of Psychiatry* 57: 406–413.

Parker, G., and Brotchie, H. (2010). "Do the Old Psychostimulant Drugs Have a Role in Managing Treatment-Resistant Depression?" *Acta Psychiatrica Scandinavia* 121: 308–314.

Patel, D. and Goldman-Levine, J. D. (2011). "Doxepine (Silenor) for Insomnia." *American Family Physician* 84: 453–454.

Patkar, A., et al. (2012). "A 6 Week Randomized Double-Blind Placebo-Controlled Trial of Ziprasidone for the Acute Depressive Mixed State." *Plos One* April, 7: e34757.

Peritogiannis, V., et al. (2009). "Duloxetine-Induced Hypomania: Case Report and Brief Review of the Literature on SNRIs-Induced Mood Switching." *Journal of Psychopharmacology* 23: 592–596.

Patkar, A., et al. (2012). "A 6 Week Randomized Double-Blind Placebo-Controlled Trial of Ziprasidone for the Acute Depressive Mixed State." *PLos One* 7(4): e34757.

Preskorn, S. H. (2009). "Treatment Options for the Patient Who Does Not Respond Well to Initial Antidepressant Therapy." *Journal of Psychiatric Practice* 15: 202–210.

Rahimi, R., and Abdollahi, M. (2012). "An Update on the Ability of St. John's wort to Affect the Metabolism of Other Drugs." *Expert Opinion on Drug Metabolism and Toxicology* 8: 691–708.

Ravindran, A. V., et al. (2000). "Treatment of Dysthymia with Sertraline: A Double-Blind, Placebo-Controlled Trial in Dysthymic Patients Without Major Depression." *Journal of Clinical Psychiatry* 61: 821–827.

Reinhold, J. A., et al. (2012). "Evidence for the Use of Vilazodone in the Treatment of Major Depressive Disorder." *Expert Opinions on Pharmacotherapeutics* 13: 2215–2224.

Richardson, J. D., et al. (2011). "Aripiprazole Augmentation in the Treatment of Military-Related PTSD with Major Depression: A Retrospective Chart Review." *BMC Psychiatry* 11:86

Rothschild, A. J., et al. (2012). "Vortioxetine (Lu AA21004) 5 mg in Generalized Anxiety Disorder: Results of an 8-week Randomized, Double-Blind, Placebo-Controlled Clinical Trial in the United States." *European Neuropsychopharmacology* 22: 858–866.

Sarris, J., et al. (2012). "St. John's wort (*Hypericum perforatum*) versus Sertraline and Placebo in Major Depressive Disorder: Continuation Data from a 26-Week RCT." *Pharmacopsychiatry* 45: 275–278.

Saveanu, R. V., and Nemeroff, C. B. (2012). "Etiology of Depression: Genetic and Environmental Factors." *Psychiatric Clinics of North America* 35: 51–71.

Schosser, A., et al. (2012). "European Group for the Study of Resistant Depression (GSRD) – Where Have We Gone So Far?: Review of Clinical and Genetic Findings." *European Neuropsychopharmacology* 22: 453–468.

Schweitzer, I., et al. (2009). "Sexual Side-Effects of Contemporary Antidepressants: Review." *Australian and New Zealand Journal of Psychiatry* 43: 795–808.

Sepede, G., et al. (2013). "Lamotrigine Augmentation in Premenstrual Dysphoric Disorder: A Case Report." *Clinical Neuropharmacology* 36: 31–33.

Sheehan, D. V., et al. (2012). "Long-Term Functioning and Sleep Quality in Patients with Major Depressive Disorder Treated with Extended-Release Quetiapine Fumarate." *International Clinical Psychopharmacology* 27: 239–248.

Sher, L. (2011). "The Role of Brain-Derived Neurotropic Factor in the Pathophysiology of Adolescent Suicidal Behavior." *International Journal of Adolescent Medicine and Health* 23: 181–185.

Sindrup, S. H., et al. (2005). "Antidepressants in the Treatment of Neuropathic Pain." *Basic and Clinical Pharmacology and Toxicology* 96: 399–409.

Singh, A. B., et al. (2012). "ABCB1 Polymorphism Predicts Escitalopram Dose Needed for Remission in Major Depression." *Translational Psychiatry* November 27;2: e198.

Singh, M. and Schwartz, T. L. (2012). "Clinical Utility of Vilazodone for the Treatment of Adults with Major Depressive Disorder and Theoretical Implications for Future Clinical Use." *Journal of Neuropsychiatric Disease and Treatment* 8: 123–130.

Sinyor, M., et al. (2010). "The Sequences Treatment Alternatives to Relieve Depression (STAR*D) Trial: A Review." *Canadian Journal of Psychiatry* 55: 126–135.

Spina, E., et al. (2008). "Clinically Relevant Pharmacokinetic Drug Interactions with Second-Generation Antidepressants: An Update." *Clinical Therapeutics* 30: 1206–1227.

Stahl, S. M., et al. (2013). "Serotonergic Drugs for Depression and Beyond." *Current Drug Targets* 14: 578–585.

Sublette, M. E., et al. (2011). "Meta-Analysis of the Effects of Eicosapentaenoic Acid (EPA) in Clinical Trials in Depression." *Journal of Clinical Psychiatry* 72: 1577–1584.

Thase, M. E., et al. (2006). "A Double-Blind Comparison Between Bupropion XL and Venlafaxine XR: Sexual Functioning, Antidepressant Efficacy, and Tolerability." *Journal of Clinical Psychopharmacology* 26: 482–488.

Tripp, A., et al. (2012). "Brain-Derived Neurotropic Factor Signaling and Subgenual Anterior Cingulate Cortex Dysfunction in Major Depressive Disorder." *American Journal of Psychiatry* 169: 1194–1202.

Undurraga, J., and Baldessarini, R. J. (2012). "Randomized, Placebo-Controlled Trials of Antidepressants for Acute Major Depression: Thirty-Year Meta-Analytic Review." *Neuropsychopharmacology* 37; 851–864.

Vieweg, W. V., et al. (2012). "Citalopram, QTc Interval Prolongation and Torsade de Pointes. How Should We Apply the Recent FDA Ruling?" *American Journal of Medicine* 125: 859–868.

Wade, A. G., et al. (2011). "Efficacy, Safety, and Tolerability of Escitalopram in Doses up to 50mg in Major Depressive Disorder (MDD): An Open-Label, Pilot Study." *BMC Psychiatry* 11:42.

Watanabe, N., et al. (2011). "Mirtazapine versus Other Antidepressant Agents for Depression." *Cochrane Database of Systematic Reviews* December 7; 12: CD006528.

CHAPTER 12 APPENDIX

Drugs for the Treatment of Obesity

Obesity is a chronic disease with significant long-term adverse consequences, including diabetes and heart disease. Bariatric surgery is remarkably effective, but pharmacological options have long been sought, with modest success and major limitations. During the past several decades, most drugs for obesity treatment initially achieved FDA approval, but when they reached commercial sale, they were subsequently withdrawn owing to serious adverse effects.

Early pharmaceuticals for the treatment of obesity were the catecholamine psychostimulants, such as amphetamine, dextroamphetamine, and phentermine (which resembles amphetamine in its structure and its actions). These drugs reduced appetite and induced weight loss over a few weeks until tolerance developed. As a result, the weight loss was not sustained and drug dependence became an issue. In 2007, the cannabinoid receptor antagonist rimonabant was marketed as effective in reducing body weight, but was withdrawn because of an increased risk of depression, anxiety, and suicidal ideation.

Drugs targeting the serotonin system also have a history of approval followed by later withdrawal. *Fenfluramine* (Pondimin) and its dextro-isomer *dexfenfluramine* (Redux) cause the release of serotonin (5-HT) by disrupting its vesicular storage, and reversing serotonin transporter function. The result is a feeling of fullness and loss of appetite. Both drugs were withdrawn because of serious adverse effects on heart valves and an increased risk of pulmonary hypertension. The combination of fenfluramine and the stimulant *phentermine* (Adipex, Ionamin) resulted in the infamous "fen-phen" combination. Recently, it has become available as Qsymia, a combination product containing phentermine and topiramate. Topiramate is an antiepileptic drug associated with weight loss (see Chapter 14).

Two other anti-obesity medications were Orlistat and Sibutramine. *Orlistat* (on prescription as Xenical and over-the counter as Alli) acts to block the absorption of fats from the human gastrointestinal tract, thereby reducing caloric intake. Weight loss is modest and GI effects include oily, loose stools. Sibutramine was withdrawn due to adverse cardiovascular events. Interestingly, sibutramine is a centrally acting serotonin-norepinephrine reuptake blocker (SNRI), although it lacks antidepressant action.

Other FDA-approved antiobesity agents include diethylpropion, benzphetamine, and phendimetrazine. *Diethylpropion* (also known generically as amfepramone; trade names include Tenuate, Tepanil, Anorex, and others) is an amphetamine-like antiobesity drug that can reduce appetite, along with increased heart rate and blood pressure. Benzphetamine (Didrex) and phendimetrazine (Adipost, Bontril) are yet two other amphetamine-like antiobesity agents, similar to amfepramone. Besides Orlistat, none of these drugs were intended for use for more than 2 or 3 weeks, due to the potential severity of side effects.

Therefore, one can readily see that most antiobesity agents resemble the structure and actions of amphetamine, acting by increasing norepinephrine and dopamine activity in the brain. Rimonabant was a cannabinoid antagonist; and sibutramine potentiated both norepinephrine and serotonin activity. However, phenfluramine and dexfenfluramine were serotonergic agonists. Indeed, when SSRIs first came on the market in the 1990s, it was thought that they might have weight-loss properties. Unfortunately, this did not occur in clinical use. This implies an involvement of serotonergic systems in feeding behavior and metabolism.

Serotonin and Weight Loss

Serotonin neurons are confined to distinct nuclei located in the midbrain and hindbrain areas (see Chapter 1). The dorsal raphe, in particular, is a midbrain nucleus that contains a significant proportion of brain serotonin, with distinct projections to the hypothalamus and other feeding-related forebrain areas. It has been hypothesized that a dysregulation of central serotonergic pathways may be involved in obesity and that stimulation of these areas may be a target for antiobesity medications. Indeed, a specific subtype of serotonin receptor, the 5-HT$_2$ family, seems to be involved. This family of receptors has at least three sub-types: 5-HT$_{2A}$, 5-HT$_{2B}$, and 5-HT$_{2C}$ (5-HT stands for 5-hydroxy-triptamine, the chemical name for serotonin). 5-HT$_{2A}$ is located in the CNS, cardiac vessels, and heart valves. 5-HT$_{2B}$ is found in the cardiovascular system. Stimulation of 5-HT$_{2B}$ receptors may cause heart failure and fibrosis of heart valves. 5-HT$_{2C}$ is almost exclusively located in the CNS and participates in controlling caloric balance. The desired objective of appetite suppression is predominantly mediated by the 5-HT$_{2C}$ receptors.

Fenfluramine and dexfenfluramine are nonspecific agonists; they activate all three sub-types of the 5-HT$_2$ receptors. The adverse cardiac and pulmonary effects likely resulted from unwanted 5-HT$_{2B}$ receptor stimulation. Needed was a more specific agonist at 5-HT$_{2C}$ receptors. Lorcaserin (Belvik) is such a drug, devoid of actions on 5-HT$_{2B}$ receptor subtypes responsible for cardiac valve damage. In several clinical trials, the drug appeared efficacious and relatively safe.

The drug received FDA approval for clinical use in 2012. In December 2012, the U.S. Drug Enforcement Agency classified lorcaserin as a Schedule IV drug because of occasional reports of LSD-like hallucinations and concern that some users could develop psychiatric dependencies on the drug. The psychedelic effects of LSD are attributed to its strong partial agonist effects at 5-HT$_{2A}$ receptors. Specific 5-HT$_{2A}$ agonists are psychedelics and 5-HT$_{2A}$ antagonists block the psychedelic activity of LSD. Exactly how this produces LSD's psychedelic effects is unknown. Concern has been that lorcaserin might share some of this LSD-like potential (even though it does not affect 5-HT$_{2A}$ receptors). Recent reviews include those by Bello and Liang (2011) and Bai and Wang (2011). Khan, et al. (2012) review agents under development.

APPENDIX REFERENCES:

Bai, B., and Wang, Y. (2011). "The Use of Lorcaserin in the Management of Obesity: A Critical Appraisal." *Drug Design, Development and Therapy* 5: 1–7.

Bello, N. T., and Liang, N. (2011). "The Use of Serotonergic Drugs to Treat Obesity – Is There Any Hope?" *Drug Discovery, Development and Therapy* 5: 95–109.

Khan, A., et al. (2012). "Current Updates in the Medical Management of Obesity." *Recent Patents on Endocrine, Metabolic and Immune Drug Discovery* 6: 117–128.

Chapter 13

Sedative-Hypnotic and Anxiolytic Medications

Anxiety and insomnia have long plagued mankind. Both have been the objects of drug therapy, probably since the discovery of alcohol as a product of fermentation. In this chapter, we discuss the pharmacological treatment of anxiety and insomnia by introducing the historically significant and still widely used medicines that were used as sedatives, hypnotics, and antianxiety medications. Other chapters in this text discuss more modern medications that are not classified as sedative/hypnotics, but nevertheless exert anxiolytic efficacy (atypical antipsychotic medications and certain antidepressants). Indeed, in the modern-day treatment of severe anxiety and insomnia, these medications can be used in place of older sedative-hypnotic agents (Julien, 2013).

Sedative-hypnotics include a chemically diverse group of medicines primarily prescribed for the treatment of anxiety, panic disorders, sleep disturbances, and seizure disorders. They are usually medically prescribed, but are commonly misused and this misuse can lead to abuse or result in the development of a substance abuse disorder or dependence. If inadequately treated, withdrawal from sedative-hypnotics can be life threatening. Alcohol is a sedative-hypnotic; however, it is not medically prescribed and it has a different cultural role in society. Therefore, it is considered separately (see Chapter 5).

Prior to the appearance of the third edition of the *Diagnostic and Statistical Manual of Mental Disorders* (DSM-III) in 1980, all anxiety disorder subtypes (as we know them today) were lumped under the single diagnostic entity "anxiety neurosis." To treat anxiety neurosis, barbiturates and several older nonbarbiturate sedatives, as well as the benzodiazepines (introduced in about 1960), were considered appropriate. The barbiturates were also early drugs used to treat epilepsy and to induce a state of general anesthesia for surgical procedures. These uses are discussed later in this chapter. Today, the most widely used sedative/anxiolytics are the benzodiazepines and their variants.

Historical Background

In the mid-nineteenth century, *bromide* and *chloral hydrate* became available as early sleep-inducing agents, as alternatives to alcohol and opium. In 1912, *phenobarbital* was introduced into medicine as a sedative drug, the first of the structurally classified group of drugs called *barbiturates* (Figure 13.1). Between 1912 and 1950, about 50 different barbiturates were marketed commercially. In the early 1950s, several other sedatives, including *meprobamate* (Equanil) and *carisoprodol* (Soma), were marketed as potentially safer alternatives, but their safety was not significantly better than that of the barbiturates.

In 1960, *chlordiazepoxide* (Librium) was marketed as the first sedative/anxiolytic of a new structural class of drugs called *benzodiazepines*. *Diazepam* (Valium), *alprazolam* (Xanax), *clonazepam* (Klonopin), and *lorazepam* (Ativan) are other commonly prescribed benzodiazepines. Several others are also available. The benzodiazepines had one major advantage over the barbiturates: they were rarely if ever fatal in overdosage, unless they were combined with alcohol. Because of improved safety, the benzodiazepine tranquilizers became incredibly popular (by physician prescription) for the treatment of anxiety and insomnia.

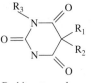

Barbiturate nucleus

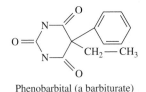

Phenobarbital (a barbiturate)

Nonbarbiturate Sedatives

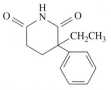
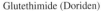

Glutethimide (Doriden)

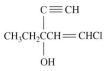

Ethchlorvynol (Placidyl)

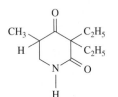

Methyprylon (Noludar)

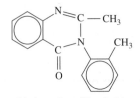

Methaqualone (Quaalude)

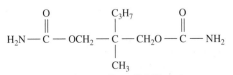

Meprobamate (Equanil, Miltown)

FIGURE 13.1 Chemical structures of classical sedatives. Barbiturates are defined by containing the barbiturate nucleus. Nonbarbiturate sedatives do not have this basic structure.

Sites and Mechanisms of Action

Historically, the sedative-hypnotic, anxiolytic, anticonvulsant, and general anesthetic actions of the barbiturates were perceived to result from a nonselective neuronal depression throughout the brain. These compounds were presumed to depress diffuse neuronal pathways both in the brain stem and in the cerebral cortex. Brainstem depression would continue as dosage was increased, accounting for the deep coma, cessation of respiration, and death that can follow drug overdosage. Today, we have much greater understanding of specific receptor-drug interactions that characterize the actions of these sedative/anxiolytic tranquilizers.

In our current era of drug development, we name new drugs not so much by their structure (as we did with barbiturates and benzodiazepines) as by the receptors that they bind to or that underlie their major clinical action (for example, a selective serotonin reuptake inhibitor, a serotonin 1_A agonist, a dopamine$_2$ blocker, and so on). If discovered today, a barbiturate or a benzodiazepine would be called a *GABA receptor agonist*. Because of what is now known of GABA receptors and because specific binding sites for both barbiturates and benzodiazepines on the GABA receptor have been identified (Figure 13.2), these and related drugs are called *benzodiazepine receptor agonists* (BZRAs). This term encompasses both the benzodiazepines and several newer nonbenzodiazepines that are widely prescribed to improve the quality of sleep in the clinical management of insomnia (Becker, 2012).

Benzodiazepines facilitate the binding of GABA to its receptor. They do not directly stimulate the GABA receptor; rather, they bind to a site adjacent to the GABA receptor,

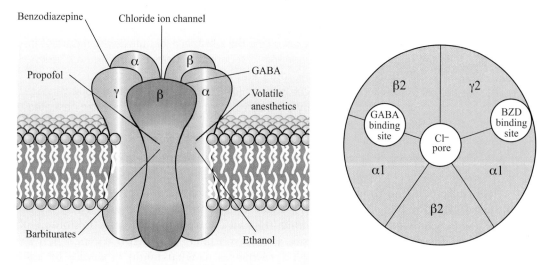

FIGURE 13.2 The GABA$_A$ receptor complex. This complex consists of several protein subunits, with each comprised further of subunit families. Different drugs bind at different sites on this complex. GABA is the normal transmitter. Benzodiazepines potentiate the influence of GABA. Other drugs, such as propofol and barbiturates potentiate GABA but also can open the channel directly. The inset is a schematic cross section of the receptor complex.

producing a three-dimensional conformational change in the receptor structure that, in turn, increases the affinity of GABA for the receptor. That action, in turn, increases the inhibitory synaptic action of GABA, facilitating the influx of chloride ions, causing hyperpolarization of the postsynaptic neuron, and depressing its excitability.

Benzodiazepines exert their anxiolytic properties by acting on GABA neurons at limbic centers. Their actions at other regions (for example, the cerebral cortex and brain stem) produce side effects such as sedation, increased seizure threshold, cognitive impairment, amnesia, and muscle relaxation. Neuroanatomically, the *amygdala, orbitofrontal cortex,* and *insula* are associated with the production of behavioral responses to fearful stimuli and the central mediation of anxiety and panic. Electrical stimulation of these structures evokes behavioral and physiological responses that are associated with fear and anxiety. Electrical lesions of the amygdala in animals result in an anxiolytic effect. PET scanning of the brain demonstrates increased amygdala blood flow concomitant with anxiety responses; MRI scanning of the brain demonstrates amygdala abnormalities in panic disorder patients.

Did You Know?

Brain's Own "Valium" Discovered

Since the 1970s, we have known that the brain produces its own natural analgesic substances (endorphins). But what about diazepam-like (Valium) anxiolytics?" Although researchers have searched for such anti-anxiety chemicals for decades, it's only now that they may finally have found one. From a practical perspective, the research may be more immediately applicable to the treatment of epilepsy than to anxiety disorders: the substance identified was important in preventing seizures in mice in a brain region that can generate them. But the authors believe that just as benzodiazepines—the class of drug that includes Valium (diazepam)—can both reduce seizure risk and relieve anxiety, the same is likely to be true for the natural version. Researchers cannot yet specifically identify the molecule involved, but the study demonstrated for the first time that either a substance called diazepam-binding inhibitor (DBI) or a protein that the brain makes from DBI behaves very much like a benzodiazepine.

Artificially blocking GABAergic function can provoke anxiety responses, with both behavioral and physiologic alterations similar to symptoms of human anxiety states. Increasing the activity of amygdala function (with lowered GABAergic inhibition of function) produces anxiogenic responses. Thus, hypofunctional GABA$_A$ receptor activity may sensitize the amygdala to anxiogenic responses to what might otherwise be considered nondistressing stimuli. This mechanism might underlie pathological emotional responses, such as chronically high levels of anxiety. The benzodiazepines may reset the threshold of the amygdala to a more normal level of responsiveness.

Recent reports offer new insights into the molecular biology of the interaction between benzodiazepines and GABA$_A$ receptor function, focusing on subtypes of the GABA$_A$ receptor (Sieghart et al., 2012; Trincavelli et al., 2012). The purpose of such study is to identify new medications that may be able to separate anxiolytic action from sedative actions and adverse cognitive impairment. For example, looking at the $GABA_A$ receptor complex (see Figure 13.2), binding to various and specific sites on the alpha-1 subunit mediates sedation, anxiolysis, and cognitive impairment. Insights into these subunits of the $GABA_A$ receptor may allow development of new therapeutic agents for the treatment of anxiety; for example, anxiolytics devoid of cognitive-impairing potential.

Did You Know?

Dogs, Humans Affected by OCD Have Similar Brain Abnormalities

Another piece of the puzzle to better understand and treat obsessive compulsive disorder (OCD) has fallen into place with new research that shows that the structural brain abnormalities of Doberman pinschers afflicted with canine compulsive disorder (CCD) are similar to those of humans with OCD. The research suggests that further study of anxiety disorders in dogs may help find new therapies for OCD and similar conditions in humans.

The causes of OCD, which affects about 2 percent of the population, are not well understood and the disorder often goes untreated or undiagnosed for decades. People with OCD often exhibit repetitive behaviors or persistent thoughts that are time consuming and interfere with daily routines. Dogs with CCD engage in repetitious and destructive behaviors such as flank- and blanket-sucking, tail chasing, and chewing. However, both OCD and CCD often respond to similar treatments.

"While the study sample was small and further research is needed, the results further validate that dogs with CCD can provide insight and understanding into anxiety disorders that affect people. Dogs exhibit the same behavioral characteristics, respond to the same medication, have a genetic basis to the disorder, and we now know have the same structural brain abnormalities as people with OCD," said Nicholas Dodman, BVMS, DACVB, professor of clinical sciences at the Cummings School of Veterinary Medicine at Tufts University.

Sedative-Induced Brain Dysfunction

High levels of alcohol (see Chapter 5) can induce a "blackout" when the level of alcohol in blood becomes extreme (e.g., a blood alcohol level of about 0.25 to 0.30 gram% or higher). A blackout is a state of *anterograde amnesia,* resulting in loss of memory for new events or actions that persist until blood alcohol falls to below the threshold level that produced the amnesia. More correctly, alcohol-induced blackout is a manifestation of a *drug-induced, reversible, organic brain syndrome* (or state of dementia) that can follow use of any sedative, including barbiturates, benzodiazepines, or other BZRAs. Therefore, any sedative, in high enough doses, can produce amnesia. This amnestic effect is clearly distinct from extreme levels that produce loss of consciousness. Therefore, a person can be in blackout, yet awake and capable of performing behavioral activities (as would be a patient with organic dementia). Indeed, these sedative-hypnotic medications now carry a FDA warning concerning a potential for inducing complex sleep-related behaviors which may include sleep-driving, making phone calls, and preparing and eating food (while a person thinks that they were asleep), and later having no memory of having done so.

This state of dementia (whether drug induced or organic) produces characteristic behavioral, intellectual, and cognitive deficits. One way to diagnose drug-induced dementia is to perform a *mental status examination* while the patient is under the influence of the drug. The examination evaluates 12 areas of mental functioning (Table 13.1). When a person is in an amnestic state, 5 of the 12 components of the mental status examination are particularly altered (sensorium, affect, mental content, intellectual function, and insight and judgment). The sensorium becomes clouded, which causes disorientation to time and place; memory becomes impaired, which is manifested by loss of ability to form short-term memory (the blackout); the intellect becomes depressed; judgment is altered. Affect becomes shallow and labile; that is, the person becomes extremely vulnerable to external stimuli and may be sullen and moody one moment and exhibit mock anger or rage the next. This kind of mental status is diagnosed as a "brain syndrome" caused by depressed nerve cell function. The reason these sedative drugs are called "date rape" drugs is that the person who takes the drug does not remember what happened during the period of intoxication. This occurs despite being in a state of wakefulness and ability to be an active participant. In medicine, this is seen when medical professionals induce a state of *"conscious sedation,"* where the patient is awake and cooperative yet does not remember the medical procedure. One example is the administration of a short-acting

---

TABLE 13.1 Mental status examination: Twelve areas of mental functioning

   1. Gentral appearance

* 2. Sensorium
      a. Orientation to time, place, and person
      b. Clear vs. clouded thinking

   3. Behavior and mannerisms

   4. Stream of talk

   5. Cooperativeness

   6. Mood (inner feelings)

* 7. Affect (surface expression of feelings)

   8. Perception
      a. Illusions (misperception of reality)
      b. Hallucinations (not present in reality)

   9. Thought processes; logical vs. strange or bizarre

* 10. Mental content (fund of knowledge)

* 11. Intellectual function (ability to reason and interpret)

* 12. Insight and judgment

---

* Characteristically altered in both organic dementia and reversible, drug-induced dementia.

benzodiazepine midazolam (Versed) so the patient does not remember a colonoscopy, despite having been awake during the procedure.

Certain people (such as the elderly) who already have some natural loss of nerve cell function are more likely to be adversely affected by these drugs; they experience increased disorientation and further clouding of consciousness. Frequently these people exhibit a state of drug-induced paradoxical excitement, which is characterized by a labile personality with marked anger, delusions, hallucinations, and confabulations (unconscious fabrication of information to fill memory gaps). Treating drug-induced memory loss requires that administration of the sedative drug (or alcohol) be stopped.

Barbiturates

In their decades of use, barbiturates were associated with thousands of suicides, deaths from accidental ingestion, widespread dependency and abuse, and many serious interactions with other drugs and alcohol. They are now rarely used; however, they remain the classic prototype of sedative-hypnotic drugs.

Pharmacokinetics

Barbiturates are all of similar structure, and classification of individual drugs is by their individual pharmacokinetics. Their half-lives can be quite short (3-minute redistribution half-life for thiopental) or as long as several days (phenobarbital). The hypnotic action of ultrashort-acting barbiturates (such as thiopental) is terminated by redistribution, while the action of other barbiturates is determined by their rate of metabolism by enzymes in the liver. Butalbital is still occasionally used in medicine and has a half-life of about 30–40 hours.

Barbiturates are well absorbed orally and well distributed to most body tissues. The ultrashort-acting barbiturates are exceedingly lipid soluble, cross the blood-brain barrier rapidly, and induce sleep within seconds following their intravenous injection. Because the longer-acting barbiturates are more water soluble, they are slower to penetrate the central nervous system (CNS). Sleep induction with these compounds, therefore, is delayed for 20 to 30 minutes, and residual hangover is prominent (since the plasma half-lives of most barbiturates are longer than that needed for 8 hours of sleep).

Pharmacological Effects

Barbiturates have a low degree of selectivity, and it is not possible to achieve anxiolysis without evidence of sedation. Barbiturates are not analgesic; they cannot be relied on to produce sedation or sleep in the presence of even moderate pain. Sleep patterns are decidedly affected by barbiturates; rapid eye movement (REM) sleep is markedly suppressed. Because dreaming occurs during REM sleep, barbiturates suppress dreaming. During drug withdrawal, dreaming becomes vivid and excessive. Such rebound increase in dreaming during withdrawal (termed "REM rebound") is one example of a withdrawal effect following prolonged periods of barbiturate ingestion. The vivid nature of the dreams can lead to insomnia, which can be clinically relieved by restarting the drug, terminating the withdrawal response.

Since barbiturates depress memory functioning, they are *cognitive inhibitors*. Drowsiness and more subtle alterations of judgment, cognitive functioning, motor skills, physical coordination, and behavior may persist for hours or days until the barbiturate is completely metabolized and eliminated. Sedative doses of barbiturates have minimal effect on respiration, but overdoses (or combinations of barbiturates and alcohol) can result in death.

Barbiturates exert few significant effects on the cardiovascular system, the gastrointestinal tract, the kidneys, or other organs until toxic doses are reached. In the liver, barbiturates stimulate the synthesis of enzymes that metabolize barbiturates as well as other drugs, an effect that produces significant tolerance to the drugs.

Psychological Effects

The behavioral, motor, and cognitive inhibitions caused by barbiturates are similar to those caused by alcohol. A person may respond to low doses either with relief from anxiety (the expected effect) or with withdrawal, emotional depression, or aggressive and violent behavior. Higher doses lead to more general behavioral depression and sleep. Mental set and physical or social setting can determine whether relief from anxiety, mental depression, aggression, or another unexpected or unpredictable response is experienced. Driving skills, judgment, insight, and memory all become severely impaired during the period of intoxication.

Clinical Uses

Use of barbiturates has declined rapidly for several reasons: (1) they are lethal in overdose; (2) they have a narrow therapeutic-to-toxic range; (3) they have a high potential for inducing tolerance, dependence, and abuse; and (4) they interact dangerously with many other drugs, sometimes fatally. Because of these disadvantages, they have largely been replaced by benzodiazepines. Occasionally, barbiturates (such as butalbital) are found in combination with other medications (such as aspirin or acetaminophen combined with caffeine in Fiorinol or Fioricet) for the treatment of migraine headache.

Adverse Reactions

Drowsiness is an inescapable accompaniment to the anxiolytic effect and is often the effect sought if the drug is intended to produce either daytime sedation or nighttime sleep. Barbiturates as cognitive inhibitors significantly impair motor and intellectual performance and judgment. It should be emphasized that all sedatives are equivalent to alcohol in their effects, that all are additive in their effects with alcohol, and that their effects persist longer than might be predicted. There are no specific antidotes with which one can treat barbiturate overdosage. Treatment is aimed at supporting the respiratory and cardiovascular system until the drug is metabolized and eliminated.

Tolerance

The barbiturates can induce tolerance by either of two mechanisms: (1) the induction of drug-metabolizing enzymes in the liver; or (2) the adaptation of neurons in the brain to the presence of the drug. With the latter mechanism, tolerance develops primarily to the sedative effects, much less to the brain-stem depressant effects on respiration. Thus, the margin of safety for the person who uses the drug decreases.

Physical Dependence

Normal clinical doses of barbiturates can induce a degree of physical dependence, usually manifested by sleep difficulties during attempts at withdrawal. Withdrawal from high doses of barbiturates may result in hallucinations, restlessness, disorientation, and even life-threatening convulsions.

Effects in Pregnancy

Barbiturates, like all psychoactive drugs, are freely distributed to the fetus. Data are limited on whether deleterious fetal abnormalities occur as a result of a pregnant woman taking barbiturates, although it has been suggested that developmental abnormalities occur. This possibility can be a concern for pregnant women who are epileptic and must take a barbiturate to prevent seizures. At a minimum, there is uncertainty concerning the risk of fetal problems associated with the ingestion of barbiturates by pregnant women (Eadie, 2008); nevertheless, barbiturates are considered to be relatively safe during pregnancy (Timmermann et al., 2009).

Nonbarbiturate Sedative-Hypnotic Drugs

In the early 1950s, several "nonbarbiturate" sedatives—*glutethimide* (Doriden), *ethchlorvynol* (Placidyl), and *methyprylon* (Noludar), for example—were introduced as anxiolytics, daytime sedatives, and hypnotics. They somewhat resembled the barbiturates (see Figure 13.2), but they did not have the exact barbiturate nucleus and could not legally be called "barbiturates," despite being pharmacologically interchangeable. These drugs offered no advantages over the barbiturates. Now considered obsolete for use in medicine, they are occasionally encountered as drugs of abuse.

Meprobamate (Equanil, Miltown) was marketed in 1955 as an alternative to the barbiturates for daytime sedation and anxiolysis. Around it developed the term *tranquilizer* in a marketing attempt to distinguish it from the barbiturates, a distinction that was not borne out in clinical practice. Like barbiturates, meprobamate produces long-lasting daytime sedation, mild euphoria, and relief from anxiety. Meprobamate is not as potent a respiratory depressant as are the barbiturates; attempted suicides from overdosage are seldom successful unless the drug is mixed with opioid narcotics such as morphine or oxycodone. Despite a continuing reduction in clinical use, abuse and dependency continue and are difficult to treat. There is a possibility that use of meprobamate during pregnancy may be associated with an increased frequency of congenital malformations.

Carisoprodol (Soma) is a precursor compound to meprobamate; after it is absorbed, it is rapidly metabolized to meprobamate, which is the active form of the drug. Currently, carisoprodol, as an intoxicant, is increasingly encountered as a drug of abuse.

Methaqualone (Quaalude) was another nonbarbiturate sedative that had little to justify its widespread use. During the late 1970s, its popularity rivaled that of marijuana and alcohol in its level of abuse. The attention was due to an undeserved reputation as an aphrodisiac (as a sedative, it was actually an *anaphrodisiac*, much like alcohol). It was, however, a "date rape" drug since, as with all these drugs, the amnestic effect occurred at doses lower than the dose required to produce incapacitation or unconsciousness. Extensive illicit use and numerous deaths led to its being banned in the United States in 1984, although illicit supplies occasionally emerge as a drug of abuse.

Chloral hydrate (Noctec) is yet another drug of historical interest, having been available clinically since the late 1800s. It is rapidly metabolized to *trichlorethanol* (a derivative of ethyl alcohol), which is a nonselective CNS depressant and the active form of chloral hydrate. The drug is an effective sedative-hypnotic, with a plasma half-life of about 4 to 8 hours. Next-day hangover is less likely to occur than with compounds having longer half-lives. Withdrawal of the drug may be associated with disrupted sleep and intense nightmares. One interesting aside is that the combination of chloral hydrate with alcohol can produce increased intoxication, stupor, and amnesia. This mixture, called a *Mickey Finn*, was an early example of a "date rape" drug combination.

Paraldehyde, introduced into medicine before the barbiturates, is a polymer of acetaldehyde, an intermediate by-product in the body's metabolism of ethyl alcohol. Administered either rectally or orally, paraldehyde was historically used to treat delirium tremens (DTs) in alcoholics undergoing detoxification. Paraldehyde is rapidly absorbed (from both rectal and oral routes), sleep ensues within 10 to 15 minutes after hypnotic doses, and the drug is metabolized in the liver to acetaldehyde. Some paraldehyde is eliminated through the lungs, producing a characteristic unpleasant breath odor.

Gamma hydroxybutyrate, (GHB, Xyrem) is a most interesting chemical and drug. It is an endogenous neurotransmitter, synthesized from glutamate, exhibiting binding to GHB receptors present on both pre- and postsynaptic neurons, inhibiting GABA release. In overdose, GHB acts both directly as a partial GABA$_B$ receptor agonist and indirectly through its metabolism to GABA (Schep et al., 2012). Absalom and coworkers (2012) discuss the complicated mechanisms of action of GHB in greater detail.

GHB was synthesized and developed in 1960 as a short-acting anesthetic. It later achieved popularity as a recreational drug and a nutritional supplement marketed to bodybuilders. As a drug of abuse, it was classified in 1990 as a Schedule 1 drug in the United States, and sales were banned.[1] However, it and its precursors, GBL (gamma butyrolactone) and 1,4-butanediol (1,4-BD) remain widely available on the Internet and alternative sources.

In 2002, sodium oxybate (a formulation of GHB) was FDA-approved for the treatment of narcolepsy and was classified as a Schedule III drug. This was the first and only time a single drug was FDA-classified in two schedules, depending on its intended use.

Its disinhibiting, hypnotic and amnestic actions have led to its identification as a "date-rape" drug, although such use is not as widespread as commonly thought (Nemeth et al., 2010).

---

[1] A Schedule I classification means that to the FDA a drug has a high potential for abuse with no therapeutic use. Schedules II through V allow for therapeutic use under varying degrees of prescription regulation.

Besides approved use in the treatment of narcolepsy, there is interest in the use of GHB in the treatment of alcoholism (Sewell and Petrakis, 2011) and perhaps treatment-resistant depression (Bosch et al., 2012). As a sedative, GHB has been abused as a purported aphrodisiac and a euphoriant. It has been sold illicitly under such names as RenewTrient, Revivarant, Blue Nitro, Remiforce, GH Revitalize, and Gamma G. It has been called "nature's Quaalude" and "Liquid Ecstasy," among a variety of other names. As a "date rape" drug, it produces alcohol-like disinhibition and amnesia, although the victim is not necessarily asleep or unconscious (Madea and Mubhoff, 2009). Often GHB is added to alcohol to produce this state.

GHB has a rapid onset (about 30 minutes) and a short half-life (about 30 minutes). The drug is rapidly metabolized to inactive metabolites and ultimately to carbon dioxide and water. It is detectable in urine for only very brief periods of time. Overdoses are characterized by stupor, delirium, unconsciousness, coma, and death. Combined with alcohol, the drug's toxic potential is greatly magnified. Acute withdrawal in a GHB-dependent person results in rapid onset of insomnia, anxiety, hallucinations, tremors, agitation, and other signs (Schep et al., 2012). Withdrawal symptoms usually resolve in about 3 to 10 days. Possible long-term adverse effects on cognitive functioning and neurotoxicity have been postulated (vanAmsterdam et al, 2012).

As stated earlier, GHB has been used intravenously for the induction of general anesthesia. This use has been supplanted by superior anesthetics. However, GHB remains useful in treating narcolepsy, a lifelong disorder characterized by fragmented sleep during the night, altered sleep patterns, and excessive sleepiness during the day. GHB is taken at bedtime and then 2.5 to 4 hours later, even if the patient has to be wakened to take the medicine. Taken in this fashion, the drug improves sleep and markedly reduces the number of daytime narcoleptic attacks.

Benzodiazepines

In the 1960s, the benzodiazepines replaced the barbiturates and quickly became the most widely used class of psychotherapeutic drugs; the terms *tranquilizer* and *anxiolytic* rapidly became synonymous with the *benzodiazepines*. These medications remain in wide use today (by prescription) and are widely abused or otherwise used inappropriately. About 2.5 percent of the adult population receives a prescribed benzodiazepine and they continue to be used despite well-recognized impairments in cognition, memory, attention, reaction time, and psychomotor functioning. Indicated only for short-term use (up to one month), their median duration of use is almost 2 years. Dependence occurs in about 10 percent of users, up to 34 percent when a comorbid depressive disorder is present (Hadley et al, 2012). They are often used or misused by opioid-dependent persons to self-medicate opioid withdrawal and anxiety, to intensify the effects of methadone (by reducing its metabolism), or to ameliorate the adverse effects of cocaine and methamphetamine.

Pharmacokinetics

Fifteen benzodiazepine derivatives remain available (see Table 13.2). They differ from one another mainly in their pharmacokinetic parameters and the routes through which they are administered. Pharmacokinetic differences include rates of metabolism to pharmacologically active intermediates and plasma half-lives of both the parent drug and any active metabolites. Twelve of the benzodiazepines are commercially available in the United States; all 12 are available in dosage forms intended only for oral ingestion, two (diazepam and lorazepam) are available for both oral use and use by injection, and one (midazolam) is available only in injectable formulation.

Absorption and Distribution. Benzodiazepines are well absorbed when they are taken orally; peak plasma concentrations are achieved in about one hour. Some (for example, oxazepam and lorazepam) are absorbed more slowly, while others (for example, triazolam) are absorbed more rapidly. Clorazepate is metabolized in gastric juice to an active metabolite (nordiazepam) that is completely absorbed.

Metabolism and Excretion. Psychoactive drugs are usually metabolized to pharmacologically inactive products, which are then excreted in urine. Although some benzodiazepines behave this way, several are first metabolized to pharmacologically active intermediates; these products, in turn, are detoxified by further metabolism before they are excreted (Figure 13.3). As can be seen from Table 13.2 and Figure 13.3, several benzodiazepines are metabolized into the long-lasting, pharmacologically active metabolite nordiazepam, the half-life of which is about 60 hours, much longer (perhaps one to two weeks) in the elderly. Thus, the long-acting benzodiazepines are long acting primarily because of the long half-life of a pharmacologically active metabolite. In contrast, the short-acting benzodiazepines are short acting because they are metabolized directly into inactive products that are then excreted in the urine.

Benzodiazepines in the Elderly. The elderly have a reduced ability to metabolize long-acting benzodiazepines and their active metabolites. In this population, the elimination half-life for diazepam and its active metabolite is about 7 to 10 days. Since it takes about six half-lives to rid the body completely of a drug, it may take an elderly patient 6 to 10 weeks to become drug-free after stopping the drug. With short-acting benzodiazepines, such as midazolam, pharmacokinetics are not so drastically altered, but the dose necessary to achieve effect is reduced by about 50 percent.

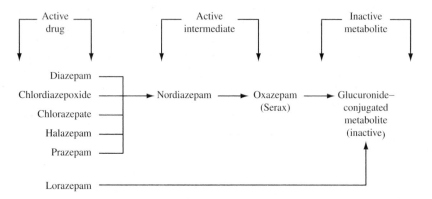

FIGURE 13.3 Metabolism of benzodiazepines. The intermediate metabolite nordiazepam is formed from many agents. *Oxazepam* (Serax) is commercially available and is also an active metabolite in the metabolism of nordiazepam to its inactive products.

TABLE 13.2 Benzodiazepines

Drug name		Dosage form		Active metabolite	Active compounds in blood	Mean elimination half-life in hours (range)
Generic	Trade	Oral	Parenteral			
LONG-ACTING AGENTS						
Diazepam	Valium	X	X	Yes	Diazepam	24 (20–50)
					Nordiazepam	60 (50–100)
Chlordiazepoxide	Librium	X		Yes	Chlordiazepoxide	10 (8–24)
					Nordiazepam	60 (50–100)
Flurazepam	Dalmane	X		Yes	Desalkylflurazepam	80 (70–160)
Halazepam	Paxipam	X		Yes	Halazepam	14 (10–20)
					Nordiazepam	
Prazepam	Centrax	X		Yes	Nordiazepam	
Chlorazepate	Tranxene	X		Yes	Nordiazepam	
INTERMEDIATE-ACTING AGENTS						
Lorazepam	Ativan	X	X	No	Lorazepam	15 (10–24)
Clonazepam	Klonopin	X		No	Clonazepam	30 (18–50)
Quazepam	Dormalin	X		Yes	Quazepam	35 (25–50)
					Desalkylflurazepam	80 (70–160)
Estazolam	ProSom	X		Yes	Hydroxyestazolam	18 (13–35)
SHORT-ACTING AGENTS						
Midazolam	Versed		X	No	Midazolam	2.5 (1.5–4.5)
Oxazepam	Serax	X		No	Oxazepam	8 (5–15)
Temazepam	Restoril	X		No	Temazepam	12 (8–35)
Triazolam	Halcion	X		No	Triazolam	2.5 (1.5–5)
Alprazolam	Xanax	X		No	Alprazolam	12 (11–18)

Because all benzodiazepines can produce cognitive dysfunction, elderly patients can become clinically demented as a result. In general, benzodiazepines should be used only with great caution (if at all) in the elderly (Weston et al., 2010). Rang and Dale (1991) stated some 25 years ago:

> At the age of 91, the grandmother of one of the authors was growing increasingly forgetful and mildly dotty, having been taking nitrazepam for insomnia regularly for years. To the author's lasting shame, it took a canny general practitioner to diagnose the problem. Cancellation of the nitrazepam prescription produced a dramatic improvement. (p. 637)

Paterniti and coworkers (2002) followed over 130 benzodiazepine-using elderly people for up to 4 years. Even periodic use was associated with prolonged decreases in cognitive performance, compared with non-drug-taking elderly. Wu and coworkers (2009) reported that long-term benzodiazepine use was associated with a more than twofold-increased risk of dementia. They postulate that this dementing action in the elderly may follow from hyperpolarization of neuronal cell membranes, possibly reducing synaptic plasticity and hindering the individual's ability to form new memories.

Increases in the incidence of falls and bone fractures constitute another significant problem with benzodiazepines in the elderly (Nurmi-Luthje et al., 2006). Atypical antipsychotic drugs, such as *quetiapine* (Seroquel) are replacing the use of benzodiazepines for sedation and treatment of agitated behaviors in the elderly.

Pharmacological Effects

All benzodiazepines are termed *pure GABA agonists* because they faithfully facilitate GABA binding at GABA receptors. GABA normally attaches to postsynaptic $GABA_A$ receptors, causing them to open chloride ion channels, slowing down neurotransmission. Benzodiazepines bind to a specific benzodiazepine modulatory site next to the $GABA_A$ receptor (see Figure 13.2) and enhance the opening of the ion channel, increasing the efficacy of endogenous GABA. This increased inhibitory influence in the brain presumably leads to antianxiety and sedative effects.

Low doses of benzodiazepines moderate anxiety, agitation, and fear by their actions on receptors located in the amygdala, orbitofrontal cortex, and insula. Mental confusion and amnesia follow action on GABA neurons located in the cerebral cortex and the hippocampus. The mild muscle relaxant effects of the benzodiazepines are probably caused both by their anxiolytic actions and by effects on GABA receptors located in the spinal cord, cerebellum, and brain stem. The antiepileptic actions seem to follow from actions on GABA receptors located in the cerebellum and the hippocampus.[2] The behavioral rewarding effects, drug abuse potential, and psychological dependency probably result from actions on GABA receptors that modulate the discharge of neurons located in the ventral tegmentum and the nucleus accumbens.

Clinical Uses and Limitations

From 1960 to the late 1990s, the benzodiazepines were the drugs of choice for the short-term pharmacological treatment of stress-related anxiety, anxious-depression, and insomnia. They are easy to use, have relatively low toxicity, and are effective in producing a "tranquil" state with reductions in anxiety. The benzodiazepines, however, are not antidepressant; in fact, they intensify depression in much the same way that alcohol intensifies depression. The cognitive impairments and potential for producing dependency are generally conceded to limit their therapeutic use to relatively short periods of time and to conditions in which short-term therapy is beneficial. For longer-term treatment of such disorders as insomnia, generalized anxiety, phobias, and panic disorder, behavioral

---

[2] A sixteenth benzodiazepine, *clobazam* (Onfi) was FDA-approved in 2011 for use in difficult-to-control epileptic seizures, as well as for short-term treatment of severe anxiety and agitation.

treatments and both antidepressant and atypical antipsychotic drugs are now preferred over benzodiazepine therapy. In instances where a combination of cognitive-behavioral therapies and benzodiazepines are used to treat anxiety, the benzodiazepines have the potential to interfere with the cognitive therapy, perhaps significantly reducing its efficacy. A cognitive inhibitor could certainly be predicted to block cognitive-based psychological therapies.[3] Benzodiazepines are generally not indicated for the treatment of obsessive-compulsive disorder (OCD) and post-traumatic stress disorder (PTSD) (Bostwick et al, 2012).

Benzodiazepines are generally not indicated for chronic use or for treating depression. When chronically used in clinical practice (such as in treating generalized anxiety disorder) there is little evidence of effectiveness, dependence develops and cognitive side effects can complicate life. They should be avoided in situations requiring fine motor or cognitive skills or mental alertness, or in situations where alcohol or other CNS depressants are used. They should be used only with great caution in the elderly, in children or adolescents, and in anyone with a history of drug misuse or ongoing abuse.

One possible indication for benzodiazepine therapy is for the short-term treatment of anxiety that is so debilitating that the patient's life-style, work, and interpersonal relationships are severely hampered. A benzodiazepine may alleviate the symptoms of nervousness, dysphoria, and psychological distress without necessarily blocking the physiological correlates accompanying the state of anxiety.

Because they are sedating, benzodiazepines can be used as hypnotics for the treatment of insomnia. Agents with rapid onset, a 2- to 3-hour half-life, and no active metabolites may be preferred to minimize daytime sedation (note that few benzodiazepines fit this profile; see Table 13.2). Use in treating insomnia is also limited by the development of habituation and dependence, as reflected by rebound increases in insomnia upon drug discontinuation.

The benzodiazepines have been used as muscle relaxants, both to directly reduce states associated with increased muscle tension and to reduce the psychological distress that can predispose to muscle tension. However, they do not directly relax muscles. They relieve only the distress associated with muscle tension (much like alcohol).

Benzodiazepines are exceedingly effective in producing anterograde amnesia (amnesia that starts at the time of drug administration and ends when the blood level of drug has decreased to a point where memory function is regained). For this use, two injectable benzodiazepines are available—lorazepam, when long-lasting amnesia is desirable, and midazolam, when shorter periods of amnesia are desirable.

Often, however, an amnestic effect is undesirable. For example, concern has been expressed about an illegally imported "date rape" drug, which turned out to be a benzodiazepine that is commercially marketed outside the United States. This drug, *flunitrazepam* (Rohypnol), is very similar to *triazolam* (Halcion; see Table 13.2); it produces anxiolysis, sedation, and amnesia, especially when taken with alcohol. When an unknowing victim ingests the drug and alcohol, the effect closely resembles the effect

---

[3] A patient is often unaware of this interaction since the long half-lives of benzodiazepines imply that a patient is seldom, if ever, free of drug. Neither the patient nor the therapist knows the patient's cognitive ability in the absence of drug.

of a Mickey Finn (chloral hydrate in alcohol), and amnesia is achieved without loss of consciousness.[4]

Panic attacks and phobias can be treated with benzodiazepines such as *alprazolam* (Xanax), although the efficacy of benzodiazepines may be less than that of the serotonin-type antidepressants, which are actually more specific anxiolytics (Moylan et al., 2012). Moreover, unlike with the benzodiazepines, SSRIs do not cause impairments in psychomotor performance, do not impair learning and cognition, do not reduce alertness, and have little or no potential for dependence and abuse. Alternatives to benzodiazepines for the treatment of generalized anxiety and panic disorders include serotonin-type antidepressants (SSRIs), dual action antidepressants (e.g., venlafaxine), and mood, stabilizing anticonvulsants such as pregabalin (Diaper et al., 2012; Feltner et al, 2011; Hadley et al., 2012; Rickels et al., 2012). The anticonvulsant *topiramate* (Topamax) has been shown effective in reducing symptoms of PTSD (Yeh et al., 2011).

Because benzodiazepines can substitute for alcohol, they are used both in treating acute alcohol withdrawal and in long-term therapy to reduce the rate of relapse to previous drinking habits. Today, however, certain of the antiepileptic mood stabilizers are viable alternatives.

Finally, all benzodiazepines exert antiepileptic actions because they raise the threshold for generating seizures. In general, however, benzodiazepines are used as secondary drugs or as adjuvants to other, more specific anticonvulsants.

In summary, perhaps the only well-accepted situation in which benzodiazepines cannot readily be replaced by other drugs is the intentional production of anterograde amnesia, for example, in hospital situations where it is desirable to block the memory for certain unpleasant or painful procedures. The newer antidepressant/anxiolytic agents continue to replace benzodiazepines for the treatment of most anxiety disorders, although the benzodiazepines may have a faster onset of effect and be efficacious for very short-term use.

Side Effects and Toxicity

Common acute side effects associated with benzodiazepine therapy are usually dose-related extensions of the intended actions, including sedation, drowsiness, ataxia, lethargy, mental confusion, motor and cognitive impairments, disorientation, slurred speech, amnesia, and induction or extension of the symptoms of dementia. At higher doses, mental and psychomotor dysfunction progress to hypnosis. Used for the treatment of insomnia, benzodiazepines are especially controversial; drugs can cause the expected sedation, or they can induce paradoxical agitation (anxiety, aggression, hostility, and behavioral disinhibition). In addition, cessation of use results in rebound increases in insomnia (*REM rebound*) and anxiety.

Impairment of motor abilities—especially a person's ability to drive an automobile—is common. In monograph form, Baselt (2011) reviews the literature on specific drugs

---

[4] Rohypnol intoxication (and the amnesia it causes) can begin within about 30 minutes, peak within 2 hours, and persist for up to 8 hours. With a combination of Rohypnol and alcohol, the amnestic and intoxicating effects can last 8 to 18 hours. Disinhibition is another widely reported effect of Rohypnol when it is ingested alone or in combination with alcohol.

and their side effects, including references for blood concentrations associated with driving impairments. In general, when viewed as a group, all benzodiazepines are capable of impairing driving, even at therapeutic concentrations.

Vindenes and coworkers (2012) recently reported impairing concentrations of benzodiazepines and several other drugs in comparison with *blood alcohol concentrations* of 0.02 gram%, 0.05 grams% and 0.12 grams%. These Norwegian authors note that in Norway, the impairment limit for alcohol is 0.02 grams% and graded sanctions are given for higher BACs, with limits corresponding to levels of 0.05 grams% and 0.12 grams%. Some countries, like Sweden, have zero-tolerance laws, with the exception of prescribed medications. Vindenes and coworkers list blood concentrations of benzodiazepines and other drugs (stimulants, THC, GHB, hallucinogens, and opioids) that cause impairment similar to the three chosen BAC concentrations.

Verster and Roth (2012) note that while group differences in concentrations were found as evidenced by significant effects of dose and time of driving since time of drug ingestion, no significant relationship between *individual* blood drug concentrations and impairment[5] was found. Therefore, for any individual charged with driving under the influence, the blood concentration must be considered in light of observed impairments and the medication history. Deficits in driving ability are compounded by the drug-induced suppression of a person's ability to assess his or her own level of physical and mental impairment.

The cognitive deficits associated with benzodiazepine use are significant. In both children and adults, benzodiazepines can significantly interfere with learning behaviors, academic performance, and psychomotor functioning. Cognitive and generalized intellectual impairments can persist even long after the benzodiazepine is discontinued, although cognitive improvements after discontinuation are the norm.

Tolerance and Dependence

When benzodiazepines are taken for prolonged periods of time, a pattern of dependence can develop. Early withdrawal signs include a return (and possible intensification) of the anxiety state for which the drug was originally given. Rebound increases in insomnia, restlessness, agitation, irritability, and unpleasant dreams gradually appear. In rare instances, hallucinations, psychoses, and seizures have been reported. Most of these withdrawal symptoms subside within one to four weeks. Hadley and coworkers (2012) discuss a protocol for gradual tapering of benzodiazepines with replacement with *pregabalin* (Lyrica) as a safe and effective method for discontinuing long-term benzodiazepine therapy and dependence.

Effects in Pregnancy

Benzodiazepines are commonly used by women of reproductive age, and hence many women are exposed to them (Enato et al, 2011). *Diazepam* (Valium) is one of the most frequently prescribed drugs in pregnancy, taken by up to 33 percent of pregnant women. During pregnancy, all benzodiazepines freely cross the placenta and accumulate in

---

[5] Impairment was measured by the standard deviation of lateral position (tracking of the vehicle while driving on a city street).

the fetal circulation. Benzodiazepines administered during the first trimester of pregnancy do not seem to be associated with an increased risk of congenital malformations (Bellantuono et al., 2013); during the entire pregnancy the odds ratio of having any form of malformation is 1.07 (95 percent confidence limits = 0.91- 1.25, mostly accounted for by a slight risk of oral cleft malformations (Enato, et al., 2011).

Near the time of delivery, if a mother is on high doses of benzodiazepines, a fetus can develop benzodiazepine dependence or even a "floppy-infant syndrome," followed after delivery by signs of withdrawal. Because benzodiazepines are excreted in breast milk and because they can accumulate in nursing infants, taking benzodiazepines while breastfeeding is not recommended.

Flumazenil: A Benzodiazepine Receptor Antagonist

Flumazenil (Romazicon) is a benzodiazepine that binds with high affinity to benzodiazepine receptors on the $GABA_A$ complex, but after binding, it exhibits no intrinsic activity. As a consequence, it competitively blocks the access of pharmacologically active benzodiazepines to the receptor, effectively reversing the antianxiety and sedative effects of any benzodiazepines administered before flumazenil.

Flumazenil is metabolized quite rapidly in the liver and has a short half-life (about 1 hour). Because this half-life is much shorter than that of most benzodiazepines, the benzodiazepine effects can reappear as flumazenil is eliminated, thus necessitating reinjection. Flumazenil is utilized as an antidote (administered by intravenous injection) when benzodiazepine overdosage is suspected, although such use is fairly rare due to fear of precipitating withdrawal seizures.

Benzodiazepine Receptor Agonist (BZRA) Hypnotics

Any drug that activates the benzodiazepine receptor is termed a *benzodiazepine receptor agonist* (BZRA). The benzodiazepines are obviously in this category, since they all work by binding to the benzodiazepine receptor and exert an agonist action to increase GABA activity. Because benzodiazepines are non-specific agonists at the $GABA_A$ receptors they exert both anxiolytic and sedative-hypnotic effects.

Three drugs that are currently available are structurally not classified as benzodiazepines but nevertheless are agonists at the benzodiazepine receptor. These *nonbenzodiazepine BZRAs* are prescribed as hypnotic drugs intended for the treatment of insomnia. They are not prescribed as anxiolytics because they more specifically bind to the alpha-1 subunit (sedative) of the $GABA_A$ receptor. These three drugs, as well as the benzodiazepines, have been implicated in behavioral activities that occur while one is amnestic (for example, driving, eating, cooking a meal, or engaging in sexual activity and not remembering having done so).

Chronic insomnia can manifest itself as difficulty falling asleep, difficulty staying asleep, waking up too early, or waking in the morning without feeling "refreshed." About 10 percent of people experience chronic insomnia. Roughly 50 percent of people with other medical or psychological conditions complain of insomnia. Consequences of insomnia include daytime fatigue, lack of energy, poor concentration and memory, moodiness and irritability, and difficulty completing tasks. Treatments can be either psychological or pharmacological. Of the psychological therapies, cognitive-behavioral therapies have been shown to be at least as effective as pharmacotherapies. Practice parameters for the psychological and behavioral treatment of insomnia are available (Morgenthaler et al., 2006). Pharmacotherapies include two types of FDA-approved insomnia medications: agonists of the benzodiazepine receptor (BZRAs) and a melatonin receptor agonist (ramelteon).

Benzodiazepine BZRAs

As discussed earlier, all benzodiazepines exhibit hypnotic properties. Five of them (flurazepam, estazolam, quazepam, temazepam, and triazolam) are formally approved for the treatment of insomnia. Triazolam has the shortest half-life, 2 to 4 hours, and is associated with the least daytime sedation. It may not provide adequate sedation through the night. Conversely, the others have longer half-lives and increase sleep maintenance, but they have adverse cognitive consequences the next day. Dependence and tolerance are potentially harmful.

Nonbenzodiazepine BZRAs

There are three drugs that are structurally not benzodiazepines but nevertheless bind to the same receptors to which benzodiazepines bind and exert the same agonist effects as the benzodiazepines (see Figure 13.4). These three drugs are referred to as *nonbenzodiazepine*

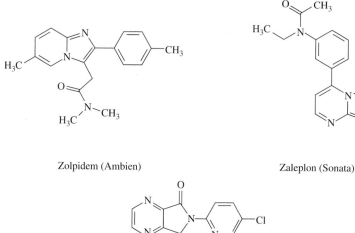

Zolpidem (Ambien)   Zaleplon (Sonata)

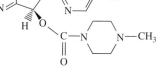

Eszopiclone (Lunesta)

FIGURE 13.4 Structural formulas of *zolpidem* (Ambien), *zaleplon* (Sonata), and *eszopiclone* (Lunesta). Note the close (but dissimilar) relationship of their basic three-ring structures to the benzodiazepine nucleus. Thus, these three compounds are nonbenzodiazepines despite similar GABAergic actions and clinical effects.

BZRAs. Because these three hypnotic agents all start with the letter Z, they are sometimes referred to as the "Z drugs."

Zolpidem. *Zolpidem* (Ambien, Ambien-CR, Edluar, Intermezzo) is marketed for the treatment of insomnia. Binding to the alpha-1 subunit of the GABA$_A$ receptor, it exhibits primarily a hypnotic rather than an anxiolytic effect. With a half-life of about 1.5 to 2.5 hours, zolpidem is often compared to *triazolam* (Halcion), a benzodiazepine with similar pharmacokinetics; at comparable doses, there appears to be little to differentiate the two drugs. A controlled-release, 2-layer formulation of *zolpidem* (Ambien CR) is available as a sublingual tablet (Edluar). Also, a new formulation (called Intermezzo) is a low-dose formulation of zolpidem (1.75 mg for women and 3.5 g for men) intended to be taken when one wakens in the middle of the night and cannot get back to sleep.[6] Because daytime impairment can be problematic, why one wants to extend the duration of action of a hypnotic remains unclear.

At doses of 5 to 10 milligrams, zolpidem produces sedation and promotes a physiological pattern of sleep in the absence of anxiolytic, anticonvulsant, or muscle relaxant effects. Memory is adversely affected as it is by benzodiazepines, and drug-induced blackouts and sleep-related activities are common.

Dose-related adverse effects of zolpidem include drowsiness, dizziness, and nausea. In doses of 5 milligrams, zolpidem exhibits minimal next-day effects on memory or psychomotor performance, such as driving; however, doses of 10 to 20 milligrams significantly impair performance and memory even 4 hours after taking the drug.

Recently, the FDA has become very concerned about zolpidem-induced "sleep-related activities" (discussed below) and later having no memory of performing such activities. The FDA has recommended limiting doses to an absolute minimum necessary for sleep maintenance.

Overdoses to 400 milligrams (40 times the therapeutic dose) have not been fatal. In the elderly, confusion, falls, memory loss, and psychotic reactions have been reported. The calculated half-life is prolonged in the elderly and, here, the extended-release preparation may further increase the risk of next-day sedation and cognitive impairment. Finally, patients with diminished function of their drug-metabolizing enzymes exhibit prolonged half-lives of the drug.

Zaleplon. *Zaleplon* (Sonata) is a second nonbenzodiazepine agonist that binds to the alpha-1 subunit of the GABA$_A$ receptor. In general, it exerts actions similar to those of zolpidem as a hypnotic agent. The half-life of zaleplon is very short (less than one hour), and only about 30 percent of the dose reaches the bloodstream; most undergoes first-pass metabolism in the liver. Because Zaleplon is poorly absorbed and short acting, it does not require predicting that insomnia will occur on a particular night. Instead, if unable to fall asleep and stay asleep without pharmacological assistance, the person has the option of taking this very short-acting agent without fear of detrimental effects the next morning.

Sleep is quite rapidly induced with zaleplon at doses of 5 to 10 milligrams, and sleep quality is improved without rebound insomnia. Zaleplon appears particularly noteworthy

---

[6] But only when one still has at least 4 hours of bedtime left.

in its lack of deleterious effects on psychomotor function and driving ability the morning following use. Allowing at least 4 hours from drug intake to driving results in few adverse effects. In fact, at 4 hours after oral administration, most of the drug is eliminated from the body. Dependence is unlikely to develop because of the short half-life: by morning, the drug is metabolized. In essence, a person taking the drug withdraws daily, and drug does not persist in the body. At extremely high doses (25 to 75 milligrams), an abuse potential comparable to that seen for *triazolam* (Halcion) is seen.

Eszopiclone. *Eszopiclone* (Lunesta) is the third BZRA approved for the treatment of insomnia. It is the active isomer of *zopiclone* (Immovane), which has been used outside the United States for many years. Eszopiclone shares all the actions of zolpidem and traditional benzodiazepines. Because of a half-life of 5 to 7 hours, eszopiclone has the most prolonged action of the nonbenzodiazepine BZRAs. Therefore, it might be preferable to the others for improving both sleep latency and sleep maintenance. However, this benefit is offset by increased risk of next-day sedation. It was the first of these agents to have data reported from long-term trials, and thus it has been approved by the FDA for longer-term use. At its highest dose level (3 milligrams), next-day memory impairments and poor performance on measures of psychomotor performance have been reported.

Partial Agonists at GABA$_A$ Receptors

"Full" BZRA agonists are effective anxiolytics and/or sedatives; however, their use is limited by rebound anxiety (on discontinuation), physical dependence, abuse potential, and side effects that include ataxia, sedation, memory impairments, and cognitive disturbances. For many years, attempts have been made to identify "partial" agonists of GABA receptors (*partial BZRAs*) in the hope of providing anxiolytics that may be equally as effective without the side effects that limit the use of the benzodiazepines. To date, several have been examined, although none are currently available. The best studied of these agents are alpidem which was briefly marketed for the treatment of anxiety. It was withdrawn, however, because of liver toxicity (Skolnick 2012). Other partial BZRAs have suffered a similar fate.

Sleep Driving and Sleep-Related Activities

In March 2007, the FDA released an advisory requesting that all manufacturers of sedative-hypnotic products that are used to induce and/or maintain sleep strengthen their product labeling to include risks of "sleep driving" and "sleep-related activities." Sleep driving is defined as driving while not fully awake after ingestion of a sedative-hypnotic product and having no memory of the event—in other words, driving while still in a drug-induced amnestic state. Sleep-related activities that can occur include making telephone calls, preparing and eating food, and engaging in sexual activity and then having no later memory of having done so (Zammit 2009). Thirteen products were listed on the FDA advisory. These included: the three nonbenzodiazepine BZRAs Ambien, Sonata, and Lunesta; the benzodiazepines Dalmane, Halcion, ProSom, and Restoril; the barbiturates Butisol, Carbrital, and Seconal; the melatonin agonist Rozerem; and two miscellaneous agents Doral and Placidyl. This advisory is not all-inclusive as all benzodiazepines can cause the same thing.

General Anesthetics

All sedatives in sufficient doses can produce amnesia and loss of consciousness. General anesthetics are drugs that are used to intentionally produce these effects for the performance of surgical procedures. The agents that are used as general anesthetics are of two types: (1) those that are administered by inhalation through the lungs; and (2) those that are injected directly into a vein.

Inhalation anesthetics in current use include one gas (nitrous oxide) and five volatile liquids (isoflurane, halothane, desflurane, enflurane, and sevoflurane). These drugs produce a dose-related depression of all functions of the CNS—an initial period of sedation followed by the onset of sleep. As anesthesia deepens, both amnesia and unconsciousness are induced. Adding an opioid narcotic (such as morphine) to a volatile anesthetic adds analgesic action to this state of unconsciousness.

Occasionally, the inhaled anesthetic agents are subject to misuse. *Nitrous oxide*, a gas of low anesthetic potency, is an example. Currently used not only in anesthesia but also as a carrier gas in whipped cream charger cans (for example, Whippets), nitrous oxide induces a state of behavioral disinhibition, analgesia, and mild euphoria. Since the inhalation of nitrous oxide dilutes the air that a person is breathing, extreme caution must be exercised to prevent hypoxia. If the nitrous oxide is mixed only with room air, hypoxia results, which could produce irreversible brain damage. Other forms of inhalant abuse are discussed in Chapter 5.

Several *injectable anesthetics* are available. *Thiopental* (Pentothal) and *methohexital* (Brevital) are ultrashort-acting barbiturates. *Propofol* (Diprovan) and *etomidate* (Amidate) are structurally unique; propofol structurally resembles the neurotransmitter GABA. Because propofol and etomidate are now generically available (and inexpensive), more expensive preparations have been marketed. *Fospropofol* (Lusedra) is a prodrug to propofol; fospropofol is rapidly converted to propofol, its active form (Bengalorkar et al., 2011). *Desmedetomidine* (Precedex) is structurally related to etomidate and likely works with identical efficacy (Mizrak et al., 2010). It is an alpha-2 agonist at the $GABA_A$ receptor and is available commercially for sedation procedures in medicine.

Ramelteon: A Selective Melatonin Receptor Agonist

Melatonin, a naturally occurring hormone secreted by the pineal gland, has been used for the treatment of insomnia since the timing of its secretion in human and most animals coincides with the increase of nocturnal sleep propensity (Srinivasan et al., 2012). It remains available as an over-the-counter drug for the treatment of insomnia. It has a short half-life, and slow-release preparations remain fairly ineffective, except perhaps on people with disrupted sleep wake-cycles, such as shift workers and people with jet lag. Neurons in the anterior hypothalamus coordinate the timing of this circadian system and maintain 24-hour periodicity, controlling the pineal gland in producing melatonin, with melatonin levels increasing as bedtime approaches, plateauing during the night, and decreasing as sleep ends in the morning. These anterior hypothalamic neurons contain a high concentration of melatonin receptors.

Ramelteon (Rozerem)(Figure 13.5) is an agonist of melatonin receptors (both melatonin-1 and melatonin-2). It has been approved by the FDA for the treatment of insomnia characterized by difficulty with sleep onset. The drug is thought to be nonaddicting

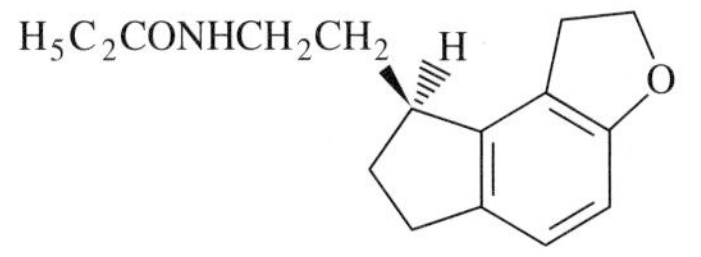

$H_5C_2CONHCH_2CH_2$

Ramelteon (Rozerem)

FIGURE 13.5 Structural formula of *ramelteon* (Rozerem).

and therefore devoid of abuse potential. Rebound insomnia following a period of nightly drug use has not been reported. In an available 8-milligram dose, it is taken 30 minutes before going to bed. A half-life of about 3 hours is thought to leave little morning drowsiness, although next morning driving performance has been reported as being impaired (Mets et al., 2011). Driving impairments appear to be similar to those of zopiclone.

In controlled trials, efficacy was quite modest, with sleep onset occurring only about 10 or 15 minutes earlier than after taking placebo and with total sleep time little affected (Liu and Wang, 2012). Efficacy trials against established anti-insomnia drugs, including the nonbenzodiazepine BZRAs, have not been reported. Therefore, its efficacy relative to other therapeutic options cannot be estimated at this time. Norris and coworkers (2012) recently studied ramelteon as an adjunct to regular psychiatric medications in patients with euthymic bipolar disorder. The authors reported that patients were only about half as likely to relapse, compared with placebo-treated patients. Brower and coworkers (2011), in a small study of five alcohol-dependent patients, noted improved insomnia scores, total sleep time, and a shorter time to fall asleep. Given its lack of abuse potential, ramelteon deserves further study in this population.

Agomelatine: Another Selective Melatonin Receptor Agonist

Like ramelteon, *agomelatine* (Valdoxan, Thymanax) is an agonist at melatonin-1 and melatonin-2 receptors; it is also an antagonist at serotonin 5-HT$_{2c}$ receptors. As such, agomelatine improves sleep patterns (the melatonin action) and it possesses clinically significant antidepressant and anxiolytic actions (Fornaro et al., 2010; Levitan et al., 2012; Tardito et al., 2012). While efficacy was modest, agomelatine was devoid of sexual side effects, weight gain, insomnia, and anxiety reactions (side effects common with serotonin antidepressants). The drug had been marketed in over forty countries; however, emerging data indicates that the drug can cause liver problems with hepatotoxicity, elevations in liver enzymes, and even liver failure. Strict guidelines for liver function testing were made in October 2012. These requirements will limit the use of the drug as well as any FDA approval in the United States.

Orexin Antagonists for Insomnia

About 20 years ago, *orexin* neuropeptide transmitters were discovered. Named *orexin-A* and *orexin-B,* they were originally thought to promote feeding behaviors (*orexis* in Greek means appetite). More recently, it had been learned that while orexin effects on feeding are less pronounced than originally thought, their effects on arousal and sleep are profound (Scammell and Winrow, 2011). Narcolepsy (one of the most common causes of sleepiness) is caused by

TABLE 13.3 Adverse effects of benzodiazepines, nonbenzodiazepine hypnotics, and sedating antidepressants and potential adverse effects of orexin antagonists.

The side effects of conventional hypnotics are well documented, but little is known about the clinical effects of orexin antagonists. Some effects such as morning sedation may depend on the particular compound's pharmacokinetics. The frequency of these effects is indicated by the following symbols: ++, common; +, occasional; −, rare.

	Benzodiazepines (e.g., clonazepam, lorazepam)	Nonbenzodiazepines (e.g., zolpidem, zaleplon)	Sedating antidepressants (e.g., trazodone, doxepin)	Orexin antagonists
Morning sedation	+	+	+	+
Hypnagogic hallucinations, sleep paralysis	−	−	−	+
Unsteady gait, falls	++	+	+	+/−
Confusion	++	+	−	−
Amnesia	+	+	−	−
Dependence and abuse	+	+/−	−	−
Rebound insomnia	+	+	−	−
Respiratory depression	+	+/−	−	−
Orthostasis	−	−	+	−
Anticholinergic effects	−	−	++/+	−

After Scammell and Winrow (2011), Table 1.

the loss of orexin-producing neurons in the hypothalamus. This has led to a search for *orexin receptor antagonists* as a novel approach for promoting sleep and treating insomnia (Coleman et al., 2011). Unlike the sedating benzodiazepines and nonbenzodiazepine "Z-drugs," these orexin antagonists are not associated with mental clouding, gait problems, or dependence (Table 13.3). Besides promoting sleep, these *orexin-A* and *orexin-B* antagonists may reduce reward associated with food and drugs of abuse and may reduce autonomic responses to stress.

   To date, at least four pharmaceutical companies are developing dual orexin-A and orexin-B antagonists, although none have yet been submitted for FDA approval. Compounds under study include suvorexant, almorexant, MK-4305, MK-6096, SB-649868, and others. To date, side effects have been modest and the future prospects are relatively hopeful. These drugs are the most promising new agents for the treatment of insomnia, with encouraging results in preliminary clinical trials (Bettica et al., 2012; Hoever et al., 2012; Ioachimescu and El-Solh, 2012; Winrow et al., 2012).

Serotonin Receptor Agonists as Anxiolytics

Anxiety may, at least in part, result from defects in serotonin neurotransmission, and drugs that augment serotonin activity are useful in the treatment of anxiety disorders. Perhaps the most widely used class of serotonin agonists are the SSRI-type antidepressants which are today considered to be drugs of first choice in the treatment of anxiety disorders. We focus here on several other agents that act through direct stimulation of the postsynaptic serotonin 5-HT$_{1A}$ receptor.

Serotonin 5-HT$_{1A}$ receptors are found in high density in the hippocampus, the septum, parts of the amygdala, and the dorsal raphe nucleus, areas all presumed to be involved in fear and anxiety responses. Activation of 5-HT$_{1A}$ receptors is thought to diminish neuronal activity. Mice selectively bred without 5-HT$_{1A}$ receptors display increased fear responses, suggesting that reductions in 5-HT$_{1A}$ receptor activity or density (presumably due to genetic deficits or environmental stressors) result in heightened anxiety.

Buspirone. Clinical interest in serotonin anxiolytics began 25 years ago with demonstration of the anxiolytic action of *buspirone* (BuSpar), a selective serotonin 5-HT$_{1A}$ agonist. Thereafter, other related agents were identified, but they have not yet been marketed. Gepirone, ipsapirone, and alnespirone are three examples of such drugs.

Buspirone (BuSpar) is a partial 5-HT$_{1A}$ agonist with demonstrable anxiolytic and antidepressant properties. It has also been recommended for patients who suffer from mixed symptoms of anxiety and depression, as well as for elderly people with agitated dementia.

Buspirone is most helpful in anxious patients who do not demand the immediate symptom relief they associate with the benzodiazepine response. Slower and more gradual onset of anxiety relief is balanced by the increased safety and lack of dependency-producing aspects of buspirone. It takes several weeks of continuous treatment to see clinical effects. Patients who have previously been taking benzodiazepines do poorly on buspirone. These slow-onset and subtle actions appear to result from the fact that only about 5 percent of orally administered drug reaches the bloodstream (much is metabolized by first-pass metabolism). Inhibition of such metabolism that occurs while the drug is being absorbed can be alleviated by concurrent drinking of grapefruit juice, which blocks enzymes responsible for buspirone's initial metabolism during its intestinal absorption (Paine et al., 2006).

Gepirone. *Gepirone* (Arisa, Variza) is another 5-HT$_{1A}$ agonist developed many years ago. It has yet to receive FDA approval in the United States either as an antidepressant or as an anxiolytic. Interestingly, some of the atypical antipsychotics like *aripiprazole* (Abilify) are also partial agonists at the 5-HT$_{1A}$ receptor and are sometimes used in low doses as augmentations to the SSRIs in poorly responsive patients.

Antiepileptic Drugs

Sedative-hypnotic drugs used for the treatment of epilepsy have been called anticonvulsants or antiepileptic drugs. The number of these drugs commercially available has more than doubled in the last 15 years. Currently 24 anticonvulsants are available, and of these five have become available since 2009 (Table 13.4). Two of the new drugs have unique

TABLE 13.4 Antiepileptic Drugs Currently Approved by the Food and Drug Administration

Before 1993	1993-2005	2009-2013
Carbamazepine	Felbamate	Vigabatrin
Clonazepam	Gabapentin	Rufinamide
Diazepam	Lamotrigine	Lacosamide
Ethosuccimide	Levetiracetam	Clobazam
Lorazepam	Oxcarbazepine	Ezogabine
Phenobarbital	Pregabalin	Perampanel
Phenytoin	Tiagabine	
Primidone	Topiramate	
Valproic acid	Zonisamide	

Modified from Sirven et al., 2012, Table 1, page 880.

mechanisms of action, offering new potential for better control of seizures. Sirven and coworkers (2012) present an introduction to understanding how these drugs work to control brain excitability and epileptic seizures.

In recent years, their uses have been expanded to treatment of bipolar disorder; treatment of explosive behavioral disorders in children, adolescents, and adults; management of alcohol withdrawal and cravings; treatment of chronic *pain*; and management of certain anxiety disorders such as posttraumatic stress disorder, generalized anxiety disorder, and even certain components of borderline personality disorder. These nonepileptic uses necessitate the terms *mood stabilizer* to cover this multitude of actions. In this section, these drugs are introduced for their original indication: antiepileptic agents or anticonvulsants. The currently available antiepileptic drugs are listed in Table 13.4.

Phenobarbital (a barbiturate) (Figure 13.6) was the first widely effective antiepileptic drug. This and other barbiturates, because of their sedative and adverse cognitive depressant effects, are today rarely used; equally effective, more specific, and less sedating antiepileptic agents are now available.

Phenytoin (Dilantin), introduced into medicine in 1938, remains a commonly used *hydantoin* anticonvulsant, producing less sedation than do the barbiturates. Phenytoin has a half-life of about 24 hours; thus, daytime sedation can be minimized if the patient takes the full daily dose at bedtime. Many bothersome side effects limit its use in favor of newer, less toxic agents. Other, older anticonvulsants included *primidone* and *ethosuximide*, introduced in the late 1950s.

Valproic acid (divalproex, Depakene, Depakote), introduced in 1974, is effective in treating *petit mal* seizure disorders in children. It acts by augmenting the postsynaptic action of GABA. Valproic acid has a short half-life (about 6 to 12 hours); it must therefore be administered two or three times a day. Common side effects include sedation and cognitive impairments. Serious side effects are rare, but liver failure has been reported. Like many of the newer anticonvulsants, valproic acid is effective in people with bipolar

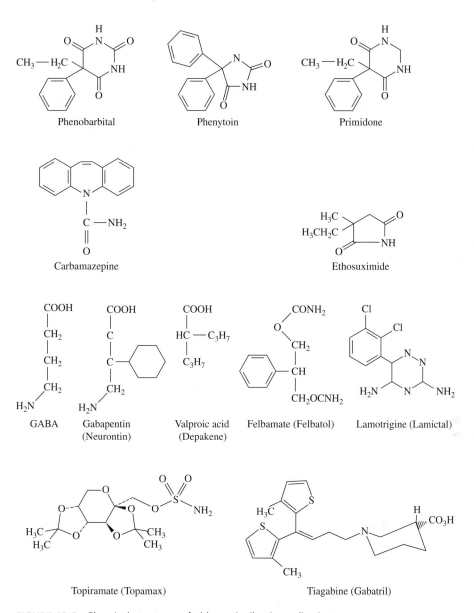

FIGURE 13.6   Chemical structures of older antiepileptic medications.

disorder, posttraumatic stress disorder, borderline personality disorder, aggressive behaviors, schizophrenia, and alcohol and cocaine dependence. A long-acting, slow-release formulation (Depakote-ER) is approved for the treatment of migraine headache.

Carbamazepine (Tegretol, Equitro), introduced in 1963, is an antiepileptic drug with a sedative effect that is perhaps less intense than that of the other antiepileptic agents. The primary limitations of carbamazepine include serious alterations in the cellular composition of blood (reduced numbers of white blood cells), presumably secondary to a depressant effect on bone marrow. Carbamazepine also increases the production of drug-metabolizing enzymes in the liver, such that both itself (*autoinduction*) as well as other drugs metabolized by the same enzymes are metabolized much faster than would normally be expected and these drugs become clinically "less effective" due to lower-than-expected blood concentrations. Often, the dose of these drugs needs to be doubled to compensate. For nonepileptic use, carbamazepine is used in the treatment of bipolar disorder, explosive behavioral disorders, pain syndromes, and alcohol withdrawal.

Gabapentin (Neurontin), introduced in 1993, is a structural analogue of GABA, was synthesized as a specific GABA-mimetic antiepileptic drug. Gabapentin is effective in treating both an anxiety disorder (phobia) and pain (reflex sympathetic dystrophy). Since then, gabapentin has been used in a wide variety of chronic pain states and psychiatric disorders, including bipolar disorder, and in the demented elderly to treat agitation and aggressive behavior. Gabapentin can be effective in treating alcohol withdrawal and for prevention of relapse. It also possesses significant anxiolytic efficacy, and therefore is used for treatment of a variety of anxiety disorders. A related drug, *pregabalin* (Lyrica) was introduced as an anticonvulsant in 2004; like gabapentin, it has multiple uses in medicine as discussed elsewhere in this text.

Lamotrigine (Lamictal), introduced into medicine in 1995, acts by inhibiting ion fluxes through sodium channels, stabilizing neuronal membranes, and inhibiting the presynaptic release of neurotransmitters, principally glutamate. First introduced as an antiepileptic drug, it has beneficial effects on mood, mental alertness, and social interactions in some epilepsy patients. An unusual and significant advantage of lamotrigine is that it improves cognitive functioning and exerts antidepressant actions (Brown, 2009). Clinically, it has been used for the treatment of resistant depression (McIntyre and Morel, 2006) as well as the depressive phase in bipolar disorder. It does not appear to cause a "manic flip" in such patients.

Oxcarbazepine (Trileptal) is a structural derivative of carbamazepine. It differs in two ways: (1) it is rapidly metabolized by a process called *reduction* to an active molecule, and (2) it has not been associated with the white blood cell toxicity associated with carbamazepine. Oxcarbazepine is being increasingly used to treat bipolar illness and other disorders for which carbamazepine is also effective.

Tiagabine (Gabitril) became clinically available in 1998 as another antiepileptic drug. The drug acts by inhibiting neuronal and glial uptake of GABA, secondary to its irreversibly inhibiting one of the GABA reuptake transporters located on the presynaptic nerve terminals of GABA-releasing neurons. This action serves to prolong GABA's synaptic action. Tiagabine appears to be less useful in the treatment of bipolar illness than are other antiepileptic drugs. It has been shown effective in the treatment of generalized anxiety disorder, although its efficacy was limited (Pollack et al., 2008).

Several other antiepileptic drugs introduced between 1993 and 2005 have found use in the treatment of bipolar illness: *topiramate* (Topamax), *levetiracetam* (Keppra), and *zonisamide* (Zonegran). Topiramate is discussed in Chapter 5 for its use in treating alcoholism. Zonisamide has been shown to be effective as an antiobesity agent when combined with a balanced low-calorie diet. It has also been used to treat binge-eating disorder.

Levetiracetam (Keppra) is effective in treating partial-onset seizures, the most common form of epilepsy. It has a unique mechanism of action (Yan et al., 2013) making it suitable for add-on therapy of epilepsy in both adults and children with refractory seizures (Mbizvo et al., 2012).

Lacosamide (Vimpat) is an anticonvulsant, introduced in 2008, that appears to act in a different way than do other anticonvulsants such as phenytoin. Traditional anticonvulsants affect a "fast action potential generation," while lacosamide interacts with sodium channels without affecting fast inactivation. It is a "novel sodium channel modulator" useful in the treatment of epilepsy (Kellinghaus, 2009). Lacosamide has also been shown to be effective in the treatment of neuropathic pain (Harris and Murphy, 2009) and anxiety disorders (Higgins et al., 2009). It may exert fewer cognitive-depressing side effects than other anticonvulsants (Higgins et al., 2010).

Vigabatrin (Sabril) has long been available in Europe, but was introduced into the United States only in 2010. Despite serious side effects, it is indicated only for two forms of severe epilepsy: infantile spasms and as add-on therapy for refractory partial epilepsy in adults when other options have failed. Because its use is associated with loss of peripheral vision and can even produce permanent loss of vision, it is available only through a single national pharmacy and with requirements for formal ophthalmologic evaluation with continuing follow-up.

Rufinamide (Banzel) is another new antiepileptic agent, structurally different from other anticonvulsants. It is FDA-approved for a specific type of epilepsy (Lennox-Gastaut syndrome). It is also effective in refractory partial seizures; it seems to have no adverse effects on cognitive functioning (Wisniewski, 2010; Besag and Patsalos, 2012).

Clobazam (Onfi) is a benzodiazepine approved in the United States in 2011 for the treatment of seizures associated with Lennox-Gastaut syndrome. It is also approved for the treatment of refractory epilepsy and for the short-term treatment of severe anxiety and agitation as seen in psychotic disorders. Like all benzodiazepines, adverse sedation and cognitive deficits are common. In long-term use tolerance to its beneficial effects may develop. In December 2013, the FDA warned of the possibility of serious skin reactions to the drug.

Ezogabine (Potiga) appears to act by opening potassium channels in the brain. Such action is unique among anticonvulsants. Dizziness, somnolence, fatigue, and confusional states have been reported with its use.

Stiripentol (Diacomit) is another new antiepileptic drug that acts by increasing GABA transmission and by limiting GABA synaptic uptake, prolonging GABA activity. It has a specific use in treating severe myoclonic epilepsy in infants. It strongly inhibits the metabolism of other drugs, making other drugs both more effective and/or toxic; dose reductions of other medications is usually required. The drug has not been FDA-approved in the United States, but it may be legally imported under an "orphan drug" status with the FDA on a "compassionate-use basis." It appears effective in a rare childhood genetic form of epilepsy called Dravet syndrome.

Eslicarbazene (Aptiom) is a prodrug that is activated to eslicarbazepine, which is the active metabolite of *oxcarbazepine* (Trileptal). Eslicarbazene therefore shares the actions of oxcarbazepine, including potential to treat not only epilepsy but bipolar disorder, and certain pain syndromes. In November 2013, the FDA approved eslicarbazene for the treatment of partial-onset seizures in adults with epilepsy.

Perampanel (Fycompa) was FDA-approved in late 2012 as the newest FDA-approved antiepileptic drug. It is unique as a blocker of the AMPA subtype of glutamate receptors, giving it a wide spectrum of anticonvulsant usefulness. Labeling contains a "black-box" warning of adverse effects including "aggression, hostility, irritability, anger, and homicidal ideation." Other adverse effects that have been reported include suicidal thoughts and behavior, dizziness, gait disturbances, somnolence, and fatigue.

Antiepileptic Drugs in Pregnancy

Approximately one million women with epilepsy in the United States are in their active reproductive years. Most require anticonvulsant medication during pregnancy, and many anticonvulsants have adverse fetal outcomes. However, most women with epilepsy will have a normal pregnancy and a favorable outcome (Klein, 2011). Antiepileptic medications are also used to treat an ever-expanding range of medical conditions including bipolar disorder, migraine headache, and chronic pain syndromes. Overall the risk to the fetus of a congenital malformation is doubled with the use of these drugs, compared to the risk seen in a nonmedicated mother. Further, when multiple anticonvulsants are prescribed during pregnancy, the risk is tripled, especially when *valproic acid* (Depakote) is included (Nadebaum et al., 2012). Problems include not only teratogenic (structural) deficits, but also neurodevelopmental deficits later in the early life of the newborn (Tomson and Battino, 2012; Wlodarczyk et al., 2012). In fact, in June 2011, the FDA issued a safety announcement on the adverse impact of valproic acid on cognitive impairments in offspring of mothers who took valproic acid during pregnancy. In 2009, the American Academy of Neurology and the American Epilepsy Society published a Practice Parameter Update on the management of pregnant women with epilepsy (Harden et al., 2009).

Antiepileptic Drugs and Risk of Suicidal Thoughts and Behavior

On December 16, 2008 (updated May 5, 2009), the FDA notified manufacturers of antiepileptic medicines that it now requires a warning that the use of these drugs may increase the risk of suicidal thoughts and behaviors (Patorno et al., 2010). The medical community received this warning with skepticism because of multiple problems related to the basis for the FDA's warning (Kanner, 2011). Multiple other factors may be involved in the increased rate of suicidality in patients taking anticonvulsants (depression, epilepsy surgery, bipolar disorder, substance abuse, and anxiety disorders) (Gibbons et al., 2009; Bagary, 2011).

Regardless, patients taking antiepileptic drugs should be carefully monitored for behavioral changes that could be precursors to emerging suicidality, including drug-induced anxiety, agitation, hostility, and mania or hypomania. Landmark and Johannessen (2012) term this *pharmacovigilance*. This warning applies whether these medicines are used to treat seizures, psychiatric disorders, migraine headaches, or other conditions. The exact risk was not considered sufficient to require a "black-box warning" (the FDA's strongest warning); however, both revised labeling and development of a medication guide were required.

STUDY QUESTIONS

1. What are the advantages of benzodiazepines over barbiturates?
2. Describe the mechanism action of benzodiazepines.
3. How do benzodiazepines resemble alcohol? How do they differ?
4. Describe the structure and function of the benzodiazepine receptor.
5. How might you describe anxiety or panic in terms of receptors or neurochemicals (at this point)?
6. List some of the clinical uses of benzodiazepines.
7. List three processes that might prolong the half-life of a benzodiazepine.
8. Why should the elderly avoid using long-acting benzodiazepines?
9. Describe the most clinically significant drug interaction that involves benzodiazepines.
10. Discuss benzodiazepine withdrawal and its treatment.
11. What is flumazenil and for what purpose can it be used?
12. Compare and contrast the mechanisms of action and clinical uses of benzodiazepines and buspirone.
13. To what benzodiazepine is zolpidem most often compared? Why?
14. Compare and contrast zolpidem, zaleplon, and eszopiclone.
15. Discuss the future treatment of anxiety disorders.

REFERENCES

Absalom, N., et al. (2012). "alpha-4/Beta-o GABA(A) receptors are High-Affinity Targets for gamma-Hydroxybutyric Acid (GHB)." *Proceedings of the National Academy of Sciences USA* 109: 13404–13409.

Bagary, M. (2011). "Epilepsy, Antiepileptic Drugs, and Suicidality." *Current Opinions in Neurology* 24: 177–182.

Baselt, R. (2011). *Disposition of Toxic Drugs and Chemicals in Man*, 9th edition. Biomedical Publications: Seal Beach California.

Becker, D. (2012). "Pharmacodynamic Considerations for Moderate and Deep Sedation." *Anesthesia Progress* 59: 28–42.

Bellantuono, C., et al. (2013). "Benzodiazepine Exposure in Pregnancy and Risk of Major Malformations: A Critical Overview." *General Hospital Psychiatry* 35: 3–8.

Bengalorkar, G. M., et al. (2011). "Fospropofol: Clinical Pharmacology." *Journal of Anaesthesiology and Clinical Pharmacology* 27: 79–83.

Besag, F., and Patsalos, P. N. (2012). "New Developments in the Treatment of Partial-Onset Epilepsy." *Neuropsychiatric Disease and Treatment* 8: 455–464.

Bettica, P., et al. (2012). "Differential Effects of a Dual Orexin Receptor Antagonist (SB-649868) and Zolpidem on Sleep Initiation and Consolidation, SWS, REM Sleep, and EEG Power Spectra in a Model of Situational Insomnia." *Neuropsychopharmacology* 37: 1224–1233.

Bosch, O. G., et al. (2012). "Reconsidering GHB: Orphan Drug or New Model Antidepressant?" *Journal of Psychopharmacology* 26: 618–628.

Bostwick, J. R., et al. (2012). "Benzodiazepines: A Versatile Clinical Tool." *Current Psychiatry* 11: 55–64.

Brower, K. J., et al. (2011). "Ramelteon and Improved Insomnia in Alcohol-Dependent Patients: A Case Series." *Journal of Clinical Sleep Medicine* 7: 274–275.

Brown, E. S. (2009). "Effects of Glucocorticoids on Mood, Memory, and the Hippocampus. Treatment and Preventive Therapy." *Annals of the New York Academy of Science* 1179: 41–55.

Coleman, P. J., et al. (2011). "Discovery of Dual Orexin Receptor Antagonists (DORAs) for the Treatment of Insomnia." *Current Topics in Medicinal Chemistry* 11: 696–725.

Diaper, A., et al. (2013). "Evaluation of the Effects of Venlafaxine and Pregabalin on the Carbon Dioxide Inhalation Models of Generalized Anxiety Disorder and Panic." *Journal of Psychopharmacology* 27: 135–145.

Eadie, M. J. (2008). "Antiepileptic Drugs as Human Teratogens." *Expert Opinion on Drug Safety* 7: 195–209.

Enato, E., et al. (2011). "The Fetal Safety of Benzodiazepines: An Updated Meta-Analysis." *Journal of Obstetrics and Gynaecology Canada* 33: 46–48.

Feltner, D. E., et al. (2011). "Efficacy of Pregabalin in Generalized Social Anxiety Disorder: Results of a Double-Blind, Placebo-Controlled, Fixed-Dose Study." *International Clinical Psychopharmacology* 26: 213–220.

Fornaro, M., et al. (2010). "A Systematic, Updated Review on the Antidepressant Agomelatine Focusing on its Melatonergic Modulation." *Current Neuropharmacology* 8: 287–304.

Gibbons, R. D., et al. (2009). "Relationship Between Antiepileptic Drugs and Suicide Attempts in Patients with Bipolar Disorder." *Archives of General Psychiatry* 66: 1354–1360.

Hadley, S. J., et al. (2012). "Switching from Long-Term Benzodiazepine Therapy to Pregabalin in Patients with Generalized Anxiety Disorder: A Double-Blind, Placebo-Controlled Trial." *Journal of Psychopharmacology* 26: 461–470.

Harden, C. I., et al. (2009). "Practice Parameter Update: Management issues for Women with Epilepsy – Focus on Pregnancy (An Evidence-Based Review)." *Neurology* 73: 142–149.

Harris, J. A., and Murphy, J. A. (2009). "Lacosamide: An Adjunctive Agent for Partial-Onset Seizures and Potential Therapy for Neuropathic Pain." *Annals of Pharmacotherapy* 43: 1809–1817.

Higgins, G. A., et al. (2009). "The Anti-Epileptic Drug Lacosamide (Vimpat) Has Anxiolytic Property in Rodents." *European Journal of Psychopharmacology* 624: 1–9.

Higgins, G. A., et al. (2010). "Comparative Study of Five Antiepileptic Drugs on a Translational Cognitive Measure in the Rat: Relationship to Antiepileptic Property." *Psychopharmacology* 207: 513–527.

Hoever, P., et al. (2012). "Orexin Receptor Antagonism. A New Sleep-Enabling Paradigm: A Proof-of-Concept Clinical Trial." *Clinical Pharmacology & Therapeutics* 91: 975–985.

Ioachimescu, O. C., and El-Solh, A. A. (2012). "Pharmacology of Insomnia." *Expert Opinion on Pharmacotherapy* 13: 1243–1260.

Julien, R. M. (2013). "Treatment of Anxiety Across the Age Span." In: *Anxiety Disorders: A Concise Guide and Casebook for Psychopharmacology and Psychotherapy Integration.* S. M. Stahl and B. A. Moore (Editors). Routledge/Taylor & Francis: Psychopharmacology and Psychotherapy in Clinical Practice Treatment Series, B.A. Moore, series editor.

Kanner, A. M. (2011). "Are Antiepileptic Drugs used in the Treatment of Migraine Associated with an Increased Risk of Suicidality?" *Current Pain and Headache Reports* 15: 164–169.

Kellinghaus, C. (2009). "Lacosamide as Treatment for Partial Epilepsy: Mechanisms of Action, Pharmacology, Effects, and Safety." *Therapeutics and Clinical Risk Management* 5: 757–766.

Klein, A. M. (2011). "Epilepsy Cases in Pregnant and Postpartum Women: A Practical Approach." *Seminars in Neurology* 31: 392–396.

Landmark, C. J. and Johannessen, S. I. (2012). "Safety Aspects of Antiepileptic Drugs: Focus on Pharmacovigilance." *Pharmacoepidemiology and Drug Safety* 21: 11–20.

Levitan, M. N., et al. (2012). "A Review of Preliminary Observations on Agomelatine in the Treatment of Anxiety Disorders." *Expert Clinical Psychopharmacology* 20: 504–509.

Liu, J. and Wang, L. N. (2012). "Ramelteon in the Treatment of Chronic Insomnia: Systematic Review and Meta-Analysis." *International Journal of Clinical Practice* 66: 867–873.

Madea, B., and Mubhoff, F. (2009). "Knock-Out Drugs: Their Prevalence, Modes of Action, and Means of Detection." *Deutsches Arztebatt International* 106: 341–347.

Mbizvo, G. K., et al. (2012). "Levetiracetam Add-On for Drug Resistant Focal Epilepsy: An Updated Cochrane Review." *Cochrane Database of Systematic Reviews* 9: CD001901.

McIntyre, J., and Morel, M. A. (2006). "Spotlight on Lamotrigine for Depression." *Drug News Perspectives* 19: 427–430.

Mets, M. A., et al. (2011). "Next-Day Effects of Ramelteon (8 mg), Zopiclone (7.5 mg), and Placebo on Highway Driving Performance, Memory Functioning, Psychomotor Performance, and Mood in Healthy Adult Subjects." *Sleep* 34: 1327–1334.

Mizrak, A., et al. (2010). "Pretreatment with Desmedetomidine or Thiopental Decreases Myoclonus After Etomidate: A Randomized, Double-Blind Controlled Trial." *Journal of Surgical Research* 159(1): e11–e16.

Morgenthaler, T., et al. (2006). "Practice Parameters for the Psychological and Behavioral Treatment of Insomnia: An Update. An American Academy of Sleep Medicine Report." *Sleep* 29: 1415–1419.

Moylan, S., et al. (2012). "The Role of Alprazolam for the Treatment of Panic Disorder in Australia." *Australia and New Zealand Journal of Psychiatry* 46: 212–224.

Nadebaum, C., et al. (2012). "Neurobehavioral Consequences of Prenatal Antiepileptic Drug Exposure." *Developmental Neuropsychology* 37: 1–29.

Nemeth, Z., et al. (2010). "The Involvement of gamma-Hydroxybutyrate in Reported Sexual Assaults: A Systematic Review." *Journal of Psychopharmacology* 24: 1281–1287.

Norris, E. R., et al. (2013). "A Double-Blind, Randomized, Placebo-Controlled Trial of Adjunctive Ramelteon for the Treatment of Insomnia and Mood Stability in Patients with Euthymic Bipolar Disorder." *Journal of Affective Disorders* 144: 141–147.

Nurmi-Luthje, I., et al. (2006). "Use of Benzodiazepines and Benzodiazepine-Related Drugs Among 223 Patients with an Acute Hip Fracture in Finland: Comparison of Benzodiazepine Findings in Medical Records and Laboratory Assays." *Drugs and Aging* 23: 27–37.

Paine, M. F., et al. (2006). "A Furanocoumarin-Free Grapefruit Juice Establishes Furanocoumarins as the Mediators of the Grapefruit Juice-Felodipine Interaction." *American Journal of Clinical Nutrition* 83: 1097–1105.

Paterniti, S., et al. (2002). "Long-Term Benzodiazepine Use and Cognitive Decline in the Elderly: The Epidemiology of Vascular Aging Study." *Journal of Clinical Psychopharmacology* 22: 285–293.

Patorno, E., et al. (2010). "Anticonvulsant Medications and the Risk of Suicide, Attempted Suicide, or Violent Death." *Journal of the American Medical Association* 303: 1401–1409.

Pollack, M., et al. (2008). "Tiagabine in Adult Patients with Generalized Anxiety Disorder: Results from 3 Randomized, Double-Blind, Placebo-Controlled, Parallel-Group Studies." *Journal of Clinical Psychopharmacology* 28: 308–316.

Rang, H. P., and Dale, M. M. (1991). *Pharmacology,* 2nd ed. Edinburgh: Churchill Livingstone.

Rickels, K., et al. (2012). "Adjunctive Therapy with Pregabalin in Generalized Anxiety Disorder Patients with Partial Response to SSRI or SNRI Treatment." *International Clinical Psychopharmacology* 27: 142–150.

Scammell, T. E. and Winrow, C. J. (2011). "Orexin Receptors: Pharmacology and Therapeutic Opportunities." *Annual Reviews of Pharmacology and Toxicology* 51: 243–266.

Schep, L. J., et al. (2012). "The Clinical Toxicology of gamma-Hydroxybutyrate, gamma-butyrate, and 1,4-Butanediol." *Clinical Toxicology* 50: 458–470.

Sewell, R. and Petrakis, I. L. (2010). "Does Gamma-Hydroxybutyrate (GHB) Have a Role in the Treatment of Alcoholism?" *Alcohol and Alcoholism* 46: 1–2.

Sieghart, W., et al. (2012). "A Novel GABA(A) Receptor Pharmacology: Drugs Interacting with the alpha(+) B(−) Interface." *British Journal of Pharmacology* 166: 476–485.

Sirven, J. I., et al. (2012). "Antiepileptic Drugs 2012: Recent Advances and Trends." *Mayo Clinic Proceedings* 87: 879–889.

Skolnick, P. (2012). "Anxioselective Anxiolytics: On a Quest for the Holy Grail." *Trends in Pharmacological Sciences* 33: 611–620.

Srinivasan, V., et al. (2012). "Melatonergic Drugs for Therapeutic Use in Insomnia and Sleep Disturbances of Mood Disorders." *CNS & Neurological Disorders - Drug Targets* 11: 180–189.

Tardito, D., et al. (2012). "Synergistic Mechanisms Involved in the Antidepressant Effects of Agomelatine." *European Neuropsychopharmacology* 22 (Supplement 3): S482–486.

Timmermann, G., et al. (2009). "Congenital Abnormalities of 88 Children Born to Mothers Who Attempted Suicide with Phenobarbital During Pregnancy: The Use of a Disaster Epidemiological Model for the Evaluation of Drug Teratogenicity." *Pharmacoepidemiology and Drug Safety* 18: 815–825.

Tomson, T. and Battino, D. (2012). "Teratogenic Effects of Antiepileptic Drugs." *Lancet Neurology* 11: 803–813.

Trincavelli, M. L., et al. (2012). "The GABAA-BZR Complex as Target for the Development of Anxiolytic Drugs." *Current Topics in Medicinal Chemistry* 12: 254–269.

vanAmsterdam, J. G., et al. (2012). "Possible Long-Term Effects of gamma-Hydroxybutyrate (GHB) Due to Neurotoxicity and Overdose." *Neuroscience & Biobehavioral Reviews* 36: 1217–1227.

Verster, J. C. and Roth, T. (2013). "Blood Drug Concentrations of Benzodiazepines Correlate Poorly with Actual Driving Impairment." *Sleep Medicine Review* 17: 153–159.

Vindenes, V., et al. (2012). "Impairment Based Legislative Limits for Driving Under the Influence of Non-Alcohol Drugs in Norway." *Forensic Science International* 219: 1–11.

Weston, A. L., et al. (2010). "Potentially Inappropriate Medication Use in Older Adults with Mild Cognitive Impairment." *Journal of Gerontology, Series A, Biological Sciences and Medical Sciences* 65A(3): 318–321 doi:10.1093/gerona/glq158.

Winrow, C. J., et al. (2012). "Pharmacological Characterization of MK-6096 – A Dual Orexin Receptor Antagonist for Insomnia." *Neuropharmacology* 62: 978–987.

Wisniewski, C. S. (2010). "Rufinamide: A New Antiepileptic Medication for the Treatment of Seizures Associated with Lennox-Gastaut Syndrome." *Annals of Pharmacotherapy* 44: 658–667.

Wlodarczyk, B. J., et al. (2012). "Antiepileptic Drugs and Pregnancy Outcomes." *American Journal of Medical Genetics-A* 158A: 2071–2090.

Wu, C. S., et al. (2009). "The Association Between Dementia and Long-Term Use of Benzodiazepines in the Elderly: Nested Case-Control Study Using Claims Data." *American Journal of Geriatric Psychiatry* 17: 614–620.

Yan, H. D., et al. (2013). "Inhibitory Effects of Levetiracetam on the High-Voltage-Activated L-Type $Ca(2+)$ Channels in Hippocampal CA3 Neurons of Spontaneously Epileptic Rat (SER)." *Brain Research Bulletin* 90: 142–148.

Yeh, M. S., et al. (2011). "A Double-Blind Randomized Controlled Trial to Study the Efficacy of Topiramate in a Civilian Sample of PTSD." *CNS Neuroscience & Therapeutics* 17: 305–310.

Zammit, G. (2009). "Comparative Tolerability of Newer Agents for Insomnia." *Drug Safety* 32: 735–748.

Chapter 14

Drugs Used to Treat Bipolar Disorder

Bipolar Disorder

Bipolar disorder (manic-depressive disorder) is one of the ten most disabling conditions in the world, with a lifetime prevalence of about 1 percent across all populations, regardless of nationality, race, or socioeconomic status (Merikangas et al., 2011). People who have the disorder lose many years of healthy functioning, in which their livelihood, marriage, social relationships, and even life may be destroyed. The illness is episodic, with alternating periods of mania and/or depression nearly half the time and intervening periods of at least some degree of recovery and sometimes remission. Although it may appear in childhood or adolescence, the diagnosis is difficult and it is still being debated (see Chapter 15). The main problems in diagnosis are that mania or hypomania may be underreported, that symptoms of unipolar and bipolar depression overlap, and that there is a high degree of comorbidity with many other psychiatric conditions (Hirschfeld, 2009). Generally, onset is between the second and third decade or later, often with a significant delay between the appearance of symptoms and a correct diagnosis and treatment. Most patients experience several episodes during the course of their lives. The risk of recurrence has been reported to be 24 percent by 6 months, 36 percent by one year, and 61 percent by 4 years (Baldassano, 2009).

There are several subtypes of the disorder. The traditional subtype, bipolar disorder I (BP-I), includes at least one episode of full-blown mania with or without an episode of major depression. The disorder is classified as bipolar II (BP-II) if the manic episode is less severe, or "hypomanic," and episodes of major depression also occur. A patient is said to be a "rapid cycler" if at least four illness episodes occur in a 12-month period. Several other bipolar subtypes have been described, exhibiting varying degrees of severity in recurrent mood swings. Together, the variants bring the prevalence of all bipolar disorders to 4.4 percent of U.S. residents (Merikangas et al., 2011).

Despite intensive care and treatment, outpatients with bipolar disorder have a considerable degree of illness-related morbidity, including a threefold greater amount of time spent depressed than time spent manic (Post et al., 2005). Those patients who have residual subsyndromal depressive symptoms following a manic episode may have a poorer outcome and more difficulty reaching functional recovery over their lifetime (Gitlin et al., 2011). And patients who have mixed episodes (i.e., symptoms of both mania and depression during the same episode, Swann et al., 2013) have been shown to have an earlier age of onset of bipolar disorder, have more frequent hospitalizations, and episodes of illness as observed in a 10-year prospective study (Gonzalez-Pinto et al., 2011). Moreover, there is a high rate of mortality (Kupfer, 2005). One of every four or five untreated or inadequately treated patients commits suicide during the course of the illness, a rate ten times that of the general population. Other predictors of mortality in bipolar patients include male gender, history of alcoholism, and poor occupational status before the index episode, as well as a history of previous episodes, psychotic features, mixed episodes, and residual affective symptoms between episodes. This speaks to the need for aggressive treatment of bipolar disorder with a goal of reaching full remission from each episode, if possible.

Did You Know?

MENTAL ILLNESS IN THE MOVIES: No Laughing Matter

The movie *Silver Linings Playbook* has earned critical acclaim and numerous award nominations, including four nods from the Golden Globes. But how accurately does it portray mental illness, a major theme in the film? In the movie, actor Bradley Cooper plays a man with bipolar disorder who is being released from a psychiatric hospital. He soon connects emotionally with a quirky young woman, played by Jennifer Lawrence, who has struggled with her own mental health issues, largely brought on by her husband's death. There has also been a lot of talk in the press about Cooper's character and whether his depiction of bipolar disorder is accurate.

Interestingly, the director (David O. Russell) has said in interviews that his son has the disorder. The movie is based on a book by Matthew Quick, who has reported that he has suffered with depression. "You're never laughing at somebody that has a mental health illness, you're laughing at the absurdity of what's going on, for all the characters involved," said Quick in an interview with the *Hollywood Reporter*. "As someone who has worked in the mental health community, I know that laughter is very important," added Quick.

Diagnostic and Treatment Issues

Bipolar versus Unipolar Depression

Similar to unipolar depression, the symptoms of bipolar depression, as described by patients, include (in decreasing order of prevalence): sadness, insomnia, feelings of worthlessness, loss of energy and ability to concentrate, inability to enjoy everyday activities, thoughts of death and suicide, and an inability to function. Manic symptoms include various aspects of behavioral and physiological hyperactivity, such as erratic sleep, increased sexual interest, emotional elation and racing thoughts, increased physical activity, impulsiveness, poor judgment, and reckless and aggressive behavior.

Comorbid substance abuse affects at least 60 percent of bipolar I and 50 percent of bipolar II patients, with reported rates for alcohol (82 percent), cocaine (30 percent), marijuana (29 percent), sedatives or amphetamines (21 percent), and opioids (13 percent). It may, at least initially, represent an attempt at self-medication for the symptoms accompanying the affective disorder. Unfortunately, substance abuse is associated with a greater risk of switching from a depressive episode to one of mania, hypomania, or a mixed mood state (Ostacher et al., 2010), sometimes referred to as a "flip" or "switch."

Although a patient with bipolar disorder may present initially with either mania or depression, most patients seek treatment for depression. As a result, many are incorrectly diagnosed with unipolar depression and consequently receive inappropriate treatment with antidepressants alone. For example, the Bipolar Disorder: Improving Diagnosis, Guidance, and Education (BRIDGE) study found that almost one-half of patients presenting with a depressive episode were mistakenly diagnosed with unipolar depression when in fact they had bipolar disorder that was detected after a more comprehensive evaluation (Angst et al., 2011). Unfortunately, while antidepressants (and electroshock treatment, Bailine et al., 2010) can be effective against depressive symptomatology, they may induce or trigger a manic episode, that is, produce a "switch," or "flip," resulting in serious adverse consequences for the patient (Goldberg 2010). The risk of such an event is apparently greater if patients have more severe manic symptoms at baseline, before addition of the antidepressant (Frye et al., 2009). Because of this risk, administration or addition of a *mood stabilizer* (MS) is the most recommended pharmacological treatment for bipolar depression (Bauer and Mitchner, 2004; Mundo et al., 2006). Unfortunately, even combinations may increase the risk of a manic flip, and the risk varies among the different antidepressants (Leverich et al., 2006; Pacchiarottia et al., 2013). Long-term treatment with antidepressant/mood stabilizer combinations may even worsen manic symptom severity (Goldberg et al., 2007) or increase the likelihood of a switch in patients who are rapid cyclers (Schneck et al., 2008). Given that maintenance treatment with antidepressants may not prevent depressive relapses, weaning patients off antidepressants 6 to 12 months after remission has been advised. Yet, considering the scarcity of definitive data, even this advice may change in the future (Amsterdam and Shults, 2010).

Obviously, because of these significant differences in recommended pharmacological treatment, it is important to be able to differentiate between unipolar and bipolar depression. Although the distinction is not always easy to make, some clinical features have been proposed to help (Perlis et al., 2006a). Unipolar depression usually develops after the age of 25 years and may be preceded by an extended period of gradually worsening symptoms. Unipolar patients usually have no history of mania or hypomania. In contrast, bipolar depression typically occurs before the age of 25 years, with a more abrupt onset of hours or days, and may be periodic or seasonal.

Bipolar disorder is highly heritable and may run in families, which makes a thorough family history a crucial component of the diagnosis. Similarly, a personal history of disruptive behavioral patterns or evidence of mania, hypomania, increased energy, or decreased need for sleep may suggest a bipolar diagnosis, as would treatment-emergent mania or hypomania during antidepressant monotherapy. It has recently been proposed that postpartum depression may also be misdiagnosed as major depressive disorder, when, in fact, more than half of patients who received a referral diagnosis of postpartum depression were later found to have bipolar disorder (Sharma et al., 2009, and references therein).

Research is underway to determine if techniques such as neuroimaging can help identify epigenetic biomarkers that can reliably predict if individuals who present in a depressed state are likely to have unipolar vs. bipolar depression which would help the clinician determine which pharmacotherapeutic strategy would have the best chance of success without risking a "flip or switch" to mania (de Almeida et al., 2013).

Overview of Pharmacotherapy.   Medications are currently available to treat acute manic/mixed states and acute bipolar depression and for the prophylactic prevention of recurrent episodes. However, the quality of evidence for efficacy in each of these phases differs among the putative mood stabilizers. Table 14.1 summarizes the

---

TABLE 14.1 Quality of Evidence for the Use of Mood Stabilizers in Bipolar Disorder

A Double-blind placebo-controlled trials with adequate samples
B Double-blind comparator studies with adequate samples
C Open trials with adequate samples
D Uncontrolled observation or controlled study with ambiguous result
E No published evidence
F Available evidence negative

	Acute mania/ Mixed	Mood stabilizer prophylaxis	Acute bipolar depression
Lithium	A+	A+	A
Valproic acid	A+	A−	D
Carbamazepine	A	B−	D
Lamotrigine	F	A+	A
Gabapentin	F	E	D
Topiramate	D	E	D
Aripiprazole	A	E	E
Haloperidol	A	E	E
Olanzapine	A+	E	A
Risperidone	A	E	D
Quetiapine	A	E	E
Ziprasidone	A	E	E
Omega-3	E	D	E

A+ is reserved for those instances when fewer than 40 studies have been reported and more than one double-blind placebo-controlled study supports the same finding. A− indicates positive outcomes on some but not all relevant measures. After G. S. Sachs, "Decision Tree for the Treatment of Bipolar Disorder," *Journal of Clinical Psychiatry* 64, Supplement 8 (2003), p. 37.

relative effectiveness of the available agents for each phase (see also Bauer, 2005). These drugs include the lithium ion, several anticonvulsant "neuromodulators," second-generation antipsychotics (SGAs), and a dietary supplement of the omega-3 fatty acids (Parker et al., 2006a).

The classic mood stabilizer is *lithium*. Although lithium may effectively control manic symptoms and reduce the recurrence of both manic and depressive episodes, its bothersome and serious side effects have necessitated a search for equally effective, safer, and more tolerable agents. Today, it is recognized that combination treatment with two or more medications is often required, preferably with adjunctive psychosocial interventions.

In 1996, the American Psychiatric Association published its first clinical practice guideline for the treatment of patients with bipolar disorder. A revision was published in 2002, emphasizing that the major objectives of intervention are to treat acute manic episodes and to reduce their frequency of recurrence. The most recent update was the result of a consensus conference in May 2004, which reinforced the general treatment goals of: (1) symptomatic remission; (2) full return of psychosocial functioning; and (3) prevention of relapses and recurrences (Suppes et al., 2005). A recent guideline for monitoring the safety of drug treatment in bipolar disorder recognizes the challenging side-effect burden of many of these drugs, as described below (Ng et al., 2009).

For less severe acute manic episodes, first-line treatment is monotherapy with lithium, valproate (divalproex), or a second-generation antipsychotic (Suppes et al., 2005). The same guidelines apply for mixed episodes, except that lithium is less efficacious for that condition. For more severe situations, the combination of either lithium or valproate (or another neuromodulator anticonvulsant) and an antipsychotic is recommended. For the special situation of patients who have a pattern of rapid cycling, a recent review of the literature concludes that rapid cycling patients have worse outcomes than patients without rapid cycling, and suggests the following: (1) there is still uncertainty of any difference in acute response to treatment between rapid cyclers and non-rapid cyclers; (2) in contrast to earlier beliefs, lithium and anticonvulsants have comparable, albeit relatively low, efficacies in rapid cyclers; (3) no consistent evidence supports combinations of anticonvulsants being better than monotherapy for rapid cycling; (4) the atypical antipsychotics aripiprazole, olanzapine, and quetiapine are effective in acute episodes of rapid cyclers and appear promising for response maintenance; (5) olanzapine is equally effective to anticonvulsants during acute treatment; and (6) there is an association between antidepressant use and the presence of rapid cycling, although a causal relationship cannot yet be established (Fountoulakis et al., 2013).

First-line treatment of less severe acute bipolar depression is monotherapy with the "third-generation" neuromodulator/anticonvulsant lamotrigine, with the addition of an antimanic agent if there is a history of severe mania. For maintenance treatment, regardless of whether the most recent episode was manic, depressed, or mixed, it is acceptable to stay on the acute-phase medication if it is well tolerated. However, if additional options are necessary, antipsychotics are recommended when the most recent episode is manic or mixed; if the most recent episode is depressed, either lithium or the combination of an antimanic and an antidepressant may be helpful.

Pathophysiology and Mechanisms of Drug Action

Identifying the therapeutic action of mood stabilizers in the treatment of bipolar disorder has been particularly challenging, and as yet there is no unifying hypothesis. It is difficult to understand how any single drug class can reduce symptoms of both mania and depression, and it has proven difficult to find a mechanism among the relevant drug classes that would account for this dual therapeutic efficacy.

Mood stabilizers may have some neurobiological actions in common with antidepressants. This conclusion comes from growing evidence of similarities between the damaging effects of depression and bipolar disorder on the brain. As discussed in Chapter 12, severe depression is associated with an increase in neuronal vulnerability to injury or trauma, including stress, which may damage neural structures and produce functional impairment. Imaging and postmortem studies have shown similar types of structural changes in the brains of patients diagnosed with bipolar disorder. As in major depressive disorder, reductions in the volume of the prefrontal cortex and hippocampus are significant (Bertolino et al., 2003); the number of neurons and glial cells in the prefrontal cortex is decreased; and levels of the neurochemical N-acetyl-aspartate, which is considered a marker of neuronal "health," are lower (Zarate et al., 2005).

Like antidepressants, mood stabilizers may reverse some of the impairments in brain structure and levels of brain-derived neurotrophic factor (BDNF) (Figure 14.1), reversals that could be relevant to the therapeutic benefit of mood stabilizers in bipolar disorder (Yasuda et al., 2009). In laboratory models, lithium was found to protect neurons against a variety of toxic agents and to promote the growth of neuronal processes; in the human brain, lithium increases levels of N-acetyl-aspartate and gray matter volume. However, in spite of their common neuroprotective effects, no universal mechanism has yet been identified to account for the therapeutic and neurobiological similarities between antidepressants and mood stabilizers. While antidepressants and antipsychotics have some common effects on neurotransmitter receptors in the brain (which could be relevant to their common antidepressant efficacy; Yatham et al., 2005), neither lithium nor the "neuromodulatory" anticonvulsants share these

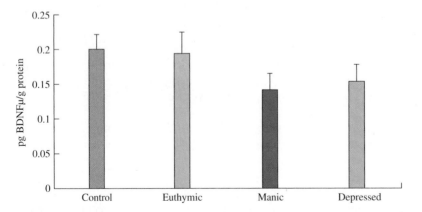

FIGURE 14.1 Serum BDNF levels in BD patients and healthy controls. Measurement is picograms of BDNF protein per microgram of total serum protein. [Data from Cunha et al., (2006), p. 216.]

mechanisms of action. That is, unlike antidepressants and antipsychotics, lithium and many of the anticonvulsants do not exert their primary effect at neuronal synapses. Rather, these drugs seem to act intracellularly to produce changes that "stabilize" neuronal membranes.

Currently, the most extensively studied putative mechanisms of mood stabilizers are the second- and third-messenger systems, that is, the intracellular biochemical processes produced by activation of G-protein-coupled receptors. It has already been established that lithium, valproate, and carbamazepine interact with various enzymes involved in these intracellular signaling pathways, especially involving glutamate neural transmission in the hippocampus (Schloesser et al., 2012). Although individual drugs may interact at different sites within the neurochemical systems, they may all ultimately produce some final common effect that is responsible for their clinical efficacy in bipolar disorder (Gould et al., 2004; Rapoport et al., 2009).[1] For example, valproic acid inactivates voltage-gated sodium channels; lamotrigine blocks both voltage-gated sodium channels and certain calcium channels; valproic acid and lamotrigine act on presynaptic transporters to enhance clearance of glutamate thus indirectly reducing excitatory neurotransmission (Schloesser et al., 2012). The target sites of the hippocampus and its connections with the prefrontal cortex and amygdala make these actions relevant for understanding some of the effects of these drugs on behaviors associated with bipolar disorder including decreased executive function (impulsivity); changes in mood polarity; and changes in cognition and memory function. Finally, there is increasing evidence of the impact of circulating glucocorticoids on mood disorders. Hypercortisolemia can produce mood changes, may occur in bipolar disorder patients and has deleterious effects on the brain. Cortisol elevation can be reversed by chronic treatment with lithium and valproic acid, suggesting new targets for drug development (Schloesser et al., 2012 and references therein).

STEP-BD Study

Progress is being made in determining the best approach for the clinical management of bipolar illness. To provide therapeutic guidelines for practitioners, a large-scale, federally funded trial, called the STEP-BD study, completed in 2005, compared pharmacological treatments for bipolar disorder in a semi-controlled, "real-world" environment.

STEP-BD stands for Systematic Treatment Enhancement Program for Bipolar Disorder; it was one of several studies funded by the National Institute of Mental Health (NIMH) designed to determine the real-world effectiveness of the major psychiatric drug classes. Like the companion studies for depression (the STAR*D trial, see Chapter 12) and schizophrenia (the CATIE trial, see Chapter 11), this investigation involved large numbers of typical patients and used few exclusion criteria in an effort to make the results more generalizable for treatment in standard clinical practice.

---

[1] One possibility is suggested by the fact that lithium and valproate, like antidepressants, increase the levels of proteins, such as cAMP response element-binding protein (CREB), which, in turn, activates genes that produce additional proteins (in particular, one called bcl-2) and a neurotrophic factor (BDNF) that are known to protect neurons from the toxic effects of injury or trauma. Because of this, the two drugs are sometimes referred to as "neuroprotective" agents. Such a broad, general effect on neuronal health may be the reason these drugs are also useful in the management of other clinical conditions, such as aggressive disorders and pain, discussed later in this chapter.

The nature, scope, and overall design of the STEP-BD study are described in Sachs et al (2003), and multiple reports of its results have been published. In brief, Perlis et al., (2006b) found that only 58.4 percent (858 patients) of a subset of 1469 patients who participated for at least 2 years achieved recovery (defined as having only two symptoms of the disorder for at least eight weeks); almost half of this group, 48.5 percent, or 416 patients, had a recurrence at some point, most commonly to a depressive episode (72 percent); recurrence was most likely in those who had residual symptoms at recovery or had an additional psychiatric illness. Unfortunately, Sachs et al. (2007) found no benefit from adding an antidepressant to a mood stabilizer. Patients who were treatment-resistant could choose to enter the last portion of the program. The 66 participants who agreed were randomly assigned one of three additional agents: the anticonvulsant *lamotrigine* (Lamictal), the antipsychotic *risperidone* (Risperdal), or inositol (a sugar, which is an isomer of glucose and is normally a component of one of the second-messenger pathways). Recovery rates were 23.8 percent, 4.6 percent, and 17.4 percent, respectively, and were not statistically different from one another (perhaps because of the small number of subjects), although the relatively poor effect of the antipsychotic was unexpected (Nierenberg et al., 2006).

One particularly important finding of the STEP-BD study was the confirmation that valproic acid may increase the risk of polycystic ovarian syndrome (PCOS); PCOS symptoms (menstrual irregularities, acne, male-pattern hair loss, elevated testosterone, and excessive body hair) were found in 9 of 86 women (10.5 percent) on valproate compared to only 2 of 144 women on another agent (1.4 percent) (Joffe et al., 2006). Valproate also increases the risk of certain birth defects and is not recommended for women who are pregnant (see Chapter 15).

Peters and his colleagues (2011) noted five main lessons from the STEP-BD study that could inform clinical practice: (1) antidepressants added to mood stabilizers are no more effective than placebo for treatment of bipolar depression; (2) antidepressants did not induce mania more frequently than placebo in bipolar depressed patients receiving mood stabilizers who had no history of antidepressant-induced mania; (3) patients with an acute depressive episode who also had subsyndromal manic symptoms did not recover any faster with the addition of antidepressants to their mood stabilizers compared to similar patients who did not receive add-on antidepressants; if anything, those who received the antidepressants were more likely to relapse or have an exacerbation of their manic symptoms; (4) lamotrigine showed benefit for treatment-resistant bipolar depression; and (5) intensive psychosocial treatments provided more rapid recovery, improved social functioning, and greater life satisfaction compared to simple collaborative care.

Mood Stabilizers: Lithium

Lithium has historically been the drug of first choice for treating bipolar disorder and reducing its rate of relapse.[2] Unfortunately, its clinical effectiveness is less than that predicted by clinical trials and relapse often occurs because of patient nonadherence to

---

[2] For a historical overview of lithium therapy and commentaries on lithium, see four related letters in *Archives of General Psychiatry* 54 (1997): 9–23.

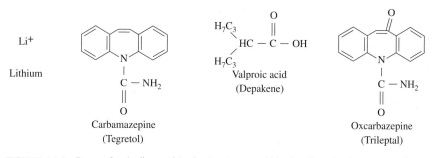

Li+

Lithium

Carbamazepine
(Tegretol)

Valproic acid
(Depakene)

Oxcarbazepine
(Trileptal)

FIGURE 14.2 Drugs classically used in the treatment of bipolar disorder. Structures of newer anticonvulsants used in bipolar disorder are shown in Figure 13.6

therapy. This problem needs to be recognized during treatment, and alternative agents considered.

Lithium (Li+) is the lightest of the alkali metals (Figure 14.2) and shares some characteristics with sodium (Na+). In nature, lithium is abundant in some alkaline mineral spring waters. Devoid of psychotropic effects in normal people, lithium is effective in treating 60 to 80 percent of acute manic and hypomanic episodes, although in the last few years its use has declined because of toxicities, side effects, nonadherence, and relapse as well as the prospect of more alternatives.

The discovery, and "rediscovery" of lithium has a long history (Shorter, 2009). The modern era begins with the Australian physician, John Cade, who noted that when lithium was administered to guinea pigs (used as a solvent in which to dissolve the drugs he was studying), the animals became lethargic. Taking an intuitive leap, Cade administered lithium to patients with acute mania and noted remarkable improvement. However, because of the earlier problems with lithium as a salt substitute resulting in some deaths, the medical community took more than 20 years to accept this agent as an effective treatment for mania. Fortunately, research in the 1970s found lithium to be clearly superior to placebo in the prophylaxis of bipolar disorder; less than a third of lithium-treated patients relapsed, compared with 80 percent of placebo-treated patients.

Many controlled studies demonstrate lithium's efficacy for acute mania, acute depressive episodes, and maintenance treatment for relapse prevention (Geddes et al., 2010). Baldessarini and Tondo (2000, p. 190) recommended lithium as a drug of first choice for both the treatment of acute manic attacks and the long-term management of bipolar disorder:

"No other proposed mood-stabilizing treatment has such substantial research evidence of long-term efficacy in both type I and type II bipolar disorders, as well as yielding a substantial reduction of mortality risk."

Although referred to as the "gold standard" of bipolar treatment, real-world experience indicates that lithium is utilized far less often now than are anticonvulsants or antipsychotic medications. It has been argued that lithium is less effective than these other agents, that requirements for routine periodic blood tests to measure lithium levels may make it inconvenient and/or costly for some patients, and that its spectrum of side effects may limit its choice for some patients. Despite these disadvantages, reviews of the

TABLE 14.2 "Signature" of a lithium responder

Essential features

Recurrent mood disorder

Episodic course of illness

Remission is complete between episodes

Indicative features

Predominance of depressive episodes

Absence of rapid-cycling pattern

Episodic course in another family member

No significant psychiatric comorbidity

"Classic" pattern of mood episodes

The features tabulated can be broadly regarded as a "signature" of potential lithium response, and although not predictive in an absolute manner, are suggestive of an increased likelihood of a response to treatment with lithium. However, when determining treatment choice, the overall clinical profile of the patient needs to be considered along with tolerability and patient preference. Features have been derived from 'Grof (2006), p. 157-178.

historical effectiveness of lithium support its stature as a first-line treatment for individuals with the more "classic" presentation of bipolar disorder (Gershon et al., 2009) (Table 14.2). When used properly in accurately diagnosed patients lithium has the greatest efficacy compared to other drugs, reducing suicidal risk, and enhancing effectiveness of antidepressants (Grof et al., 2009); and it is an effective agent for maintenance treatment (Coryell, 2009).

Pharmacokinetics

Peak blood levels of lithium are reached within 3 hours of oral administration, complete absorption by 8 hours. The drug crosses the blood-brain barrier slowly and incompletely, and, although the clinical significance of the observation is unclear, there can be a twofold variation in the concentration of lithium in the brain compared with its concentration in plasma. However, the therapeutic efficacy of lithium is directly correlated with its blood level.

Lithium is not metabolized and is excreted unchanged by the kidneys, with only small amounts excreted through the skin. About half an oral dose is eliminated within 18 to 24 hours and the rest, which is taken up by the cells of the body, is excreted over the next 1 to 2 weeks. Thus, when therapy is initiated, lithium slowly accumulates over about 2 weeks until a steady state is reached, making once-daily dosing appropriate for many patients.

Lithium has a very narrow therapeutic range below which the drug is ineffective and above which side effects and toxicity are prevalent. Usually guidelines recommend about 0.8 to 1.2 milliequivalents per liter of blood (mEq/l) for acute treatment and 0.6 to 0.8 mEq/l for maintenance. More adverse effects, increasing the likelihood of discontinuation, occur at levels above 1.5 mEq/l, and levels above 2.0 mEq/l are potentially lethal. Because lithium closely resembles table salt, when a patient lowers his or her normal salt intake or loses excessive amounts of salt, such as through sweating, lithium blood levels may rise, quickly producing toxicity. Consequently, patients taking lithium should avoid marked changes in sodium intake or excretion and replenish salts after excessive exercise or illness-induced dehydration.

Pharmacodynamics

In therapeutic concentrations, lithium has almost no discernible psychotropic effect in normal persons and, unlike many psychoactive drugs, does not produce sedation, depression, or euphoria. Although the mechanism of action has not been proved, lithium, valproate, and lamotrigine are all known to inhibit the intracellular enzyme glycogen synthase kinase-3 (GSK-3). One consequence is an increase in the level of a protein, β-catenin, that promotes cell survival and stimulates axonal growth. GSK-3 is also involved in producing amyloid-β which is a major component of the plaques that are found in Alzheimer's disease, suggesting that GSK-3 inhibitors might someday be treatments for that disorder. In that regard, a nationwide study of lithium prescription registry data from Denmark found a decreased risk of dementia in patients who continued lithium use over a 10-year period (Kessing et al., 2008).

As another example, Cui and coworkers (2007) found that lithium and valproate also protected neurons in the brains of rats (in culture) from damage due to oxidative stress. Oxidative stress occurs when intracellular enzymes cannot sufficiently reduce the levels of toxic substances produced by metabolic activity. In this environment, lithium and valproate increased the amount of the antioxidant enzyme glutathione, which plays an important role in reducing oxidative damage. Furthermore, chronic treatment with lamotrigine and carbamazepine had similar effects. Valproate also influences DNA to alter genetic processes that could protect cells from injury or toxic agents. These interactions are believed to increase levels of cellular protective proteins, such as CREB and *bcl-2* and other neurotrophic substances such as BDNF (Einat and Manji, 2006; Zarate et al., 2006).

Clinical evidence shows that the laboratory results may be relevant to the therapeutic effect of these drugs. It has been reported that levels of BDNF were significantly decreased in the blood serum of patients with bipolar disorder who were either manic or depressed compared to patients who were euthymic or to healthy controls (see Figure 14.1). Another study found that the volume of gray matter in the brains of patients on lithium was as much as 15 percent larger in areas that are critical for paying attention and controlling emotions, compared to the brain volume of people without the disorder and of bipolar patients not on lithium (Bearden et al., 2007). The possibility that lithium may affect how genes are controlled means that it might also be helpful for treating genetic disorders. Evidence for this possibility was reported by researchers working with a mouse model of a lethal neurodegenerative disease called spinocerebellar ataxia type 1. Mice with this disease that were fed lithium showed improvement in coordination and memory, although lithium did not increase their life span (Watase et al., 2007). Reviews by Beaulieu and Caron (2008) and Marmol (2008) provide thorough discussions of the history, clinical application, and neurochemistry of lithium, including evidence for its neuroprotective effects in brain injury, Parkinson's disease, Huntington's chorea, and Alzheimer's disease. Unfortunately, early reports of benefit in ALS (amyotrophic lateral sclerosis) were not confirmed (Aggarwal et al., 2010).

Another possible therapeutic target comes from a recent meta-analysis showing elevations in certain cytokines in patients, even when they are in a euthymic state (Munkholm et al., 2013). This suggests a role for immune system dysfunction in bipolar disorder.

Side Effects and Toxicity

Because of lithium's extremely narrow therapeutic range, lithium blood levels must be closely monitored. The occurrence and intensity of side effects and toxic reactions are usually related to plasma drug concentrations and involve the nervous system, the gastrointestinal (GI) tract, the kidneys, the thyroid, the cardiovascular system, and the skin.

At plasma levels of 1.5 to 2.0 mEq/l and sometimes lower, most reactions involve the GI tract, resulting in nausea, vomiting, diarrhea, and abdominal pain. Nevertheless, weight gain may be substantial during long-term therapy—up to 30 percent of patients become obese, a prevalence three times greater than in the general population that can profoundly affect adherence (Keck and McElroy, 2003).

Lithium may elicit a variety of dermatological reactions. These include rashes, acne, psoriasis, hair and nail disorders, lesions of the mucosal tissue, and other conditions (Jafferany, 2008). Chronic lithium treatment may enlarge the thyroid. As many as 60 percent of patients on lithium may experience increased thirst, water intake, and urine output (due to an impairment of renal concentrating ability). Although kidney function should be assessed periodically, permanent damage is rare (McKnight et al., 2012).

Neurological side effects include a slight tremor, lethargy, impaired concentration, dizziness, slurred speech, ataxia, muscle weakness, and nystagmus (uncontrollable, jerky eye movements in any direction). Lithium-induced tremor is very common, and more than 30 percent of patients report this reaction even at therapeutic blood levels of 0.6 to 1.2 mEq/l. A hypothyroid condition may develop, and enlargement (hypertrophy) of the gland can occur at normal doses. Adverse effects on memory and cognition are common, and patients often complain of memory problems. Consistent with these effects, some researchers found improvements in motor performance, cognition, and creative ability after lithium withdrawal. Severe cognitive deficits are seen with lithium toxicity.

At plasma lithium levels above 2.0 mEq/l, more severe side effects include fatigue, muscle weakness, slurred speech, and worsening tremors. Thyroid gland function becomes more depressed and the gland may enlarge further, resulting in goiter. Muscle fasciculations, abnormal motor movements, psychosis, and stupor may occur. Above 2.5 mEq/l, toxic symptoms include muscle rigidity, coma, renal failure, cardiac arrhythmias, and death.

Treatment of poisoning or overdose is nonspecific; there is no antidote to lithium. Usually drug administration is stopped and sodium-containing fluids are infused immediately. If toxic signs are serious, hemodialysis, gastric lavage, diuretic therapy, antiepileptic medication, and other supports may be needed. Complete recovery may be prolonged, with full return of renal and neurological function taking weeks or months. See Li (2011) for a summary of how to use lithium most effectively for clinical treatment of bipolar disorder.

Effects in Pregnancy

There is concern about the use of lithium during pregnancy, particularly in the first trimester, as there is a risk of fetal malformation of the cardiovascular system involving the tricuspid valve (Ebstein's Anomaly) (Ernst and Goldberg, 2002). However, the risk of not treating bipolar disorder is greater when considering the health and welfare of both the mother and the child. In addition, the risk of using other drugs like antiepileptic agents or even antipsychotics may be greater during pregnancy compared to lithium (Gentile, 2012). When a pregnant woman is on lithium therapy, the drug should be discontinued several days before delivery because (1) when the water breaks, acute dehydration will quickly increase lithium to toxic levels and (2) the newborn will have difficulty excreting the drug. On the other hand, it is important for the mother to restart her lithium within 24 hours of delivery to reduce the risk of relapse. Breast-feeding is also contraindicated during lithium therapy because lithium passes easily into breast milk. For a summary of the approaches to treating women with bipolar disorder before, during, and after pregnancy, (see Novosolov 2012).

Nonadherence

Nonadherence is associated with significant morbidity, recurrent episodes, and greatly increased suicide risk. Nevertheless, up to 50 percent of patients on lithium stop taking the drug against medical advice. Some years ago it was felt that discontinuation of lithium treatment would result in treatment resistance when therapy was resumed, but this does not appear to be the case.

Nonadherence seems to result primarily from intolerance of side effects, particularly memory impairment and cognitive slowing, weight gain, and the subjective feeling of reduced energy and productivity. Other reasons include missing the manic "highs," belief that the disorder has resolved and the drug is unnecessary, and feelings of stigmatism in having a psychiatric illness.

Lithium therapy reduces suicidal behaviors in bipolar patients. Unfortunately, when patients stopped taking the drug, the rate of suicide attempts increased fourteen-fold and the rate of completed suicides thirteen-fold. The prophylactic effect of lithium on mortality and morbidity was confirmed by Cipriani and coworkers (2013), who reported that lithium was effective in the prevention of suicide, and death from all causes in patients with mood disorders. It should be appreciated that reduction of suicidal behavior occurs independently of lithium's effect on mood. There is growing evidence for the effectiveness of lithium as an anti-suicide agent, even when used as an adjunct medication, in any situation in which suicide is a concern (Baldessarini et al., 2006; Cipriani et al., 2013).

Combination Therapy

Combination therapy—often lithium plus an antiepileptic or antipsychotic drug—can provide both greater therapeutic efficacy and better protection against relapse than lithium therapy alone. In fact, combination therapy has become the rule rather than the exception (Geddes et al., 2004), with lithium most effective for mania, for augmenting antidepressant efficacy in refractory patients, and for maintenance; and an anticonvulsant such as lamotrigine is often helpful against bipolar depression as well as mania

(Goodwin et al., 2004). Moreover, there is some evidence that such combinations may also exert greater neuroprotective effects on the brain (Leng et al., 2008).

LiTMUS Study

Sponsored by the National Institute for Mental Health (NIMH), the Lithium Treatment Moderate-Dose Use Study (LiTMUS) was designed using the STAR*D model used for antidepressant treatment. It was intended to answer the question of whether combining lithium with other mood stabilizers or SGAs resulted in any greater benefit, relative to the additional side effect risk, than just using the mood stabilizers or SGAs alone. Patients with either bipolar I or bipolar II disorders who were at least mildly ill and had not previously been treated with adjunctive lithium were eligible to be randomized to one of two groups and followed for 6 months. The two groups were: (1) optimized personalized treatment (OPT) which was based on the Texas Implementation of Medication Algorithm (TIMA), a decision tree approach to making medication decisions based on objective assessment of patient outcomes at each treatment visit; and (2) OPT plus adjunctive lithium. This is a naturalistic study allowing a broader range of participants including those with substance abuse and other co-morbid conditions. In fact, the few exclusion criteria were a contraindication to the use of lithium, pregnancy, age less than 18 years, and unwillingness to comply with study requirements.

The overall finding of the study was that there was no difference between the two treatment groups in the primary outcome measure of change in psychiatric symptoms as measured by a variety of symptom rating scales. That is, adding lithium to OPT did not improve outcomes. But, a secondary finding was that the OPT + lithium group was less likely to be treated with SGAs than the OPT only group, suggesting that the lithium add-on permitted less exposure to SGAs along with their potential side effects. The authors offered several possible reasons for the apparent lack of effectiveness of added lithium including the fact that the lithium doses used produced blood levels below 0.6 mEq/l (normal maintenance range would be 0.6 mEq/l to 0.8 mEq/l) suggesting that the prescribers were not being aggressive enough with the lithium treatment although they were following the study protocol (Nierenberg et al., 2013).

Mood Stabilizers: "Neuromodulator" Anticonvulsants

Only about 60 to 70 percent of patients with bipolar disorder can be adequately helped by lithium alone, both for maintenance and for relapse prevention; and lithium is even less effective in controlling episodes of rapid-cycling mania. Therefore, there is a need for alternative agents in patients who are treatment-refractory, nonadherent, or intolerant of lithium's side effects. One alternative is anticonvulsants (see Chapter 13). The variety of disorders for which these drugs are now used is much broader than their original indication for epilepsy. Their use in alcohol detoxification and relapse prevention is described in Chapter 5; Chapter 13 describes their use in the treatment of anxiety disorders and the control of emotional outbursts in such disorders as posttraumatic stress disorder (PTSD); Chapter 15 describes their use in treating aggressive and explosive behavioral disorders in children and adolescents. Treating people afflicted with this variety of disorders with an antiepileptic drug may give the wrong impression that somehow they are "epileptic." To avoid this misconception, we introduce the broader term *neuromodulator* (to be used interchangeably with *anticonvulsant*), reflecting the diverse clinical applications of these agents.

First-generation anticonvulsants included phenobarbital, other barbiturates, and phenytoin and its derivatives, none of which were useful in treating bipolar illness.[3] Second-generation anticonvulsants included *valproic acid* (Divalproex, Depakote), and *carbamazepine* (Tegretol), which have significant side effects that limit their use.

In particular, many of the antiepileptic drugs (AEDs) produce birth defects. However, there is great variability among reports. This variability may be because the baseline rate of all major congenital anomalies in newborns in the U.S. population is between 2 and 4 percent (Montouris, 2005) and because epilepsy per se is associated with an increased risk of such anomalies (Perucca, 2005). There is also agreement that the magnitude of the risk increases in offspring exposed to polypharmacy (Perucca, 2005). The most common congenital malformations from anticonvulsants are the same as the malformations in the general population, for example, heart defects, clubfoot, and cleft palate.

In addition to these concerns, the FDA issued a warning in 2008 about increased suicidal behavior related to use of anticonvulsant drugs. Despite studies questioning the increased suicide risk (Gibbons et al., 2009), the FDA warning has been supported by an analysis of individual medications based on a large dataset of more than 250,000 patients (Patorno et al., 2010). Although not all anticonvulsants were associated with an increased risk, the results showed that the class-wide warning was warranted and it remains in effect.

Carbamazepine

Studies conducted in the early 1990s indicated that carbamazepine (Tegretol; see Figure 14.2) might be as effective as lithium in preventing the recurrence of mania. However, in bipolar patients not previously treated with mood stabilizers, lithium is superior to carbamazepine in prophylactic efficacy (Hartong et al., 2003). Nevertheless, some patients who do not respond adequately to either agent alone are helped by the combination of the two drugs (Keck and McElroy, 2002). Because of the correlation between therapeutic effectiveness and plasma level, one reason patients may fail to respond to carbamazepine is inadequate blood levels. The therapeutic level for epilepsy and for bipolar disorder is estimated to be the same, between 8 and 12 µg/ml.

Several possible mechanisms have been proposed to explain carbamazepine's action in treating epilepsy and bipolar disorder. Its anticonvulsant effects may occur because it reduces neuronal excitation by blocking sodium channels and thus the ability of sodium to initiate action potentials. Its benefit for bipolar disorder may be related to the fact that carbamazepine, like lithium, inhibits enzyme activity in intracellular second-messenger systems. In the treatment of bipolar disorder, carbamazepine is useful for prophylaxis— that is, reducing the frequency of episodes—and it may be the better choice for episodes of mixed mania and rapid cycling.

---

[3] Phenytoin was never widely used as a mood stabilizer, although there are positive reports from some investigators (Bersudsky, 2005; Mishory et al., 2000).

Adverse effects of carbamazepine include GI upset, sedation, ataxia, visual distur-bances, and rare but life-threatening dermatological reactions, many of which may be caused by a metabolite, carbamazepine-epoxide. While the risk of the skin reactions is 1 to 6 per 10,000 new Caucasian users of the drug, the risk is estimated to be about 10 times higher for those of Asian ancestry. Therefore, there is an FDA requirement that manufacturers add a recommendation to the labeling of this drug that patients of Asian ancestry get a genetic blood test that would indicate whether they are in the population at risk. Although impairment of higher-order cognitive functioning is modest, some patients may be particularly sensitive to this side effect. More serious reactions involve the blood and range from a relatively benign reduction in white blood cell count (leuco-penia) to, on rare occasions, a severe reduction, called agranulocytosis. For this reason it received a "black box" warning and a recommendation for periodic blood tests.[4]

Drug interactions involving carbamazepine are common and result from drug-induced stimulation of drug-metabolizing enzymes, especially CYP-3A4 in the liver. As a result, acute blood levels may decrease, which may require increasing the dose by up to 100 percent to maintain a therapeutic blood level. This effect also extends to other drugs metabolized by the same enzyme family when combined with carbamazepine.

As stated, because carbamazepine is potentially teratogenic, it should not be admin-istered during pregnancy if at all possible.

It was approved by the FDA in 2005 for the treatment of manic and mixed episodes in an extended-release form (Equetro).

Oxcarbazepine

Oxcarbazepine (Trileptal) can be considered a safer carbamazepine, capable of replac-ing carbamazepine for all its uses with comparable efficacy and greatly improved safety. The difference is the result of a small structural variation between the two drugs (see Figure 14.2). Oxcarbazepine is essentially carbamazepine with an oxygen molecule attached to one of the rings. The liver can thus easily metabolize the drug by a process called hydroxylation. In fact, this process occurs within 5 minutes after drug absorption, and the monohydroxy derivative is the active form of the drug; oxcarbazepine is therefore an inactive "prodrug." Because of this easy metabolic process, there is no enzyme induc-tion, no alteration in liver enzymes, no white blood cell problems, no required blood monitoring, and few drug interactions.

Oxcarbazepine is approved for use in epilepsy, and it is becoming widely used to treat bipolar disorder and other disorders treatable with carbamazepine (Ghaemi et al., 2003). It has been shown to be superior to placebo in the treatment of acute mania in adults and comparable to lithium, valproate, and the antipsychotic haloperidol. However, Wagner and coworkers (2006) found no difference between oxcarbazepine and placebo in chil-dren and adolescents.

---

[4] A black box warning is an FDA-mandated list of adverse effects placed in a large black box just below the drug name on the package insert that accompanies every container of prescription medication received by a pharmacy.

Valproic Acid

Valproate (valproic acid, divalproex, Depakene, Depacon, Depakote; see Figure 14.2) is the second anticonvulsant that was systematically studied for treatment of bipolar illness, and it has been used for this disorder since its introduction in 1994. In 2008 the FDA approved a delayed-release valproate therapy in soft gel capsules (Stavzor), for BD, epilepsy, and migraine headache. In 2009 the FDA approved a generic version of Depakote extended-release (ER) tablets.

Several actions of valproic acid have been identified. First, it binds to and inhibits GABA transaminase, the enzyme that breaks down GABA. Therefore, the drug's anticonvulsant activity may be related to increased brain concentrations of GABA. Second, valproic acid may increase GABA by blocking its reuptake into glia and nerve endings. Third, valproic acid may also work by suppressing repetitive neuronal firing through inhibition of voltage-sensitive sodium channels. A fourth mechanism was proposed by Chen and coworkers (1999), who observed an effect of valproate on enzymes associated with the cellular organization of DNA. By influencing these enzymes and altering DNA function, valproate may be involved in gene transcription.

Valproate is particularly effective in the treatment of acute mania, mixed states, schizoaffective disorder, and rapid-cycling bipolar disorder. It may be more effective than other agents in treating lithium-resistant patients, producing a positive response in up to 71 percent of patients. The combination of valproate and lithium may be more efficacious than either agent alone. A two-year trial comparing the effectiveness of lithium, valproate, and their combination in preventing relapse found the combination seemed best at preventing manic episodes and lithium alone in preventing depressive episodes. Although the study had no placebo group, it was a real-world design and argues for greater use of lithium (Geddes et al., 2010).

Valproic acid has traditionally been administered in divided doses through the day. An extended-release preparation allows once-daily dosing, usually at bedtime, to improve adherence and help alleviate daytime sedation and memory impairment. Depakene comes in capsules and as a syrup, while Depacon is the intravenous solution and Depakote is the formulation of tablets or delayed-release tablets.

Side effects associated with valproate include GI upset, sedation, lethargy, hand tremor, alopecia (hair loss), and some metabolic changes in the liver. In females starting valproate before the age of 20, the drug has been associated with an 8 percent prevalence of marked obesity, polycystic ovaries, and markedly increased levels of serum androgens (increased testosterone levels). Valproate may be slightly more detrimental to cognitive function than carbamazepine.

Like lithium and carbamazepine, valproate can be teratogenic, increasing the risk of spina bifida, neural tube defects, and developmental deficits in the infant. In fact, it has been suggested that this property may be related to its interaction with DNA. Withdrawal symptoms, including irritability, jitteriness, abnormal tone, feeding difficulties, and seizures, have been described in infants whose mothers took valproate during pregnancy. Consequently, caution must be exercised in using valproate in women who may become pregnant during drug therapy. Other serious side effects of valproate, which have resulted in black box warnings, include hepatotoxicity (liver damage) and pancreatitis (inflammation of the pancreas).

An analog of valproic acid, *valnoctamide*, has been used in Europe but is not available in the U.S.; it does not go through the same metabolic pathway and its chemical structure is sufficiently different compared to valproic acid such that it is much less teratogenic; it has been tested in one controlled trial as an add-on to risperidone and compared to placebo add-on; valnoctamide was significantly more effective than placebo on all measures (Mathews et al., 2012).

Lamotrigine

The third-generation anticonvulsant neuromodulator, *lamotrigine* (Lamictal) (Figure 14.3) was equal to lithium in *preventing* relapse to any manic episode, better than lithium in *preventing* relapse to a depressive episode (Amann et al., 2011; Bowden et al., 2003), and it was less likely to cause a manic shift compared with the conventional antidepressants (Goldberg et al., 2009; Keck et al., 2003). Conversely, it is not useful for acute mania, and in five different studies lamotrigine performed no better than placebo against acute bipolar depression. Although most of these data were not published, the manufacturer, GlaxoSmithKline, has posted results of all its studies on its Web site (http://ctr.gsk.co.uk/Summary/lamotrigine/studylist.asp).

In 2003 lamotrigine was approved for the long-term maintenance of adults with bipolar I disorder, that is, for delaying the time to relapse to depressive and manic symptoms. This benefit is most evident if patients respond acutely to lamotrigine. Generic lamotrigine tablets were approved in 2008; in 2009 the chewable tablet formulation, and that same year the FDA also approved Lamictal (lamotrigine) orally disintegrating tablets for long-term treatment of BP-I .

In some studies lamotrigine may still be less effective than lithium in long-term maintenance (Kessing et al., 2012), as "add-on" medication (Kemp et al., 2012), or for bipolar depression (Bowden et al., 2012). Some of the more recent negative findings may be due to the fact that adding lamotrigine to other drugs may increase adverse reactions, or, that lamotrigine is simply not effective in refractory patients. Regardless of the reason, lamotrigine's inconsistent history, specifically for bipolar depression, has been reflected in clinical treatment guidelines' varied recommendations about where it should be placed (i.e., first line, second line, monotherapy, add-on only, etc.) as a treatment option (Tränkner et al., 2013).

Lamotrigine's major mechanism of action is blockade of voltage-dependent sodium channel conductance, which inhibits depolarization of the glutaminergic presynaptic

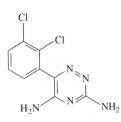

Lamotrigine
(Lamictal)

FIGURE 14.3   Chemical structure of lamotrigine (Lamictal); also shown in Figure 13.6.

membrane, and reduces glutamate release, particularly in the cortex and hippocampus. This decrease in neuronal excitability may account for its antiepileptic, mood-stabilizing, and analgesic effects (Ketter et al., 2003), and it may also have some neuroprotective effects in people who suffer traumatic brain injuries (Pachet et al., 2003).

After oral administration, lamotrigine is rapidly and completely absorbed, reaching peak plasma concentrations in 1 to 5 hours. It is metabolized before excretion, with a half-life of 26 hours, which can decrease to about 7.4 hours when used with phenytoin or carbamazepine (requiring increased doses of lamotrigine) or increase to 60 hours when used with valproate (requiring decreased doses of lamotrigine) (Hurley, 2002). Therapeutic blood concentrations of lamotrigine used to treat epilepsy are in the range of about 1.5 to 5 µg/ml (mg/L), with adverse effects increasing with higher doses (Hirsch et al., 2004). It is presumed that the same concentration range applies to treatment of bipolar disorder.

Side effects associated with lamotrigine include dizziness, tremor, somnolence, headache, nausea, and rash. The most serious side effect is rash, which conceivably may be severe enough to require hospitalization and prove fatal. Adolescents are believed to be more prone to this reaction, so the drug is not indicated for patients younger than 16 years of age. The incidence of rash is currently about 1 in 500, which may be reduced by a slow titration of dose over about six weeks (Calabrese et al., 2002). In marked contrast to other antiepileptic agents, lamotrigine can improve cognitive functioning (Khan et al., 2004).

Of all the antiepileptic drugs, lamotrigine has been found to be the safest to use in pregnancy. There has been no evidence of increased fetal malformations (Moore et al., 2012; Vajda et al., 2013).

Gabapentin and Pregabalin

Introduced in the United States in 1993 as an anticonvulsant for the treatment of partial complex seizures, *gabapentin* (Neurontin) is also used for the treatment of anxiety, neuropathic pain (Gralise), substance dependency, and behavioral dyscontrol, as well as bipolar disorder. Mechanistically, it is a GABA analogue, but it has little or no action on the GABA receptor. Although it increases GABA levels, it is not clear how much the increase contributes to its efficacy. A derivative of gabapentin, *pregabalin* (Lyrica), was approved for use in the United States in 2005 for the treatment of pain states, such as diabetic peripheral neuropathy and postherpetic neuralgia, and as adjunctive therapy in the treatment of partial seizures in adults (Beydoun et al., 2005). In June 2007 the FDA approved Lyrica for the treatment of fibromyalgia. Although moderately effective (Smith et al., 2012), cost must be considered (Lloyd et al., 2012).

The most recent hypothesis for the mechanism of action of these two drugs is that they interact with a component of the calcium channel in presynaptic neuronal membranes to decrease the influx of calcium ions. As a result, less neurotransmitter is released, which translates into antiepileptic, analgesic, and anxiolytic effects (Chiu et al., 2005).

Gabapentin has an excellent pharmacokinetic profile: it is not bound to plasma proteins; it is not metabolized; it is excreted unchanged through the kidneys, with an elimination half-life of 5 to 7 hours; and it has few pharmacokinetic drug interactions. Gabapentin is absorbed by a saturable active transport mechanism from intestine to plasma, so doses up to 1500 milligrams can be given at any one time. Like gabapentin, pregabalin is excreted unchanged, and therefore it has no effect on the liver. Because it is excreted unchanged, it can be safely used in the treatment of alcoholism (see Chapter 5). It is two to three times as potent as gabapentin and has a slightly longer half-life of 6 to 8 hours. It is clear that gabapentin and pregabalin are not effective as monotherapy for bipolar disorder. However, there is evidence that these drugs may be very beneficial for neuropathic pain and at least some types of anxiety disorders, as described below.

Topiramate

Topiramate (Topamax, Topiragen), discussed in Chapter 5 as an antiepileptic drug used to prevent relapse in people with alcoholism, is a very potent anticonvulsant and has been approved by the FDA for the treatment of migraine headaches. Structurally different from other agents in this group, it is derived from the sugar D-fructose and was initially developed as an antidiabetic drug. Topiramate has multiple mechanisms of action. It inhibits sodium conductance, decreasing the duration of spontaneous bursts and the frequency of generated action potentials; it enhances GABA by unknown mechanisms; and it blocks the AMPA subtype glutamate receptor.

The initial positive results of open-label studies of the drug to treat bipolar disorder were not supported by four clinical trials showing topiramate monotherapy to be ineffective in acute mania (Kushner et al., 2006). In addition, topiramate was no different than placebo when combined with either valproate or lithium for the treatment of bipolar I disorder (Chengappa et al., 2006). The main advantage of topiramate is that it is associated with weight loss rather than weight gain. This characteristic may make the drug useful as an adjunctive agent to offset the weight gain associated with other antimanic drugs, but due to the side effects noted below *metformin* (Glucophage) may be a better choice in this regard (Elligner et al., 2010; Mahmoudi-Gharaei et al., 2012).

Unfortunately, the cognitive impairment (especially problems in word-finding) induced by topiramate is greater than that produced by other anticonvulsants, although impairment may occur more frequently at higher doses and with rapid dose increases. Other side effects include tingling in the extremities, irritability, anxiety, and depression. However, these effects may subside within a few weeks. Studies of pregnant women taking topiramate indicated a significantly higher rate of fetal malformations, particularly oral cleft. As a result, the FDA changed topiramate's pregnancy classification to category D (evidence of teratogenicity in humans, but drug may be used if benefit outweighs risk) (Nonacs, 2012).

Topiramate is excreted unchanged and is less likely to be involved in drug interactions mediated by the liver. However, this drug has the potential to increase plasma levels of other drugs excreted by the kidneys, such as lithium. It may also increase the incidence of kidney stones. In 2009 the FDA approved generic Topamax, as topiramate tablets, and a generic version of Topamax as topiramate capsules (Sprinkle).

Zonisamide

Zonisamide (Zonegran) is an antiepileptic drug long available in Japan, and in the United States since mid-2000 for the treatment of epilepsy. Its major mechanism of action is reduction of neuronal repetitive firing by blocking sodium channels preventing the influx of calcium ions and transmitter release, and it may exert neuroprotective effects.

Zonisamide has not been shown to have any beneficial effect on reduction of bipolar symptoms compared to placebo when used as an adjunct to ongoing treatment (Dauphinais et al., 2011). Side effects include reduced white blood cell counts, elevated liver enzymes, and several drug interactions. Like topiramate, this drug may be of use in treating binge eating, but again, metformin may be a better choice.

Tiagabine

The mechanism of action of *tiagabine* (Gabitril) as an anticonvulsant involves inhibition of the active reuptake of GABA by inhibiting the GABA transporter in the hippocampus and cerebral cortex. There are no controlled studies that would support its use in the treatment of bipolar disorder.

A review of 18 randomized controlled trials of either monotherapy or combination therapy with anticonvulsants in the treatment of acute bipolar depression found that valproic acid and lamotrigine have the best evidence for being effective; however, small sample sizes in all the studies limited the strength of the findings and many anticonvulsants have not yet been subjected to RCT research (Reinares et al., 2012).

Other Uses for Anticonvulsant Mood Stabilizers

Neuropathic Pain

Patients with trigeminal neuralgia have been treated with carbamazepine for decades, and topiramate is the second antiepileptic drug, after valproate, to be approved for the prevention of migraine (in 2004). Because recommended doses are much lower than those for other indications, the cognitive side effects may not be as troublesome for migraine. Gabapentin has proven effective against neuropathic pain induced by diabetic neuropathy, postherpetic neuralgia, and spinal cord injury. Clinical studies show that *pregabalin* (Lyrica) shares this analgesic effectiveness in patients with diabetic neuropathy and fibromyalgia. Treatment of neuropathic pain is seen as the drug's leading indication. McDonald and Portenoy (2006) provide an excellent review of the use of anticonvulsants in neuropathic pain states.

Anxiety Disorders

Pregabalin has shown early onset of action and short-term and long-term efficacy in patients with generalized anxiety disorder (Feltner et al., 2003; Pande et al., 2003). A ten-week, randomized, open-label trial of tiagabine and paroxetine found that both agents significantly reduced anxiety and depressive symptoms and improved sleep quality and overall functioning (Rosenthal, 2003). In addition, topiramate has been found useful for the treatment of posttraumatic stress disorder (Berlant and van Kammen, 2002) in decreasing nightmares and flashbacks in the majority of patients. In social phobia, gabapentin was found to be superior to placebo (Pande et al., 1999), and one randomized placebo-controlled study found that gabapentin reduced panic symptoms in severe panic disorder (Pande et al., 2000).

Borderline Personality Disorder

Borderline personality disorder is characterized by emotional instability, impulsivity, and aggression and is associated with considerable morbidity and mortality. It is a common comorbid condition with bipolar disorder. All the medications routinely used in treating bipolar disorder have been shown in published studies to have some value in treating borderline personality disorder: antidepressants, mood stabilizers, and antipsychotics ameliorate the irritability and anger and reduce the tempestuousness of the relationships and the impulsive aggressiveness of these patients. However, numerous studies indicated that the neuromodulator anticonvulsants had a particular benefit in this regard, and this has recently been supported in two reviews (Lieb et al., 2010; Mercer et al., 2009) and a meta-analysis of randomized controlled trials (Ingenhoven et al., 2010). Mood stabilizers had a pronounced effect on impulsive behavioral dyscontrol, anger and anxiety; antipsychotics had a moderate effect on the various symptoms; and antidepressants were the least effective in this situation (Stoffers et al., 2010). However, the most effective treatment for this disorder is not a drug, but dialectical behavior therapy (DBT).

Atypical Antipsychotics for Bipolar Disorder

Acute Mania

For decades, traditional antipsychotic drugs were used to help control the symptoms of acute mania, predating the use of lithium by 20 years. The fact that the antimanic potency of the typical antipsychotics was positively associated with their affinity for D_2 receptors supported a "dopamine-blockade" hypothesis (Harrison-Read, 2009), consistent with the possibility that schizophrenia and BD share some common genetic origin (Lichtenstein et al., 2009).

All the second-generation antipsychotics have also shown efficacy either as monotherapy or as adjunctive agents for acute mania, and they have all been approved for this indication. In their meta-analysis, Scherk and coworkers (2007) concluded:

> SGAs as add-on medication to mood stabilizers are superior to mood stabilizers alone for acute manic symptoms, as indicated by greater reductions in mania scores, higher response rates, and fewer dropouts due to inefficacy. . . . Combination treatment with a second-generation atypical antipsychotic and a mood stabilizer should be the treatment of choice, in particular for severe manic episodes (p. 442).

Recently, clozapine was also found to have the same benefit (Nielsen et al., 2012). Among the antipsychotic drugs, a meta-analysis showed the three most effective were haloperidol, risperidone and olanzapine; when dropout rates were considered, olanzapine, risperidone, and quetiapine were better than haloperidol. Taken together (effectiveness and acceptability) olanzapine and risperidone were considered superior to all other drugs. However, the authors note that this finding only applies to the short-term acute treatment of manic symptoms and not to the long-term maintenance treatment of either bipolar mania or depression. For maintenance, lithium remains one of the most effective drugs (Cipriani et al., 2011; see also Yildiz et al., 2011). A consensus guideline on the use of aripiprazole for the treatment of mania was published in the United Kingdom (Aitchison et al., 2009).

Maintenance of Remission

Risperidone has been found effective in extension trials as monotherapy or as adjunctive treatment in sustaining remission from mania while not inducing depression (Hirschfield et al., 2006; Rendell et al., 2006). Macfadden et al. (2011) administered long-acting risperidone in depot form (Risperdal Consta) to patients who were rapid-cyclers. By the end of the 16-week study, 61.3 percent of those who completed the 16-week study qualified for remission. Olanzapine (Tohen et al., 2006), quetiapine (Calabrese et al., 2005), aripiprazole (Keck et al., 2006, 2007), and ziprasidone (Bowden et al., 2010) have all been found more effective than placebo for maintenance treatment, and olanzapine was reported comparable to lithium (Tohen et al., 2005). Quetiapine was as effective as lithium at delaying onset of subsequent mood symptoms in bipolar patients who had been previously stabilized on quetiapine. Patients maintained on quetiapine, or who were switched to lithium, had more time free of any subsequent mood symptoms compared to patients on placebo (Weisler et al., 2011).

Bipolar Depression

Olanzapine has been reported to be as effective for bipolar depression as the antidepressant fluoxetine alone, or in combination as the FDA approved drug Symbyax (Amsterdam and Shults, 2005; Corya et al., 2006). Both Symbyax and lamotrigine had an equally low risk of inducing mania, which is a serious concern with antidepressant treatment for bipolar disorder. A recent meta-analysis of Symbyax in the treatment of bipolar depression showed that the combination drug was more effective than olanzapine alone, but not better than lamotrigine. But, more adverse effects were noted with the combination compared to those seen with lamotrigine (Silva et al., 2013). Studies have examined the relative risk of three other antidepressants—sertraline, bupropion, and venlafaxine—producing a "switch" when used as adjuncts to mood stabilizers. Overall, the rate was higher for bipolar I (30.8 percent) than bipolar II (18.6 percent), although eventually only 23.3 percent of patients did not switch. However, venlafaxine was reported to be more likely than the other two antidepressants to produce a switch (Leverich et al., 2006; Post et al., 2006). These results suggest that people with bipolar II might be less vulnerable to an antidepressant-induced switch. This suggestion is supported by Altshuler and coworkers (2006), who found less switching with adjunctive selective serotonergic reuptake inhibitors in bipolar II than in bipolar I patients, and by Parker and coworkers (2006b), who successfully treated depressed bipolar II patients for 9 months with SSRIs, without any worsening of symptoms. A recent consensus report on the use of antidepressants to treat bipolar depression recommended that they be used in combination with appropriate mood stabilizers. In addition, tri- and tetracyclic antidepressants and venlafaxine carry the greatest risk for inducing pathological elevations in mood (Pacchiarottia et al., 2013).

Several studies have supported the use of quetiapine in treating bipolar depression, including a retrospective chart review (Shajahan and Taylor, 2010), two clinical trials (McElroy et al., 2010; Young et al., 2010) and an open-label study (Jeong et al., 2013). In 2009, Seroquel XR (*quetiapine fumarate*) extended-release tablets were approved by the FDA for acute treatment for depressive, manic, and mixed bipolar disorder episodes and for maintenance therapy as adjunctive treatment to lithium or divalproex. The new formulation was not approved for patients with dementia-related psychosis or for patients younger than 18 years.

One of the newest antipsychotic agents, *asenepine* (Saphris), has been shown to be effective in the short-term (three weeks) in reducing manic symptoms compared to placebo as monotherapy; was found to be equal to olanzapine in an extension study at reducing both manic and/or depressive symptoms; and when added to either lithium or valproic acid, was more effective than placebo at reducing manic symptoms (Chwieduk et al., 2011). The other two new antipsychotic drugs, iloperidone and lurasidone, have not yet been approved for use in bipolar disorders.

De Fruyt and colleagues (2012) performed a meta-analysis of studies that examined the effectiveness of SGAs in the treatment of acute bipolar depression. Of the SGAs examined, quetiapine and to a lesser extent olanzapine, but not aripiprazole (see also Tsai and colleagues, 2011) demonstrated significant improvement. But, the authors point out that adverse events like weight gain, akathisia, and sedation produced by the SGAs may have reduced overall effectiveness; the number of total studies used in the analysis was small and demonstrated clinical heterogeneity making interpretation and generalizability of the results difficult.

Although the SGAs may be less likely to elicit movement disorders than the older drugs in schizophrenic patients, there is evidence that patients with bipolar disorder may be more susceptible to these side effects (Ghaemi et al., 2006). One meta-analysis (Gao et al., 2008) concluded that bipolar patients were approximately twice as likely as schizophrenic patients to suffer movement disorders (extrapyramidal symptoms, akathisia) and an increase in anticholinergic drug treatment of these symptoms. Only olanzapine was not different from placebo, in either bipolar or schizophrenic patients, while aripiprazole was more likely to cause akathisia in bipolar patients but not schizophrenic patients.

Although considered a first generation antipsychotic (FGA) drug, loxapine more closely resembles SGAs in its activity profile. A new formulation of this drug has been approved for the treatment of agitation in adults with schizophrenia or bipolar disorder. Labeled *Adasuve* by the manufacturer, this formulation of loxapine is a powder that is aerosolized and administered via inhalation. In clinical trials the drug reduced agitation within 10 minutes. Due to the risk of causing bronchospasm, the drug can only be used under specified procedural restrictions dictated by the FDA's risk evaluation and mitigation strategy (REMS) and only in facilities that are capable of providing immediate treatment for acute bronchospasm. This drug should not be used in anyone with a compromised respiratory system, like those with COPD.

Nivoli and colleagues (2011) reviewed the available guidelines for the treatment of bipolar depression and found it difficult to make comparisons. They noted that antidepressants for bipolar depression should be avoided in the absence of mood stabilizers and they saw that SGA monotherapy was becoming more recognized as first-line treatment. One of the findings from the STEP-BD study was that using more than one SGA in the treatment of bipolar disorder does not improve response to treatment and in fact may reduce clinical outcomes (Brooks et al., 2011). For a recent review of the use of mood stabilizers and antipsychotic agents as treatments for bipolar disorder see Bourin et al. (2013).

In summary, monotherapy with either lithium or valproic acid, is considered the first line of treatment for all phases of bipolar disorder; if that approach is ineffective, the next step usually involves combining these two agents or adding lamotrigine to the monotherapy agent if the primary phase of illness is depression; then, if indicated, an SGA can be added in place of one of the mood stabilizers if response to previous treatment is less than desired; on average, most patients with bipolar disorder receive 3 or more medications (Thase, 2012).

TABLE 14.3 FDA-Approved Treatments for Bipolar Disorder in Adults				
Generic Name	Mania	Mixed	Depression	Maintenance
Aripiprazole	X	X		X
Asenapine	X	X		
Carbamazepine extended-release	X	X		
Chlorpromazine	X			
Lamotrigine				X
Lithium	X			X
Olanzapine	X	X		X
Olanzapine/fluoxetine			X	
Quetiapine	X		X	
Risperidone	X	X		
Valproate	X			
Ziprasidone	X	X		

Aripiprazole, risperidone, and quetiapine are FDA-approved for bipolar I disorder (manic, mixed) in youths aged 10 to 17 years; lithium is FDA-approved for bipolar I disorder in youths aged 12 to 17 years; olanzapine is FDA-approved for bipolar I disorder in youths aged 13 to 17 years.
Matthews, D. C., et al. "New Drug Developments for Bipolar Mania," *Psychiatric Times* Vol. 29, December 12, 2012. Copyrighted 2014. UBM Medica. 107859:314BN

Table 14.3 summarizes the current, FDA-approved treatments for bipolar disorder in adults.

Omega-3 Fatty Acids for Bipolar Disorder

In countries where the diet is rich in fish oils, the incidence of bipolar disorder is quite low (Noaghiul and Hibbeln, 2003). Therefore, it is possible that fish oils may prevent BD, perhaps by protecting the brain from the neuronal injuries now being identified in this disorder. Omega-3 fatty acids, obtained from marine or plant sources, are known to damp these signal transduction pathways in a variety of cell systems (Parker et al., 2006a).

Stoll and coworkers (1999) found that augmentation of antimanic treatment with omega-3 fatty acids compared to placebo greatly increased the time before recurrence of a bipolar episode, even in patients who were not taking any other medication. Other reviews (Parker et al., 2006a; Marengell et al., 2006) suggest there is some support for the role of omega-3 fatty acids in slowing the recurrence of episodes of bipolar and other mood disorders but the results of clinical trials have been inconsistent. Montgomery and Richardson (2008) concluded that there is still not enough evidence to say whether this treatment is useful for bipolar disorder as do Wozniak et al. (2007) in their study of omega-3 in children with bipolar disorder. A more recent meta-analysis provided moderately strong evidence (effect size = 0.34) that bipolar depressive symptoms may be improved with adjunctive omega-3; but there was no support for its effect on attenuating manic symptoms (Sarris et al., 2012). The status of omega-3 fatty acid or other agents used in complementary medicine, as interventions for bipolar disorder remains unproven (Murphy, et al., 2012; Sarris, et al., 2011)

Miscellaneous Agents

Many patients are unresponsive to or intolerant of present medications, and alternative agents are much needed.

The anticholinergic drug *scopolamine* produces some effects resembling manic symptoms, such as flight of ideas, talkativeness, and difficulties in concentration. Therefore, agents that potentiate the effect of acetylcholine might have some antimanic action. Donepezil inhibits the enzyme acetylcholinesterase; however, a double-blind placebo-controlled trial found no effect of adjunctive donepezil in patients with refractory mania (Evins et al., 2006). Another drug used to treat Alzheimer's disease, *memantine* (Namenda) which is a glutamate receptor antagonist, has been evaluated in open label studies as a possible augmenting agent in the treatment of mania with some positive findings. Further controlled trials are needed (Sanches et al., 2011).

Because lithium interferes with membrane ion function, *calcium channel blockers*, such as verapamil, have been tried, but their effectiveness remains questionable. Clonidine, an antihypertensive drug, has been tried in treatment-refractory patients with bipolar disorder but despite initial positive results, effectiveness remains unproved.

Kulkarni and colleagues (2006) reported that the hormonal agents *tamoxifen* (Cytogen) and *medroxyprogesterone acetate* (Depo-Provera) were more effective than placebo in improving the symptoms of mania in 13 women with acute bipolar affective disorder. Although most commonly used for its antiestrogenic property in the treatment of breast cancer, tamoxifen is a potent inhibitor of the enzyme protein kinase C, which is involved in intracellular signal transduction, which may be the route by which it affects bipolar disorder. Three controlled trials have shown tamoxifen, either as monotherapy or used as an adjunctive medication, to improve scores on the Young Mania Rating Scale (YMRS). But long-term use of this agent is compounded by side effects associated with estrogen receptor blockade (Sanches et al., 2011).

Allopurinol (Zyloprim) is a xanthine oxidase inhibitor used to treat gout. It affects the purinergic system that has been hypothesized to be involved in the pathophysiology of mania. This is based on an observation of increased uric acid levels in patients who were acutely manic (Salvadore et al., 2010). Some initial controlled trials have indicated it may be effective as an adjunctive agent to lithium or lithium plus haloperidol in the treatment of mania. However, the studies were very short term and additional clinical trials are ongoing (Sanches et al., 2011).

Although not considered a mood stabilizer, the wakefulness-promoting agent *modafinil* (Provigil) has been useful for alleviating fatigue accompanying many medical conditions, including depression.[5] A retrospective chart review study found modafinil effective in relieving fatigue and sleepiness in adults with unipolar or bipolar depression (Nasr et al., 2006). The authors report that no patient demonstrated a switch into mania or hypomania while on modafinil. A small prospective study (which excluded patients with a history of stimulant-induced mania) also found a significantly greater improvement in depression symptoms, and in remission, in adults with bipolar

---

[5] *Modafinil* (as Provigil) is approved by the FDA for helping persons with the disease *narcolepsy* stay awake during the day, maintaining daytime wakefulness, and promoting more tiredness at bedtime.

depression (Frye et al., 2007). When *armodafinil* (Nuvigil), the longer acting isomer of modafinil, was added to the bipolar medication treatment of bipolar patients it produced a greater improvement in their depressive symptoms compared to patients who received added placebo (Calabrese et al., 2010). But, in the second of three planned clinical trials of armodafinil in bipolar depression, the drug failed to meet statistical efficacy. The manufacturer is planning to proceed with the third Phase III clinical trial.

Riluzole, (Rilutek), an inhibitor of glutamate release, is used for the treatment of amyotrophic lateral sclerosis (ALS). In a small sample of bipolar patients who were receiving lithium, the addition of riluzole produced a significant improvement of the depressive symptoms as measured by the Montgomery Asberg Depression Rating Scale (MADRS) (Zarate et al., 2005).

Pramepexole (Mirapex) is a dopamine receptor agonist that has been evaluated as an add-on to standard mood stabilizers in patients with treatment resistant bipolar depression. Two controlled studies have shown that pramepexole reduced depressive symptoms compared to placebo (Sanches et al., 2011).

Ketamine (Ketalar), a noncompetitive NMDA antagonist has been evaluated in sub-anesthetic doses in individuals with bipolar disorder. In a double-blind, randomized, placebo-controlled crossover study, a single IV infusion of ketamine to individuals receiving lithium or valproic acid, improved depressive symptoms compared to placebo. Although the onset of the effect was within 40 minutes, the duration of the effect was short (up to 3 days). Despite the impressive results, the use of ketamine is not currently practical given the need for IV administration, the short duration of action, and the side effects associated with it being a general anesthetic (Diazgranados et al., 2010).

Based on research in animals, inflammatory processes are hypothesized to be involved in some of the behavioral manifestations of psychiatric disorders. With this evidence in mind, *celecoxib* (Celebrex), a cyclooxygenase-2 (COX-2) inhibitor was administered to adults with bipolar depression who were also taking a mood stabilizer or antipsychotic medication. A small but significant advantage for celecoxib at week one was not sustained over the remaining observation periods (Nery et al., 2008).

Agomelatine (Valdoxan) is a melatonin receptor agonist marketed as an antidepressant in Europe but not available in the United States. Used as an add-on to mood stabilizing agents, agomelatine produced significant improvement in patients with bipolar depression compared to a placebo add-on. Further studies are ongoing (Sanches et al., 2011).

Insulin has been shown to mediate a wide range of metabolic, neuromodulatory, growth regulatory, and neuroendocrine functions including modulation of CNS concentrations of neuropeptides, monoamines, and other neurotransmitters that have been implicated in the pathophysiology of psychiatric disorders. There is early evidence of elevated indices of inflammation in patients with bipolar disorder linked to leptin and insulin production (Tsai et al., 2012). Studies are under way to determine if insulin sensitizers like *rosiglitazone* (Avandia) have antidepressant effects in bipolar disorder (McIntyre et al., 2011). In one recent study, the ability of *intranasal insulin* to improve neurocognitive function was examined. Sixty-two patients with bipolar disorder were randomly selected to receive the insulin or placebo added to their regular medications. All subjects were euthymic during the time of the study. Neuropsychological testing indicated that the insulin group had significantly better performance on one measure of executive function compared to the placebo group. But, no other differences were found on any other measure of neurocognitive function (McIntyre et al., 2012).

Methylene blue, used in the treatment of methemoglobinemia and as a dye in diagnostic applications, was administered to bipolar depressed patients who were also taking lamotrigine. Significant reductions in MADRS depression scores were seen in the group who received the full dose of the drug compared to those that received a sub-therapeutic dose. However, the FDA has issued a warning about combining methylene blue with other drugs affecting the norepinephrine and serotonin systems as methylene blue is also a potent reversible MAOI and can be expected to produce adverse affects like noradrenergic crisis or serotonin syndrome when combined with those other drugs (Bender, 2011).

Finally, oxidative stress has been implicated in the pathophysiology of bipolar disorder and levels of the antioxidant glutathione have been reported to be abnormal in individuals with bipolar disorder. The production of glutathione is limited by the availability of its precursor, cysteine. *N-acetylcysteine* (NAC; Mucomyst) is a more bioavailable form of cysteine and has been given to adults with bipolar disorder as an add-on to their normal medications in a double-blind, placebo-controlled study of its effect on depressive symptoms. Results indicated that NAC alleviated depressive symptoms after 20 weeks, and improved functional measures within 8 weeks. (Berk et al., 2008). These same authors reported similar outcomes in a second study (Berk et al., 2011).

Did You Know?

Ebselen a Possible Lithium Mimic, Mouse Study Hints

The experimental drug *ebselen* may work like lithium for bipolar disorder but without lithium's side effects, according to a study in mice. Mice who were made manic with small doses of amphetamines were able to be calmed again with ebselen.

Ebselen is an experimental drug that was tested in people for stroke, and does not have the same side effects as lithium. The researchers filtered through a library of existing drugs—the U.S. National Institutes of Health Clinical Collection—that are considered safe but do not currently have a proven use. They screened the library for any drugs that blocked an enzyme that is key to lithium's success and found ebselen was a possible lithium mimic. Ebselen is an antioxidant originally developed up to late stage, or phase III, clinical trials by the Japanese firm Daiichi Sankyo for the treatment of stroke, but which never reached market and is now out of patent.

The researchers are now starting a small study in healthy human volunteers to look for effects on brain function. If that shows ebselen has similar effects to lithium, they plan to move to second stage trial in bipolar patients.

Psychotherapeutic and Psychosocial Treatments

Increasing focus on the pharmacologic treatment of bipolar disorders has sometimes led clinicians to forgo psychological interventions as an adjunctive treatment (Colom et al., 2003, p. 402). Patients with bipolar disorder suffer from the psychosocial consequences of past episodes, the ongoing vulnerability to future episodes, and the burdens of adhering to a long-term treatment plan that may involve some unpleasant side effects. In addition, many patients have clinically significant mood instability between episodes.

Successful treatment involves a social network primed to recognize the early symptoms of an episode, to seek help for patients who lack insight into their condition, and to assist with recognition of side effects and toxicities, thus aiding in compliance with therapy.

It is also important to ensure that the manic state is not being caused by medications, such as antidepressants, caffeine, herbals containing ephedrine, behavioral stimulants (including illegal drugs, such as cocaine), corticosteroids (cortisone), anabolic steroids, antiparkinsonian drugs, over-the-counter cough and cold preparations, and diet aids. One must also rule out thyroid disease because mania secondary to thyroid hyperactivity is common.

Psychotherapy with pharmacotherapy is associated with 30 to 40 percent reduction in relapse rates over 12 to 30 months (Miklowitz, 2008). Type of psychotherapy used may be based on the stage of illness. Specifically, the following evidence-based therapies are recommended as adjuncts to medication treatment of bipolar disorder: Cognitive behavior therapy (CBT) and family-focused therapy (FFT) are efficacious and interpersonal social rhythm therapy (IPSRT) possibly efficacious as adjuncts to medication in the treatment of depression. Psychoeducation (PE) is efficacious in the prevention of mania/hypomania (and possibly depression) and FFT is efficacious and IPSRT and CBT possibly efficacious in preventing bipolar episodes (Hollon et al., 2010).

STUDY QUESTIONS

1. Discuss the symptomatology of bipolar disorder, including the subtypes and the issue of unipolar versus bipolar depression; why is it important to try to differentiate them?

2. What are the major pharmacological drug categories useful in the treatment of bipolar disorder and the major drugs in each category?

3. What neurochemical actions do the drugs used to treat bipolar disorder have in common?

4. Compare and contrast the anticonvulsants that have some efficacy in treating bipolar disorder, with those that don't.

5. Besides bipolar disorder (and epilepsy), what other disorders are some of the anticonvulsants approved for?

6. Which antipsychotics have been found useful for treatment of bipolar disorder?

7. What are the difficulties in regard to using mood stabilizers in pregnant women?

8. What types of novel drugs are being studied for treatment of bipolar disorder?

REFERENCES

Aggarwal, S. P., et al. (2010). "Safety and Efficacy of Lithium in Combination with Riluzole for Treatment of Amyotrophic Lateral Sclerosis: A Randomized, Double-Blind, Placebo-Controlled Trial." *Lancet Neurology* 9: 481–488.

Aitchison. K. J., et al. (2009). "A UK Consensus on the Administration of Aripiprazole for the Treatment of Mania." *Journal of Psychopharmacology* 23: 231–240.

Altshuler, L. L., et al. (2006). "Lower Switch Rate in Depressed Patients with Bipolar II than Bipolar I Disorder Treated Adjunctively with Second-Generation Antidepressants." *American Journal of Psychiatry* 163: 313–315.

American Psychiatric Association. (2002). "Practice Guideline for the Treatment of Patients with Bipolar Disorder (Revision)." *American Journal of Psychiatry* 159, Supplement (April).

Amman, B., et al. (2011). "Lamotrigine: When and Where Does It Act in Affective Disorders? A Systematic Review." *Journal of Psychopharmacology* 25: 1289–1294.

Amsterdam, J. D., and Shults, J. (2005). "Comparison of Fluoxetine, Olanzapine, and Combined Fluoxetine plus Olanzapine Initial Therapy of Bipolar Type I and Type II Major Depression—Lack of Manic Induction." *Journal of Affective Disorders* 87: 121–130.

Amsterdam, J. D., and Shults, J. (2010). "Efficacy and Safety of Long-Term Fluoxetine versus Lithium Monotherapy of Bipolar II Disorder: A Randomized, Double-Blind, Placebo-Substitution Study." *American Journal of Psychiatry* 167: 792–800.

Angst, J., et al. (2011). "Prevalence and Characteristics of Undiagnosed Bipolar Disorders in Patients with a Major Depressive Episode: The BRIDGE Study." *Archives of General Psychiatry* 68: 791-799.

Bailine, S., et al. (2010). "Electroconvulsive Therapy Is Equally Effective in Unipolar and Bipolar Depression." *Acta Psychiatrica Scandinavica* 121: 431–436.

Baldassano, C. F. (2009). "Promoting Wellness in Patients with Bipolar Disorder: Strategies to Move Beyond Maintaining Stability and Minimizing Adverse Events in Effective Long-Term Management." *Current Psychiatry,* Supplement *Maintaining Wellness in Patients with Bipolar Disorder: Moving Beyond Efficacy to Effectiveness* (October 2009): S12–S18.

Baldessarini, R. J., et al. (2006). "Decreased Risk of Suicides and Attempts During Long-Term Lithium Treatment: A Meta-Analytic Review." *Bipolar Disorders* 8: 625–639.

Baldessarini, R. J., and Tondo, L. (2000). "Does Lithium Treatment Still Work? Evidence of Stable Responses over Three Decades." *Archives of General Psychiatry* 57: 187–190.

Bauer, M. S. (2005) "How Solid Is the Evidence for the Efficacy of Mood Stabilizers in Bipolar Disorder?" *Essential Psychopharmacology* 6: 301–318.

Bauer, M. S., and Mitchner, L. (2004). "What Is a 'Mood Stabilizer'? An Evidence-Based Response." *American Journal of Psychiatry* 161: 3–18.

Bearden, C. E., et al. (2007). "Greater Cortical Gray Matter Density in Lithium-Treated Patients with Bipolar Disorder." *Biological Psychiatry* 62: 7–16.

Beaulieu, J.-M., and Caron, M. G. (2008). "Looking at Lithium: Molecular Moods and Complex Behavior." *Molecular Interventions* 8: 230–241.

Bender, K. J. (2011). "Methylene Blue Studied for Bipolar as FDA Issues Warning." *Psychiatric Times* http://www.psychiatrictimes.com/bipolar-disorder/content/article/10168/1963962.

Berk, M., et al. (2008). "N-acetyl Cysteine for Depressive Symptoms in Bipolar Disorder: A Double-blind Randomized Placebo-controlled Trial." *Biological Psychiatry* 64: 468-475.

Berk, M., et al. (2011). "The Efficacy of N-acetylcysteine as an Adjunctive Treatment in Bipolar Depression: An Open Label Trial." *Journal of Affective Disorders* 135: 389-394.

Berlant, J., and van Kammen, D. P. (2002). "Open-Label Topiramate as Primary or Adjunctive Therapy in Chronic Civilian Posttraumatic Stress Disorder: A Preliminary Report." *Journal of Clinical Psychiatry* 63: 15–20.

Bersudsky, Y. (2005). "Phenytoin: An Anti-Bipolar Anticonvulsant?" *International Journal of Neuropsychopharmacology* 9(4): 479–484.

Bertolino, A., et al. (2003). "Neuronal Pathology in the Hippocampal Area of Patients with Bipolar Disorder: A Study with Proton Magnetic Resonance Spectroscopic Imaging." *Biological Psychiatry* 53: 906–913.

Beydoun, A., et al. (2005). "Safety and Efficacy of Two Pregabalin Regimens for Add-On Treatment of Partial Epilepsy." *Neurology* 64: 475–480.

Bourin, M., et al. (2013). "How Assess Drugs in the Treatment of Acute Bipolar Mania?" *Frontiers in Pharmacology* doi: 10.3389/fphar.2013.00004.

Bowden, C. L., et al. (2003). "A Placebo-Controlled 18-Month Trial of Lamotrigine and Lithium Maintenance Treatment in Recently Manic or Hypomanic Patients with Bipolar I Disorder." *Archives of General Psychiatry* 60: 392–400.

Bowden, C. L., et al. (2010). "Ziprasidone plus a Mood Stabilizer in Subjects with Bipolar I Disorder: A 6-Month, Randomized, Placebo-Controlled, Double-Blind Trial." *Journal of Clinical Psychiatry* 71: 130–137.

Bowden, C. L., et al. (2012). "Lamotrigine (Lamictal IR) for the Treatment of Bipolar Disorder." *Expert Opinion on Pharmacotherapy* 13: 2565-2571.

Brooks, J. O., et al. (2011). "Safety and Tolerability Associated With Second-generation Antipsychotic Polytherapy in Bipolar Disorder: Findings From the Systematic Treatment Enhancement Program for Bipolar Disorder." *Journal of Clinical Psychiatry* 72: 240–247.

Brown, E. B., et al. (2006). "A 7-Week, Randomized Double-Blind Trial of Olanzapine/Fluoxetine Combination versus Lamotrigine in the Treatment of Bipolar I Depression." *Journal of Clinical Psychiatry* 67: 1025–1033.

Calabrese, J. R., et al. (2002). "Rash in Multicenter Trials of Lamotrigine in Mood Disorders: Clinical Relevance and Management." *Journal of Clinical Psychiatry* 63: 1012–1019.

Calabrese, J. R., et al. (2005). "A Randomized, Double-Blind, Placebo-Controlled Trial of Quetiapine in the Treatment of Bipolar I or II Depression." *American Journal of Psychiatry* 162: 1351–1360.

Calabrese, J. R., et al. (2010). "Adjunctive Armodafinil for Major Depressive Episodes Associated with Bipolar I Disorder: A Randomized, Multicenter, Double-blind, Placebo-controlled, Proof-of-concept Study." *Journal of Clinical Psychiatry* 71: 1363-1370.

Chen, G., et al. (1999). "Valproate Robustly Enhances AP-1 Mediated Gene Expression." *Brain Research: Molecular Brain Research* 64: 52–58.

Chengappa, R., et al. (2006). "Adjunctive Topiramate Therapy in Patients Receiving a Mood Stabilizer for Bipolar I Disorder: A Randomized, Placebo-Controlled Trial." *Journal of Clinical Psychiatry* 67: 1698–1706.

Chiu, S. (2005). "GABApentin Treatment Response in Selective Serotonin Reuptake Inhibitor (SSRI)-Refractory Panic Disorder." *Psychiatry-Online.* http://www.priory.com/psych/gabapentin.htm.

Chwieduk, C. M., et al. (2011). "Asenapine: A Review of Its Use in the Management of Mania in Adults with Bipolar I Disorder." *CNS Drugs* 25:251-267.

Cipriani, A., et al. (2013). "Lithium in the Prevention of Suicide in Mood Disorders: Updated Systematic Review and Meta-analysis." *British Medical Journal*: 346: 1–13: doi: 10.1136/bmj.f3646.

Cipriani, A., et al. (2011). "Comparative Efficacy and Acceptability of Antimanic Drugs in Acute Mania: A Multiple-treatments Meta-analysis." *The Lancet* 378: 1306–1315.

Corya, S. A., et al. (2006). "A 24-Week Open-Label Extension Study of Olanzapine-Fluoxetine Combination and Olanzapine Monotherapy in the Treatment of Bipolar Depression." *Journal of Clinical Psychiatry* 67: 798–806.

Coryell, W. (2009). "Maintenance Treatment in Bipolar Disorder: A Reassessment of Lithium as the First Choice." *Bipolar Disorders* 11 (Suppl. 2): 77–83.

Cui, J., et al. (2007). "Role of Glutathione in Neuroprotective Effects of Mood Stabilizing Drugs Lithium and Valproate." *Neuroscience* 144: 1447–1453.

Cunha, A. B. M., et al. (2006)."Serum Brain-Derived Neurotrophic Factor Is Decreased in Bipolar Disorder During Depressive and Manic Episodes," *Neuroscience Letters* 398: 215–219.

Dauphinais, D., et al. (2011). "Zonisamide for Bipolar Disorder, Mania or Mixed States: A Randomized, Double-Blind, Placebo-Controlled Adjunctive Trial." *Psychopharmacology Bulletin* 44: 5–17.

De Almeida, J. R. C., et al. (2013). "Distinguishing Between Unipolar Depression and Bipolar Depression: Current and Future Clinical and Neuroimaging Perspectives." *Biological Psychiatry* 73: 111–118.

De Fruyt, J., et al. (2012). "Second Generation Antipsychotics in the Treatment of Bipolar Depression: A Systematic Review and Meta-analysis." *Journal of Psychopharmacology* 26: 603–617.

Diazgranados, N., et al. (2010). "A Randomized Add-on Trial of an N-methyl-d-aspartate Anatagonist in Treatment-resistant Bipolar Depression." *Archives of General Psychiatry* 67: 793–802.

Einat, H., and Manji, H. K. (2006). "Cellular Plasticity Cascades: Genes-to-Behavior Pathways in Animal Models of Bipolar Disorder." *Biological Psychiatry* 59: 1160–1171.

Ellinger, L. K., et al. (2010). "Efficacy of Metformin and Topiramate in Prevention and Treatment of Second-Generation Antipsychotic-Induced Weight Gain." *Annals of Pharmacotherapy* 44: 668–679.

Ernst, C. L., and Goldberg, J. F. (2002). "The Reproductive Safety Profile of Mood Stabilizers, Atypical Antipsychotics, and Broad-Spectrum Psychotropics." *Journal of Clinical Psychiatry* 63, Supplement 4: 42–55.

Evins, A. E., et al. (2006). "A Double-Blind, Placebo-Controlled Trial of Adjunctive Donepezil in Treatment-Resistant Mania." *Bipolar Disorders* 8: 75–80.

Feltner, D. E., et al. (2003). "High Dose Pregabalin Is Effective for the Treatment of Generalized Anxiety Disorder." *Journal of Clinical Psychopharmacology* 23: 240–249.

Fountoulakis, K. N., et al. (2013). "A Systematic Review of the Evidence on the Treatment of Rapid Cycling Bipolar Disorder." *Bipolar Disorders* 15: 115–137.

Frye, M., et al. (2007). "A Placebo-Controlled Evaluation of Adjunctive Modafinil in the Treatment of Bipolar Depression." *American Journal of Psychiatry* 164: 1242–1249.

Frye, M., et al. (2009). "Correlates of Treatment-Emergent Mania Associated with Antidepressant Treatment in Bipolar Depression." *American Journal of Psychiatry* 166: 164–172.

Gao, K., et al. (2008). "Antipsychotic-Induced Extrapyramidal Side Effects in Bipolar Disorder and Schizophrenia: A Systematic Review." *Journal of Clinical Psychopharmacology* 28: 203–209.

Geddes, J. R., et al. (2004). "Long-Term Lithium Therapy for Bipolar Disorder: Systematic Review and Meta-Analysis of Randomized Controlled Trials." *American Journal of Psychiatry* 161: 217–222.

Geddes, J. R., et al. for the BALANCE Investigators and Collaborators. (2010). "Lithium plus Valproate Combination Therapy versus Monotherapy for Relapse Prevention in Bipolar I Disorder (BALANCE): A Randomized Open-Label Trial." *Lancet* 375: 385–395.

Gentile, S. (2012). "Lithium in Pregnancy: The Need to Treat, the Duty to Ensure Safety." *Expert Opinion on Drug Safety* 11: 425–437.

Gershon, S., et al. (2009). "Lithium Specificity in Bipolar Illness: A Classic Agent for the Classic Disorder." *Bipolar Disorders* 11(Suppl. 2): 34–44.

Ghaemi, S. N., et al. (2003). "Oxcarbazepine Treatment of Bipolar Disorder." *Journal of Clinical Psychiatry* 64: 943–945.

Ghaemi, S. N., et al. (2006). "Extrapyramidal Side Effects with Atypical Neuroleptics in Bipolar Disorder." *Progress in Neuro-Psychopharmacology & Biological Psychiatry* 30: 209–213.

Gibbons, R., et al. (2009). "Relationship Between Antiepileptic Drugs and Suicide Attempts in Patients with Bipolar Disorder." *Archives of General Psychiatry* 66: 1354–1360.

Gitlin, M. J., et al. (2011). "Subsyndromal Depressive Symptoms After Symptomatic Recovery from Mania Are Associated with Delayed Functional Recovery." *Journal of Clinical Psychiatry* 72: 692–697.

Goldberg, J. F. (2010). "Antidepressants in Bipolar Disorder. 7 Myths and Realities." *Current Psychiatry* 9: 41–48.

Goldberg, J. F., et al. (2007). "Adjunctive Antidepressant Use and Symptomatic Recovery Among Bipolar Depressed Patients with Concomitant Manic Symptoms: Findings From the STEP-BD." *American Journal of Psychiatry* 164: 1348–1355.

Goldberg, J. F., et al. (2009). "Mood Stabilization and Destabilization During Acute and Continuation Phase Treatment for Bipolar I Disorder with Lamotrigine or Placebo." *Journal of Clinical Psychiatry* 70: 1273–1280.

Gonzalez-Pinto, A., et al. (2011). "Poor Long-term Prognosis in Mixed Bipolar Patients: 10-year Outcomes in the Vitoria Prospective Naturalistic Study in Spain." *Journal of Clinical Psychiatry* 72: 671–676.

Goodwin, G. M., et al. (2004). "A Pooled Analysis of Two Placebo-Controlled 18-Month Trials of Lamotrigine and Lithium Maintenance in Bipolar I Disorder." *Journal of Clinical Psychiatry* 64: 432–441.

Gould, T. D., et al. (2004). "Emerging Experimental Therapeutics for Bipolar Disorder: Insights from the Molecular and Cellular Actions of Current Mood Stabilizers." *Molecular Psychiatry* 9: 734–755.

Grof, P. (2006). "Responders to Long-term Lithium Treatment." in Bauer, M., Grof, P., Mueller-Oerlinghausen, B. Eds. *Lithium in Neuropsychiatry: The Comprehensive Guide.* London: Informa, 2006: 157–178.

Grof, P., et al. (2009). "A Critical Appraisal of Lithium's Efficacy and Effectiveness: The Last 60 Years." *Bipolar Disorders* 11 (Suppl. 2): 10–19.

Harrison-Read, P. E. (2009). "Antimanic Potency of Typical Neuroleptic Drugs and Affinity for Dopamine D2 and Serotonin 5-HT2A Receptors—A New Analysis of Data from the Archives and Implications for Improved Antimanic Treatments." *Journal of Psychopharmacology* 23: 899–907.

Hartong, E. G., et al. (2003). "Prophylactic Efficacy of Lithium versus Carbamazepine in Treatment-Naïve Bipolar Patients." *Journal of Clinical Psychiatry* 64: 144–151.

Hirsch, L. J., et al. (2004). "Correlating Lamotrigine Serum Concentrations with Tolerability in Patients with Epilepsy." *Neurology* 28: 1022–1026.

Hirschfield, R. M., et al. (2006). "An Open-Label Extension Trial of Risperidone Monotherapy in the Treatment of Bipolar I Disorder." *International Journal of Clinical Psychopharmacology* 21: 11–20.

Hirschfeld, R. M. A. (2009). "Making Efficacious Choices: The Integration of Pharmacotherapy and Nonpharmacologic Approaches to the Treatment of Patients with Bipolar Disorder." *Current Psychiatry*, Supplement *Maintaining Wellness in Patients with Bipolar Disorder: Moving Beyond Efficacy to Effectiveness* (October 2009): S6–S11.

Hollon, S. D., et al. (2010). "A Review of Empirically Supported Psychological Therapies for Mood Disorders in Adults." *Depression and Anxiety* 27: 891–932.

Hurley, S. C. (2002). "Lamotrigine Update and Its Use in Bipolar Disorders." *Annals of Pharmacotherapy* 36: 860–873.

Ingenhoven, T., et al. (2010). "Effectiveness of Pharmacotherapy for Severe Personality Disorders: Meta-Analyses of Randomized Controlled Trials." *Journal of Clinical Psychiatry* 71: 14–25.

Jafferany, M. (2008). "Lithium and Skin: Dermatologic Manifestations of Lithium Therapy." *International Journal of Dermatology* 47: 1101–1111.

Jeong, J-H., et al. (2013). "Efficacy of Quetiapine in Patients With Bipolar I and II Depression: A Multicenter, Prospective, Open-label, Observational Study." *Neuropsychiatric Disease and Treatment* 9: 197–204.

Joffe, H., et al. (2006). "Valproate Is Associated with New-Onset Oligoamenorrhea with Hyperandrogenism in Women with Bipolar Disorder." *Biological Psychiatry* 59: 1078–1086.

Keck, P. E., et al. (2003). "Advances in the Pharmacological Treatment of Bipolar Depression." *Biological Psychiatry* 53: 671–679.

Keck, P. E., et al. (2006). "A Randomized, Double-Blind, Placebo-Controlled 26-Week Trial of Aripiprazole in Recently Manic Patients with Bipolar I Disorder." *Journal of Clinical Psychiatry* 67: 626–637.

Keck, P. E., et al. (2007) "Aripirazole Monotherapy for Maintenance Therapy in Bipolar I Disorder: A 100 Week, Double-Blind Study versus Placebo." *Journal of Clinical Psychiatry* 68: 1480–1491.

Keck, P. E., and McElroy, S. L. (2002). "Carbamazepine and Valproate in the Maintenance Treatment of Bipolar Disorder." *Journal of Clinical Psychiatry* 63, Supplement 10: 13–17.

Keck, P. E., and McElroy, S. L. (2003). "Bipolar Disorder, Obesity, and Pharmacotherapy-Associated Weight Gain." *Journal of Clinical Psychiatry* 64: 1426–1435.

Kemp, D. E., et al. (2012). "Lamotrigine as Add-on Treatment to Lithium and Divalproex: Lessons Learned From a Double-blind, Placebo-controlled Trial in Rapid-cycling Bipolar Disorder." *Bipolar Disorders* 14: 780–789.

Kessing, L. V., et al. (2008). "Lithium Treatment and Risk of Dementia." *Archives of General Psychiatry* 65: 1331–1335.

Kessing, L. V., et al. (2012). "An Observational Nationwide Register Based Cohort Study on Lamotrigine Versus Lithium in Bipolar Disorder." *Journal of Psychopharmacology* 26: 644–652.

Ketter, T. A., et al. (2003). "Potential Mechanisms of Action of Lamotrigine in the Treatment of Bipolar Disorders." *Journal of Clinical Psychopharmacology* 23: 484–495.

Kulkarni, J., et al. (2006). "A Pilot Study of Hormone Modulation as a New Treatment for Mania in Women with Bipolar Affective Disorder." *Psychoneuroendocrinology* 31: 543–547.

Kupfer, D. J. (2005). "The Increasing Medical Burden in Bipolar Disorder." *Journal of the American Medical Association* 293: 2528–2530.

Kushner, S. F., et al. (2006). "Topiramate Monotherapy in the Management of Acute Mania: Results of Four Double-Blind Placebo-Controlled Trials." *Bipolar Disorders* 8: 15–27.

Leng, Y., et al. (2008). "Synergistic Neuroprotective Effects of Lithium and Valproic Acid or Other Histone Deacetylase Inhibitors in Neurons: Roles of Glycogen Synthase Kinase-3 Inhibition." *Journal of Neuroscience* 28: 2576–2588.

Leverich, G. S., et al. (2006) "Risk of Switch in Mood Polarity to Hypomania or Mania in Patients with Bipolar Depression During Acute and Continuation Trials of Venlafaxine, Sertraline, and Bupropion as Adjuncts to Mood Stabilizers." *American Journal of Psychiatry* 163: 232–239.

Li, D. (2011). "Using Lithium in Bipolar Disorder: A Primer." *The Carlat Psychiatry Report* 9: 1–3.

Lichtenstein, P., et al. (2009). "Common Genetic Determinants of Schizophrenia and Bipolar Disorder in Swedish Families: A Population-Based Study. *Lancet* 373: 234–239.

Lieb, K., et al. (2010). "Pharmacotherapy for Borderline Personality Disorder: Cochrane Systematic Review of Randomised Trials." *British Journal of Psychiatry* 196: 4–12.

Lloyd, A., et al. (2012). "The Cost-effectiveness of Pregabalin in the Treatment of Fibromyalgia: US Perspective." *Journal of Medical Economics* 15: 481–492.

Macfadden, W., et al. (2011). "Adjunctive Long-acting Risperidone in Patients With Bipolar Disorder Who Relapse Frequently and Have Active Mood Symptoms." *Biomed Central Psychiatry* 11:171.

Mahmoudi-Gharaei, J., et al. (2012). "Topiramate Versus Valproate Sodium as Adjunctive Therapies to a Combination of Lithium and Risperidone for Adolescents with Bipolar I Disorder: Effects on Weight and Serum Lipid Profiles." *Iranian Journal of Psychiatry* 7: 1–10.

Marengell, L. B., et al. (2006). "Omega-3 Fatty Acids in Bipolar Disorder: Clinical and Research Considerations." *Prostaglandins Leuokotrienes and Essential Fatty Acids* 75: 315–321.

Marmol, F. (2008). "Lithium: Bipolar Disorder and Neurodegenerative Diseases Possible Cellular Mechanisms of the Therapeutic Effects of Lithium." *Progress in Neuro-Psychopharmacology & Biological Psychiatry* 32: 1761–1771.

Mathews, D. C., et al. (2012). "New Drug Developments for Bipolar Mania." *Psychiatric Times* 29: http://www.psychiatrictimes.com/bipolar-disorder/content/article/10168/2119724.

McDonald, A. A., and Portenoy, R. K. (2006). "How to Use Antidepressants and Anticonvulsants as Adjuvant Analgesics in the Treatment of Neuropathic Cancer Pain." *Journal of Supportive Oncology* 4: 43–52.

McElroy, S. L., et al. (2010). "A Double-Blind Placebo-Controlled Study of Quetiapine and Paroxetine as Monotherapy in Adults with Bipolar Depression (EMBOLDEN II)." *Journal of Clinical Psychiatry* 71: 163–174.

McIntyre, R. S., et al. (2011). "Novel Treatment Avenues for Bipolar Depression." *Psychiatric Times* 28: http://www.psychiatrictimes.com/bipolar-disorder/content/article/10168/1846994?_EXT_4_comsort=of.

McIntyre, R. S., et al. (2012). "A Randomized, Double-blind, Controlled Trial Evaluating the Effect of Intranasal Insulin on Neurocognitive Function in Euthymic Patients with Bipolar Disorder." *Bipolar Disorders* 14: 697–706.

McKnight, R. F., et al. (2012). "Lithium Toxicity Profile: A Systematic Review and Meta-analysis." *The Lancet* 379: 721–728.

Mercer, D., et al. (2009). "Meta-Analyses of Mood Stabilizers, Antidepressants and Antipsychotics in the Treatment of Borderline Personality Disorder: Effectiveness for Depression and Anger Symptoms." *Journal of Personality Disorders* 23: 156–174.

Merikangas, K. R., et al. (2011). "Prevalence and Correlates of Bipolar Spectrum Disorder in the World Mental Health Survey Initiative." *Archives of General Psychiatry* 68: 241–251.

Miklowitz, D. J. (2008). "Adjunctive Psychotherapy for Bipolar Disorder: State of the Evidence." *American Journal of Psychiatry* 165: 1408–1419.

Mishory, A., et al. (2000). "Phenytoin as an Antimanic Anticonvulsant: A Controlled Study." *American Journal of Psychiatry* 157: 463–465.

Montgomery, P., and Richardson, A. J. (2008). "Omega-3 Fatty Acids for Bipolar Disorder." *Cochrane Database of Systematic Reviews* Issue 2. Art. No.: CD005169. DOI: 10.1002/14651858.CD005169.pub2.

Montouris, G. (2005). "Safety of the Newer Antiepileptic Drug Oxcarbazepine During Pregnancy." *Current Medical Research Opinion* 21: 693–701.

Moore, J. L., et al. (2012). "Lamotrigine Use in Pregnancy." *Expert Opinion on Pharmacotherapy* 13: 1213–1216.

Mundo, E., et al. (2006). "Clinical Variables Related to Antidepressant-Induced Mania in Bipolar Disorder." *Journal of Affective Disorders* 92: 227–230.

Munkholm, K., et al. (2013). "Cytokines in Bipolar Disorder: A Systematic Review and Meta-analysis." *Journal of Affective Disorders* 144: 16–27.

Murphy, B. L., et al. (2012). "Omega-3 Fatty Acid Treatment, With or Without Cytidine, Fails to Show Therapeutic Properties in Bipolar Disorder: A Double-blind, Randomized Add-on Clinical Trial." *Journal of Clinical Psychopharmacology* 32: 699–703.

Nasr, S., et al. (2006). "Absence of Mood Switch with and Tolerance to Modafinil: A Replication Study from a Large Private Practice." *Journal of Affective Disorders* 95: 111–114.

Nery, F. G., et al. (2008). "Celecoxib as an Adjunct in the Treatment of Depressive or Mixed Episodes of Bipolar Disorder: A Double-blind, Randomized, Placebo-controlled Study." *Human Psychopharmacology* 23: 87–94.

Ng, F., et al. (2009). "The International Society for Bipolar Disorders (ISBD) Consensus Guidelines for the Safety Monitoring of Bipolar Disorder Treatments." *Bipolar Disorders* 11: 559–595.

Nielsen, J., et al. (2012). "Real-world Effectiveness of Clozapine in Patients With Bipolar Disorder: Results From a 2-year Mirror-image Study." *Bipolar Disorders* 14: 863–869.

Nierenberg, A. A., et al. (2006). "Treatment-Resistant Bipolar Depression: A STEP-BD Equipoise Randomized Effectiveness Trial of Antidepressant Augmentation with Lamotrigine, Inositol, or Risperidone." *American Journal of Psychiatry* 163: 210–216.

Nierenberg, A. A., et al. (2013). "Lithium Treatment Moderate-Dose Use Study (LiTMUS) for Bipolar Disorder: A Randomized Comparative Effectiveness Trial of Optimized Personalized Treatment With and Without Lithium." *American Journal of Psychiatry* 170: 102–110.

Nivoli, A. M. A., et al. (2011). "New Treatment Guidelines for Acute Bipolar Depression: A Systematic Review." *Journal of Affective Disorders* 129: 14–26.

Noaghiul, S., and Hibbeln, J. R. (2003). "Cross-National Comparisons of Seafood Consumption and Rates of Bipolar Disorder." *American Journal of Psychiatry* 160: 2222–2227.

Nonacs, R. (2012). "Topiramate (Topamax) Associated With an Increased Risk of Oral Clefts." *Massachusetts Center for Women's Mental Health* http://www.womensmentalhealth.org/posts/topiramate-topamax-associated-with-an-increased-risk-of-oral-clefts/.

Novosolov, F. (2012). "Treating Bipolar Disorder During Pregnancy and Lactation." *The Carlat Report-Psychiatry* 10: 1–2, 4–5).

Ostacher, M. J., et al. (2010). "Impact of Substance Use Disorders on Recovery from Episodes of Depression in Bipolar Disorder Patients: Prospective Data from the Systematic Treatment Enhancement Program for Bipolar Disorder (STEP-BD)." *American Journal of Psychiatry* 167: 289–297.

Pacchiarottia, I., et al. (2013). "The International Society for Bipolar Disorders (ISBD) Task Force Report on Antidepressant Use in Bipolar Disorders." *American Journal of Psychiatry* 170: 1249–1262.

Pachet, A., et al. (2003). "Beneficial Behavioural Effects of Lamotrigine in Traumatic Brain Injury." *Brain Injury* 17: 715–722.

Pande, A. C., et al. (1999). "Treatment of Social Phobia with Gabapentin: A Placebo-Controlled Study." *Journal of Clinical Psychopharmacology* 19: 341–348.

Pande, A., et al. (2000). "Placebo-Controlled Study of GABApentin Treatment of Panic Disorder." *Journal of Clinical Psychopharmacology* 20: 467–471.

Pande, A., et al. (2003). "Pregabalin in Generalized Anxiety Disorder: A Placebo-Controlled Trial." *American Journal of Psychiatry* 160: 533–540.

Parker, G., et al. (2006a). "Omega-3 Fatty Acids and Mood Disorders." *American Journal of Psychiatry* 163: 969–978.

Parker, G., et al. (2006b) "SSRIs as Mood Stabilizers for Bipolar II Disorder? A Proof of Concept Study." *Journal of Affective Disorders* 92: 205–214.

Patorno, E., et al. (2010). "Anticonvulsant Medications and the Risk of Suicide, Attempted Suicide, or Violent Death." *Journal of the American Medical Association* 303: 1401–1409.

Perlis, R. H., et al. (2006a). "Clinical Features of Bipolar Depression versus Major Depressive Disorder in Large Multicenter Trials." *American Journal of Psychiatry* 163: 225–231.

Perlis, R. H., et al. (2006b). "Predictors of Recurrence in Bipolar Disorder: Primary Outcomes from the Systematic Treatment Enhancement Program for Bipolar Disorder (STEP-BD)." *American Journal of Psychiatry* 163: 217–224.

Perucca, E. (2005). "Birth Defects After Prenatal Exposure to Antiepileptic Drugs." *Lancet Neurology* 4: 781–786.

Peters, A. T., et al. (2011). "Stepping Back to Step Forward: Lessons From the Systematic Treatment Enhancement Program for Bipolar Disorder (STEP-BD)." *Journal of Clinical Psychiatry* 72: 1429–1431.

Post, R. M., et al. (2005). "The Impact of Bipolar Depression." *Journal of Clinical Psychiatry* 66, Supplement 5: 5–10.

Post, R. M., et al. (2006). "Mood Switch in Bipolar Depression: Comparison of Adjunctive Venlafaxine, Bupropion and Sertraline." *British Journal of Psychiatry* 189: 124–131.

Rapoport, S. I., et al. (2009). "Bipolar Disorder and Mechanisms of Action of Mood Stabilizers." *Brain Research Reviews* 61: 185–209.

Reinares, M., et al. (2012). "A Systematic Review on the Role of Anticonvulsants in the Treatment of Acute Bipolar Depression." *International Journal of Neuropsychopharmacology* 16: 485–496.

Rendell, J. M., et al. (2006) "Risperidone Alone or in Combination for Acute Mania." *Cochrane Database of Systematic Reviews* CD004043.

Rosenthal, M. (2003). "Tiagabine for the Treatment of Generalized Anxiety Disorder: A Randomized, Open-Label, Clinical Trial with Paroxetine as a Positive Control." *Journal of Clinical Psychiatry* 64: 1245–1249.

Sachs, G. S., et al. (2003). "Rationale, Design, and Methods of the Systematic Treatment Enhancement Program for Bipolar Disorder (STEP-BD)." *Journal of Clinical Psychiatry* 53: 1028–1042.

Sachs, G. S., et al. (2007). "Effectiveness of Adjunctive Antidepressant Treatment for Bipolar Depression." *New England Journal of Medicine* 356: 1711–1722.

Salvadore, G., et al. (2010). "Increased Uric Acid Levels in Drug-naïve Subjects With Bipolar Disorder During a First Manic Episode." *Progress in Neuro-psychopharmacology & Biological Psychiatry* 34: 19–21.

Sanches, M., et al. (2011). "New Drugs for Bipolar Disorder." *Current Psychiatry Reports* 13: 513–521.

Sarris, J., et al. (2011). "Bipolar Disorder and Complementary Medicine: Current Evidence, Safety Issues, and Clinical Considerations." *Journal of Alternative and Complementary Medicine* 17: 881–890.

Sarris, J., et al. (2012). "Omega-3 for Bipolar Disorder: Meta-Analyses of Use in Mania and Bipolar Depression." *Journal of Clinical Psychiatry* 73: 81–86.

Scherk, H., et al. (2007). "Second-Generation Antipsychotic Agents in the Treatment of Acute Mania." *Archives of General Psychiatry* 64: 442–455.

Schloesser, R. J., et al. (2012). "Mood-stabilizing Drugs: Mechanisms of Action." *Trends in Neuroscience* 35: http://dx.doi.org/10.1016/j.bbr.2011.03.031.

Schneck, C. D., et al. (2008). "The Prospective Course of Rapid-Cycling Bipolar Disorder: Findings from the STEP-BD." *American Journal of Psychiatry* 165: 370–377.

Shajahan, P., and M. Taylor (2010). "The Uses and Outcomes of Quetiapine in Depressive and Bipolar Mood Disorders in Clinical Practice." *Journal of Psychopharmacology* 24: 565–572.

Sharma V., et al. (2009). "Bipolar II Postpartum Depression: Detection, Diagnosis, and Treatment." *American Journal of Psychiatry* 166: 1217–1221.

Shorter, E. (2009). "The History of Lithium Therapy." *Bipolar Disorders* 11 (Suppl. 2): 4–9.

Silva, M. T., et al. (2013). "Olanzapine Plus Fluoxetine for Bipolar Disorder: A Systematic Review and Meta-analysis." *Journal of Affective Disorders* 146: 310–318.

Smith, M. T., et al. (2012). "Pregabalin For the Treatment of Fibromyalgia." *Expert Opinion on Pharmacotherapy* 13: 1527–1533.

Stoffers J, et al. (2010). "Pharmacological Interventions for Borderline Personality Disorder." *Cochrane Database of Systematic Reviews* Issue 6. Art. No.: CD005653. DOI: 10.1002/14651858.CD005653.pub2.

Stoll, A. L., et al. (1999). "Omega-3 Fatty Acids in Bipolar Disorder: A Preliminary Double-Blind, Placebo-Controlled Trial." *Archives of General Psychiatry* 56: 407–412.

Suppes, T., et al. (2005). "The Texas Implementation of Medication Algorithms: Update to the Algorithms for Treatment of Bipolar I Disorder." *Journal of Clinical Psychiatry* 66: 870–886.

Swann, A. C., et al. (2013). "Bipolar Mixed States: An International Society for Bipolar Disorders Task Force Report of Symptom Structure, Course of Illness, and Diagnosis." *American Journal of Psychiatry* 170: 31–42.

Thase, M. E. (2012). "Bipolar Disorder Maintenance Treatment: Monitoring Effectiveness and Safety." *Journal of Clinical Psychiatry* 73.4: e15.

Tohen, M., et al. (2005). "Olanzapine versus Lithium in the Maintenance Treatment of Bipolar Disorder: A 12-Month, Randomized, Double-Blind, Controlled Clinical Trial." *American Journal of Psychiatry* 162: 1281–1290.

Tohen, M., et al. (2006). "Randomized, Placebo-Controlled Trial of Olanzapine as Maintenance Therapy in Patients with Bipolar I Disorder Responding to Acute Treatment with Olanzapine." *American Journal of Psychiatry* 163: 247–256.

Tränkner, A., et al. (2013). "A Critical Review of the Recent Literature and Selected Therapy Guidelines Since 2006 On the Use of Lamotrigine in Bipolar Disorder." *Neuropsychiatric Disease and Treatment* 9: 101–111.

Tsai, A. C., et al. (2011). "Aripiprazole in the Maintenance Treatment of Bipolar Disorder: A Critical Review of the Evidence and Its Dissemination into the Scientific Literature." *PLoS Medicine* 8: e1000434. doi: 10.1371/journal.pmed.1000434.

Tsai, Y. S., et al. (2012). "Inflammatory Markers and Their Relationships with Leptin and Insulin from Acute Mania to Full Remission in Bipolar Disorder." *Journal of Affective Disorders* 136: 110–116.

Wagner, K. D., et al. (2006). "A Double-Blind, Randomized, Placebo-Controlled Trial of Oxcarbazepine in the Treatment of Bipolar Disorder in Children and Adolescents." *American Journal of Psychiatry* 163: 1179–1186.

Wajda, F. J. E., et al. (2013). "Lamotrigine in Epilepsy, Pregnancy and Psychiatry - A Drug for All Seasons?" *Journal of Clinical Neuroscience* 20: 13–16.

Watase, K., et al. (2007) "Lithium Therapy Improves Neurological Function and Hippocampal Dendritic Arborization in a Spinocerebellar Ataxia Type 1 Mouse Model." *PLoS Med* 4(5): e182. doi:10.1371/journal.pmed.0040182.

Weisler, R. H., et al. (2011). "Continuation of Quetiapine Versus Switching to Placebo or Lithium for Maintenance Treatment of Bipolar I Disorder (Trial 144: A Randomized Controlled Study)." *Journal of Clinical Psychiatry* 72: 1462–1464.

Wozniak, J., et al. (2007). "Omega-3 Fatty Acid Monotherapy for Pediatric Bipolar Disorder: A Prospective Open-Label Trial." *European Neuropsychopharmacology* 17: 440–447.

Yasuda, S., et al. (2009). "The Mood Stabilizers Lithium and Valproate Selectively Activate the Promoter IV of Brain-Derived Neurotrophic Factor in Neurons." *Molecular Psychiatry* 14: 51–59.

Yatham, L. N., et al. (2005). "Atypical Antipsychotics in Bipolar Depression: Potential Mechanisms of Action." *Journal of Clinical Psychiatry* 66, Supplement 5: 40–48.

Yildiz, A., et al. (2011). "Efficacy of Antimanic Treatments: Meta-analysis of Randomized, Controlled Trials." *Neuropsychopharmacology* 36: 375–389.

Young, A. H., et al. (2010). "A Double-Blind, Placebo-Controlled Study of Quetiapine and Lithium Monotherapy in Adults in the Acute Phase of Bipolar Depression (EMBOLDEN I)." *Journal of Clinical Psychiatry* 71: 150–162.

Zarate, C. A., et al. (2005). "Molecular Mechanisms of Bipolar Disorder." *Drug Discovery Today: Disease Mechanisms* 2: 435–445.

Zarate, C.A., et al. (2005). "An Open-label Trial of the Glutamate-modulating Agent Riluzole in Combination with Lithium for the Treatment of Bipolar Depression." *Biological Psychiatry* 57: 430–432.

Zarate, C. A., et al. (2006). "Cellular Plasticity Cascades: Targets for the Development of Novel Therapeutics for Bipolar Disorder." *Biological Psychiatry* 59: 1006–1020.

PART 4

Special Populations and Integration

In this last part, the remaining chapters will present information about the use of the psychotropic drugs presented in Part 3 in the special populations of children and adolescents (Chapter 15) and the elderly (Chapter 16). It is important to understand how treatment approaches vary based on the consideration of age and the associated physiological changes that occur with aging. In Chapter 15, information about the treatment of mental disorders during pregnancy is discussed and includes consideration of the risk of breast-feeding while taking psychotropic medications. The use of psychotropic medications is becoming more prevalent in the very young, even pre-school age children. It is important to understand the risks of this exposure versus the evidence of benefit for disorders detected at this age. The continuing use of stimulants for the treatment of attentional disorders in children and adolescents is an ongoing area of research. And the use of psychotropic medications for the treatment of the behavioral disorders of children and adolescents with autism spectrum disorders will be of significance since the prevalence of these disorders is rising based on increased awareness and methods for early detection. In Chapter 16, the authors discuss the use of psychotropic medications in the elderly and how changing physiology, natural course of mental disorders, and response to these agents have an impact on approaches to treatment.

Finally, in Chapter 17 (Challenging Times for Mental Health), a variety of topics are discussed that are not directly related to the pharmacology of drugs, but which none the less have a significant influence on how and whether they are used. Policy changes at the federal, state, and local levels of government can affect access to medications, and budgetary decisions can determine utilization. Changes in nosology influence indications for medications and the recent implementation of the new DSM-5 will be discussed in that regard. There is also continuing concern about the difficulty of demonstrating that the newer psychotropic drugs are any better than older drugs, including evidence that in many trials, new drugs fail to exceed the effects of placebo. Shifting priorities influence drug development in new areas such as treatments for dementia. At the same time, the pipeline for development of new drugs in all psychotropic classes has been declining over the last several years. Finally, it is important to recognize that drug treatment alone rarely produces remission or can maintain recovery. Most studies show that the combination of pharmacotherapy and evidence-based psychotherapy not only promotes a greater chance of reaching remission, but also increases the probability that an individual will sustain their recovery over a longer period of time.

Chapter 15

Child and Adolescent Psychopharmacology

The United States is currently experiencing a silent epidemic of mental illness among youth and teenagers. According to a new Centers for Disease Control and Prevention report (2013), 13 to 20 percent of children between the ages of 3 and 17 years experience a mental disorder in a given year. Half of all lifetime adult psychiatric illnesses start by 14 years of age, and three-fourths of them are present by 25 years of age. Delays between initial diagnosis and treatment are common. The median delay across disorders is nearly a decade; the longest delays are 20 to 23 years for anxiety disorders and 10 years for patients with mood disorders. However, the majority of mental illnesses in young people go unrecognized and untreated, leaving youth vulnerable to emotional, social, and academic impairments during a critical phase in their lives. In total, about 14 to 25 percent of youths during their upbringing endure a mental disorder; yet among youth and adolescents with mental health service needs, 67 percent receive no services, diagnosis, or treatment, at least until the disorder is deeply entrenched and much more difficult to treat (Costello et al., 2007). One in eight children had a mental health disorder at the time of the survey, but only half were treated (Merikangas et al., 2010). All this despite the fact that mental health disorders are the chronic disorders of young people! Indeed, data are quite clear that youth with untreated childhood and adolescent mental health disorders carry the disorder into adulthood and function poorly as adults.

Disorders affecting children and adolescents include anxiety disorders, depression, attention deficit/hyperactivity disorder (ADHD), schizophrenia, bipolar disorder, eating disorders, and autism spectrum disorders. While focus traditionally has been on the effects of prescribed medications on school-aged children and adolescents, increasing focus is on preschool-aged children and on intrauterine effects when a pregnant female takes medication for her own mental health disorder. Therefore, this chapter will be presented in three parts:

1. Pregnancy and Psychotropic Drugs
2. Preschool Psychopharmacology
3. Child and Adolescent Psychopharmacology

PREGNANCY AND PSYCHOTROPIC DRUGS

> It should be kept in mind that no psychotropic drug is approved by the FDA for use during pregnancy. Furthermore, no decision (to treat or not to treat) is risk-free and no decision is perfect. (Cohen, 2007, pp. 4–5)

In 2008, the American College of Obstetricians and Gynecologists (ACOG) published a clinical guideline on the use of psychoactive medications during pregnancy and lactation (ACOG Committee on Practice Bulletins-Obstetrics, 2008). They noted that more than 500,000 pregnancies in the United States each year involve women who have a psychiatric illness that either predates or emerges during pregnancy, and one-third of all pregnant women are exposed to a psychotropic medication at some point during their pregnancy. If the mother takes psychoactive medicines with frequency, is there a potential for such medication to injure the fetus (resulting in birth defects or, later in life, in developmental problems)? On the other hand, are there fetal developmental problems that might follow from the mother experiencing untreated mental health disorders? Such is the conundrum about the decision to treat pregnant women with serious mental health disorders. By definition, a psychoactive medication crosses the blood-brain barrier and reaches the brain. The blood-brain barrier is the most resistant of all physiological barriers to drug distribution, and the placental barrier is the easiest to cross. Therefore, as a general rule, *the fetus will have about the same blood level of drug as does the mother*. Therefore, risks of using medication during pregnancy include:

- Risk of potential teratogenic (structural) damage to the fetus
- Risk of postnatal behavioral abnormalities in the child exposed to medication *in utero*
- Risk of perinatal syndromes or neonatal toxicity in the child if the mother continues medications while breast-feeding

On the other hand, untreated maternal mental illness may result in:

- Poor compliance with prenatal care
- Inadequate nutrition
- Exposure to undesired drugs, medications, or herbals
- Increased alcohol, caffeine, and tobacco use
- Deficits in mother-infant bonding
- Neglect of proper postnatal infant care
- Disruptions in the family environment

TABLE 15.1 Impact of untreated mental health illnesses on pregnancy outcome			
Disorder	Obstetric	Neonatal	Options
Anxiety disorders	Long labor, fetal distress, preterm labor, spontaneous abortion	Reduced developmental scores, slowed mental development	Fluoxetine Psychological therapies
Depression and dysthymia	Low birth weight, reduced fetal growth, postnatal complications Hippocampus shrinks	Increased stress hormone levels, reduced bonding, small size and low weight, etc.	SSRIs Psychological therapies Omega-3 fatty acids ECT
Bipolar disorder	Similar to major depression	Similar to major depression	Lithium Lamotrigine Atypical Antipsychotics Omega-3 fatty acids
Schizophrenia	Preterm, low weight, small Placenta abnormalities	Increased rate of postnatal death	Antipsychotics

Table 15.1 lists some of the complications of a mother's untreated mental illness on pregnancy outcome.

Certainly, cigarettes (U.S. Preventive Services Task Force, 2009a) and alcohol (Sayal, et al., 2009) are contraindicated during pregnancy because of adverse fetal outcomes. Even caffeine is problematic, with intake as low as 100–200 mg/day (1–3 cups of coffee) can result in fetal growth restriction (CARE Study Group, 2008). Sowell and coworkers (2010) demonstrated the neonatal toxicity associated with maternal use of methamphetamine. Kousik and coworkers (2012) and Kiyatkin (2013) review the effects of psychostimulants (methamphetamine, Ecstasy, cocaine, and nicotine) on blood-brain barrier structure, accounting for much of the neurotoxicity of these drugs, an effect that presumably can also occur *in utero*.

Did You Know?

Doubling of Deaths Among Sick Moms-To-Be Amid Poor Evidence On Drug Safety in Pregnancy

The lack of hard data on the safety and effectiveness of a wide range of drugs in pregnancy has hindered the treatment of pregnant women, contributing to a doubling of deaths among moms-to-be with an underlying health problem over the past 20 years, argues an editorial in the Drug and Therapeutics Bulletin (DTB). It's time to include pregnant women in drug trials so that they can get the medical treatment they need, says DTB.

In the absence of reliable information on the pros and cons of treatment during pregnancy, and haunted by the specter of thalidomide, doctors are reluctant to prescribe, while pregnant women are wary of taking drugs that might harm their developing baby, contends the editorial.

Yet an estimated 1 in 10 moms-to-be has a long-term condition that requires medication, while around 4 out of 10 develop new health problems during their pregnancy. And it's going to get worse, the editorial warns, with the increasing trend for older age at childbirth and the expanding girth of the nation, both of which are pushing up the numbers of women requiring drug treatment during their pregnancy. *DTB* 2013;**51**:61 doi:10.1136/dtb.2013.6.0182

Antidepressants in the Pregnant Female and Neonatal Outcomes

Depressive and anxiety disorders are common in women of childbearing age. Many of these women are treated with antidepressant medication, primarily of the SSRI-type. Given that 50 percent of pregnancies are unplanned, the safety of these medications on the developing fetus, especially in the first 3 months of pregnancy is a major public health concern.

In 2009, a collaborative effort by ACOG and the American Psychiatric Association resulted in development of algorithms for the treatment of women with depression who either are contemplating pregnancy or are already pregnant (Yonkers, et al., 2009). They concluded that adequate treatment is essential, preferably beginning before conception. Women with severe, recurrent depression who stop medication are at high risk for relapse, and depression during pregnancy raises the risk of postpartum depression. As reported by Cohen and coworkers (2006), women who discontinued their antidepressant medication relapsed significantly more frequently over the course of their pregnancy, compared with women who stayed on their medication (Figure 15.1). This was recently confirmed by Roca and coworkers (2013). Pregnancy is not protective against either depression or dysthymia (Parry, 2009; Wisner et al., 2009). Untreated major depression often results in severe depressive disorders as well as substance abuse, both of which can be detrimental to the developing fetus.

In total, about eight percent of pregnant women will be exposed to antidepressants during their pregnancy. This raises questions as to the teratogenicity[1] of antidepressants as well as the possibility of adverse long-term neurobehavioral outcomes. By the year 2000, most SSRI-type antidepressants were thought to be nonteratogenic. However, in January 2006, the FDA issued a warning that *paroxetine* (Paxil) used in the first trimester might increase the incidence of congenital malformations, primarily cardiac defects. In December 2006, ACOG advised against using paroxetine during pregnancy. Pedersen and coworkers (2009) extended this warning to *sertraline* (Zoloft) and *citalopram* (Celexa), although the increases in the number affected were small, becoming significant only when the mother was taking more than one antidepressant. Fluoxetine had the smallest increase in incidence. Ramos and coworkers (2008), in examining the extensive literature

---

[1] Teratogenicity refers to structural defects in the neonate as a result of maternal drug intake.

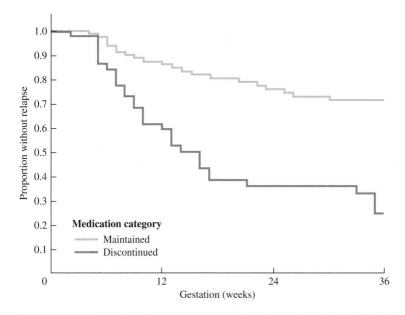

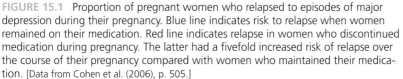

FIGURE 15.1 Proportion of pregnant women who relapsed to episodes of major depression during their pregnancy. Blue line indicates risk to relapse when women remained on their medication. Red line indicates relapse in women who discontinued medication during pregnancy. The latter had a fivefold increased risk of relapse over the course of their pregnancy compared with women who maintained their medication. [Data from Cohen et al. (2006), p. 505.]

on this matter, concluded that data *"do not support an association between duration of antidepressant use during the first trimester of pregnancy and major congenital malformations in the offspring of women with psychiatric disorders"* (p. 344). Aside from a possible association of paroxetine use and heart defects, SSRIs appear to be relatively safe during the first trimester of pregnancy. Questions about possible association between SSRIs and slower rates of fetal growth remain unanswered, but any risk is thought to be small (Marroun et al, 2012; Wisner et al., 2013). SSRI use late in pregnancy has been associated with a slightly increased risk of pulmonary hypertension in the newborn (Kieler et al., 2011). Finally, Stephansson and coworkers (2013) concluded that there was no significant association between SSRI use during pregnancy and infant mortality.

Newly identified, as a result of using SSRI-type antidepressants in the *third* trimester of pregnancy, have been reports of SSRI-discontinuation syndrome in the newborn (Alwan and Friedman, 2009). Here, following delivery, as the neonate metabolizes drug received via the mother's blood, classic signs of SSRI-withdrawal can be observed: irritability with constant crying, sleep disturbances, hyperactive reflexes, breathing and feeding difficulties, and so on. This might be misdiagnosed as severe colic. One suggestion is to switch the mother from other SSRIs to fluoxetine (the SSRI with the longest half-life) as soon as pregnancy is confirmed and then stop the fluoxetine at about seven months of gestation, allowing the infant to detoxify *in utero*. During this period (7–9 months), the mother can be treated with intensive psychological interventions. Likely, tricyclic antidepressants and clomipramine should be avoided (Horst et al., 2012).

In sum, as stated by Parry (2009), *"from the evidence available to date, the risks of an untreated maternal depression are far greater than the risks of serious adverse sequelae from antidepressant medication"* (p. 512). It is now quite clear that untreated maternal depression is a larger threat to offspring than antidepressants; however, antidepressant medication during pregnancy should be used only if the indication is compelling (Nulman et al., 2012; Steiner, 2012). Recent reviews by Byatt et al. (2013) and Chaudron (2013) update research into these controversies.

Finally, Rifkin-Graboi and coworkers (2013) demonstrated antenatal maternal depression was associated with amygdalar microstructural abnormalities in newborns born to these mothers. This was consistent with prenatal transmission of vulnerability of depression from mother to newborn and that interventions targeting maternal depression begin early in pregnancy.

Mood Stabilizers in the Pregnant Female and Neonatal Outcomes

Freeman (2007) stated:

> Untreated maternal mood disorders during pregnancy are serious risk factors for the fetus. . . . Untreated mania poses clear risks to the individual due to impulsivity and impaired judgment. Mania often results in poor self-care, which is dangerous to both mother and child. (p. 1771)

Indeed, untreated bipolar disorder in the pregnant female is associated with relapse to drug and alcohol abuse, manic episodes, interpersonal life disruptions, and early postpartum mania, depression and psychosis (DiFlorio et al., 2013). Viguera and coworkers (2007a) reported on pregnant women who either continued or stopped their medications. They found that the overall the risk of a bipolar episode during pregnancy was 71 percent regardless of whether they stayed on medication or not, but the risk was twofold greater if one discontinues medication. If medication is stopped, the time to first recurrence is four times shorter than if she stays on medication, and the proportion of weeks in bipolar illness was five times greater (Figure 15.2). If medication is necessary, what is known of the teratogenicity of mood stabilizer medications?

Lithium is recognized as a modest teratogen, with a potential for cardiac malformations greater than that in the general population (Nguyen et al., 2009). If absolutely necessary during pregnancy, doses should be minimized and the fetus closely followed by echocardiography. During periods of breast-feeding, some lithium is transferred to the infant. Maternal serum, breast milk, and infant concentrations of lithium averaged 0.76, 0.35, and 0.16 mEq/L respectively, each lithium level lower than the preceding level by approximately one-half (Viguera et al., 2007b). No significant adverse outcomes were reported.

Valproic acid (Depakote) is associated with the highest rate of major congenital malformations, with a relative risk estimated to be up to 16 percent (compared to about 2.9 percent in nonmedicated females (Nguyen et al., 2009; Tomson and Battino, 2009).

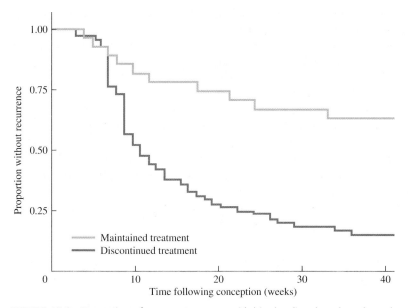

FIGURE 15.2   Proportion of pregnant women with bipolar disorder who relapsed to bipolar episodes during their pregnancy. Blue line indicates risk to relapse when women remained on their medication. Red line indicates relapse in women who discontinued medication during pregnancy. Mean time to first recurrence from the date of conception was greater than 41 weeks when treatment was maintained; and only 9 weeks when treatment was discontinued. [Data from Viguera et al. (2007a), p. 1821.]

In addition, use of valproic acid during pregnancy has been associated with impaired cognitive functioning at 3 years of age in offspring, with an IQ (intelligence coefficient) 9 points lower than children exposed to lamotrigine, 7 points lower than those exposed to phenytoin, and 6 points lower than children exposed to carbamazepine (Banach, et al., 2010; Meador et al., 2013). Finally, evidence has been reported that exposure to valproic acid by the fetus may increase the risk for autism spectrum disorders (Bromley, et al., 2008; Christensen, et al., 2013). Incidence rates for autism spectrum disorders ranged from <1 percent in control children to 2 percent with lamotrigine monotherapy, and 6 percent with valproic acid monotherapy. The FDA has concluded that women of childbearing potential should only use valproic acid if it is essential to manage their medical condition and only if they have been adequately warned of its potential for causing harm.

Carbamazepine (Tegretol, Equitro) is considered to be slightly teratogenic, increasing the incidence of adverse fetal outcomes by about 3 percent over nonmedicated females. Interestingly, abnormal effects on postnatal growth and development have not been reported by its close structural derivative oxcarbazepine.

Lamotrigine (Lamictal) is not considered to be a major teratogen, although a slightly increased incidence of cleft lips and cleft palates has been reported. The mean lamotrigine concentration in breast milk was 41 percent of the maternal level: the mean fetal blood concentration was 18 percent of the maternal level and about 50 percent of the concentration in breast milk. No adverse events were observed in breast-fed infants (Newport et al., 2008a). Newport and coworkers (2008b) concluded:

> Discontinuing mood stabilizer treatment presents high risks of bipolar recurrence among pregnant women. Lamotrigine may afford protective effects in pregnancy, and its reported fetal safety compares favorably to other agents used to manage bipolar disorder. (p. 432)

Topiramate (Topamax), whether used in the treatment of epilepsy, bipolar disorder, borderline personality disorder, or migraine headache, has been associated with an increase in major congenital malformations, although the numbers of pregnancies studied is small (Hunt et al., 2008). Oral clefts and penile malformations (in male infants) occurred at a rate of about 11 times the control rate. Larger sample numbers are needed before more broad interpretations can be made.

Limited data to date on *gabapentin* (Neurontin) and *pregabalin* (Lyrica) have not reported them to be major teratogens (Einarson and Boskovic, 2009).

Atypical Antipsychotics in the Pregnant Female and Neonatal Outcomes

Atypical antipsychotic drugs are used to treat schizophrenia, bipolar disorder, borderline personality disorder, PTSD, and other mental health disorders, many of which occur in women of childbearing years and who might be exposed to these drugs during their pregnancy. Use of atypical antipsychotics during pregnancy is rapidly increasing, with 0.72 percent of pregnant women receiving such medication anytime from 60 days before pregnancy through delivery (Toh et al., 2013). This represents a twofold increase from 2001 through 2007, with depression being the most common mental health diagnosis.

Newham and coworkers (2008) compared offspring of mothers who ingested either *clozapine* (Clozaril) or *olanzapine* (Zyprexa) during pregnancy with offspring of mothers who ingested first-generation antipsychotic medicines during their pregnancy. Thirty-one percent of infants exposed to clozapine or olanzapine were large for gestational age and had birth weights heavier than those exposed to first generation agents. These infants were thought to be at risk or predisposed to heavy weight and perhaps to diabetes later in life.

Coppola and coworkers (2007) studied the delivery outcome of infants exposed to *risperidone* (Risperdol) during pregnancy. The incidence of congenital malformations and spontaneous abortions paralled the rates in control persons. When exposed to risperidone in the third trimester of pregnancy, the majority of the infants displayed tremor, jitteriness, irritability, feeding problems, and somnolence. This may represent a discontinuation syndrome. The authors concluded that risperidone should only be used during pregnancy if the benefits outweigh the potential risks.

To date, only scattered case reports address the issue of newer atypical antipsychotics in pregnancy. In 2011, the FDA issued an advisory concerning the possibility of extrapyramidal (motor) movements and discontinuation symptoms in newborns whose mothers took these medications during pregnancy. Peng and coworkers (2013) studied outcomes in women exposed to atypical antipsychotics during pregnancy. Only minor effects were noted and by 1 year of age, even these had dissipated. Sadowski and coworkers (2013) found that *in utero* exposure to monotherapy involving atypical antipsychotics resulted in little risk to the fetus, whereas polydrug therapy was associated with adverse outcomes for both the mother and the child. Certainly, polytherapy should be avoided if at all possible.

Gentile (2008) reviews the issue of safety in infants who breast-fed from mothers who were taking atypical antipsychotic medicines. The American College of Obstetricians and Gynecologists (ACOG) clinical guideline on the use of psychoactive medications during pregnancy and lactation (ACOG Committee on Practice Bulletins-Obstetrics, 2008), concluded:

> There is little evidence to suggest that atypical antipsychotics are associated with elevated risks for neonatal toxicity or somatic teratogenesis. No long-term neurobehavioral studies of exposed children have yet been conducted. Therefore, their routine use during pregnancy and lactation cannot be recommended. (p. 1010)

Did You Know?

FDA Warns Against Valproate to Prevent Migraine in Pregnancy

The U.S. Food and Drug Administration (FDA) has strengthened warnings against the use of valproate products as a preventive measure against migraine in women who are pregnant.

The new contraindication is based on recently published data from the Neurodevelopmental Effects of Antiepileptic Drugs (NEAD) study showing further evidence that exposure to valproate products during pregnancy can lead to reduced IQ scores in children.

"Valproate medications should never be used in pregnant women for the prevention of migraine headaches because we have even more data now that show the risks to the children outweigh any treatment benefits for this use," said Russell Katz, MD, director of the Division of Neurology Products in the FDA's Center for Drug Evaluation and Research. http://consumer.health day.com/disabilities-information-11/misc-birth-defect-news-63/fda-warns-pregnant-women-about-migraine-drugs-676158.html

---

PRESCHOOL PSYCHOPHARMACOLOGY

Prior to the year 2007, there were scant research or practice guidelines for the use of psychopharmacology for very young children. In 2007, Gleason and coworkers (2007) reviewed the topic and described recommended algorithms for medication use in children aged 5 and younger. The goal was *"to promote responsible treatment of young children, recognizing that this will sometimes involve the use of medication."* Preschool children with severe mental health problems present a dilemma for prescribers when they do not respond to non-medication interventions (Luby, 2010). A professional must weigh the potential risks of medication with the risks of not intervening. The focus is on young children with moderate to severe symptoms and functional impairments.

Psychopharmacological interventions are not indicated for preschoolers with only mild symptoms or impairment. In the algorithms presented in the Gleason and coworkers (2007) review, step one of each algorithm begins with a diagnostic assessment, step 2 is diagnosis (which generally drives treatment planning), step 3 is development of non-pharmacological treatments, and step 4 is consideration of pharmacological treatment.

Medications for Treating Attention Deficit/Hyperactivity Disorder (ADHD) in Very Young Children

ADHD has been well studied in school aged children, adolescents, and adults. Only recently has there been focus on ADHD in preschoolers (Tandon et al., 2011). Certainly, ADHD is a highly heritable disorder with early developmental risk factors also involved. ADHD can present during the preschool years and does persist into adulthood (Cherkasova et al., 2013). Accurate diagnosis requires adaptation of the current diagnostic criteria to account for differences in symptomatology across the life span. Before consideration of medication, nonpharmacological interventions should be tried (Ghuman and Ghuman, 2013). Indeed, Charach and coworkers (2013) note that parent behavior training has greater evidence of efficacy than methylphenidate for treatment of preschoolers at risk of ADHD.

Also, before medicating, other comorbid diagnoses should be entertained. Indeed, in a study of 303 preschoolers (3–5.5 years of age) with moderate to severe ADHD, 70 percent experienced comorbid disorders, with oppositional defiant disorder, communication disorders, or anxiety disorders being most common (Posner et al., 2007). The differential diagnosis of ADHD and the pattern of psychiatric comorbidity vary with each age group and complicate diagnosis and management. To maximize outcomes, clinicians must be able to accurately identify ADHD in preschoolers, and develop comprehensive, collaborative treatment plans.

The Preschool ADHD Treatment Study (PATS) first demonstrated the potential utility of methylphenidate for treating ADHD in preschoolers (Greenhill et al., 2006). At an average daily dose of 14 mg, immediate-release methylphenidate (range = 7.5–30 mg/day, divided into three daily increments) immediate-release methylphenidate produced significant reduction on scores on ADHD symptom scales, although efficacy was less than that cited for school-age children (Abrikoff et al., 2009). In a 10-month continuation phase of the PATS study, with gradual dose increases, efficacy could be maintained, but significant variability was observed with many subjects dropping out of the study for adverse effects or behavioral worsening (Vitiello, et al., 2007).

Recently, Riddle and coworkers (2013) reported on a 6-year follow-up of the original PATS participants. Symptom severity initially decreased from baseline to year 3, but then remained relatively stable and in the moderate to severe range through year 6 of treatment. Overall, 89 percent met ADHD symptoms and impairment criteria. The authors concluded: *"The course (of ADHD over 6 years) is generally chronic, with high symptom severity and impairment, in very young children with moderate-to-severe ADHD, despite treatment with medication."* (p. 264). Obviously, these data are discouraging, and more effective treatment strategies are needed. Some possible medication alternatives are discussed later in this chapter.

Medications for Treating Disruptive Behaviors in Very Young Children

Hirshfeld-Becker and coworkers (2007) studied behavioral disinhibition in preschoolers and described it as a temperamental antecedent of disruptive behavioral disorders and their comorbidity with mood disorders in middle childhood, which may be targeted for preventive intervention. Belden and coworkers (2012) noted that preschoolers diagnosed with preschool-onset psychiatric disorders were three times as likely as healthy preschoolers to be classified as aggressors, victims, or aggressive victims; children diagnosed with preschool-onset disruptive, depressive, and/or anxiety disorders were at least six times more likely to become aggressive-victims during elementary school as are normal preschoolers. Nevels and coworkers (2010) discuss medication use in children, including treatment of aggression comorbid with ADHD.

Currently, there is evidence for efficacy of risperidone in preschoolers with obsessive-compulsive disorder, conduct disorder, or disruptive behavioral disorders (DBD) in children who otherwise demonstrate normal development (Ercan et al., 2011; Loy, et al., 2012). The use of antipsychotic drugs in very young children was reviewed by Olfson and coworkers (2010), with an editorial by Egger (2010). Not endorsed is medication without accompanying psychotherapy, use of medications as chemical restraints, or use of medication "as needed." In discussing their results, Olfson and coworkers (2010) noted that fewer than one-half (40 percent) of antipsychotic-treated young children received a mental health assessment, a psychotherapy visit (41 percent), or visit with a psychiatrist (42 percent). Further, the authors stated:

> It is widely recommended that children presenting for mental health care receive comprehensive and developmentally sensitive mental health assessments and trials of relevant psychosocial treatments before consideration is given to psychotropic medications. . . . However, most very young children in the present study did not receive a mental health assessment, a psychiatrist visit, or a single session of psychotherapy during the year in which they received antipsychotic medications. (p. 21)

Medications for Treating Depression in Very Young Children

Childhood depression is a serious and relapsing psychiatric disorder. However, until recently, studies have focused on school-aged children and adolescents. In a study of 306 preschoolers, age 3 to 6 years, depression symptoms were common and in 40 percent of young children persisted for the 24 months of follow-up study (Luby et al., 2009a, b). Depression was most common in children with a depressed mother, mothers who had other mood disorders, or who had experienced a traumatic event. Young children were not too emotionally immature to experience it. Depressed children appear sad even when playing; games may have themes of death or other somber topics; there are also appetite loss, sleep problems, and temper tantrums, grumpiness, and high levels of shame and maladaptive guilt. The authors did not address treatment: psychotherapy is the first choice over medication.

Chapter 12 presented current concepts of brain pathology underlying depression. This included hippocampal damage that resulted from the lack of neurotropic proteins. Rao and coworkers (2010) reported that similar pathology occurs in youths and places one at risk of developing depressive disorder. The authors concluded: *"early-life adversity may interact with genetic vulnerability to induce hippocampal changes, potentially increasing the risk for depressive disorder"* (p. 357). Luby and coworkers (2012) found that early supportive parenting in preschoolers exerted positive effects on hippocampal volume and later positive cognitive and socio-emotional outcomes, including reducing depression severity. Conversely, Suzuki and coworkers (2013) demonstrated abnormal brain circuitry in the hippocampus, amygdala, and prefrontal cortex in children with preschool depression. Gaffrey and coworkers (2012) noted a clinically relevant "brain-behavior" relationship between atypical functional connectivity of the posterior cingulate and disruptions in emotional regulation in preschoolers with depression.

Neither antidepressant drugs nor atypical antipsychotics have yet been evaluated in preschool depression (Nevels et al., 2010).

Medications for Treating Bipolar Disorder in Very Young Children

Bipolar disorder is well described in school-aged children and adolescents; there is increasing thought that it also occurs in preschoolers. Irritability, not elevated mood, seems to be the core feature (Parry and Levin, 2012). Clinically, it tends to be associated with aggressive medication therapies, often with poor diagnosis and without psychotherapeutic/social assistance. Safest are psychotherapeutic interventions such as Parent-Child Interaction Therapy (Luby et al., 2009c).

Psychopharmacological interventions might be considered in cases of significant impairment and distress associated with signs of serious mood and behavioral dysregulation. Recent studies have reported the efficacy of aripiprazole (Findling et al., 2012) and quetiapine (Joshi et al., 2012) in preschool-onset bipolar disorder. Seida and coworkers (2012) reviewed the safety and efficacy of second generation antipsychotic medications in children and young adults.

Medications for Treating Anxiety Disorders in Very Young Children

Guidelines for treating preschool anxiety disorders tend to group together situational anxiety disorder, generalized anxiety disorder, selective mutism and specific phobias. Posttraumatic stress disorder (PTSD) and obsessive-compulsive disorder (OCD) are treated individually. For non-PTSD, non-OCD anxiety disorders in preschoolers, behavioral therapy techniques, cognitive therapies, and internalizing prevention programs are valuable (Dougherty et al., 2013; Rapee, 2013). Preschool anxiety has a longitudinal course (Bufferd et al., 2012) and such children who show anxiety are inhibited, have overinvolved mothers, and mothers with their own anxiety disorder and are at increased risk for development and maintenance of such a disorder (Hudson and Dodd, 2012). For non-PTSD, non-OCD anxiety disorders in preschoolers, few case reports are available. Fluoxetine may be the preferred medication should pharmacological treatment of preschool anxiety be considered necessary. A trial of discontinuation after 6–9 months of therapy has been suggested. Benzodiazepines (because of cognitive impairments) are not recommended except for short medical/dental procedures.

PTSD is common in preschoolers and is difficult to treat. This includes children exposed to intimate partner violence (Graham-Bermann et al., 2012). There is strong evidence in support of psychotherapeutic intervention in preschool PTSD (Gillies et al., 2012; Weems and Scheeringa, 2013). The experts do not endorse medication, however, only 11 percent of providers reported that they *do not* use medication for preschool PTSD (thus, 89 percent did). Here, experts differ from practitioners. Again, benzodiazepines are not recommended.

There is little research on *OCD* in preschoolers. However, OCD may emerge in preschool children as early as 2 years of age, being more common in males (Coskun, et al., 2012). It has a chronic course and occurs comorbid with other psychological disorders. Psychoeducation, cognitive therapies, and exposure therapies are useful. Later in this chapter, we will discuss the Pediatric Obsessive-Compulsive Treatment Study (POTS), and extrapolate that SSRIs are efficacious and can be combined with cognitive therapies. However, one should consider SSRIs as treatment of last resort and SSRI treatment should always occur in the context of ongoing cognitive and/or behavioral interventions.

Medications for Treating Autism Spectrum Disorders in Very Young Children

Autism must present before age 3 and other autism spectrum disorders are typically recognized by 3 years of age. Treatment is multimodal and multidisciplinary, with early intervention necessary (Eapen et al., 2013). A 40-child study (2–9 years of age) with risperidone showed a 63 percent positive response rate in controlling irritability and behaviors associated with autism. Risperidone is now FDA-approved for children ages 5 and over for behaviors associated with autism. The pharmacological treatment of school age children with autism and similar disorders is discussed below.

CHILD AND ADOLESCENT PSYCHOPHARMACOLOGY

In 2009, the American Academy of Child and Adolescent Psychiatry published a clinical practice guideline on the use of psychotropic medication in children and adolescents (Waldkup, and the American Academy of Child and Adolescent Psychiatry, 2009). Some of the principles delineated include:

- Before initiating pharmacotherapy, a psychiatric evaluation is completed
- Treatment involves history and medical evaluation when appropriate
- Treatment involves communication with other professionals for history and sets the stage for monitoring outcome and side effects
- Before prescribing, develop psychosocial and medication plan
- Develop a plan for outcome monitoring, both short and long term
- Proceed with caution if no monitoring is possible
- Educate all about the treatment plan
- Document assent of the child and consent of parents
- Focus on risks and benefits of medications and alternatives to medication
- Implement a medication trial using adequate dose for an adequate duration
- Reassess treatment plan if no response to initial trial of medication
- A medication discontinuation trial requires a specific plan

Medications for Treating Autism Spectrum Disorders (ASD)

Autism is a pervasive developmental disorder characterized by severe impairment in several areas of development, including deficits in social interactions, communication skills, and the presence of stereotyped behavior, interests, and activities. The incidence of diagnosed cases of autism is increasing, affecting about 1 percent of children. The use of psychotropic drugs targeted to possible neurochemical systems involved in the pathophysiology of autism have been often shown to reduce aggression, self-injurious behaviors, anxiety, repetitive behaviors, mood dysregulation, hyperactivity, impulsiveness, and other maladaptive behaviors. Physical aggression and self-injurious behaviors are especially problematic in adolescents whose large size and physical strength create additional danger. Medications can be quite useful in reducing the intensity and frequency of these behaviors (Propper and Orlik, 2011).

Medications, however, do not cure ASD, but may be effective in treating various behavioral symptoms that interfere with daily life and may cause impairment or distress (Kumar et al., 2012). FDA-approved medications include risperidone and aripiprazole; other medications may be effective in ASD-related symptoms such as hyperactivity, lack of attention, agitation, insomnia, aggression, self-injury, irritability, repetitive and compulsive behaviors, and anxiety.

Historically, antidepressants were used in attempts to reduce the anxiety, agitation, and compulsiveness associated with autism (Doyle and McDougle, 2012). Indeed, SSRIs had been frequently used, at least until the demonstration of the efficacy of risperidone. Lack of efficacy, accompanied by a high incidence of side effects, such as behavioral activation and agitation limit their use. Clomipramine may have some efficacy for the treatment of repetitive behaviors, stereotypies, and obsessiveness in some persons with ASD.

Atypical antipsychotic drugs are clinically the most effective drugs for reducing aggression, irritability, and severe tantrums in youth with autism (Doyle and McDougle, 2012). Indeed, risperidone and aripiprazole are currently considered first-line therapy in child and adolescent autism (Figure 15.3) and are FDA-approved for the treatment of irritability, aggression, and self-injurious behaviors. Paliperidone (the active metabolite of risperidone) has also been shown to be effective (Stigler, et al., 2012). Weight gain, glucose intolerance, prolactin increases, and hyperlipidemia are limiting and are serious considerations in children and adolescents. Relevant reviews of note include those by Marcus, et al. (2011), Ching and Pringsheim (2012), Elbe and Lalani (2012), Kirino (2012), and Pringsheim and Gorman (2012).

In the treatment of hyperactivity, impulsiveness and attention deficit associated with ASD, traditional anti-ADHD medications (including methylphenidate, atomoxetine, guanfacine, and clonidine) have demonstrated modest efficacy (Doyle and McDougle, 2012). Side effects, mostly irritability, often limit therapeutic use. Multiple other medications are being evaluated. One of these, bumetanide, a diuretic and chloride channel antagonist, has recently been shown to be effective (Lemonnier et al., 2012).

Improved efficacy of medication treatment and longer-term outcomes likely will involve medication plus parent training, CBT, and other complimentary efforts (Storch et al., 2013). One of the most commonly used complimentary medicines are the omega-3 fatty acids. While evidence of efficacy in autism is contradictory, supplemental omega-3-fatty acid therapy might be helpful, does not cause harm, and can be administered without significant side effects (Meiri et al., 2009).

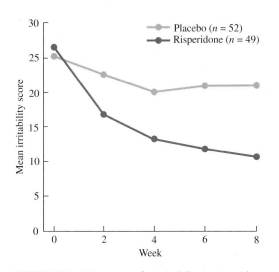

FIGURE 15.3   Mean score for irritability in risperidone- and placebo-treated children with autism. Total number of subjects studied = 101. Higher scores on the irritability subscale of the Aberrant Behavior Checklist indicate greater irritability. [Data from McDougle et al. (2003). "Treatment of Aggression in Children and Adolescents with Autism and Conduct Disorder." *Journal of Clinical Psychiatry* 64, Supplement 4, p. 17.]

Medications for Treating Behavioral or Aggressive Disorders

Severe childhood aggression is one of the most challenging disorders to treat. Nonpharmacological treatments have advantages over medication treatment, but efficacy is variable. Once these nonpharmacological approaches have been tried and found inadequate, the second choice is medication. Disruptive behavioral disorders include conduct disorder, oppositional defiant disorder, and disruptive behavior NOS. ADHD (discussed next) is frequently associated with disruptive behavioral disorder as demonstrated by aggression and severe behavioral problems. About 50 percent of youth with behavioral disruptive disorders progress to antisocial personality disorder as adults suggesting that their externalizing disruptive symptoms in childhood can be a marker for more pervasive psychopathology as adults.

Currently, there is a marked increase in the use of atypical antipsychotic drugs in this population of young persons, either as monotherapy or adjunctive therapy to anti-ADHD medications. Research has focused predominantly on 4 classes of medications: psychostimulants, atypical antipsychotics, mood stabilizers, and alpha-2 agonists (Farmer et al., 2011).

Psychostimulants such as methylphenidate and amphetamine products (discussed below) are commonly used to treat ADHD. These drugs may ameliorate aggression, but comorbidity with conduct disorder is less responsive.

Mood stabilizers, such as lithium and anticonvulsants such as lamotrigine and valproic acid, reduce aggressive behaviors in children with explosive tempers and mood lability (Pappadopulos et al., 2011). Requirements for frequent blood testing with some of these drugs may be unappealing to many patients and providers. Donovan and coworkers (2000) studied 20 youths (10–18 years, 80% male) with conduct or oppositional defiant disorder as well as explosive temper and mood lability. Subjects received 6 weeks of valproic acid or placebo: 8 of 10 on valproate responded positively. None of the subjects responded to placebo.

Saxena and coworkers (2006) studied the use of valproic acid in youth (average age 11 years) who had parents with bipolar disorder and who displayed irritability, rapid mood shifts, and aggression. Valproate (dosed to a blood concentration of 50 to 120 micrograms per milliliter) improved both mood and aggressive symptoms, and over 75 percent of the young people studied were considered "responders." Khanzode and coworkers (2006) reexamined the use of valproic acid in incarcerated youths diagnosed with severe conduct disorders. High doses (500 to 1500 milligrams per day) produced improvements in depression and impulse control but no improvement in other emotional states. The researchers suggested that an integrated approach combining pharmacotherapy with psychotherapy may be needed to achieve overall improvement.

Alpha-2 agonists (clonidine and *guanfacine)* can be used to treat ADHD, although generally less successfully than the psychostimulants (Nevils et al., 2010).

Atypical antipsychotic medications are currently the mainstay in the treatment of aggressive disorders in children and adolescents (Findling 2008; Loy et al., 2012). Risperidone and olanzapine (see Farmer et al., 2011) have been used to target aggressive behaviors, but they tend to cause weight gain and other adverse metabolic effects. Aripiprazole can be used and has a better side effect profile (Ercan et al., 2012; Frye et al., 2008; Scheltema and deHaan, 2010).

Polypharmacy is becoming increasingly utilized in disruptive behaviors only as a partial response to single-medication therapy. Conceptually, combining medications with differing profiles of side effects make sense, such as combining a psychostimulant (weight loss, poor feeding, insomnia) with an atypical antipsychotic (weight and appetite gain and sedation) might be particularly appealing. To study polypharmacy, the NIH has funded a multisite study termed "Treatment Of Severe Child Aggression (TOSCA)" (Farmer et al., 2011). This study began by administering methylphenidate to children 6–12 years old with ADHD and comorbid aggression (oppositional defiant disorder or conduct disorder). Children whose behaviors were not normalized received a second medication (risperidol or placebo) by random assignment. This is the first carefully performed evaluation of polypharmacy in the treatment of comorbid ADHD and behavioral aggression in children and adolescents.

In summary, although aggressive and rage behaviors are highly prevalent in child and adolescent psychiatry, there are few guidelines for treating them. In addition, children and adolescents referred for treatment for behavioral and aggressive disorders are likely to show several other problems (for example, ADHD, pervasive developmental disorders, depression, and substance abuse) that raise their own separate challenges. Parents and siblings of children referred for therapies for conduct disorder often themselves show significant impairment (psychiatric disorder, marital discord, family stress, dysfunctional relationships, abusive parenting, and so on). All these problems need to be addressed as drug prescription is being considered. Currently, off-label use of atypical antipsychotics, especially aripiprazole, is most promising. As always in child and adolescent psychopharmacology, risks must be weighed against possible benefits. Also, the chronicity of illness may necessitate long-term use of these agents. No studies of long-term use of atypical antipsychotic therapy in children have been reported. Despite this, the severity of disease may necessitate a trial of pharmacotherapy.

Medications for Treating ADHD

Attention deficit/hyperactivity disorder (ADHD) is the most extensively studied of the pediatric mental disorders, a disorder that has a longitudinal continuum through adolescence and adulthood. On average, one in every ten children in the United States has been diagnosed with the disorder and about one-half of these are on stimulant medication: most commonly the stimulants methylphenidate and amphetamine. Increasingly, non-stimulant options are being investigated. Sonuga-Barke and coworkers (2013) recently addressed these issues in a critical review.

Currently an estimated 3.5 percent of children in the United States receive stimulant medication (Zuvekas and Vitiello, 2012). Alarmingly, a diagnosis of ADHD indicates co-morbidity with many neurodevelopmental conditions (Larson et al., 2011). Parents report that 46 percent of children with ADHD had a learning disability versus 5 percent without ADHD; 27 percent versus 2 percent had a conduct disorder, 18 percent versus 2 percent anxiety, 14 percent versus 1 percent depression, and 12 percent versus 3 percent speech problems. Comorbid disorders are common with 33 percent having one, 16 percent having two, and 18 percent having three or more. The risk for three or more comorbidities is 3.8 percent times higher for poor versus affluent children. Mahajan and coworkers (2012) discuss the treatment of ADHD in children with autism spectrum disorders.

Much has been written on possible genetic versus environmental contributions to ADHD behaviors. Genetic influences underlying the disorder may involve variances in the D_4 subtype of the dopamine receptor complex (Gonzalez et al., 2012). Indeed, disruption of dopamine reward pathways may be associated with motivational deficits seen in ADHD, and possible later increases in substance abuse disorders (Lee et al., 2011; Pingault et al., 2013), even though exposure to stimulant medication by itself has little effect on later substance abuse (Harty et al., 2011).

Alterations in dopaminergic activity in the prefrontal cortex (PFC) of the brain seems to be important in ADHD. The PFC is critical for the regulation of behavior, attention, and cognition. The PFC reduces the effect of distraction and divided attention. Lesions to the PFC produce a profile of distractibility, forgetfulness, impulsivity, poor planning, and locomotor hyperactivity (all prominent in ADHD). Optimal levels of norepinephrine and dopamine are essential for proper PFC control of behavior and attention. Genetic alterations in norepinephrine or dopamine receptors or systems contribute to dysregulation of PFC circuits in ADHD. Stimulant medications tend to augment deficient dopaminergic (or norepinephrine) systems, optimizing PFC regulation of behavior and attention. As noted above, this may involve genetic alterations in the dopamine D_4 receptor complex.

In addition to dopamine being involved in the PFC, dopamine is a major transmitter in the *nucleus accumbens* (NAc), the so-called "pleasure center" in the brain. Augmentation of dopaminergic activity in the NAc by stimulants appears to account for the emotional stimulation, pleasure response, and attractiveness of these drugs that leads to compulsive abuse.

Medication treatment of ADHD is not new. Amphetamines (such as *Benzedrine* and *dextroamphetamine*) were used to treat ADHD as early as 1937; *methylphenidate* (Ritalin) was introduced in the United States in 1955 and formally approved by the FDA for use in children in 1961. Since then, multiple formulations of stimulants have been marketed (Table 15.2) and a few non-stimulant products have appeared (e.g., atomoxetine, extended-release guanfacine, and extended-release clonidine).

TABLE 15.2 Stimulant medications currently available clinically for the treatment of ADHD

Medication (trade name)	Mode of delivery	Generic	Maximum dose per day	Duration of action, hours
Methylphenidate (Ritalin)	Immediate release	Yes	60 mg	4
Methylphenidate (Methylin)	Immediate release	Yes	60 mg	4
d-Methylphenidate (Focalin)	Immediate release	Yes	20 mg	4
Mixed amphetamine salts (Adderall)	Immediate release	Yes	40 mg	8
Amphetamine (Dexedrine)	Immediate release	Yes	40 mg	8
Amphetamine (Dextrostat)	Immediate release	Yes	40 mg	8
Methylphenidate (Ritalin SR)—pulse	Gradually released from wax matrix	Yes	60 mg	Up to 8
Methylphenidate (Metadate ER)—pulse	Gradually released from wax matrix	Yes	60 mg	7–8
Methylphenidate (Methylin ER)—pulse	Gradually released from wax matrix	Yes	60 mg	7–8
Methylphenidate (Metadate CD)—pearls	Beaded delivery system—30% immediate release and 70% 3 h later	Yes	60 mg	8–9
Methylphenidate (Ritalin LA)—pearls	Beaded delivery system—50% immediate release and 50% 4 h later	Yes	60 mg	7–9

Guidelines for Management of ADHD

In July 2007, a clinical practice parameter for the assessment and treatment of children and adolescents with ADHD was published (American Academy of Child & Adolescent Psychiatry, 2007). The guideline is both practical and evidence-based. Diagnostic criteria, behavioral rating assessment scales, and medication options are discussed in detail. This guideline was updated in 2012. The American Academy of Pediatrics also published a 2011 guideline with expanded coverage of the diagnosis and treatment of ADHD in children ages 4–18 years as well as expanded discussion of behavioral interventions (American Academy of Pediatrics, 2011a). Extensive supplemental information is available, including a listing of currently available FDA-approved medications, dosing considerations and pharmacokinetics (American Academy of Pediatrics, 2011b).

Table 15.2 continued

Medication (trade name)	Mode of delivery	Generic	Maximum dose per day	Duration of action, hours
d-Methylphenidate (Focalin XR)-pearls	Beaded delivery system—50% immediate release and 50% 4 h later	Yes	30 mg	Up to 12
Methylphenidate (Concerta)—pump	OROS delivery system—22% immediate release and 78% gradually released osmotically	Yes	72 mg	Up to 12
Methylphenidate (Daytrana)—patch	Patch worn up to 9 h per day, gradually releasing methylphenidate	No	30 mg	12
Mixed amphetamine salts (Adderall XR)—pearls	Beaded delivery system—50% immediate release and 50% 4 h later	Yes	30 mg	10
Amphetamine (Dexedrine Spansule)—pearls	Beaded delivery system—initial dose released immediately and remainder gradually released	Yes	40 mg	10
Lisdexamfetamine (Vyvanse)—prodrug	Amphetamine with lysine attached, activated in gastrointestinal tract when lysine is cleaved	No	70 mg	10
Atomoxetine (Strattera)	10–100 mg capsules	No	1.4 mg/kg	10–12
Extended-release guanfacine (Intuniv)	1–4 mg tablets	No	4 mg	10–12
Extended-release clonidine (Kapvay)	0.1 to 2 mg tablets	No	0.4 mg	10–12

Modified from J. M. Daughton and C. J. Kratochvil, "Review of ADHD Pharmacotherapies: Advantages, Disadvantages, and Clinical Pearls," *Journal of the American Academy of Child and Adolescent Psychiatry* 48 (2009): 243–244.

Stimulant Treatment for ADHD

Stimulant medications are well known to improve attention and concentration in ADHD-diagnosed children. Children treated with stimulants show improvements in parent- and teacher-rated ADHD symptoms, but unfortunately often make little or no improvements in functional impairment (Epstein, et al., 2010). Therefore, use of stimulant medication in isolation may only resolve symptoms, and *"collaboration with other mental health or educational services in addition to medication appears warranted"* (Epstein et al., 2010, p. 160). Despite this limitation, the treatment of ADHD with psychostimulants has become one of the most broadly effective drug therapies of the twenty-first century.

More recently, however, it is becoming clear that these medications do not normalize the ability to learn and apply knowledge (Advokat, 2010). Indeed, academic underachievement and less-than-optimal educational outcomes are persistent. Therefore, these drugs are not true "cognitive enhancers," as ADHD-diagnosed young adults are more likely to report academic problems and are less likely to graduate from college, regardless of whether or not they received medication. Despite this poor long-term outcome, stimulant medication is widely used in the short-term treatment of of hyperactivity and inattention. Whether that is sufficient to justify long-term use is debatable.

In December 1999, results of the Multimodal Treatment Study of Children with Attention-Deficit/Hyperactivity Disorder (MTA Cooperative Group, 1999) were published. In the study, a cohort of 579 children with ADHD was assigned to 14 months of medication management, intensive behavioral treatment, and the two combined, or standard community care. Carefully structured medication management resulted in a better outcome than did intensive behavioral treatment, and combined treatment yielded an outcome that was better than the outcome of behavioral treatment but equivalent to the outcome of medication management. As stated:

> Carefully crafted medication management was superior to behavioral treatment and to routine community care that included medication. Combined treatment did not yield significantly greater benefits than medication management for core ADHD symptoms, but it may have provided modest advantages for non-ADHD symptoms and positive functioning outcomes. (p. 1073)

A 24-month follow-up of the MTA study (MTA Cooperative Group, 2004) revealed that cessation of drug therapy was associated with clinical deterioration, continued drug therapy was associated with only mild deterioration, and stimulant initiation (in the group not receiving stimulants in the early study) was associated with clinical improvements.

The participants in the original MTA study have now been followed for 8 years (Molina et al., 2009). At eight years, 33 percent of the original participants were still receiving medication, usually stimulants (83 percent). While improvements seen at the end of the 14 month study were generally maintained, MTA participants were not "normalized" at eight years, with 30 percent still meeting the criteria for ADHD. Clinically significant antisocial behavior was present in 25–30 percent of MTA participants; 25 percent met criteria for oppositional defiant disorder or conduct disorder; 27 percent had been arrested at least one time; and 30 percent reportedly had moderate to serious delinquent behavior. Academically, medicated children with ADHD had significant improvements in mathematics and reading scores over untreated children with ADHD, but these improvements were insufficient to eliminate the test-score gap between children with ADHD and those without (Barnard-Brak and Brak, 2011; Scheffler et al., 2009). Perhaps of importance in ADHD treatment is a child's relative age compared with other children in the same class. Here, younger children tend to perform at a lower level, have a higher rate of ADHD diagnosis, and a higher rate of stimulant treatment (Figure 15.4). Thus, these children may be at a maturity disadvantage that can have a negative effect on health and personal achievement (Morrow et al., 2012; Zoega et al., 2012).

Methylphenidate

Currently, methylphenidate preparations account for 90 percent of the prescribed medication for ADHD. Because it is so widely used and because no one dosage regimen is ideal, multiple different dosage forms and methods of delivering the drug to the bloodstream

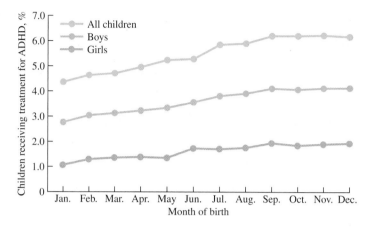

FIGURE 15.4 Percentage of children aged 6 to 12 years receiving pharmacologic treatment for ADHD, by month of birth. In this Canadian study, the cut-off date of birth that allows entry into kindergarten or first grade is December 31st. Consequently, children born in December are the youngest in the grade. [Data from Morrow et al. (2012), Figure 1, p. 757.]

have been devised (see Table 15.2). *Methylphenidate* (as Ritalin) is of rapid onset and short duration; thus, it must be administered two or three times daily. It is not administered in the evening to permit the blood level to drop, allowing normal sleep. The short half-life is a problem in some children who experience an end-of-dose rebound in dysfunctional behavior. The beneficial effect of methylphenidate in children extends into clinical use in adults.

Early extended-release preparations of methylphenidate were disappointing. Recently, more dependable extended-release preparations have become available. The prototype was Concerta, an osmotic-release preparation that delays absorption and extends duration up to 12 hours. The product is prepared with 22 percent of the drug in a coating on the outside of the capsule (immediate release drug), with 78 percent delivered by an "osmotic pump" that releases drug over a 10-hour period in gradually increasing serum concentrations. One daily dose of Concerta yields about the same plasma concentrations as three daily doses of immediate-release methylphenidate with essentially equal efficacy. Other new formulations of methylphenidate for oral administration are of two types:

1. Single pulse, sustained-release formulations (Ritalin-SR, Metadate ER, Methylin CD) use a wax matrix to prolong release. Their duration of action is about 8 hours, but may be unreliable compared with other preparations

2. Beaded double-pulse products (Ritalin LA, Focalin XR, Metadate CD) use an extended release formulation with bi-modal release.

   – Ritalin LA and Focalin XR = 50 percent in immediate release and 50 percent in enteric coated, delayed release beads

   – Metadate CD = 30 percent immediate-release beads and 70 percent delayed-release beads that are released 4 hours later, eliminating lunch-time dose

TABLE 15.3 Recommended titration schedule for the methylphenidate transdermal "Daytrana" skin patch

	Upward titration, if response is not maximized			
	Week 1	Week 2	Week 3	Week 4
Patch size	12.5 cm^2	18.75 cm^2	25 cm^2	37.5 cm^2
Nominal delivered dose* (mg/9 hours)	10 mg	15 mg	20 mg	30 mg
Delivery rate*	(1.1 mg/hr)*	(1.6 mg/hr)*	(2.2 mg/hr)*	(3.3 mg/hr)*

*Nominal in vivo delivery rate in pediatric subjects aged 6–12 when applied to the hip, based on a 9-hour wear period.

Comparing Concerta and Focalin XR showed behavioral improvement superior to that achieved with Focalin-XR at 0.5 and 5 hours, but Concerta was superior over Focalin XR at 11 and 12 hours. Using this data, prescribers and parents can find an appropriate preparation of methylphenidate, depending on the desired time of maximal effect and duration of action.

In 2007, a transdermal methylphenidate delivery system (a "skin patch" sold under the trade name Daytrana) was introduced. The patch is applied daily, has a clinical onset of effect within 2 hours, and is worn for a maximum of 9 hours. Following removal, the effects of the methylphenidate continue for another 3 hours. Patches containing 10, 15, 20, and 30 milligrams are available (Table 15.3). If removed before 9 hours, less drug is absorbed and therefore duration of action is decreased. Bukstein and coworkers (2009), in a four-week study in 164 children who received *extended release, oral methylphenidate preparations* (Ritalin LA, Concerta, or Metadate CD) and then switched to the methylphenidate patch found improved ADHD behavior and quality of life. Caregivers (mostly parents) reported high satisfaction with the patch, improved behavior, and less worry about missed doses.

Recently, a liquid suspension formulation of *methylphenidate* (Quillivant XR) was FDA approved for ADHD. Efficacy was recently reported by Wigal et al. (2013) in a study in 45 children, aged 6–12 years. ADHD symptoms were reduced beginning at 45 minutes and continuing for 12 hours post dose.

Also commercially available is *dexmethylphenidate* (d-methylphenidate or Focalin), the active D-isomer of methylphenidate. This isomer has twice the potency of methylphenidate, so the dose of dexmethylphenidate is one-half the dose of methylphenidate. Focalin is available in an extended-release formulation (Focalin XR).

Amphetamines

Since about 1937, amphetamines have been used for the treatment of ADHD. Available amphetamines include *dextroamphetamine* (Dexedrine), *mixed amphetamine salts* (Adderall), an *extended-release formulation of Adderall* (Adderall XR), and *lisdexamfetamine* (Vyvanse). A transdermal amphetamine preparation is currently under development; study results have not yet been published. Adderall is called "mixed amphetamine salts," and pharmacologically was the same as Benzedrine from 1937. In lisdexamfetamine, a molecule of dextroamphetamine is bonded to L-lysine, a naturally occurring amino acid, resulting in a molecule lacking biological activity (a pro-drug). When taken orally, the bond is broken by gastrointestinal enzymes, releasing the amphetamine, which is then absorbed. If crushed and injected, the bond is only slowly broken; thus diversion may theoretically be reduced. Doses of 10, 30, and 70 milligrams of lisdexamfetamine result in bioavailability of about 5 to 30 milligrams of dextroamphetamine (Goodman, 2010; Faraone et al., 2012).

Once-daily Adderall appears to be similar to twice-daily methylphenidate and is therapeutically equivalent or even superior to generic methylphenidate for improving a relatively wide range of behavior problems commonly displayed by children with ADHD. The issue of comparative equivalence remains unclear, as head-to-head comparisons of Concerta and Adderall in treating ADHD have not been reported.

Alternative Medications for Treating ADHD

About 10 to 30 percent of ADHD patients do not respond adequately to stimulants and are considered to be treatment-resistant. In addition, some children and their parents may desire that stimulants not be used. Therefore, there is a need for treatment alternatives. Some of these are now FDA approved for use in ADHD.

Atomoxetine (Strattera). In 2003, the FDA approved atomoxetine for the treatment of child and adult ADHD. In 2008, the FDA expanded its approval to include indication for the maintenance treatment of ADHD in children and adolescents. This is the first selective norepinephrine reuptake inhibitor (SNRI) antidepressant approved for use in treating ADHD in children 6 years of age and older as well as in adults. At a daily dose of about 1.4–1.8 mg/Kg/day, the drug is effective in reducing ADHD symptoms (Kratochvil et al., 2011; Bushe and Savill, 2013). The drug appears to be tolerable and relatively safe when used in children over a period of up to 4 years (Donelly et al., 2009). A British study of 201 children with ADHD reported that atomoxetine was more effective in treatment-naive patients than in patients who had been previously treated with stimulant medication (Prasad et al., 2007), suggesting a trial of atomoxetine prior to initiation of stimulants. Abuse potential appears to be minimal (Upadhyaya et al., 2013).

Guanfacine-ER and clonidine-ER. Two CNS-acting antihypertensive (blood pressure-lowering) dopaminergic agonists in extended release formulation—*clonidine* (Kapvay) and *guanfacine* (Intuniv)—are FDA-approved for the treatment of ADHD, either as monotherapy or used concomitly with a stimulant. This may relate to increased alpha-2-receptor stimulation in the prefrontal cortex. Bukstein and Head (2012) report that guanfacine-ER works better as an adjunct to stimulants, rather than as a sole agent. Jain, et al. (2011) detailed the efficacy of extended-release clonidine (0.2 and 0.4 mg/day) in reducing inattention scores and hyperactivity/impulsivity scores.

These two drugs are generally considered to be second-line medications. Guanfacine-ER has a longer half-life than does clonidine and is less sedating. Guanfacine ER has modest efficacy at a dose of 2–4 mg/day; sedation and fatigue being common side effects, but these were not limiting and sedation seems to decrease with increasing duration of treatment (Farone and Glatt, 2010).

Tricyclic antidepressants (especially *nortriptyline;* see Chapter 12) have been studied and have occasionally been reported to be effective. However, cognitive impairments, limited efficacy, and rare cases of potentially fatal cardiac toxicities associated with tricyclic antidepressant use in children and adolescents pose considerable limitations.

Initial reports on other medications indicate some usefulness of the antidepressant *fluoxetine* (Prozac) and the anxiolytic *buspirone* (BuSpar), although the effects were not robust. Quintana and coworkers (2007), however, demonstrated a more robust effect of fluoxetine in ADHD with comorbid nonbipolar mood disorders in children and adolescents aged 6 to 18 years. Symptoms of inattention, overactivity, aggression, defiance, and depression were improved in 47 percent of participants. *Duloxetine* (Cymbalta) has been reported effective in adults with ADHD, depression, and anxiety (Bilodeau, et al., 2012). Of additional interest is the dopaminergic antidepressant *bupropion SR* (Wellbutrin-SR); the drug has been reported effective in adults with ADHD and in both adults and adolescents with ADHD comorbid with other disorders such as depression or substance abuse.

Modafinil (Provigil) is a nonstimulant drug that is FDA-approved for the maintenance of daytime wakefulness in the treatment of narcolepsy, in shift-work sleep disorders, and in sleep apnea. Although possibly efficacious, it is not approved for use in child and adolescent ADHD, in part because of potentially serious skin toxicity (Kumar, 2008).

Modafinil had been thought to be distinct from stimulants and has not been classified as a stimulant. It was thought not to have abuse potential. However, Volkow and coworkers (2009) demonstrated that modafinil increases dopamine in the nucleus accumbens and may therefore have potential for abuse. This may account for some of the increasing use of the drug.

Metadoxine-ER is a non-stimulant shown effective in adults with ADHD (Manor et al., 2012). Side effects are low and tolerable. The drug is currently in clinical trial; comparative studies are not yet reported. Metadoxine has long been used for the treatment of alcoholism (Leggio et al., 2011).

EB-1020 is an experimental dopamine/norepinephrine reuptake inhibitor shown to be effective in an animal model of ADHD (Bymaster et al., 2012). This drug may have both antidepressant and anti-ADHD activity.

Side Effects of Stimulant Medications

Common side effects of stimulant medications include nighttime wakefulness (insomnia), elevations in blood pressure and heart rate, reductions in appetite, and possible growth suppression. With proper care, these usually can be well managed. Other potential side effects include adverse psychiatric problems, including new or worsening behavioral and thought problems, new or worsening bipolar illness, new or worsening aggressive or hostility problems, and in children and teenagers, new psychiatric symptoms, including hearing voices, believing things that are not true, increased suspiciousness, or new manic symptoms. All these effects are predictable consequences seen in some people using any psychostimulant, whether for therapeutic purposes or for abuse purposes.

More serious effects of stimulant medications involve cardiac (heart) safety and reports of sudden deaths among children and adolescents receiving these medications for treatment of ADHD. Concerns that stimulants may increase the risk of sudden unexplained deaths in children surfaced from case reports since the early 1990s. In 2006, the FDA requested that package inserts of stimulant medications contain a warning that stimulant products generally should not be used in children or adolescents with known serious structural cardiac abnormalities, cardiomyopathy, serious heart rhythm abnormalities, or other serious heart problems that may place them at increased vulnerability to the stimulant effects of the drug.

Current labeling instructions emphasize that children should receive a physical examination and a review of personal and family history for relevant cardiac events prior to starting stimulant treatment. If abnormalities are suspected, careful cardiac evaluation likely should be performed. The rarity of sudden, unexplained deaths confounds recommendations. For example, one study found no events in an examination of over 125,000 person-years of use (Gould et al., 2009). Similarly, serious cardiovascular events were not found by Habel and coworkers (2011), Schelleman and coworkers (2011), Cooper and coworkers (2011), and Olfson and coworkers (2012). Stimulants and atomoxetine are certainly not innocuous medications and all side effects, including elevations in blood pressure and preexisting heart disease, need to be taken into account before and during prescription.

One other concern with ADHD medication is whether exposure to stimulants might increase future stimulant abuse. Humphreys and coworkers (2013) reviewed studies on this topic and concluded that children with ADHD treated with stimulants were no more or less likely to abuse stimulants as adults than children with ADHD not treated with stimulants.

Medications and Medical Issues in Treating Depression

Perhaps the greatest controversy in child and adolescent psychopharmacology is that surrounding the use of antidepressant medication to treat major depressive disorders in children and adolescents. Do these medications even work? Do they increase the risk of suicide? Is their cost-benefit ratio worth the risks involved? These and other questions plague prescribers, let alone parents and patients. In essence, controversy surrounds the balance between expected benefits (effectiveness in relieving depression) versus potential risks (possibility of increasing the risk of suicide). To understand this controversy, a bit of history is in order. First, research conducted in the late 1990s and early 2000s demonstrated several important points:

- There was a high prevalence of suicidal ideation and completed suicides among untreated children and adolescents with depressive disorders.
- Sixty-two percent of children with depression had experienced childhood adversity, with traumatic events (35 percent) and bullying victimization (29 percent) most commonly reported (Tunnard et al., 2014).
- Not only does depression exist in adolescence, but adolescence is the period of highest risk for onset of depression.
- Adolescent depression has a protracted, longitudinal course with persistence into adult life (adolescents do not "grow out of it"), which results in ongoing disruption of interpersonal relationships, risk for substance abuse, early pregnancy, low educational achievement, poor occupational functioning, unemployment, and continued risk of suicide.
- Untreated childhood and adolescent depression is associated with later development of serious personality disorders in early adulthood; dependent, antisocial, passive-aggressive, substance abuse, and histrionic personality disorders.

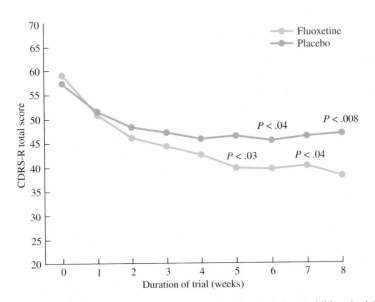

FIGURE 15.5   Weekly Children's Depression Rating Scale in 96 child and adolescent outpatients (aged 7 to 17 years) with nonpsychotic major depressive disorder treated with fluoxetine or placebo and evaluated weekly for 8 consecutive weeks. [Data from Emslie et al. (1997), p. 1035.]

These data compelled clinicians to intervene aggressively to prevent teenagers from developing into troubled and dysfunctional adults. A partial answer was discovered in 1997 when Emslie and coworkers demonstrated that *fluoxetine* (Prozac) was superior to placebo treatment in lowering scores on the Children's Depression Rating Scale—Revised (Figure 15.5). This led to widespread off-label use of fluoxetine for child and adolescent depression, culminating in the NIMH-funded TADS (Treatment for Adolescents with Depression Study) research, the first phase of which was published in 2004 [Treatment for Adolescents with Depression Study (TADS) Team, 2004]. The 12-week TADS study compared usual clinical management with fluoxetine (10 to 40 milligrams per day) alone, cognitive-behavioral therapy (CBT) alone, or the combination of CBT and fluoxetine. Response to combination treatment (71 percent) was significantly greater than to fluoxetine alone (61 percent), CBT alone (43 percent), and placebo (usual clinical management, 35 percent). Fluoxetine monotherapy was superior to placebo and to CBT alone. This study set the standard that the best treatment of child and adolescent depression is a combination of fluoxetine and CBT.

Subsequent to this initial study, results of longer-term phases of the TADS study have appeared. In general, over the past decade, combination therapy (CBT plus fluoxetine) has emerged as therapy of choice for child and adolescent depression:

- Patients in all treatment groups tended to improve even more after three years of therapy, although about one-third of patients will be resistant to therapy.
- At least 9 months of treatment likely is needed for the average patient; longer times of treatment are associated with persistence of benefits for at least 1 year following medication discontinuation [Treatment for Adolescents with Depression Study (TADS) Team, 2009].

- About 9 months of combination therapy should be the modal treatment from a public health perspective as well as to maximize benefits and minimize harms for individual patients (March and Vitiello, 2009).

- Recurrence is to be expected, occurring in about 50 percent of recovered adolescents, with higher probability in females. Adding CBT to fluoxetine therapy minimizes persistent suicidal ideation and treatment-emergent suicidal events (discussed below) and enhances treatment safety (Vitiello, 2009).

- While combination therapy (CBT plus fluoxetine) is more expensive per year than fluoxetine alone, improved outcomes may justify combination therapy as cost effective; CBT alone is not cost effective (Domino et al., 2009; Lynch, et al., 2011).

- The long half-life of fluoxetine seems to account for its superiority over other medications (Smith, 2009).

- Resistance to combination therapy remains a significant problem, indicating that Treatment Of Resistant Depression In Adolescents (the TORDIA trial) needs addressing (Curtis and Fairman, 2008).

- Adolescents resistant to a combination of fluoxetine alone or combined with CBT may react positively to a combination of CBT and a different SSRI (Brent et al., 2008; Kennard et al., 2009), although citalopram use has been associated with increased suicidality (Shoval et al., 2011). Augmentation strategies (e.g., added to CBT and fluoxetine) have not been systematically reported to date.

Alternative Medications and Treatments

Until recently, *fluoxetine* was the only drug whose antidepressant effect has been clearly established in a pediatric population and the only drug approved in the United States for the treatment of depression in children and adolescents. In 2009, the FDA gave approval for the use of *escitalopram* (Lexapro) for the treatment of depression in adolescents, ages 12–17 years. This approval was based on three studies on citalopram and escitalopram, the last study reporting that scores on the Child Depression Rating Scale were reduced by 22 points compared with a 19 point reduction in the placebo-treated group (Emslie et al., 2009). Whether this is clinically significant is yet unknown. No head-to-head comparisons between fluoxetine and escitalopram have been reported. It does, however, provide clinicians with a second FDA-approved medication. The possible increase in suicidality with citalopram remains a problem (Ahn et al., 2011).

Emslie and coworkers (2007) performed an open-label trial of *venlafaxine* extended release (Effexor-XR) in child and adolescent depression (no placebo group for comparison). While efficacy was demonstrated, serious side effects occurred in about 8 percent of patients; including suicide attempts, hostility, and hallucinations. Brent and coworkers (2009) reported that venlafaxine treatment was associated with a higher rate of self-harm adverse events in those with higher suicidal ideation. As venlafaxine in adults with bipolar depression is associated with "manic flips," one wonders whether some of this toxicity represents an unmasking of bipolarity in some adolescents suffering these side effects. In a meta-analysis of the literature, Bridge and coworkers (2007) found poor efficacy for venlafaxine. In this same meta-analysis, *paroxetine* (Paxil) was also relatively ineffective in treating child and adolescent depression and was associated with serious side effects, including suicidal ideation.

As discussed earlier, *atomoxetine* (Strattera) is the first commercially available drug in the new class of SNRI-type antidepressants. Atomoxetine is approved for treatment of ADHD in children and adolescents, and it is likely effective in child and adolescent depression. Atomoxetine likely is effective in situations of depression comorbid with ADHD or anxiety disorders, especially since, unlike fluoxetine, SNRIs may be better at increasing social functioning; they may improve patient motivation, energy, and self-perception.

Finally, adjunctive use of benzodiazepines (in depressed children) was associated with higher rates of both suicidal and nonsuicidal self-harm adverse events (Brent et al., 2009). Cognitive and behavioral activating side effects also limit use (Eapen and Crncec, 2012).

Adjuvant Medications. Two additional classes of drugs are being evaluated to see whether they can be used as adjuvant medication to improve the efficacy of fluoxetine in child and adolescent depression. First, *lamotrigine* (Lamictal) is now FDA-approved for the treatment of resistant depression in adults. Studies on the use of lamotrigine as an augmenting agent in children and adolescents with resistant unipolar depression have not been reported, despite its use in treatment-resistant bipolar depression in young persons.

Second, the atypical antipsychotic drugs *aripiprazole* (Abilify) and *quetiapine* (Seroquel) have antidepressant properties and are FDA-approved as augmenting agents in adults with inadequate response to SSRI therapy. As aripiprazole and quetiapine are widely used in the treatment of various behavioral disorders in children and adolescents, it is likely that they will be studied as augmenting agents for child and adolescent depression only partially responsive or unresponsive to fluoxetine therapy. More on the use of these three medicines in child and adolescent depression should be forthcoming.

Complementary Treatments. Parslow and coworkers (2008) reviewed evidence of efficacy of complementary *and self-help treatments* for depression in children and adolescents. Relevant evidence was available for glutamine, S-adenosylmethionine, St John's wort, vitamin C, omega-3 fatty acids, light therapy, massage, art therapy, bibliotherapy, distraction techniques, exercise, and relaxation therapy and sleep deprivation. However, the evidence was limited and generally of poor quality. The only treatment with reasonable supporting evidence was *light therapy* for winter depression.

Antidepressants and Suicidal Ideation

The issue of potential suicidal ideation and behaviors (but rarely completed suicides) has become so contentious that a *PubMed* search[2] by this author in 2013 using the two words "antidepressant" and "suicide" returned over 12,892 separate research article "hits" in the medical literature. Some points follow:

• In 2002, 264 children and adolescents ages 5–14 years died by suicide in the United States, the fifth leading cause of death in this age group. The FDA report linked many of these deaths to SSRI treatment. Based on this finding [regarding SSRI use and the possibility of drug-caused increases in suicidal ideation (Gibbons et al., 2007)] the FDA

---

[2] The medical literature can be accessed at www.ncbi.nlm.gov/sites/entrez or more simply by typing *PubMed* on an Internet search engine.

published a warning in 2003 and required a "black box" warning in 2005. This well-intended warning (to reduce suicide deaths presumably caused by SSRI antidepressants), resulted in reductions in SSRI prescriptions for depression (Libby et al., 2009).

- Unexpectedly, the reduction in antidepressant use (as a result of FDA warnings) resulted not only in reduced SSRI prescriptions, but a possible increase in suicides (Gibbons et al., 2007). This indicated that perhaps SSRI therapy was indeed effective in the long-term treatment of depression and an overall reduction in suicides.
- Vitiello and coworkers (2009) noted that most suicidal events occurred in the context of persistent depression and insufficient improvement without evidence of medication-induced behavioral activation as a precursor. Severity of self-rated suicidal ideation and depressive symptoms predicted emergence of suicidality during treatment.
- As discussed above, adding CBT to fluoxetine therapy enhances the safety of medication therapy.
- It is now generally conceded that antidepressant therapy reduces suicide risk *in adults* by reducing depression severity. In children and adolescents, there is a strong association between depression severity and suicide risk. Fluoxetine therapy is not related to suicide risk (Gibbons et al., 2012).

> Since there is continuing controversy over the use of antidepressants in children and adolescents and the FDA maintains a black box warning about increased risk of suicide when antidepressants are prescribed to children and adolescents, it is important for the prescriber to provide all of the available information to the patient and their caregivers so that they may make an informed decision about chosing treatments. Clearly, for severe depression, the risk of initially increasing suicidal thought/behaviors may be less than the eventual benefit to the child/adolescent in reducing their depression and decreasing those suicidal thoughts/behaviors with continued treatment. For more minor levels of depression, the risk/benefit analysis may favor nonpharmacological interventions. If the choice is made to treat the child/adolescent with antidepressant medication, then the prescriber would be wise to clearly document their decision process and the risk/benefit analysis; the consent of the parents/caregiver and assent of the child/adolescent; the safety plan, and to closely monitor the response to the medication with frequent phone calls and office visits initially. It would also be important to document the education of the family on the signs/symptoms of worsening depression and early signs of suicidal thought/behaviors and what to do if these are detected.

Considering the above material, we offer the following for consideration:

Guidelines for Adolescent Depression for Primary Care (GLAD-PC)

In 2007, clinical practice guidelines were published to assist primary care physicians in the treatment of adolescent depression (Cheung et al., 2007; Zuckerbrot et al., 2007). These guidelines emphasize identification of youth at risk, assessment procedures, patient and family psychoeducation, community links, and establishment of a safety plan. They make specific recommendations for collaborative care between prescriber and therapist. These guidelines are essential reading for all who care for these patients.

Thapar and coworkers (2012) present a readable and logical introduction to the treatment of depression in adolescence, emphasizing much of what has been written above.

Calls for Widespread Screening for Youth at Risk

The prevalence of current or recent depression among children is 3 percent and among adolescents is 6 percent. Lifetime prevalence in adolescents may be as high as 20 percent. Child- and adolescent-onset depression is associated with persistent sadness, social isolation, increased risk of death by suicide, suicide attempts, recurrent depression in young adulthood, early pregnancy, poor school and occupational performance, and impaired work, social, and family functioning during young adulthood. Mass screening in schools and primary care offices may help identify missed cases and increase the proportion of depressed youth who might receive appropriate care, hopefully to help prevent the otherwise disastrous long-term effects of untreated depression. Of note, the majority of depressed youth today do not receive any type of treatment, despite the availability of depression-screening tools that are feasible for use in school and clinical settings. In a follow-up, the US Preventive Services Task Force (2009b) issued a call to "screen adolescents (12–18 years of age) for major depressive disorder when systems are in place to ensure accurate diagnosis, psychotherapy (cognitive-behavioral or interpersonal), and follow-up." They further stated that "the current evidence is insufficient to warrant a recommendation to screen children (7–11 years of age) for major depressive disorder" (p. 1223).

Table 15.4 summarizes these recommendations. As more data concerning the efficacy of treatment of younger children accumulates, further recommendations will undoubtedly follow.

Medications for Treating Anxiety Disorders

Anxiety disorders are common in children and cause substantial impairment in school, in family relationships, and in social functioning. Such disorders also predict adult anxiety disorders and major depression. Efficacious treatments are available; however, anxiety disorders in childhood remain underrecognized and undertreated, often being misdiagnosed as ADHD or depression. The prevalence of any anxiety disorder in children and adolescents ranges in various studies from 6.0 percent to as high as 17.7 percent. A reasonable estimate is that about 13 percent of 15-year-olds meet diagnostic criteria for having an anxiety disorder. Bridge and coworkers (2007), in their meta-analysis of antidepressant efficacy, found considerable benefit when these drugs were used to treat both OCD and non-OCD anxiety disorders. Indeed, it is now generally agreed that psychotherapy and pharmacotherapy are effective in improving clinical impairments from anxiety disorders and maintaining these improvements (Kodish et al., 2011; Rynn et al., 2011).

A clinical practice parameter for the treatment of children and adolescents with anxiety disorders is available (Connolly et al., 2011). This practice parameter emphasizes treatment with a combination of pharmacotherapy and psychotherapy. With increasing recognition of childhood anxiety as a serious illness with potentially life-long consequences, interest has risen about the use of psychopharmacologic interventions. On the other hand, this has been accompanied by concern over potential over-diagnosis, overtreatment of youths (Correll et al., 2011), and potential for medication-induced suicidal thoughts or actual suicides. Regarding suicidality with SSRIs, anxiety alone does

Population	Adolescents (12–18 y)	Children (7–11 y)
Recommendation	Screen (when systems for diagnosis, treatment, and follow-up are in place)	No recommendation
	Grade B[b]	Grade I[c]
Risk assessment	Risk factors for major depressive disorder (MDD) include parental depression, having comorbid mental health or chronic medical conditions, and having experienced a major negative life event.	
Screening tests	The following screening tests have been shown to do well in teens in primary care settings: • Patient Health Questionnaire for Adolescents (PHQ-A) • Beck Depression Inventory—Primary Care version (BDI-PC)	Screening instruments perform less well in younger children.
Treatments	Among pharmacotherapies, fluoxetine, a selective serotonin reuptake inhibitor (SSRI), has been found efficacious. However, because of risk of suicidality, SSRIs should be considered only if clinical monitoring is possible. Various modes of psychotherapy, and pharmacotherapy combined with psychotherapy, have been found efficacious.	Evidence on the balance of benefits and harms of treatment of younger children is insufficient for a recommendation.

TABLE 15.4 Summary and recommendations from the U.S. Preventive Services Task Force (USPSTF) for broad screening of children and adolescents for depressive disorders[a]

[a] Also included are the listings of the USPSTF for risk assessment, screening tests, and treatments for depression.
[b] Grade "B" in the recommendation means that the USPSTF recommends the action. Also, there is high certainty that the net benefit is moderate or there is moderate certainty that the net benefit is moderate to substantial. The USPSTF suggests public health workers to offer or provide this service.
[c] The grade "I" means that there is insufficient evidence to assess the balances and harms of the service.

not appear to be a predictive factor; however, these medications can at the beginning of administration as monotherapy have pro-suicidal effects in vulnerable patients by increasing the intensity of already present suicide risk factors, such as dysphoria, impulsiveness, agitation, and so forth. If depression is suspected, appropriate diagnosis and interventions should be undertaken before SSRI treatment is initiated. Finally, anxiety disorders in youths often do not present as a single disorder; comorbidity is common and must be carefully sought (Kendall et al., 2010).

Generalized Anxiety Disorder (GAD), Separation Anxiety Disorder (SAD), and Social Phobia (SoP)

In clinical trials, GAD, SAD, and SoP are often grouped together because of the high degree of overlap in symptoms and the distinction from other anxiety disorders (e.g., obsessive-compulsive disorder). GAD, SAD, and SoP are characterized by excessive anxiety, worry, restlessness, fatigue, concentration difficulty, irritability, muscle tension, or sleep disturbances of 6 months duration or that cause functional disturbances. The child may experience tension, apprehension, need for reassurance, and negative self-image, and may have physical complaints. He or she may appear overly mature, perfectionistic, and sensitive to criticism. He or she may tend to seek reassurance for worries and self-doubt. Many of these youth with GAD, SAD, or SoP have a comorbid depressive disorder (the converse is also true), second anxiety disorder, or ADHD. GAD, SAD, and SoP have a high familial association: 40 percent of parents of children with GAD, SAD, or SoP have had the disorder themselves during their childhood.

Treatment of GAD, SAD, and SoP usually involves a combination of pharmacotherapy and psychotherapy (cognitive-behavioral therapy, social skills training, and exposure therapy). In 2008, Waldkup and coworkers, in a 12-week study, reported the effects of sertraline, CBT, and a combination of both on GAD, SAD, and SoP in 488 children and adolescents (7 to 17 years of age). The percentage of participants who were rated as much improved or very much improved (on the Clinical Global Impression-Improvement scale) were 80.7 percent for the combination therapy group, 59.7 percent for the CBT group, and 54.9 percent for the sertraline group, and 23.7 percent in the placebo drug group. Results on the Pediatric Anxiety Rating Scale were of similar magnitude (Figure 15.6).

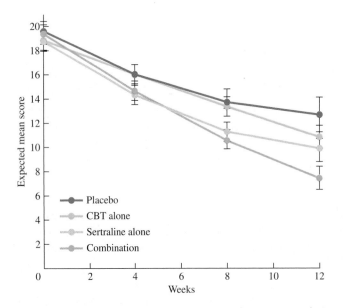

FIGURE 15.6   Scores on the Pediatric Rating Scale For Anxiety during 12 weeks of therapy with placebo, cognitive-behavioral therapy (CBT), *sertraline* (Zoloft) alone, or a combination of CBT and sertraline. Scores >13 are consistent with moderate levels of anxiety and a diagnosis of an anxiety disorder. Mean scores and confidence levels shown. [Data from Walkup et al. (2008), Figure 2.]

The authors concluded that CBT alone, sertraline alone, or the combination are all efficacious short-term treatments for childhood anxiety disorders. Combination therapy is most efficacious and "provides the best chance for a positive outcome." Any of the three treatments can be recommended, taking into consideration the family's treatment preferences, treatment availability, cost, and time burden.

Recommended starting doses for SSRI treatment of childhood anxiety are as follows: fluvoxamine 25 mg/day, fluoxetine 10 mg/day, and sertraline 25 mg/day, though lower starting doses can be used. Doses can be increased as needed and tolerated. Continuation treatment is recommended for about 1 year following remission in symptoms as some symptoms of anxiety persist, even among those children showing improvement after 12 weeks of treatment (Ginsburg et al., 2011). When discontinuing medication, one should choose a stress-free time of the year. If symptoms return, medication re-initiation should be seriously considered. As reviewed by Connolly and coworkers (2011):

> CBT has been extensively studied and has shown good efficacy in the treatment of child-hood anxiety disorders. A combination of CBT and medication may be required for moderate to severely impairing anxiety disorders and may improve functioning better than either intervention alone. SSRIs are currently the only medications that have consistently shown efficacy. Despite this, the availability of CBT in the community is limited. Current research is focusing on early identification of anxiety disorders in community settings, increasing the availability of evidence-based interventions, and modification of interventions for specific populations. (p. 99)

Obsessive-Compulsive Disorder

Obsessive-compulsive disorder (OCD) is now estimated as the fourth most common psychiatric disorder in adolescents, with an incidence of 2–3.6 percent (American Academy of Child & Adolescent Psychiatry, 2007). Pharmacotherapy with SSRIs is usually indicated as part of multimodal therapy. As stated in a recent POTS II study (Pediatric OCD Treatment Study II) (Franklin et al., 2011):

> Partial response to SSRIs is the norm and augmentation with short-term OCD-specific CBT provides additional benefit (Franklin et al, 2011); 68% of OCD youths receiving medication management plus CBT strategy were considered responders, which was superior to 34% in the CBT group and 30% in the medication-only group. (p. 1224)

This POTS II study concluded:

> addition of CBT by a psychologist to medication management compared with medication management alone resulted in a significantly greater response rate, whereas, augmentation of medication management with the addition of instructions in CBT by the psychiatrist did not.

Discouragingly, perhaps 30 percent of youth with OCD will be resistant to SSRI plus CBT therapy. Augmentation strategies are therefore necessary. Here, a focus has been on the use of atypical antipsychotics in such youth. In a study by Masi and coworkers (2010), 39 adolescents (mean age 12 years) were titrated to a final dose of 12 mg of aripiprazole per day and the drug was effective in more than 50 percent of patients resistant to continuing SSRI therapy. For recent analyses, see the Brown University Child and Adolescent Psychopharmacology Update (2011), and Pessina et al. (2009).

Posttraumatic Stress Disorder (PTSD)

Posttraumatic Stress Disorder (PTSD) is relatively common in children and adolescents, often as a result of early age traumas. Despite this, little has been reported on the efficacy of pharmacological interventions. A recent practice parameter for child and adolescent PTSD includes little on psychopharmacologic treatment. Strawn and coworkers (2010) performing a meta-analysis of published literature noted that the data do not support the use of SSRIs as first-line treatments for PTSD in children and adolescents. For example, sertraline (Zoloft) was ineffective in a placebo-controlled study in 131 youths (6–17 years) with PTSD (Robb et al., 2010). Limited evidence notes that atypical antipsychotics and several mood stabilizers may attenuate some symptoms, such as intrusive thoughts. Antiadrenergic agents (e.g., clonidine, guanfacine, prazosin) can reduce symptoms such as hyperarousal, intrusive symptoms, and impulsivity. Other medications may be needed to target various associated PTSD symptoms such as depression, affect instability, disruptive behavior, and dysregulated attachment.

Again, it must be stated that cognitive inhibitors are not indicated for use in children and adolescents. This greatly limits the use of benzodiazepines, lithium, and tricyclic antidepressants. Currently, it is thought that prolonged exposure therapy and CBT are more effective in treating PTSD than is an SSRI or no treatment (Rothbaum et al., 2012).

Panic Disorder

Little is known about the treatment of panic disorder (PD) in children and adolescents. A recent guideline on the subject in adults held little on pediatric PD (Stein et al., 2009). Small studies suggest SSRI therapy as appropriate medication. CBT and other therapies (e.g., exposure therapy) may be efficacious.

Medications for Treating Bipolar Disorder

Pediatric bipolar disorder is a chronic and debilitating psychiatric illness associated with many short-term and long-term complications, including poor academic and social performance, legal problems, and increased risk of suicide. In addition, it is often complicated by and confused with other serious psychiatric disorders such as ADHD, oppositional defiant disorder (ODD), conduct disorder (CD), and substance abuse disorders. Luby and Navsaria (2010) discuss bipolar prodromal symptoms and early markers for the eventual development of the disorder. Indeed, more than half of children with bipolar disorder experienced a prodromal period of greater than one year, and another 44 percent demonstrated a short-lasting, subacute prodrome. Symptoms included agitation, anxiety, appearing stubborn, bold and bossy behavior, decreased concentration, changes in sleep and mood, excitability, grandiosity, high energy, mood lability, and somatic complaints. Perhaps, early psychotherapeutic prevention programs might address these prodromes and guide early care. Galanter and coworkers (2009) identify these and other clinical characteristics that lead to a diagnosis of bipolar disorder in children. With a 40-fold increase in diagnosis over the last 15 years, it is commonly agreed that juvenile bipolar disorder is probably over diagnosed, with other disorders such as ADHD, conduct disorder, oppositional defiant disorder, severe mood dysregulation/disruptive mood dysregulation disorder, and temper dysregulation disorder with dysphoria all frequently misdiagnosed as bipolar disorder (Hauser and Correll, 2013).

In 1997, the American Academy of Child and Adolescent Psychiatry published the first clinical practice parameters for the assessment and treatment of bipolar disorder in children and adolescents. This report was updated in 2005 (Kowatch et al., 2005) and again in 2007 (McClellan et al., 2007). In the 2007 edition, the authors state:

> The presentation of bipolar disorder in youth, especially children, is often considered atypical compared with that of the classic adult disorder, which is characterized by distinct phases of mania and depression. Children who receive a diagnosis of bipolar disorder in community settings typically present with rapid fluctuations in mood and behavior, often associated with comorbid ADHD and disruptive behavioral disorders. Thus, at this time it is not clear whether the atypical form of the disorder represents the same illness. The question of diagnostic continuity has important treatment and prognostic implications. Although more controlled trials are needed, mood stabilizers and atypical antipsychotic agents are generally considered the first line of treatment. Behavioral and psychosocial therapies are also generally indicated for juvenile mania to address disruptive behavior problems and the impact on family and community functioning. (p. 107)

Early studies on medication for pediatric bipolar disorder primarily studied lithium and anticonvulsants such as valproic acid. Newer studies focus on new generation antipsychotic drugs. Geller and coworkers (2012), in a multicenter study, compared lithium, valproic acid, and risperidone in a trial termed Treatment of Early Age Mania (TEAM). The response rate for risperidone (68 percent) was significantly higher than the rate for lithium (36 percent) or valproic acid (24 percent). Quetiapine and aripiprazole, from other studies, are at least as effective as risperidone. These newer antipsychotic drugs differ mainly in their respective side effect profiles, particularly weight gain and metabolic abnormalities. Also, it is rarely a decision whether to treat or not to treat; when a youth is manic, the question is which medication to use rather than whether to use a medication (Goldstein, 2012). Risperidone, aripiprazole, quetiapine, and olanzapine are all FDA-approved for the treatment of bipolar youth, as well as for the treatment of disruptive and aggressive behaviors. Clinical trials with *ziprasidone* (Geodon) have been cancelled. Doey (2012) reviewed clinical trials with *aripiprazole* (Abilify). Findling, et al. (2013) recently published results of a 26 week study of aripiprazole in 210 youths (10–17 years old) with bipolar I with or without psychotic features. Joshi and coworkers (2013) recently reported on the efficacy of paliperidone. Pathak and coworkers (2013) reported on the efficacy of quetiapine.

While the use of valproic acid has been decreasing in youth with bipolar disorder, the use of *lamotrigine* (Lamictal) has been increasing (Tran et al., 2012). Biederman and coworkers (2010) demonstrated the efficacy of lamotrigine in a 12-week, open study in 39 children with bipolar disorder. Skin rashes did occur in some children, but resolved with cessation of drug treatment. Interestingly, lamotrigine use in pediatric bipolar disorder is associated with cognitive improvements, especially in the areas of working and verbal memory (Pavuluri et al., 2010).

SSRI antidepressant therapy is generally discouraged in pediatric bipolar disorder. Occasionally a SSRI might be used following mood stabilization with a mood stabilizer and if depression persists.

Wozniak and coworkers (2007) demonstrated that a high eicosopentanoic acid (EPA) omega-3 fatty acid supplement was effective for children with ADD, ADHD, bipolar disorder, and other educational and behavioral problems. The OmegaBrite D supplement of omega-3 fatty acids was evaluated for efficacy and safety over an 8-week period in 20 boys and girls (ages 6 to 17 years) with bipolar disorder. Half of the youths experienced a rapid 30 percent reduction in symptoms in the absence of side effects.

Medications for Treating Psychotic Disorders

Schizophrenia and its related conditions are considered quite rare in children, and when it occurs it presents significant challenges to clinicians. Early detection and treatment of young persons at risk for psychosis is regarded as a promising strategy in fighting the devastating consequences of psychotic disorders (Schimmelmann et al., 2013). Guidelines for treatment are urgently needed (Pagsberg, 2013; Starling et al., 2013). About one in three patients with schizophrenia develops symptoms of psychosis between the ages of 10 and 20 years. Since childhood and adolescent schizophrenia are generally associated with a poor long-term outcome, effective treatments are needed for children and adolescents with psychotic disorders or, more hopefully, who are in a prodromal phase that precedes first-episode psychosis.

Atypical antipsychotics are currently first-line treatments for early onset psychosis and schizophrenia spectrum disorders. Crespo-Facorro and coworkers (2013) compared aripiprazole, ziprasidone, and quetiapine in a short (6-week) trial in first-episode psychosis. Quetiapine was perhaps less effective. Younis and coworkers (2013) reported on the use of paliperidone for the treatment of adolescent schizophrenia. This area of research is expected to rapidly expand.

Amminger and coworkers (2010) studied the effects of omega-3 polyunsaturated fatty acids (1.2 grams/day in 81 adolescents and young adults, 13–25 years of age) with subthreshold psychosis and at ultra-high risk of psychotic disorder. A 12-week treatment period was followed by a 40-week monitoring period. At cessation of monitoring (12 months), 2 of 41 individuals (4.9 percent) in the omega-3 group and 11 of 40 (27.5 percent) in the placebo group had transitioned to psychotic disorder. The authors concluded that omega-3 fatty acid treatment markedly reduced the risk of progression to psychotic disorder and "may offer a safe and efficacious strategy for indicated prevention in young people with subthreshold psychotic states" (p. 146). Finally, Gracious and coworkers (2012) note that vitamin D deficiency is highly prevalent in adolescents with psychotic disorders. No doubt both omega-3s and vitamin D will be subject to further investigation.

STUDY QUESTIONS

1. What is meant by an "off-label" use of a drug?

2. Why are psychotherapeutic drugs usually used "off-label" in children and adolescents?

3. Defend early therapeutic interventions in treating psychological disorders in children.

4. Which classes of psychotherapeutic drugs might be used to treat aggressive disorders in children and adolescents? Which might be of the most benefit?

5. Which classes of psychotherapeutic drugs might be useful in treating autism and other pervasive developmental disorders?

6. How might one of these classes be chosen over another?

7. Besides stimulant medications, what other classes of drugs might be considered for use in treating ADHD? Compare and contrast them with psychostimulants.

8. How does methylphenidate compare and contrast with cocaine?

9. Should depression in children be treated? Defend your answer.

10. Compare and contrast the tricyclic antidepressants and the SSRIs in childhood and adolescent depression.

11. What conditions might be comorbid with generalized anxiety disorder in children? How might this comorbidity affect therapy?

12. Compare and contrast the benzodiazepines and the SSRIs in the treatment of anxiety disorders in children and adolescents.

13. Compare and contrast the neuromodulator mood stabilizers and the atypical antipsychotics in the treatment of bipolar disorder in children and adolescents.

14. Discuss the relevant issues in the treatment of schizophrenia, schizoaffective disorder, and the prodromal phase of schizophrenia in children and adolescents.

REFERENCES

ACOG Committee on Practice Bulletins - Obstetrics (2008): "Use of Psychotropic Medications During Pregnancy and Lactation." *Obstetrics and Gynecology* 92: 1001–1020.

Advokat, C. (2010). "What are the Cognitive Effects of Stimulant Medications? Emphasis on Adults with Attention-Deficit/Hyperactivity Disorder" (ADHD). *Neuroscience and Biobehavioral Reviews* 34: 1256–1266.

Ahn, J. H., et al. (2011). "Escitalopram for the Treatment of Major Depressive Disorder in Youth." *Expert Opinion on Pharmacotherapy* 12: 2235–2244.

Alwan, S. and Friedman, J. M. (2009). "Safety of Selective Serotonin Reuptake Inhibitors in Pregnancy." *CNS Drugs* 23: 493–509.

American Academy of Child & Adolescent Psychiatry (2007). "Practice Parameter for the Assessment and Treatment of Children and Adolescents with Attention-Deficit-Hyperactivity Disorder." *Journal of the American Academy of Child & Adolescent Psychiatry* 46: 894–921.

American Academy of Child & Adolescent Psychiatry (2009). "Practice Parameter for the Assessment and Treatment of Children and Adolescents with Obsessive-Compulsive Disorder." *Journal of the American Association of Child & Adolescent Psychiatry* 51: 98–113.

American Academy of Child & Adolescent Psychiatry (2012). "Practice Parameter for the Assessment and Treatment of Children and Adolescents with Attention-Deficit-Hyperactivity Disorder." *Journal of the American Academy of Child & Adolescent Psychiatry* 46: 894–921.

American Academy of Pediatrics (2011a). "ADHD: Clinical Practice Guideline for the Diagnosis, Evaluation, and Treatment of Attention-Deficit/Hyperactivity Disorder in Children and Adolescents." *Pediatrics* 128: 1007–1021.

American Academy of Pediatrics (2011b). "Implementing the Key Action Statements: An Algorithm and Explanation for Process of Care for the Evaluation, Diagnosis, and Monitoring of ADHD in Children and Adolescents." *Pediatrics* 128: S11–S120.

Amminger, G. P., et al. (2010). "Long-Chain Omega-3 Fatty Acids for Indicated Prevention of Psychotic Disorders: A Randomized, Placebo-Controlled Trial." *Archives of General Psychiatry* 67: 146–154.

Banach, R., et al. (2010). "Long-Term Developmental Outcome of Children of Women with Epilepsy, Unexposed or Exposed Prenatally to Antiepileptic Drugs: A Meta-Analysis of Cohort Studies." *Drug Safety* 33: 73–79.

Barnard-Brak, L. and Brak, V. (2011). "Pharmacotherapy and Academic Achievement Among Children with Attention-Deficit Hyperactivity Disorder." *Journal of Child & Adolescent Psychopharmacology* 21: 597–603.

Belden, A. C., et al. (2012). "Relational Aggression in Children with Preschool-Onset Psychiatric Disorders." *Journal of the American Academy of Child and Adolescent Psychiatry* 51: 889–901.

Biederman, J., et al. (2010). "A Prospective Open-Label Trial of Lamotrigine Monotherapy in Children and Adolescents with Bipolar Disorder." *CNS Neuroscience & Therapeutics* 16: 91–102.

Bilodeau, M., et al. (2012). "Duloxetine in Adults with ADHD: A Randomized, Placebo-Controlled Pilot Study." *Journal of Attentional Disorders* 18: 169–175.

Brent, D. A., et al. (2008). "Switching to Another SSRI or to Venlafaxine With or Without Cognitive Behavioral Therapy for Adolescents with SSRI-Resistant Depression." *Journal of the American Medical Association* 299: 901–913.

Brent, D. A., et al. (2009). "Predictors of Spontaneously and Systematically Assessed Suicidal Adverse Events in the Treatment of SSRI-Resistant Depression in Adolescents (TORDIA) Study." *American Journal of Psychiatry* 166: 418–426.

Bridge, J., et al. (2007). "Clinical Responses and Risk for Reported Suicidal Ideation and Suicide Attempts in Pediatric Antidepressant Treatment: A Meta-Analysis of Randomized Controlled Trials." *Journal of the American Medical Association* 297: 1683–1696.

Bromley, R. L., et al. (2008). "Autism Spectrum Disorders Following *in utero* Exposure to Antiepileptic Drugs." *Neurology* 71: 1923–1924.

Brown University Child & Adolescent Psychopharmacology Update (2011). Adding full CBT shows Best Response in Pediatric SRI-partial Responders with OCD. *The Brown University Child & Adolescent Psychopharmacology Update* 13(11), November, 1–4.

Bufferd, S. J., et al. (2012). "Psychiatric Disorders in Preschoolers: Continuity from Ages 3 to 6." *American Journal of Psychiatry* 169: 1157–1164.

Bukstein, O. G., et al. (2009). "Does Switching from Oral Extended-Release Methylphenidate to the Methylphenidate Transdermal Patch Affect Health-Related Quality-of-Life and Medication Satisfaction for Children with Attention-Deficit/Hyperactivity Disorder?" *Child and Adolescent Psychiatry and Mental Health* 3:39.

Bukstein, O. G. and Head, J. (2012). "Guanfacine ER for the Treatment of Adolescent Attention-Deficit Hyperactivity Disorder. *Expert Opinion on Pharmacotherapy* 13: 2207–2213.

Bushe, C. J. and Savill, N.C. (2013). "Systematic Review of Atomoxetine Data in Childhood and Adolescent Attention-Deficit Hyperactivity Disorder 2009–2011: Focus on Clinical Efficacy and Safety." *Journal of Psychopharmacology* doi: 10.1177/0269881113478475

Byatt, N., et al. (2013). "Antidepressant Use in Pregnancy: A Critical Review Focused on Risks and Controversies." *Acta Psychiatrica Scandinavica* 127: 94

Bymaster, F. P., et al. (2012). "Pharmacological Characterization of the Norepinephrine and Dopamine Reuptake Inhibitor EB-1020: Implications for Treatment of Attention-Deficit/Hyperactivity Disorder." *Synapse* 66: 522–532.

CARE Study Group. (2008). "Maternal Caffeine Intake During Pregnancy and Risk of Fetal Growth Restriction: A Large Prospective Observational Study." *British Medical Journal* 337: a2332

Centers for Disease Control and Prevention (2013). "Mental Health Surveillance Among Children – United States, 2005–2011." Available at www.cdc.gov/mmwr/preview/mmwrhtml/su6202a1.htm?s_cid=su6202a1_w

Charach, A., et al. (2013). "Interventions for Preschool Children at High Risk for ADHD: A Comparative Effectiveness Review." *Pediatrics* 131, May 1, pp. e1584–e1604.

Chaudron, L. H. (2013). "Complex Challenges in Treating Depression During Pregnancy." *American Journal of Psychiatry* 170: 12–20.

Cherkasova, M., et al. (2013). "Developmental Course of Attention Deficit Hyperactivity Disorder and its Predictors." *Journal of the Canadian Academy of Child and Adolescent Psychiatry* 22: 47–54.

Cheung, A. H., et al. (2007). "Guidelines for Adolescent Depression in Primary Care (GLAD-PC): II. Treatment and Ongoing Management." *Pediatrics* 120: e1313–e1326.

Ching, H. and Pringsheim, T. (2012). "Aripiprazole for Autism Spectrum Disorders (ASD)." *Cochrane Database of Systematic Reviews* 16: CD009043.

Christensen, J., et al. (2013). "Prenatal Valproate Exposure and Risk of Autism Spectrum Disorders and Childhood Autism." *Journal of the American Medical Association* 309: 1696–1703.

Cohen, L. S. (2007). "Treatment of Bipolar Disorder During Pregnancy." *Journal of Clinical Psychiatry* 68 (Supplement 9): 4–9.

Cohen, L. S., et al. (2006). "Relapse of Major Depression During Pregnancy in Women Who Maintain or Discontinue Antidepressant Treatment." *Journal of the American Medical Association* 295: 499–507.

Connolly, S. D., et al. (2011). "Assessment and Treatment of Anxiety Disorders in Children and Adolescents." *Current Psychiatric Reports* 13, 99–110.

Cooper, W. O., et al. (2011). "ADHD Drugs and Serious Cardiovascular Events in Children and Young Adults." *New England Journal of Medicine* 365: 1896–1904.

Coppola, D., et al. (2007). "Evaluating the Postmarketing Experience of Risperidone Use During Pregnancy: Pregnancy and Neonatal Outcomes." *Drug Safety* 30: 247–264.

Correll, C. U., et al. (2011). "Developments in Pediatric Psychopharmacology: Focus on Stimulants, Antidepressants, and Antipsychotics." *Journal of Clinical Psychiatry* 72, 655–670.

Coskun, M., et al. (2012). "Phenomenology, Psychiatric Comorbidity and Family History in Referred Preschool Children with Obsessive-Compulsive Disorder." *Child & Adolescent Psychiatry and Mental Health* 6: 36–44.

Costello, E. J., et al. (2007). "Service Costs of Caring for Adolescents with Mental Illness in a Rural Community, 1993–2000." *American Journal of Psychiatry* 164: 36–42.

Crespo-Facorro, B., et al. (2013). "Aripiprazole, Ziprasidone, and Quetiapine in the Treatment of First-Episode Nonaffective Psychosis: Results of a 6-Week, Randomized, Flexible-Dose, Open-Label Comparison." *Journal of Clinical Psychopharmacology* 33: 215–220.

Curtis, F. R. and Fairman, K. A. (2008). "Switching Antidepressant Drug Therapy Helps Some Patients Some of the Time – What TORDIA, STAR*D, and Observational Research Taught Us About Resistant Depression." *Journal of Managed Care Pharmacy* 14:468–473.

Di Florio, A., et al. (2013). "Perinatal Episodes Across the Mood Disorder Spectrum." *JAMA Psychiatry* 70: 168–175.

Doey, T. (2012). "Aripiprazole in Pediatric Psychosis and Bipolar Disorder: A Clinical Review." *Journal of Affective Disorders* 138, Supplement: S15–S21.

Domino, M. E., et al. (2009). "Relative Cost-Effectiveness of Treatments for Adolescent Depression." *Journal of the American Academy of Child and Adolescent Psychiatry* 48: 711–720.

Donelly, C., et al. (2009). "Safety and Tolerability of Atomoxetine Over 3 to 4 Years in Children and Adolescents with ADHD." *Journal of the American Academy of Child & Adolescent Psychiatry* 48: 176–185.

Donovan, S. J., et al. (2000). "Divalproex Treatment for Youth with Explosive Temper and Mood Lability: A Double-Blind, Placebo-Controlled Crossover Design." *American Journal of Psychiatry* 157: 818–820.

Dougherty, L. R., et al. (2013). "Preschool Anxiety Disorders: Comprehensive Assessment of Clinical Demographic, Tempermental, Familial, and Life Stress Correlates." *Journal of Child and Adolescent Psychology* 42: 577–589.

Doyle, C. A. and McDougle, C. J. (2012). "Pharmacologic Treatments for the Behavioral Symptoms Associated with Autism Spectrum Disorders Across the Lifespan." *Dialogues in Clinical Neuroscience* 14: 263–279.

Eapen, V., et al. (2013). "Clinical Outcomes of an Early Intervention Program for Preschool Children with Autism Spectrum Disorder in a Community Group Setting." *BMC Psychiatry* 13: 3.

Eapen, V. and Crncec, R. (2012). "Strategies and Challenges in the Management of Adolescent Depression." *Current Opinions in Psychiatry* 25: 7–13.

Egger, H. (2010). "A Perilous Disconnect: Antipsychotic Drug Use in Very Young Children." *Journal of the American Academy of Child & Adolescent Psychiatry* 49: 3–6.

Einarson, A. and Boskovic, R. (2009). "Use and Safety of Antipsychotic Drugs During Pregnancy." *Journal of Psychiatric Practice* 15: 183–192.

Elbe, D. and Lalani, Z. (2012). "Review of the Pharmacotherapy of Irritability of Autism." *Journal of the Canadian Academy of Child & Adolescent Psychiatry* 21: 130–146.

Emslie, G. J., et al. (1997). "A Double-Blind, Randomized, Placebo-Controlled Trial of Fluoxetine in Children and Adolescents with Depression." *Archives of General Psychiatry* 54: 1031–1037.

Emslie, G. J., et al. (2007). "Long-Term, Open-Label Venlafaxine Extended-Release Treatment in Children and Adolescents with Major Depressive Disorder." *CNS Spectrums* 12: 223–233.

Emslie, G., et al. (2009). "Escitalopram in the Treatment of Adolescent Depression: A Randomized, Placebo-Controlled Multisite Trial." *Journal of the American Academy of Child & Adolescent Psychiatry* 48: 721–729.

Epstein, J. N., et al. (2010). "Attention-Deficit/Hyperactivity Disorder Outcomes for Children Treated in Community-Based Pediatric Settings." *Archives of Pediatric and Adolescent Medicine* 164: 160–165.

Ercan, E. S., et al. (2011). "Risperidone in the Treatment of Conduct Disorder in Preschool Children without Intellectual Disability." *Child and Adolescent Psychiatry and Mental Health* 5: 10.

Ercan, E. S., et al. (2012). "Aripiprazole in Children and Adolescents with Conduct Disorder: A Single-Center, Open-Label Study." *Pharmacopsychiatry* 45: 13–19.

Faraone, S. V., et al. (2012). "Dose Response Effects of Lisdexamfetamine Dimesylate Treatment in Adults with ADHD: An Exploratory Study." *Journal of Attention Disorders* 16: 118–127.

Faraone, S. V. and Glatt, S. J. (2010). "Effects of Extended-Release Guanfacine on ADHD Symptoms and Sedation-Related Events in Children with ADHD." *Journal of Attention Disorders* 13: 532–538.

Farmer, C. A., et al. (2011). "The Treatment of Severe Child Aggession (TOSCA) Study: Design Challenges." *Child and Adolescent Psychiatry and Mental Health* 5: 36–47.

Findling, R. L. (2008). "Atypical Antipsychotic Treatment of Disruptive Behavior Disorders in Children and Adolescents." *Journal of Clinical Psychiatry* 69 (Supplement 4): 9–14.

Findling, R. L., et al. (2012). "Double-Blind, Randomized, Placebo-Controlled, Long-Term Maintenance Study of Aripiprazole in Children with Bipolar Disorder." *Journal of Clinical Psychiatry* 73: 57–63.

Findling, R. L., et al. (2013). "Aripiprazole for the Treatment of Pediatric Bipolar Disorder: A 30-Week Randomized, Placebo-Controlled Study." *Bipolar Disorder* 15: 138–149.

Franklin, M. E., et al. (2011). Cognitive Behavior Therapy Augmentation of Pharmacotherapy in Pediatric Obsessive-Compulsive Disorder: The Pediatric OCD Treatment Study II (POTS II) Randomized Controlled Trial. *Journal of the American Medical Association*, 306, 1224–1232.

Freeman, M. P. (2007). "Bipolar Disorder and Pregnancy: Risks Revealed." *American Journal of Psychiatry* 164: 1771–1773.

Frye, M. A., et al. (2008). "Aripiprazole Efficacy in Irritability and Disruptive Aggressive Symptoms: Young Mania Rating Scale Line Analysis from Two, Randomized, Double-Blind, Placebo-Controlled Trials." *Journal of Clinical Psychopharmacology* 28: 243–245.

Gaffrey, M. S., et al. (2012). "Default Mode Network Connectivity in Children with a History of Preschool Onset Depression." *Journal of Child and Adolescent Psychiatry* 53: 964–972.

Galanter, C. A., et al. (2009). "Symptoms Leading to a Bipolar Diagnosis: A Phone Survey of Child and Adolescent Psychiatrists." *Journal of Child & Adolescent Psychopharmacology* 19: 641–647.

Geller, B., et al. (2012). "A Randomized Controlled Trial of Risperidone, Lithium, or Divalproex Sodium for Initial Treatment of Bipolar I Disorder, Manic or Mixed Phase, in Children and Adolescents." *Archives of General Psychiatry* 69: 515–528.

Gentle, S. (2008). "Infant Safety with Antipsychotic Therapy in Breast-Feeding: A Systematic Review." *Journal of Clinical Psychiatry* 69: 666–673.

Ghuman, J. K. and Ghuman, H. S. (2013). "Pharmacologic Intervention for Attention-Deficit Hyperactivity Disorder in Preschoolers: Is It Justified?" *Paediatric Drugs* 15: 1–8.

Gibbons, R. D., et al. (2006). "The Relationship between Antidepressant Prescription Rates and Rate of Early Adolescent Suicide." *American Journal of Psychiatry* 163: 1898–1904.

Gibbons, R. D., et al. (2007). Relationship Between Antidepressants and Suicide Attempts: An Analysis of the Veterans Health Administration Data Sets." *American Journal of Psychiatry* 164: 1044–1049.

Gibbons, R. D., et al. (2012). "Suicidal Thoughts and Behavior with Antidepressant Treatment." *Archives of General Psychiatry* 69: 580–587.

Gillies, D., et al. (2012). "Psychological Therapies for the Treatment of Post-Traumatic Stress Disorder in Children and Adolescents."*Cochrane Database of Systematic Reviews* 12: CD006726.

Ginsburg, G. S., et al. (2011). "Remission After Acute Treatment in Children and Adolescents with Anxiety Disorders: Findings from the CAMS." *Journal of Consulting and Clinical Psychology* 79: 806–813.

Gleason, M. M., et al. (2007). "Psychopharmacological Treatment for Very Young Children: Contexts and Guidelines." *Journal of the American Academy of Child & Adolescent Psychiatry* 46: 1532–1572.

Goldstein, B. I. (2012). "Pharmacologic Treatment of Youth with Bipolar Disorder: Where to Next?" *The Carlat Report: Child Psychiatry* 3(December): 1–12.

Gonzalez, S., et al. (2012). "Dopamine D_4 Receptor, But Not the ADHD-Associated $D_{4.7}$ Variant, forms Functional Heteromers with the Dopamine D_{2S} Receptor in the Brain." *Molecular Psychiatry* 17: 650–662.

Goodman, D. W. (2010). "Lisdexamfetamine Dimesylate (Vyvanse), a Prodrug Stimulant for Attention-Deficit Hyperactivity Disorder." *Pharmacy & Therapeutics* 35: 273–287.

Gould, M. S., et al. (2009). "Sudden Death and Use of Stimulant Medications in Youths." *American Journal of Psychiatry* 166: 992–1001.

Gracious, B. L., et al. (2012). "Vitamin D Deficiency and Psychotic Features in Mentally Ill Adolescents: A Cross-Sectional Study." *BMC Psychiatry* 12: 38.

Grahan-Bermann, S. A., et al. (2012). "The Impact of Intimate Partner Violence and Additional Traumatic Events on Trauma Symptoms and PTSD in Preschool-Aged Children." *Journal of Trauma and Stress* 25: 393–400.

Greenhill, L. L., et al. (2006). "Efficacy and Safety of Immediate-Release Methylphenidate Treatment for Preschoolers with ADHD." *Journal of the American Academy of Child & Adolescent Psychiatry* 45: 1284–1293.

Habel, L. A., et al. (2011) "ADHD Medicines and Risk of Serious Cardiovascular Events in Young and Middle-Aged Adults." *Journal of the American Medical Association* 306: 2673–2683.

Harty, S. C., et al. (2011). "The Impact of Conduct Disorder and Stimulant Medication on Later Substance Use in an Ethnically Diverse Sample of Individuals with Attention-Deficit/Hyperactivity Disorder in Childhood." *Journal of Child and Adolescent Psychopharmacology* 21: 331–339.

Hauser, M. and Correll, C. U. (2013). "The Significance of At-Risk or Prodromal Symptoms for Bipolar I Disorder in Children and Adolescents." *Canadian Journal of Psychiatry* 58: 22–31.

Hirshfeld-Becker, D. R., et al. (2007). "Clinical Outcomes of Laboratory-Observed Preschool Behavioral Disinhibition at Five-Year Follow-Up." *Biological Psychiatry* 62: 565–572.

Horst, P., et al. (2012). "Clomipramine Concentration and Withdrawal Symptoms in 10 Neonates." *British Journal of Clinical Pharmacology* 73: 295–302.

Hudson, J. L. and Dodd, H. E. (2012). "Informing Early Intervention: Preschool Predictors of Anxiety Disorders in Middle Childhood." *PLoS One* 7: e42359.

Humphreys, K. L. H., et al. (2013). "Stimulant Medication and Substance Use Outcomes." *JAMA Psychiatry* 70: 740–749.

Hunt, S., et al. (2008). "Topiramate in Pregnancy: Preliminary Experience from the UK Epilepsy and Pregnancy Register." *Neurology* 71: 272–276.

Jain, R., et al. (2011). "Clonidine Extended-Release Tablets for Pediatric Patients with Attention-Deficit/Hyperactivity Disorder." *Journal of the American Academy of Child & Adolescent Psychiatry* 50: 171–179.

Joshi, G., et al. (2012). "A Prospective Open-Label Trial of Quetiapine Monotherapy in Preschool and School Age Children with Bipolar Spectrum Disorder." *Journal of Affective Disorders* 136: 1143–1153.

Joshi, G., et al. (2013). "A Prospective Open-Label Trial of Paliperidone Monotherapy for the Treatment of Bipolar Spectrum Disorders in Children and Adolescents." *Psychopharmacology* 227: 449–458.

Kendall, P. C., et al. (2010). "Clinical Characteristics of Anxiety Disordered Youth." *Journal of Anxiety Disorders* 24: 360–365.

Kennard, B. D., et al. (2009). "Effective Components of TORDIA Cognitive-Behavioral Therapy for Adolescent Depression: Preliminary Findings." *Journal of Consulting and Clinical Psychiatry* 77: 1033–1041.

Khanzode, L. A., et al (2006). "Efficacy Profiles of Psychopharmacology: Divalproex Sodium in Conduct Disorder." *Child Psychiatry and Human Development* 37: 55–64.

Kieler, H., et al. (2011). "Selective Serotonin Reuptake Inhibitors During Pregnancy and Risk of Persistent Pulmonary Hypertension in the Newborn: Population Based Cohort Study from the Five Nordic Countries." *British Medical Journal* 12: 344.

Kirino, E. (2012). "Efficacy and Safety of Aripiprazole in Child and Adolescent Patients." *European Child and Adolescent Psychiatry* 21: 361–368.

Kiyatkin, E. A. (2013). "The Hidden Side of Drug Action: Brain Temperature Changes Induced by Neuroactive Drugs." *Psychopharmacology* 225: 765–780.

Kodish, I., et al. (2011). "Pharmacotherapy for Anxiety Disorders in Children and Adolescents." *Pediatric Clinics of North America* 58, 55–72.

Kousik, S. M., et al. (2012). "The Effects of Neurostimulant Drugs on Blood Brain Barrier Function and Neuroinflammation." *Frontiers in Pharmacology* 3: article 121.

Kowatch, R. A., et al. (2005). "Treatment Guidelines for Children and Adolescents with Bipolar Disorder: Child Psychiatric Workgroup on Bipolar Disorder." *Journal of the American Academy of Child & Adolescent Psychiatry* 44: 213–235.

Kratochvil, C. J., et al. (2011). "A Double-Blind, Placebo-Controlled Study of Atomoxetine in Young Children with ADHD." *Pediatrics* 127: e862–e868.

Kumar, R. (2008). "Approved and Investigational Uses of Modafinil: An Evidenced-Based Review." *Drugs* 68: 1803–1839.

Kumar, B., et al. (2012). "Drug Therapy in Autism: A Present and Future Perspective." *Pharmacological Reviews* 64: 1291–1304.

Larson, K., et al. (2011). "Patterns of Cormorbidity, Functioning, and Service Use for US Children with ADHD, 2007." *Pediatrics* 127: 462–470.

Lee, S. S., et al. (2011). "Prospective Association of Childhood Attention-Deficit/Hyperactivity Disorder (ADHD) and Substance Use and Abuse/Dependence: A Meta-Analytic Review." *Clinical Psychology Reviews* 31: 328–341.

Leggio, L., et al. (2011). "Preliminary Findings on the Use of Metadoxine for the Treatment of Alcohol Dependence and Alcoholic Liver Disease." *Human Psychopharmacology* 26: 554–559.

Lemonnier, E., et al. (2012). "A Randomised Controlled Trial of Bumetanide in the Treatment of Autism in Children." *Translational Psychiatry* 2: e202.

Libby, A. M., et al. (2009). "Persisting Decline in Depression Treatment after FDA Warnings." *Archives of General Psychiatry* 66: 633–639.

Loy, J. H., et al. (2012). "Atypical Antipsychotics for Disruptive Behavior Disorders in Children and Youths." *Cochrane Database of Systematic Reviews* 9: CD008559.

Luby, J. L. (2010). "The Use of Psychotropic Agents in Preschool Children: Issues in Practice, Research and Public Policy." *Child and Adolescent Psychopharmacology News* 14: Number 4, pp. 1–5.

Luby, J. L., et al. (2009a). "Preschool Depression: Homotypic Continuity and Course over 24 Months." *Archives of General Psychiatry* 66: 897–905.

Luby, J. L., et al. (2009b). "The Clinical Significance of Preschool Depression: Impairment in Functioning and Clinical Markers of the Disorder." *Journal of Affective Disorders* 112: 111–119.

Luby, J. L., et al. (2009c). "Preschool Bipolar Disorder." *Child and Adolescent Psychiatric Clinics of North America* 18: 391–403.

Luby, J. L., et al. (2012). "Maternal Support in Early Childhood Predicts Larger Hippocampal Volumes at School Age." *Proceedings of the National Academy of Sciences* 109: 2854–2859.

Luby, J. L. and Navsaria, N. (2010). "Pediatric Bipolar Disorder: Evidence for Prodromal States and Early Markers." *Journal of Child Psychology and Psychiatry* 51: 459–471.

Lynch, F. L., et al. (2011). "Incremental Cost-Effectiveness of Combined Therapy vs Medication Only for Youth with Selective Serotonin Reuptake Inhibitor-Resistant Depression: Treatment of SSRI-Resistant Depression in Adolescents Trial Findings." *Archives of General Psychiatry* 68: 253–262.

Mahajan, R., et al. (2012). "Clinical Practice Pathways for Evaluation and Medication Choice for Attention-Deficit/Hyperactivity Disorder Symptoms in Autism Spectrum Disorders." *Pediatrics* 130, Supplement 2: S125–S138.

Manor, I., et al. (2012). "A Randomized, Double-Blind, Placebo-Controlled, Multicenter Study Evaluating the Efficacy, Safety, and Tolerability of Extended-Release Metadoxine in Adults with Attention-Deficit/Hyperactivity Disorder." *Journal of Clinical Psychiatry* 73: 1517–1523.

March, J. S. and Vitiello, B. (2009). "Clinical Messages from the Treatment for Adolescents with Depression Study (TADS)." *American Journal of Psychiatry* 166: 1118–1123.

Marcus, R. N., et al. (2011). "Safety and Tolerability of Aripiprazole for Irritability in Pediatric Patients with Autistic Disorder: A 52-Week, Open-Label, Multicenter Study." *Journal of Clinical Psychiatry* 72: 1270–1276.

Marroun, H., et al. (2012). "Maternal Use of Selective Serotonin Reuptake Inhibitors, Fetal Growth, and Risk of Adverse Birth Outcomes." *Archives of General Psychiatry* 69: 706–714.

Masi, G., et al. (2010). "Aripiprazole Augmentation in 39 Adolescents with Medication-Resistant Obsessive-Compulsive Disorder." *Journal of Clinical Psychopharmacology* 30, 688–693.

McClellan, J., et al. (2007). "Practice Parameter for the Assessment and Treatment of Children and Adolescents with Bipolar Disorder." *Journal of the American Academy of Child & Adolescent Psychiatry* 46: 107–125.

Meador, K. J., et al. (2013). "Fetal Antiepileptic Drug Exposure and Cognitive Outcomes at Age 6 Years (NEAD Study): A Prospective Observational Study." *Lancet Neurology* 12: 244–252.

Meiri, G., et al. (2009). "Omega-3 Fatty Acid Treatment in Autism." *Journal of Child and Adolescent Psychopharmacology* 19: 449–451.

Merikangas, K., et al. (2010). "Prevalence and Treatment of Mental Disorders Among U.S. Children in the 2001–2004 NHANES." *Pediatrics* 125: 75–81.

Molina, B. S., et al. (2009). "The MTA at 8 Years: Prospective Follow-Up of Children Treated for Combined-Type ADHD in a Multisite Study." *Journal of the American Academy of Child & Adolescent Psychiatry* 48: 484–500.

Morrow, R. L., et al. (2012). "Influence of Relative Age on Diagnosis and Treatment of Attention-Deficit/Hyperactivity Disorder in Children." *Canadian Medical Association Journal* 184: 755–762.

MTA Cooperative Group (1999). "A 14-Month Randomized Clinical Trial of Treatment Strategies for Attention-Deficit/Hyperactivity Disorder." *Archives of General Psychiatry* 56: 1073–1086.

MTA Cooperative Group (2004). "National Institute of Mental Health Multimodal Treatment Study of ADHD Follow-Up: Changes in Effectiveness and Growth After the End of Treatment." *Pediatrics* 113: 762–769.

Nevels, R. M., et al. (2010). "Psychopharmacology of Aggression in Children and Adolescents with Primary Neuropsychiatric Disorders: A Review of Current and Potentially Promising Treatment Options." *Experimental and Clinical Psychopharmacology* 18: 184–201.

Newham, J. J., et al. (2008). "Birth Weight of Infants After Maternal Exposure to Typical and Atypical Antipsychotics: Prospective Comparison Study." *British Journal of Psychiatry* 192: 333–337.

Newport, D. J., et al. (2008a). "Lamotrigine in Breast Milk and Nursing Infants: Determination of Exposure." *Pediatrics* 122: e223–e231.

Newport, D. J., et al. (2008b). "Lamotrigine in Bipolar Disorder: Efficacy During Pregnancy." *Bipolar Disorder* 10: 432–436.

Nguyen, H. T., et al. (2009). "Teratogenesis Associated with Antibipolar Agents." *Advances in Therapeutics* 6: 281–294.

Nulman, I., et al. (2012). "Neurodevelopment of Children Following Prenatal Exposure to Venlafaxine, Selective Serotonin Reuptake Inhibitors, or Untreated Maternal Depression." *American Journal of Psychiatry* 169: 1165–1174.

Olfson, M., et al. (2010). "Trends in Antipsychotic Drug Use by Very Young, Privately Insured Children." *Journal of the American Academy of Child & Adolescent Psychiatry* 49: 13–23.

Olfson, M., et al. (2012). "Stimulants and Cardiovascular Events in Youth with Attention-Deficit/Hyperactivity Disorder." *Journal of the American Academy of Child & Adolescent Psychiatry* 51: 147–156.

Pagsberg, A.K. (2013). "Schizophrenia Spectrum and Other Psychotic Disorders." *European Child & Adolescent Psychiatry* 22, Supplement 1: 3–9.

Pappadopulos, E., et al. (2011). "Experts' Recommendations for Treating Maladaptive Aggression in Youth." *Journal of Child and Adolescent Psychopharmacology* 21: 505–515.

Parry, B. L. (2009). "Assessing Risk and Benefit: To Treat or Not to Treat Major Depression During Pregnancy with Antidepressant Medication." *American Journal of Psychiatry* 166: 512–514.

Parry, P. I. and Levin, E. C. (2012). "Pediatric Bipolar Disorder in an Era of 'Mindless Psychiatry'." *Journal of Trauma & Dissociation* 13: 51–68.

Parslow, R., et al. (2008). "Effectiveness of Complementary and Self-Help Treatments for Anxiety in Children and Adolescents." *Medical Journal of Australia* 17: 355–359.

Pathak, S., et al. (2013). "Efficacy and Safety of Quetiapine in Children and Adolescents with Mania Associated with Bipolar I Disorder: A 3-Week, Double-Blind, Placebo-Controlled Trial." *Journal of Clinical Psychiatry* 74: e100–109.

Pavuluri, M. N., et al. (2010). "Enhanced Working and Verbal Memory after Lamotrigine Treatment in Pediatric Bipolar Disorder." *Bipolar Disorder* 12: 213–220.

Pedersen, L. H., et al. (2009). "Selective Serotonin Reuptake Inhibitors in Pregnancy and Congenital Malformations: Population Based Cohort Study." *British Medical Journal* 339: b3569.

Pediatric OCD Treatment Study (POTS) Team (2004). "Cognitive-Behavior Therapy, Sertraline, and Their Combination for Children and Adolescents with Obsessive-Compulsive Disorder: The Pediatric OCD Treatment Study (POTS) Randomized Controlled Trial." *Journal of the American Medical Association* 292: 1969–1976.

Peng, M., et al. (2013). "Effects of Prenatal Exposure to Atypical Antipsychotics on Postnatal Development and Growth of Infants: A Case-Controlled, Prospective Study." *Psychopharmacology* 228: 577–584.

Pessina, E., et al. (2009). "Aripiprazole Augmentation of Serotonin Reuptake Inhibitors in Treatment-Resistant Obsessive-Compulsive Disorder: A 12-Week, Open-Label Preliminary Study." *International Clinical Psychopharmacology* 24: 265–269.

Pingault, J. B., et al. (2013). "Childhood Trajectories of Inattention, Hyperactivity and Oppositional Behaviors and Predictions of Substance Abuse/Dependence: A 15-Year Longitudinal Population-Based Study." *Molecular Psychiatry* 18: 806–812.

Posner, K., et al. (2007). "Clinical Presentation of Attention-Deficit/Hyperactivity Disorder in Preschool Children: The Preschoolers with Attention-Deficit/Hyperactivity Disorder Treatment Study (PATS)." *Journal of Child & Adolescent Psychopharmacology* 17: 547–562.

Prasad, S., et al. (2007). "A Multi-Centre, Randomized, Open-Label Study of Atomoxetine Compared with Standard Current Therapy in UK Children and Adolescents with Attention-Deficit/Hyperactivity Disorder." *Current Medical Research and Opinion* 23: 379–394.

Pringsheim, T. and Gorman, D. (2012). "Second-Generation Antipsychotics for the Treatment of Disruptive Behavior Disorders in Children: A Systematic Review." *Canadian Journal of Psychiatry* 57: 722–727.

Propper, L. and Orlik, H. (2011). "Pharmacotherapy of Severe Disruptive Behavioral Symptoms Associated with Autism." *Child & Adolescent Psychopharmacology News* 16 (3): 1–8.

Quintana, H., et al. (2007). "Fluoxetine Monotherapy in Attention-Deficit/Hyperactivity Disorder and Comorbid Non-Bipolar Mood Disorders in Children and Adolescents." *Child Psychiatry and Human Development* 37: 241–253.

Ramos, E., et al. (2008). "Duration of Antidepressant Use During Pregnancy and Risk of Major Congenital Malformations." *British Journal of Psychiatry* 19: 344–350.

Rao, U., et al. (2010). "Hippocampal Changes Associated with Early-Life Adversity and Vulnerability to Depression." *Biological Psychiatry* 67: 357–364.

Rapee, R. M. (2013). "The Preventative Effects of a Brief, Early Intervention for Preschool-Aged Children at Risk for Internalizing: Follow-up into Middle Adolescence." *Journal of Child and Adolescent Psychiatry* 54: 780–788.

Riddle, M. A., et al. (2013). "The Preschool Attention-Defecit/Hyperactivity Disorder Treatment Study (PATS) 6-Year Follow-Up." *Journal of the American Academy of Child & Adolescent Psychiatry* 52: 264–278.

Rifkin-Graboi, A., et al. (2013). "Prenatal Maternal Depression Associates with Microstructure of Right Amygdala in Neonates at Birth." *Biological Psychiatry*, 74: 837–844.

Robb, A. S., et al. (2010). Sertraline Treatment of Children and Adolescents with Posttraumatic Stress Disorder: A Double-Blind, Placebo-Controlled Trial. *Journal of Child and Adolescent Psychopharmacology* 20, 463–471.

Roca, A., et al. (2013). "Unplanned Pregnancy and Discontinuation of SSRIs in Pregnant Women with Previously Treated Affective Disorder." *Journal of Affective Disorders*, 150: 807–813.

Rothbaum, B. O., et al. (2012). "Early Intervention may Prevent the Development of Posttraumatic Stress Disorder: A Randomized Pilot Civilian Study with Modified Prolonged Exposure." *Biological Psychiatry* 72: 957–963.

Rynn, M., et al. (2011). Advances in Pharmacotherapy for Pediatric Anxiety Disorders. *Depression and Anxiety* 28, 76–87.

Sadowski, A., et al. (2013). "Pregnancy Outcomes Following Maternal Exposure to Second-Generation Antipsychotics Given with Other Psychotropic Drugs: A Cohort Study." *BMJ Open* 3: e003062.

Saxena, K., et al. (2006). "Divalproex Sodium Reduces Overall Aggression in Youth at High Risk for Bipolar Disorder." *Journal of Child and Adolescent Psychopharmacology* 16: 252–259.

Sayal, K., et al. (2009). "Binge Pattern of Alcohol Consumption During Pregnancy and Childhood Mental Health Outcomes: Longitudinal Population-Based Study." *Pediatrics* 123: e289-e296.

Scheffler, R. M., et al. (2009)."Positive Association Between Attention-Deficit/ Hyperactivity Disorder Medication Use and Academic Achievement During Elementary School." *Pediatrics* 123: 1273–1279.

Schelleman, H., et al. (2011). "Cardiovascular Events and Death in Children Exposed and Unexposed to ADHD Agents." *Pediatrics* 127: 1102–1110.

Scheltema, B. A. and deHaan, L. (2010). "Off-Label Second Generation Antipsychotics for Impulse Regulation Disorders: A Review." *Psychopharmacology Bulletin* 43: 45081.

Schimmelmann, B. G., et al. (2013). "The Significance of At-Risk Symptoms for Psychosis in Children and Adolescents." *Canadian Journal of Psychiatry* 58: 32–40.

Seida, J. C., et al. (2012). "Antipsychotics for Children and Young Adults: A Comparative Effectiveness Review." *Pediatrics* 129: e771-e784.

Shoval, G., et al. (2011). "Effectiveness and Safety of Citalopram in Hospitalized Adolescents with Major Depression: A Preliminary, 8-Week, Fixed-Dose, Open-Label, Prospective Study." *Clinical Neuropharmacology* 34: 182–185.

Smith, E. G. (2009). "Association Between Antidepressant Half-Life and the Risk of Suicidal Ideation or Behavior Among Children and Adolescents: Confirmatory Analysis and Research Implications." *Journal of Affective Disorders* 114: 143–148.

Sonuga-Barke, E., et al. (2013). "Nonpharmacological Interventions for ADHD: Systematic Review and Meta-Analysis of Randomized Controlled Trials of Dietary and Psychological Treatments." *American Journal of Psychiatry* 170: 275–289.

Sowell, E. R., et al. (2010). "Differentiating Prenatal Exposure to Methamphetamine and Alcohol versus Alcohol and Not Methamphetamine Using Tensor-Bases Brain Morphometry and Discriminant Analysis." *Journal of Neuroscience* 30: 3876–3885.

Starling, J., et al. (2013). "The Presentation of Early-Onset Psychotic Disorders." *Australian and New Zealand Journal of Psychiatry* 47: 43–50.

Stein, M. B., et al. (2009). "Practice Guideline for the Treatment of Patients with Panic Disorder, Second Edition." *American Journal of Psychiatry* 166, Supplement 2: 42–44.

Steiner, M. (2012). "Prenatal Exposure to Antidepressants: How Safe are They?" *American Journal of Psychiatry* 169: 1130–1133.

Stephansson, O., et al. (2013). "Selective Serotonin Reuptake Inhibitors During Pregnancy and Risk of Stillbirth and Infant Mortality." *Journal of the American Medical Association* 309: 48–54.

Stigler, K. A., et al. (2012). "Paliperidone for Irritability in Adolescents and Young Adults with Autistic Disorder." *Psychopharmacology* 223: 237–245.

Storch, E. A., et al. (2013). "The Effect of Cognitive-Behavioral Therapy versus Treatment as Usual for Anxiety in Children with Autism Spectrum Disorders: A Randomized, Controlled Trial." *Journal of the American Academy of Child & Adolescent Psychiatry* 52: 132–142.

Strawn, J. R., et al. (2010). Psychopharmacological Treatment of Posttraumatic Stress Disorder in Children and Adolescents: A Review. *Journal of Clinical Psychiatry* 71 (7), 932–941.

Suzuki, H., et al. (2013). "Structural-Functional Correlations Between Hippocampal Volume and Cortico-Limbic Emotional Responses in Depressed Children." *Cognitive, Affective, and Behavioral Neuroscience* 13: 135–151.

Tandon, M., et al. (2011). "Preschool Onset Attention-Deficit/Hyperactivity Disorder: Course and Predictors of Stability over 24 Months." *Journal of Child and Adolescent Psychopharmacology* 21: 321–330.

Thapar, A., et al. (2012). "Depression in Adolescence." *Lancet* 379: 1056–1067.

Toh, S., et al. (2013). "Prevalence and Trends in the Use of Antipsychotic Medications During Pregnancy in the U.S., 2001–2007: A Population-Based Study of 585,615 Deliveries." *Archives of Women's Mental Health* 16: 149–157.

Tomson, T. and Battino, D. (2009). "Teratogenic Effects of Antiepileptic Medications." *Neurology Clinics* 27: 993–1002.

Tran, A. R., et al. (2012). "National Trends in Pediatric Use of Anticonvulsants." *Psychiatric Services* 63: 1095–1101.

Treatment for Adolescents with Depression Study (TADS) Team (2004). "Fluoxetine, Cognitive-Behavioral Therapy, and Their Combination for Adolescents with Depression: Treatment for Adolescents with Depression Study (TADS) Randomized Controlled Trial." *Journal of the American Medical Association* 292: 807–820.

Treatment for Adolescents with Depression Study (TADS) Team, et al. (2009). "The Treatment for Adolescents with Depression Study (TADS): Outcomes over 1-Year of Naturalistic Follow-Up." *American Journal of Psychiatry* 166:1141–1149.

Tunnard, C., et al. (2014). "The Impact of Childhood Adversity on Suicidality and Clinical Course in Treatment-Resistant Depression." *Journal of Affective Disorders* 152: 122–130.

U.S. Preventive Services Task Force (2009a). "Counseling and Interventions to Prevent Tobacco-Caused Disease in Adults and Pregnant Women: U.S. Preventive Services Task Force Reaffirmation Recommendation Statement." *Annals of Internal Medicine* 150: 551–555.

U.S. Preventive Services Task Force (2009b). "Screening and Treatment for Major Depressive Disorder in Children and Adolescents: U.S. Preventive Services Task Force Recommendation Statement." *Pediatrics* 123: 1223–1228.

Upadhyaya, H. P., et al. (2013). "A Review of the Abuse Potential Assessment of Atomoxetine: A Nonstimulant Medication for Attention-Deficit Hyperactivity Disorder." *Psychopharmacology* 226: 189–200.

Viguera, A. C., et al. (2007a): "Risk of Recurrence in Women with Bipolar Disorder During Pregnancy: Prospective Study of Mood Stabilizer Discontinuation." *American Journal of Psychiatry* 164: 1817–1824.

Viguera, A. C., et al. (2007b). "Lithium in Breast Milk and Nursing Infants: Clinical Implications." *American Journal of Psychiatry* 164: 342–345.

Vitiello, B., et al. (2007). "Effectiveness of Methylphenidate in the 10-Month Continuation Phase of the Preschoolers with Attention-Deficit/Hyperactivity Disorder Treatment Study (PATS)." *Journal of Child & Adolescent Psychopharmacology* 17: 593–604.

Vitiello, B. (2009). "Combined Cognitive-Behavioral Therapy and Pharmacotherapy for Adolescent Depression: Does it Improve Outcomes Compared with Monotherapy?" *CNS Drugs* 23: 271–280.

Vitiello, B., et al. (2009). "Suicidal Events in the Treatment of Adolescents with Depression Study (TADS). *Journal of Clinical Psychiatry* 70: 741–747.

Vitiello, B., et al. (2011). "Long-Term Outcome of Adolescent Depression Initially Resistant to SSRI Treatment." *Journal of Clinical Psychiatry* 72: 388–396.

Volkow, N. D., et al. (2009). "Effects of Modafinil on Dopamine and Dopamine Transporters in Male Human Brain: Clinical Implications." *Journal of the American Medical Association* 301: 1148–1154.

Walkup, J. T., et al. (2008). "Cognitive Behavioral Therapy, Sertraline, or a Combination in Childhood Anxiety." *New England Journal of Medicine* 359: 2753–2766.

Walkup, J. T. and the American Association of Child & Adolescent Psychiatry (2009). "Practice Parameter on the Use of Psychotropic Medication in Children and Adolescents." *Journal of the American Association of Child & Adolescent Psychiatry* 48: 961–973.

Weems, C. F. and Scheeringa, M. S. (2013). "Maternal Depression and Treatment Gains Following a Cognitive Behavioral Intervention for Posttraumatic Stress in Preschool Children." *Journal of Anxiety Disorders* 27: 140–146.

Wigal, S. B., et al. (2013). "NWP06, An Extended-Release Oral Suspension of Methylphenidate, Improved Attention-Deficit Hyperactivity Disorder Symptoms Compared with Placebo in a Laboratory Classroom Study." *Journal of Child and Adolescent Psychopharmacology* 23: 3–10.

Wisner, K. L., et al. (2009). "Major Depression and Antidepressant Treatment: Impact on Pregnancy and Neonatal Outcomes." *American Journal of Psychiatry* 166: 557–566.

Wisner, K. L., et al. (2013). "Does Fetal Exposure to SSRIs or Maternal Depression Impact Infant Growth?" *American Journal of Psychiatry* 170: 485–493.

Wozniak, J., et al. (2007). "Omega-3 Fatty Acid Monotherapy for Pediatric Bipolar Disorder: A Prospective Open-Label Trial." *European Neuro-Psychopharmacology* 17: 440–447.

Yonkers, K. A., et al. (2009). "The Management of Depression During Pregnancy: A Report from the American Psychiatric Association and the American College of Obstetricians and Gynecologists." *Obstetrics and Gynecology* 114: 703–713.

Younis, I. R., et al. (2013). "An Integrated Approach for Establishing Dosing Recommendations: Paliperidone for the Treatment of Adolescent Schizoprenia." *Journal of Clinical Psychopharmacology* 33: 152–156.

Zoega, H., et al. (2012). "Age, Academic Performance, and Stimulant Prescribing for ADHD: A Nationwide Cohort Study." *Pediatrics* 130: 1012–1018.

Zuckerbrot, R. A., et al. (2007). "Guidelines for Adolescent Depression in Primary Care (GLAD-PC): I. Identification, Assessment, and Initial Management." *Pediatrics* 120: e1299-e1312.

Zuvekas, S. H. and Vitiello, B. (2012). "Stimulant Medication Use Among U.S. Children: A Twelve-Year Perspective." *American Journal of Psychiatry* 169: 160–166.

Chapter 16

Geriatric Psychopharmacology

This chapter will review how the drugs discussed in earlier chapters are applied to the treatment of disorders and disruptive behavior in geriatric populations including treatment of: depression, anxiety disorders, behavioral agitation and aggression, Parkinson's disease, and Alzheimer's disease. First, however, we present several general principles concerning the actions and effects of psychoactive drugs administered to elderly patients:

- Lower doses of medication are often as effective in the elderly as higher doses in younger people.
- When initiating drug therapy in the elderly, it is wise to "start low and go slow."
- Elimination half-lives are often prolonged in the elderly, sometimes to about twice as long as half-lives in younger people due to pharmacokinetic changes that occur with aging such as decreased liver enzyme activity. These physiological changes require adjustment of total daily doses and frequency of dosing of many medications.
- Sedative-hypnotic drugs, especially the long-half-life benzodiazepines, can be quite "dementing" in the elderly, causing marked and often prolonged cognitive impairment presenting as memory deficiencies.
- Sedative-hypnotic drugs can also induce psychomotor incoordination, resulting in an increased incidence of falls, altered driving behaviors, and so on.
- Depression and comorbid anxiety and depression are common in the elderly and need to be addressed and treated.
- Psychological therapies can be used effectively to treat anxiety disorders, sleep disorders, and other psychological disorders for which drugs are often prescribed.
- Inappropriate drug use in the elderly is a common problem with potentially tragic consequences.
- Substance abuse in the elderly often goes undetected and therefore untreated leading to broader psychological, psychiatric, and physiological morbidities.

Inappropriate Drug Use in the Elderly

The elderly are frequently prescribed medication that they do not need or that cause them significant problems either because of extensions of expected pharmacological effects or through adverse interactions with other medications. Inappropriate medication use in the elderly is a major functional and safety issue and may cause a substantial proportion of drug-related hospital or care-center admissions (Laroche et al., 2007). While only 13 percent of Americans are aged 65 years or older, this group represents the largest per capita consumers of prescription medications. A recent survey of 3,500 community-dwelling adults found that over 29 percent take five or more prescription medications, 42 percent at least one or more over-the-counter medications, and 49 percent at least one or more dietary supplements (Page et al., 2010 and references therein). To help bring attention to the inappropriate drug use in the elderly, M. H. Beers in 1997 developed specific criteria for inappropriate use, which included a list of drugs that were either ineffective or posed unnecessarily high risks for people over 65 years of age. This list is updated periodically and the most recent version (2012) can be found on the American Geriatrics Society Web site: http://www.americangeriatrics.org.

In addition, workers in different health care systems have developed modifications of the Beers criteria designed to fit their specific population. Examples include: the Medication Appropriateness Index (Steinman et al., 2006) and the HEDIS measures. The National Committee for Quality Assurance (NCQA) publishes the Healthcare Effectiveness Data and Information Set (HEDIS) and incorporates the Beers criteria into one of its quality measures: Potentially Harmful Drug-Disease Interactions in the Elderly. This quality measure is updated in concert with updates in the Beers criteria and can be found on the NCQA Web site: http://www.ncqa.org. There is also the Zhan modification of the Beers criteria for community dwelling elderly (Barnett et al., 2006); and the Improved Prescribing in the Elderly Tool (Ryan et al., 2009). All attempt to identify medicines commonly considered of more risk than benefit to the elderly. All agree that the extent of inappropriate prescription use is common, with a rate between 20 and 40 percent. In elderly patients taking eight or more medications, the incidence of inappropriate drug use rises to well over 60 percent. Among the psychoactive medicines, long-acting benzodiazepines are most commonly inappropriately prescribed, followed by drugs with anticholinergic side effects (for example, tricyclic antidepressants), then antihistamines, skeletal muscle relaxants, and opioid narcotics. For example, looking at the use of benzodiazepines in the elderly, studies have found that continued use of these agents can increase the subsequent risk of dementia by 50 percent (Billioti de Gage et al., 2010). Another problematic situation is concomitant use of two or more psychotropic medicines of the same therapeutic class. Inappropriate drug use can lead to suboptimal care that is not consistent with evidence-based clinical practice.

All the lists of criteria for inappropriate drug use in the elderly recommend avoiding drugs that produce *cognitive inhibition* (with drug-induced dementia as the most severe manifestation), *unwanted sedation* (leading to falls and hip fractures), or *bizarre behaviors and/or drug-induced delirium*. Tricyclic antidepressants (or other drugs with anticholinergic properties), and sedating antihistamines are prominent drugs of concern along with the benzodiazepines and opiates (Tannenbaum et al., 2012). Indeed, discontinuing such medications can lead to improvements in psychomotor and cognitive functioning, including memory and attention (Carnahan, 2010; Nishtala et al., 2009; Tsunoda et al., 2010).

Control of Agitated and Aggressive Behaviors in the Elderly

Atypical antipsychotic medications (see Chapter 11) had become the standard of care for behavioral and psychological symptoms of dementia (BPSD). These medicines were thought to control agitated and aggressive behaviors in the elderly, especially residents of care centers. However, in 2005, the Food and Drug Administration (FDA) issued a public health advisory warning indicating a 1.7-fold risk of all-cause mortality from these medicines compared to placebo. The FDA subsequently issued a black box warning on the use of any antipsychotic, first, second, or third generation, for the treatment of agitation and psychosis in dementia patients. This advisory has been controversial because other studies have failed to verify any increased risk of death (Elie et al., 2009; Simoni-Wastila et al., 2009). But, other studies confirm some degree of increased risk of mortality in individuals with dementia who are treated with antipsychotic medication (Meeks, 2010); the risk may vary depending on the drug used (greater for haloperidol and least for quetiapine) (Huybrechts et al., 2012; Kales et al., 2012); for dementia patients treated with antipsychotic drugs, the risk for myocardial infarction (MI) was found to be double that of the rate in individuals not receiving APs (Pariente et al., 2012). Despite this advisory and controversy, the use of atypical antipsychotics to treat elderly persons with BPSD continues, especially in long-term care settings (Connelly et al., 2009). But, Dorsey and coworkers (2010) reported that this use of atypical antipsychotic medicines is decreasing in the elderly with dementia. This has been confirmed through additional studies that attribute the decline to the FDA's initial healthcare warning followed by the black box warning (Kales et al., 2011; Ventimiglia et al., 2010). In a national survey of prescriptions within nursing home facilities, Briesacher et al. (2013) found that during 2009 to 2010, 22 percent of residents received at least one antipsychotic medication during their stay; of the antipsychotics prescribed the two most frequently administered were quetiapine and risperidone, accounting for 55.5 percent of all of the antipsychotics prescribed (Table 16.1). The 22 percent figure is a decrease from 2006 statistics indicating that 29 percent of nursing facility residents received at least one antipsychotic medication (Chen et al., 2010).

Another factor in the declining use of antipsychotic medications in the elderly in nursing facilities is an initiative by the federal Centers for Medicare and Medicaid Services (CMS) to target excessive use of these drugs in the absence of an appropriate diagnosis or documentation of medical necessity. This initiative called the ((Partnership to Improve Dementia Care)) began in May of 2012 and involves special training for nursing facility staff on humane methods for addressing BPSD; publishing data on use of antipsychotics on the Nursing Home Compare public Web site; revising staffing patterns, activities, and pain management detection and treatment; and use of antipsychotics will be part of the CMS quality review of nursing facilities.

These medicines were proposed to relieve various core symptoms that arise in the course of dementia (Omelan 2006):

- Agitation (pacing, wandering, restlessness, inability to sit long enough to eat)
- Aggression (verbal and physical), which might be directed at staff or other residents
- Physical resistance and noncompliance with care

TABLE 16.1 Most Commonly Prescribed Antipsychotic Medications in Nursing Homes

Generic drug name	Number of patients prescribed drug	Percent of total prescriptions
Quetiapine fumarate	1,356,223	31.1
Risperidone	1,061,897	24.4
Olanzapine	570,453	13.1
Haloperidol	402,077	9.2
Aripiprazole	347,900	8.0
Clozapine	232,125	5.3
Ziprasidone	138,881	3.2
Chlorpromazine	65,159	1.5
Fluphenazine	54,867	1.3
All others[a]	109,141	2.9

[a]Includes paliperidone, perphenazine, thiothixene, loxapine, trifluoperazine, combination of olanzapine and fluoxetine, asenapine, lloperidone, molindone, pimozine, trilafon, loxitane, and mesoridazine.
Adapted from B. A. Briesacher et al., "Antipsychotic Use Among Nursing Home Residents," *Journal of the American Medical Association* 309 (2013): 440–442.

- Psychosis (hallucinations, delusions)
- Depressive symptoms (apathy, lack of interest)
- Inappropriate sexual behaviors (verbal and physical)
- Sleep disturbances (day/night reversal)

In some cases, although agitation and aggression apparently may be reduced by administering an atypical antipsychotic drug, there is little evidence of drug efficacy against the core symptoms of dementia. According to Omelan (2006), certain behaviors should not be expected to improve (wandering, pacing, entering rooms uninvited, disruptive vocalizations). Initially, *risperidone* (Risperdal) and *olanzapine* (Zyprexa) were used most frequently, but *quetiapine* (Seroquel) has rapidly gained favor, perhaps because quetiapine seems to cause less undesired weight gain and has less propensity to induce type 2 diabetes. Unfortunately, Paleacu and coworkers (2008) reported results from a six-week, double-blind, placebo-controlled study of 44 patients with dementia and BPSD showing that quetiapine, in quite large doses, was only modestly more effective than placebo in reducing behavioral symptoms. However, a few patients showed a positive and sustained response. In another study of risperidone in the treatment of agitation and psychosis in patients with AD, Devanand et al. (2012) found that patients had a modest reduction in target symptoms, but this was not maintained and only some of the patients responded. Those who responded after 16 weeks of treatment were randomized to: continue treatment with risperidone for 32 weeks; or continue treatment with risperidone for 16 weeks and switched to placebo for 16 weeks; or switched to placebo for 32 weeks. The results indicated that for those that derived some benefit from risperidone, there was an increase in relapse rates for those switched to placebo compared to those continuing with risperidone treatment, indicating that the risperidone was of some benefit.

Streim and coworkers (2008) reported on the efficacy of *aripiprazole* (Abilify) in the treatment of psychosis in nursing home patients with Alzheimer's disease. The drug did not confer specific benefits for the treatment of psychotic symptoms, but BPSD symptoms—including agitation, anxiety, and depression—were significantly improved, with a low risk of side effects. De Deyn et al. (2013) also found some efficacy of aripiprazole for treatment of psychosis and agitation in patients with AD, although the effect was modest and the drug produced a high degree of sedation. They recommend only using the drug in selected patient populations who are resistant to nonpharmacological treatment and/or have persistent, severe psychotic symptoms and/or agitation leading to significant morbidity. Although aripiprazole is capable of reducing anxiety and agitation, it can also produce these same symptoms as side effects in about 8 to 10 percent of patients at doses of about 10 milligrams per day (Coley et al., 2009).

Despite these positive findings of the efficacy of SGAs on BPSD, not all studies have shown them to be beneficial. Jin and colleagues (2013) conducted a study in which the subjects and their treatment providers could choose to be assigned to one of several SGAs; despite this flexibility in choosing treatments, they found a high discontinuation rate of SGAs when used to treat older individuals with dementia and that one half of the patients remained on the study medication for less than 6 months; in addition, there was a high incidence of metabolic syndrome (36 percent), and serious (24 percent) and nonserious (51 percent) adverse events; and there was no improvement in psychotic symptoms. The authors point out that the overall risk-benefit ratio for the atypical antipsychotics in patients over age 40 was not favorable, regardless of diagnosis or drug; but they caution that the results do not suggest that SGAs should not be used in older patients with psychosis, only that there are no safe and effective treatment alternatives and short-term use may be necessary for controlling severe psychotic symptoms in some patients.

Therefore, at this point, despite the FDA's public health advisory, an atypical antipsychotic remains a cautious optional choice for the treatment of severe BPSD in the elderly with dementia. However, the use of SGAs for BPSD must be weighed against the risk not only of increased mortality for which the FDA has issued its black box warning, but also against the increased morbidity of worsening cognitive decline. One of the findings from the 36-week Clinical Antipsychotic Trials of Intervention Effectiveness-Alzheimer's Disease (CATIE-AD) indicated that compared to placebo, use of SGAs (olanzapine, risperidone, or quetiapine) "are associated with greater rates of decline in cognitive function in Alzheimer's patients with psychotic or aggressive behavior and that the magnitude of this additional decline is clinically relevant, reaching at least as great a magnitude as the effect of cholinesterase inhibitors but in the negative direction" (Vigen et al., 2011, p. 837). In the dementia antipsychotic withdrawal trial (DART-AD), long-term care residents with AD were randomized to continue their antipsychotic regimen or to be switched to placebo and then followed for 12 months; the authors found no significant difference between groups on level of cognitive symptoms or neuropsychiatric symptoms, both of which worsened (Ballard et al., 2008; also see Meeks, 2010).

In agitated, aggressive, anxious elderly with dementia, the benefits of behavioral improvement, if it occurs, may allow the patient to remain in a less-structured and less-confining environment than otherwise would be possible. Thus, the humanitarian benefits of trying antipsychotic medications may outweigh any increase in risk in some patients. But, given the current literature suggesting minimal to weak effects, these agents should be used with discretion, close monitoring, and only as part of a nonpharmacological, environmental, and behavioral intervention package (Omelan, 2006).

Undertreatment of the Elderly: Focus on Depression

Untreated depression in the elderly can seriously reduce both the quality and length of life. However, depression in the elderly remains underdiagnosed and often poorly or inadequately treated. According to 2010 statistics from the CDC, the highest rate of suicide deaths for males and females combined is in the 50 to 54 age group at 19.85 deaths per 100,000 population; next highest is in the 55 to 59 age group at 19.12 deaths per 100,000 population. Males in all age groups have higher rates of death compared to females and the highest rate is in males who are 85 years of age or older; their rate is 47.33 deaths per 100,000 population. Adults 65 years of age and older have a rate of death by suicide of 15.3 per 100,000 population which is higher than the national average of 12.4 deaths per 100,000 population. In addition, it has been observed that of the individuals with some mental health disorder, about 41 percent perceive the need for help and seek it and about 16 percent seek it from a mental health professional; the problem is that most older adults with mental health issues do not perceive the need for help such that less than 8 percent of those who are 65 years or older sought help in the previous year of this study (Mackenzie et al., 2010).

Although most older adults prefer to receive their mental health services from their primary care provider, that may not be the most effective intervention for this population. It has been suggested that a team approach to treating depression in the elderly can be quite successful. One team approach program is called IMPACT (Improving Mood: Promoting Access to Collaborative Treatment). Results from the IMPACT research have recently been updated by Van Leeuwen and coworkers (2009). IMPACT involves a team including a depression case manager (psychologist, social worker or a nurse), a primary care physician, and a consulting psychiatrist. Hunkeler and coworkers (2006) stated:

> Tailored collaborative care actively engages older adults in treatment for depression and delivers substantial and persistent long-term benefits. Benefits included less depression, better physical functioning, and an enhanced quality of life. The IMPACT model may show the way to less depression and healthier lives for older adults. (p. 259)

Information about the IMPACT model, tools, and summary of research on effectiveness can be found on the IMPACT website: http://impact-uw.org.

In support of this collaborative care model, Reynolds and coworkers (2006) studied 116 patients over the age of 70 who had been diagnosed with major depression. Here, they compared the efficacy of placebo medication, medication alone, psychological therapy alone, and combined medication and psychological therapy. The medication chosen was *paroxetine* (Paxil); the psychological therapy chosen was weekly interpersonal psychotherapy. Combination therapy improved the percentage of patients achieving remission from 35 percent with either alone to 58 percent, a remarkable improvement.

Results indicated that depression in the elderly is best treated by a combination of anti-depressant medication and psychological interventions. Not all studies, however, have found that communication between mental health professionals and primary care providers is a necessary component for the effectiveness of collaborative care interventions for the treatment of depression in the elderly (Chang-Quan et al., 2009).

Antidepressants to Treat Depression in the Elderly

Paroxetine was effective in the Reynolds study as well as in a study by Dombrovski and coworkers (2007). Kasper and coworkers (2006) demonstrated the efficacy of *escitalopram* (Lexapro) in the elderly (mean age 74 years; 82 percent female); escitalopram was later noted to be less efficacious for the treatment of generalized anxiety disorder in the elderly (Lenze et al., 2009).

Nelson and coworkers (2006) reported results on the use of *mirtazepine* (Remeron) to treat major depression in 50 patients aged 85 and older residing in nursing homes. In 45 percent of patients, mirtazepine (average dose 18 milligrams per day) was effective in decreasing the average Hamilton Rating Scale for Depression score from 17 at baseline to 7 at end point. Sedation and weight gain were prominent side effects. Administering the drug at bedtime made the sedation a positive effect. Weight gain was also seen as a positive effect in this age group, where maintaining adequate body weight is often a concern. Concern is always present when using sedative medication at bedtime in the elderly. In this study, the incidence of falls did not seem to increase; however, a control (placebo) group was not employed, so the incidence of falls could not be determined with certainty. Kok et al. (2011) analyzed the results of eight double-blind, randomized controlled trials of antidepressant (first and second generation) continuation treatment of depression in the elderly using relapse as an outcome indicator. They found that continuation of antidepressant treatment resulted in fewer relapses/recurrences when compared to placebo, suggesting that continued treatment with antidepressants is efficacious in maintaining remission / recovery from depression in the elderly. There was no difference in effectiveness between first and second generation antidepressants. But, there is also concern about the use of ADs with the elderly. Some of the concerns include the low rate of response to AD treatment by the elderly and increased risk for morbidity and mortality, including stroke, myocardial infarction, increased risk of suicide, seizures, and falls (Coupland et al., 2011). Other authors have also found that use of SSRIs in treating depression in the elderly with dementia led to a significant increase in falls; the risk of falling was related to the dose of the SSRI. (Sterke et al., 2012a).

The presence of an anxiety disorder comorbid with a depressive disorder correlates with poorer outcome for depression treatment (Lenze et al., 2005). Similarly, a high pretreatment level of anxiety increases the risk of nonresponse to antidepressant treatment as well as the risk of recurrence in the first 2 years of maintenance treatment (Andreescu et al., 2007). These results indicate that depressed elderly patients should be screened for anxiety disorders and treated for them, if they are present, as aggressively as for the depressive disorder.

In a small study of older patients with unipolar depression who were resistant to selective serotonin reuptake inhibitors (SSRIs), Rutherford and coworkers (2007) reported that *aripiprazole* (Abilify) augmentation of citalopram therapy resulted in a 50 percent rate of remission in formerly resistant elderly. This outcome was verified by Lenze and coworkers (2008), who also noted that remission was sustained in all 24 patients during 6 months of continuation treatment. The authors added:

> Incomplete response in the treatment of late-life depression is a large public health challenge: at least 50 percent of older people fail to respond adequately to first-line antidepressant pharmacotherapy, even under optimal treatment conditions. Treatment-resistant late-life depression increases risk for early relapse, undermines adherence to treatment for coexisting medical disorders, amplifies disability and cognitive impairment, imposes greater burden on family caregivers, and increases the risk for early mortality, including suicide. (p. 419)

Parkinson's Disease

Parkinson's disease (PD) is the second most common neurodegenerative disease after Alzheimer's disease. PD occurs in about 0.5 to 1 percent of people 65 to 69 years of age (about 1.5 million Americans and 6 million people worldwide), rising to 1 to 3 percent of people 80 years of age and older. More than 60,000 new cases are diagnosed in the United States each year. Although the cause of PD remains unknown, its symptoms are thought to follow from a deficiency in the number and function of dopamine-secreting neurons located primarily in the substantia nigra (a subthalamic area) of the brain. Progressive loss of these neurons is a feature of normal aging; however, most people do not lose the huge number of dopamine neurons required to cause the symptoms of PD.

Chapter 11 discussed the first-generation, or traditional, antipsychotic agents (haloperidol and the phenothiazines) used to treat schizophrenia. The most prominent side effects of those drugs are movement disorders that resemble those seen in idiopathic Parkinson's disease. Mechanistically, these side effects result from drug-induced blockade of dopamine-2 receptors, resulting in a hypodopaminergic state. PD is similarly associated with a hypodopaminergic state, characterized by a progressive loss of dopamine neurons. Currently there are no effective neuroprotective therapies. Patients are currently treated with a combination of dopamine replacement therapies (discussed here) or receive deep brain electrical stimulation to combat behavioral symptoms (Williams et al., 2010). The ideal candidate therapy would be one that prevents neurodegeneration of dopamine neurons in the brain, and specific neurotropic factors are being researched. Transplantation of dopaminergic stem cells into the brains of persons with PD has not yet met with success (Olanow et al., 2009a). The most common approach to therapy of PD is through dopamine replacement interventions designed to maintain dopaminergic function and (hopefully) slow the effect of the loss of dopamine neurons.

Regardless of the etiology of neuronal loss in PD, the clinical features emerge when about 80 percent of dopamine neurons are lost. The clinical syndrome of PD has several cardinal features:

- Bradykinesia (slowness and poverty of movement)
- Muscle rigidity (especially a "cogwheel" rigidity)
- Resting tremor, which usually abates during voluntary movement

- Impairment of postural balance, leading to disturbances of gait and falling
- Without treatment, progression over 5 to 10 years to a state of severe rigidity and loss of movement in which patients cannot care for themselves (depicted in the movie *Awakenings*)

The availability of effective treatments for the symptoms of PD has radically altered the prognosis of this disease. In most cases, good functional mobility can be maintained for many years, and the life expectancy of an affected person has been greatly extended. Replacement of the dopamine or the administration of either dopaminergic agonists or inhibitors of dopamine breakdown can restore function and ameliorate much of the symptomatology. These three approaches—dopamine replacement therapy, administration of a dopaminergic agonist, and administration of dopamine breakdown inhibitors—underlie much of today's treatment of the disease. Increasing dopamine in the brain, however, does bring with it some untoward effects, including impulse control disorders such as pathological gambling, binge eating, reckless driving and hypersexuality (Abler et al., 2009; Weintraub et al., 2010) as well as dyskinetic movement disorders.

Levodopa

Levodopa, a precursor drug to dopamine, continues to be the mainstay of therapy for Parkinson's disease, although today it is usually used in combination with other medications. Because a loss of dopamine is the primary problem in patients who have PD, replacement of the dopamine would be expected to ameliorate the symptoms of the disease. It does, but not by itself, because dopamine poorly crosses the blood-brain barrier from plasma into the central nervous system (CNS). However, the precursor compound in the biosynthesis of dopamine from the amino acid tyramine, a substance called *dihydroxyphenylalanine,* or *dopa* (Figure 16.1), crosses the blood-brain barrier and in the CNS is converted into dopamine, replacing the dopamine that is absent. Therefore, today, levodopa (the *levo* isomer being more active than the *dextro* isomer) is the most effective treatment for the motor disability, and many practitioners consider an initial beneficial response an important criterion for the diagnosis of parkinsonism.

Mechanism of Action. Administered orally, levodopa is rapidly absorbed into the bloodstream, where most of it (about 95 percent) is converted to dopamine in the plasma. Although only a small amount (about 1 to 5 percent) of levodopa crosses the blood-brain barrier and is converted to dopamine in the brain, it is enough to alleviate the symptoms of PD. In the CNS, levodopa is converted to dopamine, primarily within the presynaptic terminals of dopaminergic neurons in the basal ganglia.

One problem with this therapy is that, when levodopa is administered by itself, it is converted to dopamine in the body, resulting in undesirable side effects such as nausea. One approach to solving the problem is to reduce the high levels of dopamine in the systemic circulation while maintaining sufficient quantities in the brain. To do so, the biosynthetic pathway that leads to dopamine (see Figure 16.1) must be examined. Since the enzyme *dopa decarboxylase* is responsible for converting dopa to dopamine by inhibiting this enzyme in the systemic circulation but not in the brain, systemic biotransformation of the drug should be reduced, with a concomitant

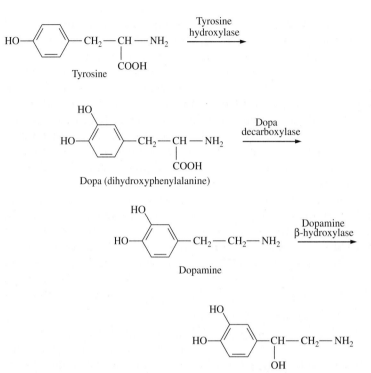

FIGURE 16.1   Synthesis of dopamine from tyrosine.

reduction in blood levels of dopamine and therefore in side effects. The drug would need a unique characteristic: it would have to be active in the body but not cross the blood-brain barrier into the brain. Thus, the metabolic conversion would occur in the CNS but not in the periphery.

An example of such a drug is *carbidopa*, available in combination with levodopa (the combination is marketed as Sinemet; also comes in rapidly dissolving tablets [Parcopa]; and an extended release version [Sinemet CR]). By combining carbidopa with levodopa, the dose of levodopa is reduced by 75 percent, with a concomitant reduction in side effects and no loss of CNS therapeutic effect. The current treatment of PD relies heavily on the use of Sinemet. The combination of levodopa and carbidopa provides near maximal therapeutic benefit with the fewest side effects.

Limitations of Levodopa Therapy.   Unfortunately, as time goes on, each dose of levodopa becomes less effective and the patient's symptoms fluctuate dramatically between doses, eventually developing into the "on-off" phenomenon. During the "on" phase, symptoms are under good control but as the medication effect "wears off" between doses, symptoms become more evident and this is referred to as the "off" phase. Part of the phenomenon is due to the short half-life of levodopa and can be minimized by increasing the dose and/or by decreasing the interval between doses. This adjustment, however, risks the development of levodopa-induced movement disorders (dyskinesia), which can be as uncomfortable and disabling as the rigidity and akinesia of parkinsonism. Indeed, within about 5 years after initiating levodopa treatment, over 50 percent of patients develop these disabling motor disorders. Stocchi and Marconi (2010) discuss a new formulation (Sirio, a combination of melevodopa and carbidopa) to reduce this "on-off" phenomenon through the use of a highly soluble form of L-dopa (melevodopa) that reduces the pulsatile peaks and troughs in blood levels seen with Sinemet. The FDA has not approved this formulation and there are no current clinical trials underway.

Does levodopa therapy adversely accelerate the course of PD? One theory of the disease is that the metabolism of dopamine produces free radicals that contribute to the death of the dopamine-releasing neurons. Oxidative stress may therefore be an important precipitating mechanism, and neuroprotective drugs might eventually be of more use in prevention of the disease. For the present, however, there is continuing concern that by ameliorating symptoms, we may be aggravating the disease. Also, since levodopa is effective for only about 5 years, therapy is often delayed until the symptoms of PD cause an unacceptable degree of functional impairment.

COMT Inhibitors

A newer advance in the PD therapeutic regimen involves an enzyme called *catechol-o-methyltransferase* (COMT). Even with the Sinemet combination, much of an oral dose of levodopa is wasted. COMT in the vasculature of the gastrointestinal tract and liver converts levodopa to an inactive metabolite with no clinical benefit. The half-life and clinical effects of Sinemet can be increased with the addition of a COMT-inhibitory drug. In 1998, the first of these drugs—*tolcapone* (Tasmar)—was introduced; it blocks the COMT enzyme, increasing the half-life of levodopa and prolonging its effect. Unfortunately, tolcapone caused a few cases of serious liver toxicity, so in late 1998 it was withdrawn from the market in Canada and in Europe. In the United States, its use is restricted to cases where all other adjunctive therapies have failed, and close monitoring of liver function is required.

A second COMT inhibitor, *entacapone,* became available in 2001 under the trade name Comtan; entacapone has not yet been associated with liver toxicity. Like tolcapone, entacapone inhibits peripheral COMT; it does not alter central COMT. Inhibition of peripheral degradation of levodopa increases central levodopa and, therefore, central dopamine concentrations. Co-administration of entacapone with levodopa plus carbidopa potentiates the effects of levodopa in patients with PD and reduces the so-called "on-off" phenomenon. In 15 to 20 percent of patients, the "on-off" phenomenon may be extreme and disabling: doses that originally were effective for 8 hours last for only 1 or 2 hours.

In 2004, the FDA approved a fixed combination product containing levodopa, carbidopa, and entacapone (available under the trade name Stalevo). As noted, the carbidopa increases the amount of dopamine in the brain while the entacapone inhibits the degradation of dopamine through inhibition of its degradative enzyme COMT. The combination provides more dopamine to the brain for a longer period of time, providing more "on" time and less "off" time associated with each dose of the drug (Hauser, 2009). The FDA is currently evaluating data from a meta-analysis of clinical trials comparing Stalevo versus Sinemet for evidence of possible increased risk of cardiovascular events with Stalevo. However, the FDA is not recommending that patients discontinue their use of Stalevo, as they are still evaluating the data.

Dopamine Receptor Agonists

Between 1 and 5 years after the start of levodopa therapy, most patients gradually become less responsive. One hypothesis for this effect is that the progression of PD may be associated with an increasing inability of dopamine neurons to synthesize and store dopamine. To relieve this problem, attempts have been made to identify drugs that directly stimulate postsynaptic dopamine receptors in the basal ganglia. These drugs do not depend on the ability of existing dopaminergic neurons to synthesize dopamine. In addition, if the free radical theory described in the previous subsection is accepted, these drugs would avoid the biotransformation of dopamine into potentially neurotoxic metabolites. As a result, they are increasingly being advocated for use in early stages of PD, especially in patients younger than about 65. These drugs might also be effective in the later stages of PD, when dopamine neurons are largely absent or nonfunctional.

Several dopamine receptor agonists are available in the United States for the treatment of PD (Figure 16.2): *bromocriptine* (Parlodel), *pergolide* (Permax), *pramipexole* (Mirapex), and *ropinirole* (Requip). Apomorphine (Apokyn) is an old drug that can be used as an adjunctive treatment for the sudden appearance of the "off" phase. However, it causes significant nausea and must be taken with anti-nausea medication. Others have been introduced and are not clinically used because of side effects (*cabergoline*, or Dostinex) or problems with manufacture (*rotigotine*, or Neupro, developed as a transdermal skin patch; removed from the U.S. market in 2008).

Bromocriptine has been available since 1978 and pergolide since 1989; both have structures that closely resemble that of dopamine. They are only marginally effective, and they have a number of potentially serious side effects. For example, pergolide has been associated with damage to the heart valves, involving 20 percent of the patients who have taken the drug. In March 2007, the manufacturers of pergolide voluntarily removed the drug from sale in the United States.

Pramipexole and ropinirole were marketed in 1997. Unlike the older two drugs, pramipexole and ropinirole are indicated for use in early-onset PD; their efficacy and safety profile is much better than that of the two older drugs. Both can increase quality of life in the early stages of the disease by improving motor problems and decreasing fluctuations in response to levodopa. Pramipexole also exerts a beneficial antidepressant effect (Fernandez and Merello, 2010). Their long half-lives may at least partially explain the reduction in the "on-off" phenomenon of levodopa therapy. Side effects of dopamine agonists include somnolence, dizziness, nausea, hallucinations, insomnia, and impulse control disorders (such as compulsive gambling, buying sprees, overeating, reckless driving, and hypersexuality (see Weintraub et al., 2010 and references therein).

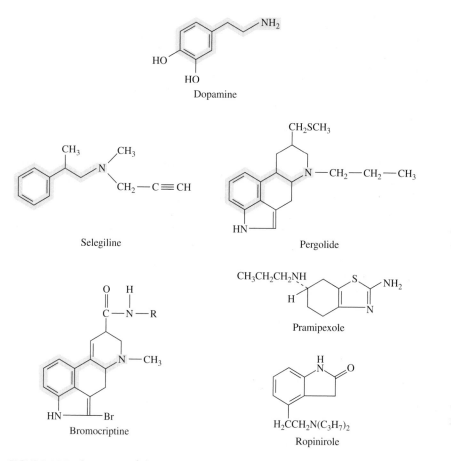

FIGURE 16.2 Structures of dopamine, selegiline, and four dopamine receptor agonists that are used to treat parkinsonism. The shaded portions, which are shared by selegiline, bromocriptine, and pergolide, resemble dopamine. The two newer dopamine receptor agonists are structurally unique and have greater affinity for dopamine-3 receptors than do older dopamine receptor agonists (which stimulate dopamine-2 receptors).

Selective Monoamine Oxidase-B Inhibitors

Selegiline (Eldepryl; and as a rapidly dissolving tablet [Zelapar]) (see Figure 16.2) reduces the symptoms of PD through a unique mechanism. The enzyme monoamine oxidase (MAO) exists in two forms (isoenzymes): MAO-A and MAO-B. Both are present in the brain; MAO-A is more closely involved with norepinephrine and serotonin nerve terminals, while MAO-B has preferential affinity for dopamine neurons located in the substantia nigra. Selegiline selectively and irreversibly inhibits MAO-B.[1] As a result, selegiline

---

[1] In Chapter 12, selegiline was discussed as the antidepressant transdermal skin patch marketed under the trade name Emsam.

inhibits the local breakdown of dopamine, thus preserving the small amounts of dopamine that are present. Both actions enhance the therapeutic effect of levodopa. Unlike the older nonselective MAO inhibitors used as clinical antidepressants (see Chapter 12), selegiline does not inhibit peripheral metabolism of levodopa; thus, it can safely be taken with levodopa. Selegiline also exhibits fewer drug/food interactions, at least at the lowest dose commercially available (6 mg daily). Unfortunately, in PD, selegiline's usefulness is limited.

Approved by the FDA in May 2006, *rasagiline* (Azilect) is the second selective MAO-B inhibitor for PD. Olanow and coworkers (2009b) reported a possibly beneficial effect of the early use of rasagiline at a 1mg/day dose, but negative findings at a 2 mg/day dose. Rasagiline may also possess a potential neuroprotective effect against the progression of PD (Malaty and Fernandez, 2009; Naoi and Maruyama, 2009). Recent studies have confirmed a beneficial effect of rasagiline in the treatment of Parkinson's disease (Leegwater-Kim and Bortan, 2010; Lew et al., 2010) and some authors suggest that MAO-B drugs should be used as the initial treatment for PD due to their safety profile and by using them first, providers can save the use of L-dopa until PD symptoms become more severe and disabling (Löhle and Reichmann, 2011).

Muscarinic Receptor Antagonists

Although widely used before the introduction of levodopa, certain anticholinergic (anti-ACh) agents (muscarinic antagonists) are now used much less often and are considered second-tier agents for the treatment of symptoms of PD. The use of these drugs was based on an understanding of the control of fine motor movements through the nigro-striatal system. The normal control of movement requires a 'balance' between dopamine and acetylcholine transmission within this system, hence the 'dopamine-acetylcholine balance theory' of movement disorders. Any shift in this balance through an increase or decrease in one neurotransmitter relative to the other results in hypo- or hyper- kinetic movement disorders. In PD, the dopamine-producing cell bodies in the substantial nigra are being destroyed and dopamine output is decreasing which produces a functional imbalance in the dopamine-acetylcholine transmission in favor of acetylcholine. To restore balance, you can either increase the dopamine transmission (by using one of the methods described above: replacement; post-synaptic stimulation; or inhibition of breakdown) or decrease the effect of acetylcholine (by using anti-ACh drugs).

Occasionally, anticholinergic drugs are used as an adjunct to L-dopa in patients with difficult-to-control tremors. Anticholinergic drugs relieve tremor in about 50 percent of patients, but they do not reduce rigidity or motor slowing. However, anti-ACh drugs can produce cognitive dysfunction that limits their use, especially in the elderly, who may already have an underlying cognitive disorder. Representative agents include *trihexyphenidyl* (Artane), *procyclidine* (Kemadrin), *biperiden* (Akineton), *ethopropazine* (Parsidol), and *benztropine* (Cogentin). Occasionally, the antihistaminic drug *diphenhydramine* (Benadryl) is also used (Benadryl has significant anticholinergic properties).

Amantadine and Memantine

Amantadine (Symmetrel) is an antiviral agent (used to treat viral influenza) with modest antiparkinsonian actions. Its mechanism of action in PD is unclear; it may alter dopamine release or reuptake, or it may have anticholinergic properties. Amantadine and a related drug, *memantine,* are active at NMDA-type glutaminergic receptors; this action perhaps offers a degree of "brain protection" that may contribute to its effects. Side effects are usually mild and reversible. A possible cognitive-enhancing effect of memantine might slow the cognitive decline that may accompany PD and Alzheimer's disease in the elderly (Burn, 2010).

New Approaches in the Pipeline

Research continues to look for better treatments for PD, especially looking for interventions that could arrest or even reverse the damage being done to the dopamine cell bodies. A summary of recent research in this area can be found on the Web site of the Parkinson's Disease Foundation at http://www.pdf.org/en/pubs_scientists/b_treatments. Some of the more recent approaches include:

- Evaluation of CERE-120, a gene-therapy product that delivers the neurotrophic factor, neurturin, to the degenerating or dying dopamine neurons; initial studies were not encouraging as several patients developed tumors (Marks et al., 2010).
- Studies involving the use of drugs to inhibit the phosphodiesterase type I (PDEI) enzyme that is stimulated by the dying dopamine cell bodies and associated nerve terminals; the PDEI inhibitors are hypothesized to restore DA function in the striatum.
- Drugs that inhibit hydroxyphenylpyruvate dioxygenase (HPPD), an enzyme responsible for the catabolism of tyrosine, the precursor to dopamine.
- Drugs that inhibit the metabotropic glutamate receptor 5 (mGluR5) which would reduce glutamate signaling; excessive glutamatergic signaling results from loss of dopamine cells and may be involved in L-dopa induced dyskinesia; mGluR5 inhibitors would be used to treat these dyskinesia side effects.
- Studies involving small molecule inducers of neurotrophic factors, like Cogane™, to enhance function of damaged nerve cells and protect intact cells from damage.
- Studies of an inhalation formulation of apomorphine for the treatment of the sudden appearance of the "off" phase.
- Drugs that stimulate Nurr1 receptors, a nuclear hormone receptor that plays a role in the growth, maintenance, and survival of dopamine neurons.
- Animal studies examining drugs that target the mitochondria of cells and boost their function by activating the PGC-1 alpha (or 'master regulator gene') gene; drugs like *pioglitazone* (Actos) used to treat diabetes and the nutrient, coenzyme Q10, are examples.

- Studies of antagonists of the adrenergic alpha-2 receptor, like fipamezole, that would enhance noradrenergic function and reduce L-dopa induced dyskinesia; amantadine extended release is being examined also for the treatment of L-dopa induced dyskinesia.

- A variety of drugs/compounds are being suggested or studied as neuroprotective agents like caffeine, nicotine (including substances found in peppers) (Nielsen et al., 2013), uric acid, vitamins, nutrients, antioxidants, and others that are summarized by Seidl and Potashkin (2011) and Huynh (2011).

- Lithium is being suggested as a neuroprotective agent.

- Studies of safinimide, which is thought to be a reversible inhibitor of MAO-B, an antagonist of activity-dependent channels, and a blocker of glutamate release.

- Clinical studies of GM1 ganglioside that is found in the outer covering of nerve cells and plays a role in neuronal development and survival, including "rescuing" damaged neurons and increasing dopamine levels.

- Clinical trials of vaccines against the neurotoxic protein, alpha-synuclein, have been attempted, but early studies found that some patients developed inflammation of the brain; studies are continuing with variations in vaccine content to minimize inflammatory risk (see Dolgin, 2012).

- Studies of pimavanserin, an antagonist/inverse agonist on $5HT_{2A}$ receptors, to treat psychosis in PD.

- Animal studies of a protein that protects cells against apoptosis normal cell death.

- Clinical studies of tozadenant, an adenosine 2-alpha receptor antagonist for reducing "off" time; and the norepinephrine prodrug, droidopa, for treatment of some adrenergic side effects (blood pressure changes, for example) of loss of dopamine neurons in PD.

Alzheimer's Disease

Alzheimer's disease (AD) is the most common neurodegenerative disease and accounts for the majority of all cases of dementia. AD is a progressive neurodegenerative disease that results in the irreversible loss of cholinergic neurons, particularly in the cerebral cortex and hippocampus. Onset occurs generally after 60 years of age but is being increasingly reported in people younger than 65. Upwards of 10 million Americans who are part of the baby-boom demographic will develop AD unless science finds a way to effectively treat and prevent this debilitating and tragic disease. In fact, authors are now referring to the upcoming dementia "epidemic" (Larson et al., 2013). By 2025, the number of people age 65 and older with Alzheimer's disease is estimated to reach 7.1 million—a 40 percent increase from the 5 million age 65 and older currently affected. By 2050, the number of people age 65 and older with Alzheimer's disease may nearly triple, from 5 million to a projected 13.8 million, barring the development of medical breakthroughs to prevent, slow or stop the disease. In addition to the slightly more than 5 million Americans living with AD, there are about another 500,000 Americans younger than age 65 who have either early-onset AD or another form of dementia. In 2013, Alzheimer's cost the nation $203 billion. This number is expected to rise to $1.2 trillion by 2050 (Alzheimer's Association, 2013).

Did You Know?

Map: Alzheimer's Disease Death Rate Per 100K Population by U.S. State, 1999–2010

In March 2013, the U.S. government reported the death rate for Alzheimer's disease rose 39 percent from 2000 through 2010. The highest rate among U.S. states was in Washington. In fact, from 1999 through 2010, Washington state had the highest age-adusted average annual death rate from Alzheimer's disease in the United States at 39.75 per 100,000 population. Rounding out the top ten U.S. states in 1999–2010, age-adjusted death rates per 100,000 population after Washington are North Dakota (32.70), Arizona (30.82), South Carolina (30.76), Tennessee (30.68), Maine (29.75), Louisiana (29.38), Alabama (28.80), Oregon (28.50), and Colorado (28.35). The CDC says the most closely correlated risk factors for Alzheimer's are age and genetics but that high blood pressure, high cholesterol, and diabetes may also contribute.

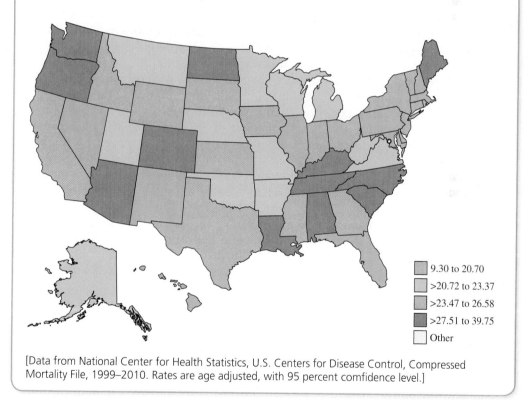

9.30 to 20.70
>20.72 to 23.37
>23.47 to 26.58
>27.51 to 39.75
Other

[Data from National Center for Health Statistics, U.S. Centers for Disease Control, Compressed Mortality File, 1999–2010. Rates are age adjusted, with 95 percent comfidence level.]

Time between symptom onset and death may span 8 to 10 years. Alzheimer's disease is the sixth leading cause of death in the United States. The gradual and continuous decline caused by AD is characterized by cognitive deterioration, changes in behavior, loss of functional independence, and increasing requirements for care. Hallmarks of AD include progressive impairment in memory, judgment, decision-making, orientation to physical surroundings, and language. Dementia (defined as cognitive impairment with the inability to form new memory) is the critical feature of AD. Diagnosis is based on neurological examination and the exclusion of other causes of dementia. A combined workgroup from the National Institute on Aging (NIA) and the Alzheimer's Association has established guidelines for the diagnosis of AD (Jack et al., 2011; McKhann et al., 2011). A definitive diagnosis can be made only at autopsy, where neuronal loss and accumulation of deposits of protein plaques (amyloid-β) and neurofibrillary tangles, composed of abnormal microtubules (tau), are observed. It is currently not known whether the plaques and tangles cause AD, are inactive by-products of the disease process, or may actually be protective. Much research is devoted to this area (Rhein et al., 2009), but, to date, results from studies of potential interventions affecting amyloid have been disappointing (Green et al., 2009).

The drugs currently used for treating AD patients act on brain neurotransmitters, although it is well recognized that they do not alter the course of the disease. The fact that some of the symptoms of AD are thought to be due to a deficiency of acetylcholine neurotransmission has given rise to a cholinergic-deficiency theory of AD. Therefore, reinforcing cholinergic function by inhibiting the enzyme that breaks down acetylcholine in the synapse (see Chapter 1) is a widespread therapy. These drugs, called acetylcholinesterase inhibitors (AChE-Is), do not alter the course of the dementia, but they can slow cognitive decline. As AD progresses and fewer cholinergic neurons remain functional, the effects of these drugs diminish. The pharmacology of the four available cholinesterase inhibitors was recently reviewed by Shah and coworkers (2010).

Memantine, discussed earlier in the section on Parkinson's disease, is not an acetylcholinesterase inhibitor but is also used for AD treatment (and is approved by the FDA for this use); it may act through effects exerted at specific subtypes of glutamate neurons thought be important for memory formation. Neither the AChE-Is nor memantine attack the root cause of AD, which is believed to involve brain proteins and peptides rather than neurotransmitters. So they may forestall further functional decline for a limited time, but they have not been shown to slow the disease progression or avoid the ultimate outcome.

AD is associated not only with cognitive impairments but with a myriad of bothersome mood alterations and behavioral symptoms that pose further challenges to treatment:

- Depression associated with AD is common. Some estimates are that between 30 percent and 50 percent of patients with AD have comorbid depression (Aboukhatwa et al., 2010). Depression in this population should be treated with antidepressant medications that lack anticholinergic side effects. Thus, SSRIs are most commonly used rather than the tricyclic agents (see Chapter 12) because they are better tolerated and produce fewer adverse cognitive effects; in addition, these antidepressants can be combined with drugs used to treat AD with few adverse interactions (Aboukhatwa et al., 2010).

- Apathy may be a prominent behavioral feature of AD that could be mistaken for depression. Approaches to treatment for this symptom include use of the psychostimulants, the antidepressant bupropion, the dopamine receptor agonist bromocriptine, and the antiparkinsonian agent amantadine and/or memantine.

- Psychosis, agitation, and other behavioral disturbances may require treatment with a newer atypical antipsychotic agent (discussed above) for BPSD. But the use of these agents have their own risk of side effects including oversedation, metabolic syndrome including exacerbation or onset of diabetes, movement disorders, akathisia, and falls (Sterke et al., 2012b).

- Some studies have shown a possible benefit of the antiepileptic mood stabilizers in treating behavioral symptoms—although valproic acid has not been found to be useful in managing agitation in AD (Tariot et al., 2011). In addition the sedating antidepressants trazodone and mirtazepine, and the SSRIs have also been shown to be helpful with behavioral symptoms. However, other studies indicate little benefit and high risks of adverse events when using drugs like antipsychotics, anticonvulsants, and anticholinesterase inhibitors (Seitz et al., 2013).

- Many drugs/compounds have been tried based on theories of AD, but they have not been shown to be effective including hormone replacement therapy (HRT); vitamin E; nonsteroidal anti-inflammatory drugs (NSAIDs) (Jaturapaptporn et al., 2012); and the herbal ginkgo biloba. In fact, after more that ten thousand patients have been involved in trials of ginkgo, there is no reported benefit (Vellas et al., 2012).

On a positive note, Schaefer and coworkers (2006) demonstrated that a diet rich in fish oils, primarily the omega-3 fatty acid decosahexaenoic acid (DHA), resulted in a 47 percent reduction in the incidence of AD in a large population of British elderly. More recent studies indicate that low blood levels of DHA are related to an increased risk of AD (Pauwels et al., 2009), likely because DHA may be neuroprotective against dementia, reducing the production and accumulation of the beta-amyloid peptide and the microtubule-associated protein tau that may promote production of the neurofibrillary tangles (Cole et al., 2009). In addition, DHA was found to have beneficial effects against age-related cognitive decline (Yurko-Mauro et al., 2010). Based on some of these findings, it has been thought that taking omega-3 fatty acid supplements or eating foods rich in omega-3s might be a good prophylactic intervention for AD. But, not all studies show such an effect. A large group of cognitively healthy elderly were randomly assigned to receive a combination of eicosapentaenoic acid (EPA) and DHA and followed for 2 years along with a group receiving placebo. At the end of the 2-year period, there was no difference between the two groups in cognitive status; i.e., cognitive status did not decline in either group (Dangour et al., 2010). Other studies have failed to find that DHA could reduce the rate of cognitive decline in AD (Quinn et al., 2010).

Much effort is being directed toward new drugs that may block the formation of amyloid plaques. Hopefully, these agents may lead to disease modification rather than merely symptom reduction. Among early attempts at this target are the use of *tramiprosate* and *tarenflurbil*. However, neither of these experimental medicines has demonstrated sufficient efficacy (Sabbagh 2009), although in a preliminary study, Wilcock and coworkers (2008) reported positive effects in a one-year study of taren-flurbil on global functioning and activities of daily living in patients with mild AD, but not in patients with moderate AD. The drug had no significant effect on cognitive functioning. In fact, one drug company has discontinued all trials with gamma secretase inhibitors like tarenflurbil due to lack of efficacy and increased risk of skin cancer (British Association for Psychopharmacology, 2011). Panza and coworkers (2009) and Frisardi and coworkers (2010) reviewed research targeting anti-amyloid drugs as disease-modifying agents in AD. But, this approach of targeting amyloid deposition may not be fruitful if it cannot be established that there is a relationship between amyloid formation and cognitive decline in the disease. In fact, some research indicates that the amyloid deposition has already occurred and reached a plateau well before even mild cognitive impairment (MCI) or frank dementia can be detected making pharmacological intervention at this point ineffective for reducing the progressive rate of cognitive decline (Chetelat et al., 2010). This finding speaks to the need to discover biological markers for the disorder so that individuals with a high risk for AD can be treated as soon as possible, well before incident symptoms occur (Selkoe, 2011). Some work is being done in this area. Roe and colleagues (2013) used a range of available biomarkers for AD to predict which individuals would develop AD symptoms. After following these individuals for several years, they were able to predict with a fair degree of accuracy who would develop the disorder and they found that any of the biomarkers were as good as any other for this prediction. They found that by combining the biomarker data with certain demographic information from the patients, they could enhance the predictive value. Vos and colleagues (2013) have been working on a system for identifying which cognitively normal individuals will develop symptoms of Alzheimer's and how rapidly their brain function will decline based on stages demarcated by changes in central biomarkers and results of neuropsychological testing. Although it is not ready to be used for clinical application, it is hoped that if this system is determined to be reliable, then it can be used to target early treatment interventions for those individuals who are most likely to develop AD.

Despite some of the more positive findings on biomarkers, the FDA has been concerned about the reliance on the use of biomarkers and imaging as outcome indicators for trials of Alzheimer treatment drugs. They have issued a guidance document that states that they will no longer accept biomarker changes or imaging data as outcome measures; they are now requiring researchers to use measures that reflect a benefit in patients' cognition and/or ability to function as the primary outcome measures for drug studies. But, more recently, the FDA has had to reconsider this guidance. For studies that attempt to identify at-risk individuals before there is evidence of any cognitive or functional decline, it would be hard for drug companies/researchers to meet this new standard since they could not demonstrate an improvement in cognition and/or function if those functions have not yet been impaired. So, the FDA is asking for public comment on relaxing the benchmark requirements for early intervention studies to allow these studies to use the original benchmarks of biomarker changes and/or imaging data. For a summary of the current status of prevention studies and rational strategies for ongoing research, see Gandy and Dekosky (2013).

Did You Know?

An Olive Oil Compound That Makes Your Throat Itch May Prevent Alzheimer's

Doctors and nutritionists have long associated the Mediterranean diet with human health benefits, including a lower risk of Alzheimer's disease.

Previously, researchers assumed this benefit came from extra virgin olive oil's high concentration of monounsaturated fatty acids. But in 2005 scientists discovered that oleocanthal—the naturally occurring compound that elicits a peppery, burning sensation in the back of the throat—seemed to produce effects strikingly similar to those of ibuprofen, which tamps down inflammation. Since then, investigators have turned their attention to the potential benefits of this particular compound.

Some studies have shown that oleocanthal interferes with the formation of characteristic neurofibrillary tangles and beta-amyloid plaques, both of which play principal roles in Alzheimer's neurological devastation. Researchers applied different concentrations of oleocanthal over 3 days to mouse brain cell cultures. They also administered oleocanthal to live mice—the first time such an experiment has been done—every day for 2 weeks. In both trials, levels of two proteins that play major roles in transporting beta-amyloid out of the brain as well as enzymes that degrade beta-amyloid, increased significantly, after administering oleocanthal.

The researchers also introduced beta-amyloid to the live mice brains. Compared with control groups, the mice that were given oleocanthal showed significantly enhanced clearance and degradation of the beta-amyloid peptides.

Acetylcholinesterase Inhibitors (AChE-Is)

As discussed, deficits in the functioning of acetylcholine-secreting neurons (cholinergic deficits) are correlated with the cognitive impairments of AD. Originally this idea stemmed from the observation that drugs that block the actions of acetylcholine (for example, scopolamine) are intense cognitive inhibitors. Therefore, drugs that increase acetylcholine levels might be cognitive enhancers and slow the rate of progression of cognitive decline seen in AD. Consistent with this idea is the observation that patients with severe AD show ACh levels that are 60 to 85 percent lower than normal, which implies very little residual ACh in the cortex—a condition that is still compatible with life but no longer optimal for brain function.

The most successful effort to increase cholinergic functioning has targeted the AChE enzyme, inhibition of which increases levels of acetylcholine in the brain. Four of these AChE-I medications have been approved by the FDA for the treatment of AD: *tacrine* (Cognex), *donepezil* (Aricept), *rivastigmine* (Exelon), and *galantamine* (Razadyne). Each improves cholinergic neurotransmission by preventing the synaptic breakdown of acetylcholine in the brain. These drugs can produce modest improvements in cognition and activities of daily living, but their side effects include nausea, diarrhea, abdominal cramping, and anorexia. The side effects result from inhibition of AChE in the periphery, not from the elevations of acetylcholine in the brain. In small numbers of patients receiving AChE-I medication, drug-induced increases in aggressive behaviors may be seen (Coco and Cannizaro, 2010); these behaviors are reversible with drug discontinuation (or dosage reductions), and treatment with antipsychotic drugs (without stopping the AChE-I) may be sometimes helpful. The modest efficacy combined with these side effects tends to limit the therapeutic usefulness of these agents.

Tacrine was the first of these agents to be approved; it is now the least used of the four, primarily because it needs frequent administration and can cause a reversible toxicity to the liver. Liver toxicity has not been associated with donepezil, rivastigmine, and galantamine.

Donepezil appears to be selective for AChE in the brain more than in the periphery. It has a long half-life and produces fewer gastrointestinal side effects. It is much more tolerable than tacrine. Petersen and coworkers (2005) reported that donepezil may slow the progression of cognitive decline in early AD but that the protective effect was lost after 18 months of treatment. Winblad and coworkers (2006) reported that donepezil improved cognitive ability and helped preserve patient functioning. Burns and coworkers (2007) reported that, over 24 weeks of treatment, donepezil produced positive effects on cognition, but that effect was lost over 132 weeks of study. Furthermore, if treatment was discontinued, benefits were not regained after treatment restart. Finally, Doody and coworkers (2009) reported that, in a 48-week study, donepezil was no better than placebo in elderly patients with mild cognitive impairment (MCI). Persons with such mild cognitive impairments are expected to progress to AD within about 6 years. In 2010, the FDA approved a new 23 milligram dose of donepezil for moderate to severe AD. There has been controversy over this approval; the data on which it was based did not show any clinically meaningful difference between the 23 milligram dose and the original 5 milligram or 10 milligram tablets; but, side effects were much greater with the 23 milligram tablet, indicating a greater risk for little to no benefit for the higher dose. The FDA is reviewing an application for a transdermal (patch) formulation of donepezil.

Rivastigmine is clinically effective, producing modest improvements in cognitive functioning and activities of daily living (Olin et al., 2010). It is better tolerated than tacrine but somewhat less so than donepezil. In contrast to the other three agents, rivastigmine causes a very slow reversible inhibition of AChE, prolonging its therapeutic action. Also available is a rivastigmine transdermal patch (Exelon Patch). Oral administration of cholinesterase inhibitors is limited by wide fluctuations in blood concentrations. With the patch, 24-hour concentrations remain relatively stable. Several recent articles attest to the superiority of the patch over oral administration of capsules (Grossberg et al., 2009; Sadowsky et al., 2010; Darreh-Shori and Jelic, 2010). Caregivers prefer the patch to the capsule (Grossberg et al., 2009); however, to avoid toxicity, only one patch at a time should be used.

Galantamine appears to have a safety and efficacy profile similar to that of rivastigmine in measures of both cognitive functioning and functional ability. In a study of quite elderly patients (average age 84 years) with severe AD, Burns and coworkers (2009) reported that galantamine moderately improved cognitive functioning but failed to significantly improve measures of overall activities of daily living.

These data imply that cholinesterase inhibitors have modest but positive effects compared with placebo in the treatment of AD, affecting cognition, function, and behavioral outcomes. They are effective in mild to moderate disease, and data with galantamine suggest that this effect can also be seen in severe disease as well.

There are limitations to these medications, however, because although stabilization occurs, there is typically only a modest improvement from baseline. Additionally, the effects are not sustained indefinitely, and the disease continues to progress even while patients are receiving treatment with cholinesterase inhibitors. Adverse effects are manageable and, with careful titration, patients can tolerate increases quite well; however, side effects can include diarrhea, nausea, vomiting, dyspepsia, asthenia, dizziness, headache, weight loss, and even anorexia—sometimes to such an extreme that patients must discontinue treatment. Hopefully, the patch delivery system may reduce some of these side effects. Additional therapies for AD need to be developed that include highly tolerable agents with alternative mechanisms of action and broader efficacy to delay disease onset, arrest the disease, and even reverse the progression of the disease entirely. Until these new therapies are developed, the cholinesterase inhibitors will remain important treatments for AD.

Recently interest has been expressed in a naturally occurring AChE-I called *huperzine A*. This substance, derived from the moss *Huperzia serrata*, has been used for centuries as a Chinese folk medicine. It has modest AChE-I activity, and it may be useful as an alternative medication for the treatment of AD (Desilets et al., 2009; Li et al., 2008). There is a lack of evidence at this point for any benefit of huperzine in AD (Rafii et al., 2011); but studies are ongoing. A limiting factor in studies up to this point is lack of availability of large amounts of huperzine. The extraction process from the native plant is complex and results in a product that is very expensive. Recently, scientists have developed a method for synthesizing huperzine in large quantities that should facilitate its use in additional studies in AD.

Memantine

As discussed in Chapter 1, *glutamate* is the principal excitatory neurotransmitter in the brain. Glutaminergic overactivity may result in neuronal damage, a phenomenon termed *excitotoxicity*. Excitotoxicity ultimately leads to neuronal calcium overload and has been implicated in neurodegenerative disorders. In addition, glutaminergic NMDA receptor activity appears to be important in memory processes, dementia, and the pathogenesis of AD. Glutaminergic overstimulation at NMDA receptors is thought to be toxic to neurons, and prevention of this neurotoxicity affords a degree of brain protection to limit further deterioration.

Memantine (Namenda; Namenda XR) is a moderate-affinity noncompetitive NMDA receptor antagonist that has been shown to reduce clinical deterioration in patients with moderate to severe AD, a phase associated with significant distress for patients and caregivers alike and for which no other treatments are available (Aarsland et al., 2009). It appears to have therapeutic potential without the undesirable side effects associated with high-affinity NMDA antagonists such as ketamine (see Chapter 8). Some studies have found that it delays clinical worsening in moderate to severe AD (Hellweg et al., 2012); but other studies have not found strong evidence of any benefit from memantine in mild AD and only meager evidence for efficacy in moderate AD (Schneider et al., 2011). It has not been shown to be effective in reducing agitation associated with AD (Fox et al., 2012; Herrmann et al., 2013). Available in Germany since 1982, memantine became available for use in the United States in 2004.

Tariot (2006) and Cummings and coworkers (2006) all reported improved cognition, patient functioning, and behaviors, as well as amelioration of agitation and other negative behaviors, in AD patients treated with a combination of an AChE-I and memantine. It is thought that the combination may delay nursing home placement, a step that can be exceedingly distressing to patients with AD and their caregivers (Rountree et al., 2013; see also Atri et al., 2013; Gauthiera and Molinuevo, 2013; Zhu et al., 2013 for effects of combining AChE-Is with memantine); although not all studies find that adding a second AD drug produces any additional benefit (Howard et al., 2012).

As with other NMDA antagonists, high brain concentrations of memantine can inhibit glutaminergic mechanisms of synaptic plasticity that are believed to underlie learning and memory. In other words, at high doses, memantine can produce the same amnestic effects as does ketamine. At lower, clinically relevant doses, however, memantine seems to promote cellular plasticity, can preserve or enhance memory, and can protect against the excitotoxic destruction of cholinergic neurons. As a "weak" NMDA antagonist, memantine may reduce overactive NMDA receptor activity that would be neurotoxic while sparing the synaptic responsiveness required for normal behavioral functioning, cognition, and memory.

Although there may be some evidence for the use of AchE-Is and memantine in the treatment of the cognitive decline associated with dementia of the Alzheimer's type, it should be noted that there is no evidence that they are of any clinical value in the treatment of cognitive decline associated with other types of dementia (i.e., Lewy body; vascular; frontotemporal) or reducing the risk of developing dementia following MCI (O'Brien and Burns, 2011). In fact, a Cochran review of the literature concludes that there is little evidence that AchE-Is or memantine affect progression to dementia from MCI; and this weak evidence is overshadowed by the greater risk of adverse events, particularly GI; thus AchE-Is should not be recommended for treatment of MCI (Russ and Morling, 2012; Tricco et al., 2013).

New Treatment Approaches: The Pipeline

Drugs targeting amyloid-β formation: bapineuzumab and solanezumab both failed in large clinical trials; a third drug, crenezumab will be tested in a large Colombian family that has a rare form of AD that develops in a high proportion of family members by middle age (Callaway 2012); other drugs/compounds that limit amyloid-β formation by blocking β-secretase activity are still under investigation; similar drugs that inhibit the γ-secretase enzyme which contributes to the formation of amyloid-β, like semagacestat, have not shown any benefit in AD and in some cases have accelerated the cognitive and functional deterioration and increased risk of skin cancer; although studies with semagacestat have been stopped, studies with other γ-secretase inhibitors are ongoing.

- *Latrepirdine* (Dimebon) an old antihistamine drug used in Russia was assessed in several trials of individuals with mild-to-moderate AD; the trials were considered failed trials; the drug did not separate from placebo; latrepirdine was never approved for use in the United States.

- PBT2 from Prana Biotechnology is a drug that is proposed to work by preventing the interaction of synaptic zinc and copper with amyloid-β to prevent the amyloid-β from becoming toxic; continues in clinical trials.

- Intravenous immunoglobulin (IVIG) in mild-to-moderate severity AD; IVIG contains antibodies to amyloid-β protein; measurement of growth rate of ventricular space showed less ventricular expansion (less brain shrinkage) compared to a placebo group; the study was not designed as an effectiveness study, so no conclusions about the results on cognitive function can be made; a rash and hemolytic anemia developed in 21 percent of the study patients; clinical trials are ongoing; other trials of vaccines, like AN1792, were stopped due to significant brain inflammation; however, other studies of vaccines with less risk for inflammation are ongoing, despite negative outcomes from all prior studies thus far.

- Selective alpha-7 nicotinic receptor agonists are being studied in individuals with mild-to-moderate AD.

- Based on a finding of zinc deficiency in AD, patients are being treated in clinical trials with dietary supplements of oral zinc cysteine; hippocampal zinc modulates the NMDA receptor and in absence of modulation by zinc, excess neuroexcitation can lead to cell death; administration of zinc would be expected to maintain modulation of the NMDA receptor activity; outcomes examine zinc and copper levels and performance on cognitive tests.

- Antioxidants that also prevent aggregation, neurotoxicity, and deposition of amyloid-β are in clinical trials.

- Drugs that regulate glucose and lipid metabolism but also suppress inflammation are being tested; two such agents, *pioglitazone* (Actos) and *rosiglitazone* (Avandia), are used to treat diabetes and are being studied for their efficacy in AD; so far results have been unimpressive; another diabetes drug being studied in this regard is *metformin* (Glucophage); insulin itself is being tested as an agent that suppresses the expression of amyloid precursor protein (APP) from which amyloid-β is derived.

- Drugs that block the formation of tumor necrosis factor (TNF) which in turn reduces inflammation are being studied as neuroprotective agents that prevent the onset of AD; anti-TNF drugs are normally used to treat rheumatoid arthritis (RA); other drugs used to treat RA like prednisone, sulfasalazine, and rituximab were not associated with lower risk for AD.

- Cotinine, a compound derived from tobacco that is nontoxic and longer lasting than nicotine, is being studied in animal models of AD; in mice, the compound reduced the deposits of amyloid plaques and seemed to block their formation.

- A red dye, orcein, derived from lichens and used to color fabrics and food has been shown to reduce small toxic protein aggregates in AD; orcein binds to small amyloid aggregates that are toxic and converts them into large, mature plaques that are considered nontoxic to neuronal cells; the dye, methylene blue, is also being clinically tested in AD based on the same mechanism of action.

- *Bexarotene* (Targretin), a drug approved for the treatment of cancer, is being studied in animal models of AD; ApoE, the main cholesterol carrier in the brain, facilitates clearance of amyloid-β from the brain; bexarotene increases ApoE expression, which in turn increases the removal of amyloid-β from the brain; it has been shown in mice to not only arrest the progression of memory deficits, but in some cases reverse the AD pathology (Cramer et al., 2012); but, recently, four other labs reported they could not replicate this finding (see Fitz et al., 2013; Price et al., 2013; Tesseur et al., 2013; Veeraraghavalu et al., 2013); other cancer drugs like *erlotinib* (Tarceva) and *fefitinib* (Iressa) are being studied in fruit flies based on drugs' ability to block the epidermal growth factor receptor (EGFR) which is active in many cancers; it is thought that EGFR activation also exacerbates memory loss and amyloid-β formation, thus drugs that block EGFR should improve memory and block amyloid-β formation.
- Studies of a nutrient "cocktail" called Souvenaid showed limited improvement on one neuropsychological test while failing to demonstrate any improvement on a host of secondary measures of neuropsychological function; the cocktail consists of omega-3 fatty acids, uridine, choline, selenium, folic acid, and the vitamins B6, B12, C, and E; it was thought that this combination of nutrients would promote the formation of new nerve synapses.
- Clinical studies have been conducted with a selective $5HT_6$ receptor antagonist as an adjunctive agent to ongoing treatment with an AChE-I; initial positive results support moving forward with additional studies.
- Peptides related to angiotensin IV, a blood pressure modulator, were observed to reverse learning deficits in animal models of dementia; to prevent it from rapid metabolism in the periphery, scientists have produced a smaller molecule named Dihexa which can cross the blood-brain barrier; the developers have stated that this compound is seven times more potent than brain-derived neurotrophic factor (BDNF), which is a growth-promoting protein associated with brain development and stimulation of neuronal connections; clinical trials will be some time down the road as basic safety of the compound must be demonstrated first.
- Clinical trials are being conducted using a formulation of caprylic triglyceride (a medium chain triglyceride and fatty acid) designed to improve cognitive function in mild-to-moderate AD.
- A novel alpha-2_c adrenoreceptor antagonist has shown initial positive results in a clinical trial of AD patients as an add-on therapy to existing treatment with AChE-Is; the alpha-2_c adrenoreceptor is thought to regulate dopamine and serotonin activity in the brain.
- Sodium phenylbutyrate (Buphenyl) is an FDA-approved drug to treat elevated ammonium levels; it is being studied as a stimulator of neuronal growth and as a neuroprotective agent.
- Two compounds found in cinnamon, are being examined for their ability to reduce tau tangles and act as antioxidants: cinnamaldehyde can reduce tau tangles and epicatechin can serve as an antioxidant; such properties are also found in blueberries (See the following "Did You Know" Box).

> ## Did You Know?
>
> ### Cinnamon Compound Has Potential Ability to Prevent Alzheimer's
>
> Two compounds found in cinnamon — cinnamaldehyde and epicatechin — are showing some promise in the effort to fight the disease. The compounds have been shown to prevent the development of the filamentous "tangles" found in the brain cells that characterize Alzheimer's.
>
> The use of cinnamaldehyde, the compound responsible for the bright, sweet smell of cinnamon, has proven effective in preventing the tau knots. By protecting tau from oxidative stress, the compound, an oil, could inhibit the protein's aggregation. To do this, cinnamaldehyde binds to two residues of an amino acid called cysteine on the tau protein. The cysteine residues are vulnerable to modifications, a factor that contributes to the development of Alzheimer's.
>
> While it can protect the tau protein by binding to its vulnerable cysteine residues, it can also come off, which can ensure the proper functioning of the protein.
>
> Epicatechin, which is also present in other foods, such as blueberries, chocolate, and red wine, has proven to be a powerful antioxidant. Not only does it quench the burn of oxidation, it is actually activated by oxidation so the compound can interact with the cysteines on the tau protein in a way similar to the protective action of cinnamaldehyde.

Principles of Care for Patients with Alzheimer's Disease

In 2008, the American College of Physicians and the American Academy of Family Physicians published a clinical practice guideline for the pharmacological treatment of dementia (Qaseem et al., 2008; Raina et al., 2008).

In 2006, the American Association for Geriatric Psychiatry outlined minimal care standards and principles for patients with AD and their caregivers. The association issued a position statement calling on clinicians to treat AD as part of their typical practice (Lyketsos et al., 2006). The statement focuses on the following five important areas of therapy:

- Disease therapies for AD, targeting aspects of the current pathophysiological understanding of the disease
- Symptomatic therapies for cognitive symptoms
- Symptomatic therapies for other neuropsychiatric symptoms
- Interventions targeted at and the provision of supportive care for patients
- Interventions targeted at and the provision of supportive care for caregivers

These principles still apply today. Disease therapies (item 1) include therapies aimed at preventing deposits of amyloid plaques and preventing excitotoxic neuronal damage. Therapies for cognitive symptoms include the AChE-I drugs and memantine. Therapies for other symptoms might include treatments for depression, agitation, aggression, and delusions, among other symptoms; therapies can be both nonpharmacological and pharmacological. Supportive care for patients and caregivers should be tailored to the condition, circumstances, and progression of functional and cognitive decline. Caregivers need to be educated about AD and how their services are essential. They especially need to be given emotional support and respite.

STUDY QUESTIONS

1. What is Parkinson's disease?
2. List the various ways that dopaminergic action in the brain might be augmented or potentiated.
3. Explain how carbidopa potentiates the action of levodopa.
4. Explain how a COMT inhibitor potentiates the action of levodopa.
5. Differentiate the newer from the older dopamine receptor agonists.
6. How does selegiline work in the treatment of Parkinson's disease?
7. Besides treatment with drugs, how might parkinsonism be managed? List the nonpharmacological options.
8. What is the currently accepted hypothesis for the genesis of Alzheimer's disease?
9. What are the currently available medications used to treat Alzheimer's disease?
10. Differentiate cholinesterase inhibitors from one another and from memantine.
11. How is glutamate involved in the action of memantine and how does this involvement relate to neuroprotection?

REFERENCES

Aarsland, D., et al. (2009). "Memantine in Patients with Parkinson's Disease Dementia or Dementia with Lewy Bodies: A Double-Blind, Placebo-Controlled, Multicentre Trial." *Lancet Neurology* 8: 613–618.

Abler, B., et al. (2009). "At-Risk for Pathological Gambling: Imaging Neural Reward Processing Under Chronic Dopamine Agonists." *Brain* 132: 2396–2402.

Aboukhatwa, M., et al. (2010). "Antidepressants Are a Rational Complementary Therapy for the Treatment of Alzheimer's Disease." *Molecular Neurodegeneration* 5: 1–17: http://www.molecularneuro degeneration.com/content/5/1/10.

Alzheimer's Association. (2013). "2013 Alzheimer's Disease Facts and Figures." The Alzheimer's Association. *Facts and Figures*. Available at www.alz.org.

Andreescu, C., et al. (2007). "Effect of Comorbid Anxiety on Treatment Response and Relapse Risk in Late-Life Depression: Controlled Study." *British Journal of Psychiatry* 190: 344–349.

Atri, A., et al. (2013). "Memantine in Patients With Alzheimer's Disease Receiving Donepezil: New Analyses of Efficacy and Safety for Combination Therapy." *Alzheimers Research & Therapy* 5: 1–11, http://alzres.com/content/5/1/6.

Ballard, C., et al. (2008). "A Randomised, Blinded, Placebo-controlled Trial in Dementia Patients Continuing or Stopping Neuroleptics (The DART-AD Trial)." *PLoS Medicine* 5(4): e76. doi:10.1371 /journal.pmed.0050076.

Barnett, M. J., et al. (2006). "Comparison of Rates of Potentially Inappropriate Medication Use According to the Zhan Criteria for VA versus Private Sector Medicare HMOs." *Journal of Managed Care Pharmacy* 12: 362–370.

Billioti de Gage, S., et al. (2010). "Benzodiazepine Use and Risk of Dementia: Prospective Population Based Study." *British Medical Journal* 345: e6231 doi: 10.1136/bmj.e6231.

Briesacher, B. A., et al. (2013). "Antipsychotic Use Among Nursing Home Residents." *Journal of the American Medical Association* 309: 440–442.

British Association for Psychopharmacology. (2011). "Updated Consensus Statement on Antidementia Drugs in Clinical Practice." *The Brown University Psychopharmacology Update* 22: 1, 6–7.

Burn, D. J. (2010). "The Treatment of Cognitive Impairment Associated with Parkinson's Disease." *Brain Pathology* 20: 672–678.

Burns, A., et al. (2007). "Efficacy and Safety of Donepezil over 3 Years: An Open-Label, Multicentre Study in Patients with Alzheimer's Disease." *International Journal of Geriatric Psychiatry* 22: 806–812.

Burns, A., et al. (2009). "Safety and Efficacy of Galantamine (Reminyl) in Severe Alzheimer's Disease (the SERAD Study): A Randomized, Placebo-Controlled, Double-Blind Trial." *Lancet Neurology* 8: 39–47.

Callaway, E. (2012). "Alzheimer's Drugs Take a New Tack." *Nature* 489: 13–14.

Carnahan, R. M. (2010). "How to Manage Your Patient's Dementia by Discontinuing Medications." *Current Psychiatry* 9: 34–37.

Chang-Quan, H., et al. (2009). "Collaborative Care Interventions for Depression in the Elderly: A Systematic Review of Randomized Controlled Trials." *Journal of Investigative Medicine* 57: 446–455.

Chen, Y., et al. (2010). "Unexplained Variation Across US Nursing Homes in Antipsychotic Prescribing Rates." *Archives of Internal Medicine* 170: 89–95.

Chetelat, G., et al. (2010). "Relationship Between Atrophy and β-amyloid Deposition in Alzheimer Disease." *Annals of Neurology* 67: 317–324.

Coco, D. L., and Cannizaro, E. (2010). "Inappropriate Sexual Behaviors Associated with Donepezil Treatment: A Case Report." *Journal of Clinical Psychopharmacology* 30: 221–222.

Cole, G. M., et al. (2009). "Omega-3 Fatty Acids and Dementia." *Prostaglandins, Leukotrienes, and Essential Fatty Acids* 81: 213–221.

Coley, K. C., et al. (2009). "Aripiprazole Prescribing Patterns and Side Effects in Elderly Psychiatric Inpatients." *Journal of Psychiatric Practice* 15: 150–153.

Connelly, P. J., et al. (2009). "Fifteen Year Comparison of Antipsychotic Use in People with Dementia Within Hospital and Nursing Home Settings: Sequential Cross-Sectional Study." *International Journal of Geriatric Psychiatry* 25: 160–165.

Coupland, C. A. C., et al. (2011). "A Study of the Safety and Harms of Antidepressant Drugs for Older People: A Cohort Study Using a Large Primary Care Database." *Health Technology Assessment* 15: 1–202; i–xii: DOI: 10.3310/hta15280.

Cramer, P. E., et al. (2012). "ApoE-Directed Therapeutics Rapidly Clear β-Amyloid and Reverse Deficits in AD Mouse Models." *Science* 335: 1503–1506.

Cummings, J. L., et al. (2006). "Behavioral Effects of Memantine in Alzheimer's Disease Patients Receiving Donepezil Treatment." *Neurology* 67: 57–63.

Dangour, A. D., et al. (2010). "Effect of 2-y n-3 Long-chain Polyunsaturated Fatty Acid Supplementation on Cognitive Function in Older People: A Randomized, Double-blind, Controlled Trial." *American Journal of Clinical Nutrition* 91: 1725–1732.

Darreh-Shori, T., and Jelic, V. (2010). "Safety and Tolerability of Transdermal and Oral Rivastigmine in Alzheimer's Disease and Parkinson's Disease Dementia." *Expert Opinion on Drug Safety* 9: 167–176.

De Deyn, P. P., et al. (2013). "Aripiprazole in the Treatment of Alzheimer's Disease." *Expert Opinion on Pharmacotherapy* 14: 459–474.

Desilets, A. R., et al. (2009). "Role of Huperzine-A in the Treatment of Alzheimer's Disease." *Annals of Pharmacotherapeutics* 43: 514–518.

Devanand, D. P., et al. (2012). "Relapse Risk after Discontinuation of Risperidone in Alzheimer's Disease." *New England Journal of Medicine* 367: 1497–1507.

Dolgin, E. (2012). "First Therapy Targeting Parkinson's Proteins Enters Clinical Trials." *Nature Medicine* 18: 992–993.

Dombrovski, A. Y., et al. (2007). "Maintenance Treatment for Old-Age Depression Preserves Health-Related Quality of Life: A Randomized, Controlled Trial of Paroxetine and Interpersonal Psychotherapy." *Journal of the American Geriatrics Society* 55: 1325–1332.

Doody, R. S., et al. (2009). "Donepezil Treatment of Patients with MCI: A 48-Week Randomized, Placebo-Controlled Trial." *Neurology* 72: 1555–1561.

Dorsey, E. R., et al. (2010). "Impact of FDA Black Box Advisory on Antipsychotic Medication Use." *Archives of Internal Medicine* 170: 96–103.

Elie, M., et al. (2009). "A Retrospective, Exploratory, Secondary Analysis of the Association Between Antipsychotic Use and Mortality in Elderly Patients with Delirium." *International Psychogeriatrics* 21: 588–592.

Fernandez, H. H., and Merello, M. (2010). "Pramipexole for the Treatment of Depressive Symptoms in Patients with Parkinson's Disease: Can We Kill Two Birds with One Stone?" *Lancet Neurology,* 9: 556–557.

Ferreira, J. J., et al. (2006). "Sleep Disruption, Daytime Somnolence, and 'Sleep Attacks' in Parkinson's Disease: A Clinical Survey in PD Patients and Age-Matched Healthy Volunteers." *European Journal of Neurology* 13: 209–214.

Fitz, N. F., et al. (2013). "Comment on 'ApoE-Directed Therapeutics Rapidly Clear β-Amyloid and Reverse Deficits in AD Mouse Models'." *Science* 340: 924.

Fox, C., et al. (2012). "Efficacy of Memantine for Agitation in Alzheimer's Dementia: A Randomized Double-blind Placebo Controlled Trial." *PLoS ONE* 7: e35185; doi: 10.1371/journal.pone.0035185.

Frisardi, V., et al. (2010). "Towards Disease-Modifying Treatment of Alzheimer's Disease: Drugs Targeting Beta-Amyloid." *Current Alzheimer's Research* 7: 40–55.

Gandy, S., and Dekosky, S. T. (2013). "Toward the Treatment and Prevention of Alzheimer's Disease: Rational Strategies and Recent Progress." *Annual Review of Medicine* 64: 367–383.

Gauthiera, S., and Molinuevo, J. L. (2013). "Benefits of Combined Cholinesterase Inhibitor and Memantine Treatment in Moderate–Severe Alzheimer's Disease." *Alzheimer's & Dementia* 9: 326–331.

Green, R. C., et al. (2009). "Effect of Tarenflurbil on Cognitive Decline and Activities of Daily Living in Patients with Mild Alzheimer Disease." *Journal of the American Medical Association* 302: 2557–2564.

Grossberg, G., et al. (2009). "Safety and Tolerability of the Rivastigmine Patch: Results of a 28-Week Open-Label Extension." *Alzheimer Disease & Associated Disorders* 23: 158–164.

Hauser, R. A. (2009). "Levodopa: Past, Present, and Future." *European Neurology* 62: 1–8.

Hellweg, R., et al. (2012). "Efficacy of Memantine in Delaying Clinical Worsening in Alzheimer's Disease (AD): Responder Analyses of Nine Clinical Trials With Patients With Moderate to Severe AD." *International Journal of Geriatric Psychiatry* 27: 651–656.

Herrmann, N., et al. (2013). "A Randomized, Double-blind, Placebo-controlled Trial of Memantine in a Behaviorally Enriched Sample of Patients With Moderate-to-Severe Alzheimer's Disease." *International Psychogeriatrics* 25: 919–927.

Howard, R., et al. (2012). "Donepezil and Memantine for Moderate-to-Severe Alzheimer's Disease." *New England Journal of Medicine* 366: 893–903.

Hunkeler, E. M., et al. (2006). "Long-Term Outcomes from the IMPACT Randomized Trial for Depressed Elderly Patients in Primary Care." *British Medical Journal* 332: 259–263.

Huybrechts, K. F., et al. (2012). "Differential Risk of Death in Older Residents in Nursing Homes Prescribed Specific Antipsychotic Drugs: Population Based Cohort Study." *British Medical Journal* 344: e977 doi: 10.1136/bmj.e977.

Huynh, T. (2011). "The Parkinson's Disease Market." *Nature Reviews* 10: 571–572.

Jack, C. R., et al. (2011). "Introduction to the Recommendations From the National Institute on Aging-Alzheimer's Association Workgroups on Diagnostic Guidelines for Alzheimer's Disease." *Alzheimer's & Dementia* 7: 257–262.

Jaturapatporn, D., et al. (2012). "Aspirin, Steroidal and Non-steroidal Anti-inflammatory Drugs for the Treatment of Alzheimer's Disease." *Cochrane Database of Systematic Reviews*, Issue 2. Art. No.: CD006378. DOI: 10.1002/14651858.CD006378.pub2.

Jin, H., et al. (2013). "Comparison of Longer-term Safety and Effectiveness of 4 Atypical Antipsychotics in Patients Over Age 40: A Trial Using Equipoise-stratified Randomization." *Journal of Clinical Psychiatry* 74: 10–18.

Kales, H. C., et al. (2011). "Trends in Antipsychotic Use in Dementia 1999–2007." *Archives of General Psychiatry* 68: 190–197.

Kales, H. C., et al. (2012). "Risk of Mortality Among Individual Antipsychotics in Patients With Dementia." *American Journal of Psychiatry* 169: 71–79.

Kasper, S., et al. (2006). "Escitalopram in the Long-Term Treatment of Major Depressive Disorder in Elderly Patients." *Neuropsychobiology* 54: 152–159.

Kok, R. M., et al. (2011). "Continuing Treatment of Depression in the Elderly: A Systematic Review and Meta-analysis of Double-blinded Randomized Controlled Trials With Antidepressants." *American Journal of Geriatric Psychiatry* 19: 249–55.

Laroche, M. L., et al. (2007). "Is Inappropriate Medication Use a Major Cause of Adverse Drug Reactions in the Elderly?" *British Journal of Clinical Pharmacology* 63: 177–186.

Larson, E. B., et al. (2013). "New Insights into the Dementia Epidemic." *New England Journal of Medicine* DOI: 10.1056/NEJMp1311405.

Leegwater-Kim, J., and Bortan, E. (2010). "The Role of Rasagiline in the Treatment of Parkinson's Disease." *Clinical Interventions in Aging* 5: 149–156.

Lenze, E. J., et al. (2005). "Efficacy and Tolerability of Citalopram in the Treatment of Late-Life Anxiety Disorders: Results from an 8-Week, Randomized, Placebo-Controlled Trial." *American Journal of Psychiatry* 162: 145–150.

Lenze, E. J., et al. (2008). "Incomplete Response in Later-Life Depression: Getting to Remission." *Dialogues in Clinical Neurosciences* 10: 419–430.

Lenze, E. J., et al. (2009). "Escitalopram for Older Adults with Generalized Anxiety Disorder." *Journal of the American Medical Association* 301: 295–303.

Lew, M. F., et al. (2010). "Long-Term Efficacy of Rasagiline in Early Parkinson's Disease." *International Journal of Neuroscience* 120: 404–408.

Li, J., et al. (2008). "Huperzine A for Alzheimer's Disease." *Cochrane Database of Systematic Reviews* 16: CD005592.

Löhle, M., and Reichmann, H. (2011). "Controversies in Neurology: Why Monoamine Oxidase B Inhibitors Could Be a Good Choice For the Initial Treatment of Parkinson's Disease." *BMC Neurology* 11: 1–7: http://www.biomedcentral.com/1471-2377/11/112.

Lyketsos, C. G., et al. (2006). "Position Statement of the American Association for Geriatric Psychiatry Regarding Principles for Care of Patients with Dementia Resulting from Alzheimer's Disease." *American Journal of Geriatric Psychiatry* 14: 561–572.

Mackenzie, C. S., et al. (2010). "Correlates of Perceived Need for and Use of Mental Health Services by Older Adults in the Collaborative Psychiatric Epidemiology Surveys." *American Journal of Geriatric Psychiatry* 18: 1103–1115.

Malaty, I. A., and Fernandez, H. H. (2009). "Role of Rasagiline in Treating Parkinson's Disease: Effect on Disease Progression." *Therapeutics and Clinical Risk Management* 5: 413–419.

Marks, W. J., et al. (2010). "Gene Delivery of AAV2-neurturin for Parkinson's Disease: A Double-blind, Randomised, Controlled Trial." *Lancet Neurology* 9: 1164–1172.

McKhann, G. M., et al. (2011). "The Diagnosis of Dementia Due to Alzheimer's Disease: Recommendations From the National Institute on Aging-Alzheimer's Association Workgroups on Diagnostic Guidelines for Alzheimer's Disease." *Alzheimer's & Dementia* 7: 263–269.

Meeks, T. (2010). "Drugs, Death, and Disconcerting Dilemmas." *Psychiatric Times* 27: 1–7: http://www.psychiatrictimes.com/display/article/10168/1633418.

Naoi, M., and Maruyama, W. (2009). "Functional Mechanism of Neuroprotection by Inhibitors of Type B Monoamine Oxidase in Parkinson's Disease." *Expert Reviews in Neurotherapeutics* 9: 1233–1250.

Nelson, J. C., et al. (2006). "Mirtazepine Orally Disintegrating Tablets in Depressed Nursing Home Residents 85 Years of Age and Older." *International Journal of Geriatric Psychiatry* 21: 898–901.

Nielsen, S. S., et al. (2013). "Nicotine from Edible Solanaceae and Risk of Parkinson Disease." *Annals of Neurology* doi: 10.1002/ana.23884.

Nishtala, P. S., et al. (2009). "Anticholinergic Activity of Commonly Prescribed Medications and Psychiatric Adverse Effects in Older People." *Journal of Clinical Pharmacology* 49: 1176–1184.

O'Brien, J. T., and Burns, A. (2011). "Clinical Practice With Anti-dementia Drugs: A Revised (Second) Consensus Statement from the British Association for Psychopharmacology." *Journal of Psychopharmacology* 25: 997–1019.

Olanow, C. W., et al. (2009a). "Dopaminergic Transplantation for Parkinson's Disease: Current Status and Future Prospects." *Annals of Neurology* 66: 591–596.

Olanow, C. W., et al. (2009b). A Double-Blind, Delayed-Start Trial of Rasagiline in Parkinson's Disease." *New England Journal of Medicine* 361: 1268–1278.

Olin, J. T., et al. (2010). "Rivastigmine in the Treatment of Dementia Associated with Parkinson's Disease: Effects on Activities of Daily Living." *Dementia and Geriatric Cognitive Disorders* 29: 510–515.

Omelan, C. (2006). Approaches to Managing Behavioural Disturbances in Dementia." *Canadian Family Physician* 52: 191–199.

Page, R. L., et al. (2010). "Inappropriate Prescribing in the Hospitalized Elderly Patient: Defining the Problem, Evaluation Tools, and Possible Solutions." *Clinical Interventions in Aging* 5: 75–87.

Paleacu, D., et al. (2008). "Quetiapine Treatment for Behavioural and Psychological Symptoms of Dementia in Alzheimer's Disease Patients: A 6-Week, Double-Blind, Placebo-Controlled Study." *International Journal of Geriatric Psychiatry* 23: 393–400.

Panza, F., et al. (2009). "Disease-Modifying Approach to the Treatment of Alzheimer's Disease: From Alpha-Secretase Activators to Gamma-Secretase Inhibitors and Modulators." *Drugs and Aging* 26: 537–555.

Pariente, A., et al. (2012). "Antipsychotic Use and Myocardial Infarction in Older Patients With Treated Dementia." *Archives of Internal Medicine* 172: 648–653.

Pauwels, E. K., et al. (2009). "Fatty Acid Facts, Part IV: Docosahexaenoic Acid and Alzheimer's Disease. A Story of Mice, Men and Fish." *Drug News and Perspectives* 22: 205–213.

Petersen, R., et al. (2005). "Vitamin E and Donepezil for the Treatment of Mild Cognitive Impairment." *New England Journal of Medicine* 352: 2379–2388.

Price, A. R., et al. "Comment on 'ApoE-Directed Therapeutics Rapidly Clear β-Amyloid and Reverse Deficits in AD Mouse Models'." *Science* 340: 924.

Qaseem, A., et al. (2008). "Current Pharmacologic Treatment of Dementia: A Clinical Practice Guideline from the American College of Physicians and the American Academy of Family Physicians." *Annals of Internal Medicine* 148: 370–378.

Quinn, J. F., et al. (2010). "Docosahexaenoic Acid Supplementation and Cognitive Decline in Alzheimer Disease." *Journal of the American Medical Association* 304:1903–1911.

Rafii, M. S., et al. (2011). "A Phase II Trial of Huperzine A in Mild to Moderate Alzheimer Disease." *Neurology* 76: 1389–1394.

Raina, P., et al. (2008). "Effectiveness of Cholinesterase Inhibitors and Memantine for Treating Dementia: Evidence Review for a Clinical Practice Guideline." *Annals of Internal Medicine* 148: 379–397.

Reynolds, C. F., et al. (2006). "Maintenance Treatment of Major Depression in Old Age." *New England Journal of Medicine* 354: 1130–1138.

Rhein, V., et al. (2009). "Amyloid-Beta and Tau Synergistically Impair the Oxidative Phosphorylation System in Triple Transgenic Alzheimer's Disease Mice." *Proceedings of the National Academy of Science* 106: 20057–20062.

Roe, C. M., et al. (2013). "Amyloid Imaging and CSF Biomarkers in Predicting Cognitive Impairment Up to 7.5 Years Later." *Neurology* 80: 1784–1791.

Rountree, S. D., et al. (2013). "Effectiveness of Antidementia Drugs in Delaying Alzheimer's Disease Progression." *Alzheimer's & Dementia* 9: 338–345.

Russ, T. C., and Morling, J. R. (2012). "Cholinesterase Inhibitors for Mild Cognitive Impairment." *Cochrane Database of Systematic Reviews*, Issue 9. Art. No.: CD009132. DOI: 10.1002/14651858. CD009132.pub2.

Rutherford, B., et al. (2007). "An Open Trial of Aripiprazole Augmentation for SSRI Non-Remitters with Late-Life Depression." *International Journal of Geriatric Psychiatry* 22: 986–991.

Ryan, C., et al. (2009). "Appropriate Prescribing in the Elderly: An Investigation of Two Screening Tools, Beers Criteria Considering Diagnosis and Independent of Diagnosis and Improved Prescribing in the Elderly Tool to Identify Inappropriate Use of Medicines in the Elderly in Primary Care in Ireland." *Journal of Clinical Pharmacy and Therapeutics* 34: 369–376.

Sabbagh, M. N. (2009). "Drug Development for Alzheimer's Disease: Where Are We Now, and Where Are We Headed?" *American Journal of Geriatric Pharmacotherapy* 7: 167–185.

Sadowsky, C. H., et al. (2010). "Safety and Tolerability of Rivastigmine Transdermal Patch Compared with Rivastigmine Capsules in Patients Switched from Donepezil: Data from Three Clinical Trials." *International Journal of Clinical Practice* 64: 188–193.

Schaefer, E. J., et al. (2006). "Plasma Phosphatidylcholine Docosahexaenoic Acid Content and Risk of Dementia and Alzheimer's Disease." *Archives of Neurology* 63: 1545–1550.

Schneider, L. S., et al. (2011). "Lack of Evidence for the Efficacy of Memantine in Mild Alzheimer Disease." *Archives of Neurology* 68: 991–998.

Seidl, S. E., and Potashkin, J. A. (2011). "The Promise of Neuroprotective Agents in Parkinson's Disease." *Frontiers in Neurology* 2: 1–12: doi: 10.3389/fneur.2011.00068.

Seitz, D. P., et al. (2013). "Pharmacological Treatments for Neuropsychiatric Symptoms of Dementia in Long-term Care: A Systematic Review." *International Psychogeriatrics* 25: 185–203.

Selkoe, D. J. (2011). "Resolving Controversies on the Path to Alzheimer's Therapeutics." *Nature Medicine* 17: 1060–1065.

Shah, D., et al. (2010). "Medications for Treating Alzheimer's Dementia." *The Carlat Psychiatry Report* 8(4): 1–3.

Simoni-Wastila, L., et al. (2009). "Association of Antipsychotic Use with Hospital Events and Mortality Among Medicare Beneficiaries Residing in Long-Term Care Facilities." *American Journal of Geriatric Psychiatry* 17: 417–427.

Steinman, M. A., et al. (2006). "Polypharmacy and Prescribing Quality in Older People." *Journal of the American Geriatric Society* 54: 1516–1523.

Sterke, C. S., et al. (2012a). "Dose–response Relationship Between Selective Serotonin Re-uptake Inhibitors and Injurious Falls: A Study in Nursing Home Residents With Dementia." *British Journal of Clinical Pharmacology* 73: 812–820.

Sterke, C. S., et al. (2012b). "New Insights: Dose-Response Relationship Between Psychotropic Drugs and Falls: A Study in Nursing Home Residents With Dementia." *Journal of Clinical Pharmacology* 52: 947–955.

Stocchi, F., and Marconi, S. (2010). "Factors Associated with Motor Fluctuations and Dyskinesia in Parkinson's Disease: Potential Role of a New Melovodopa Plus Carbidopa Formulation (Sirio)." *Clinical Neuropharmacology* 33: 198–203.

Streim, J. E., et al. (2008). "A Randomized, Double-Blind, Placebo-Controlled Study of Aripiprazole for the Treatment of Psychosis in Nursing Home Patients with Alzheimer Disease." *American Journal of Geriatric Psychiatry* 16: 537–550.

Tannenbaum, C., et al. (2012). "A Systematic Review of Amnestic and Non-Amnestic Mild Cognitive Impairment Induced by Anticholinergic, Antihistamine, GABAergic and Opioid Drugs." *Drugs & Aging* 29: 639–658.

Tariot, P. N. (2006). "Contemporary Issues in the Treatment of Alzheimer's Disease: Tangible Benefits of Current Therapies." *Journal of Clinical Psychiatry* 67, Supplement 3: 15–22.

Tariot, P. N., et al. (2011). "Chronic Divalproex Sodium to Attenuate Agitation and Clinical Progression of Alzheimer's Disease." *Journal of Clinical Psychiatry* 68: 853–861.

Tesseur, I., et al. (2013). "Comment on 'ApoE-Directed Therapeutics Rapidly Clear β-Amyloid and Reverse Deficits in AD Mouse Models.'" *Science* 340: 924.

Tricco, A. C., et al. (2013). "Efficacy and Safety of Cognitive Enhancers for Patients With Mild Cognitive Impairment: A Systematic Review and Meta-analysis." *Canadian Medical Association Journal* doi:10.1503/cmaj.130451.

Tsunoda, K., et al. (2010). "Effects of Discontinuing Benzodiazepine-Derivative Hypnotics on Postural Sway and Cognitive Functions in the Elderly." *International Journal of Geriatric Psychiatry* 25: 1259–1265.

Van Leeuwen, W. E., et al. (2009). "Collaborative Depression Care for the Old-Old: Findings from the IMPACT Trial." *American Journal of Geriatric Psychiatry* 17: 1040–1049.

Veeraraghavalu, K., et al. (2013). "Comment on 'ApoE-Directed Therapeutics Rapidly Clear β-Amyloid and Reverse Deficits in AD Mouse Models.'" *Science* 340: 924.

Vellas, B., et al. (2012). "Long-term Use of Standardised Ginkgo Biloba Extract for the Prevention of Alzheimer's Disease (GuidAge): A Randomised Placebo-controlled Trial." *Lancet Neurology* 11: 851–859.

Ventimiglia, J., et al. (2010). "An Analysis of the Intended Use of Atypical Antipsychotics in Dementia." *Psychiatry* 7: 14–17.

Vigen, C. L. P., et al. (2011). "Cognitive Effects of Atypical Antipsychotic Medications in Patients With Alzheimer's Disease: Outcomes From CATIE-AD." *American Journal of Psychiatry* 168: 831–839.

Vos, S. J. B., et al. (2013). "Preclinical Alzheimer's Disease and Its Outcome: A Longitudinal Cohort Study." *Lancet Neurology*; http://dx.doi.org/10.1016/S1474-4422(13)70194-7.

Weintraub, D., et al. (2010). "Impulse Control Disorders in Parkinson's Disease: A Cross-Sectional Study of 3,090 Patients." *Archives of Neurology* 67: 589–595.

Wilcock, G. K., et al. (2008). "Efficacy and Safety of Tarenflurbil in Mild to Moderate Alzheimer's Disease: A Randomized Phase II Trial." *Lancet Neurology* 7: 483–493.

Williams, A., et al. (2010). "Deep Brain Stimulation Plus Best Medical Therapy versus Best Medical Therapy Alone for Advanced Parkinson's Disease (PD SURG Trial): A Randomized, Open-Label Trial." *Lancet Neurology*, 9: 681–681.

Winblad, B., et al. (2006). "Donepezil in Patients with Severe Alzheimer's Disease: Double-Blind, Parallel-Group, Placebo-Controlled Study." *Lancet* 367: 1057–1065.

Yurko-Mauro, K., et al. (2010). "Beneficial Effects of Docosahexaenoic Acid on Cognition in Age-related Cognitive Decline." *Alzheimer's & Dementia* 6: 456–464.

Zhu, C. W., et al. (2013). "Long-term Associations Between Cholinesterase Inhibitors and Memantine Use and Health Outcomes Among Patients with Alzheimer's Disease." *Alzheimer's & Dementia* 9: 733–740.

Chapter 17

Challenging Times for Mental Health

"Psychopharmacology is in crisis" (Fibiger, 2012). During the last 30 years no new fundamentally novel drugs for mental illness have been developed, and the usefulness of even current medications is being challenged. Efforts to develop an effective drug for Alzheimer's disease have not been successful. Even the criteria by which psychiatric disorders are diagnosed have been revised. Many pharmaceutical companies are abandoning their psychotropic research programs. And all of this is occurring at a time of diminished public resources when the economy has suffered a severe downturn. This chapter provides an overview of the dramatic changes taking place in psychopharmacology and its effect on the relationship between psychiatry and psychology.

Did You Know?

Mortality Gap Widens for Mentally Ill

The life expectancy gap between the mentally ill and the general population has widened, largely because of comorbidities like cardiovascular disease and cancer. During a 20-year period the gap increased by more than 2 years for both men and women so that mentally ill men had a life expectancy that was about 16 years shorter than that of the general population and women with mental illness had a lifespan that was 12 years shorter.

Epidemiological Developments

SAMHSA's (Substance Abuse and Mental Health Services Administration) 2010 *National Survey on Drug Use and Health: Mental Health Findings* defines mental illness among adults 18 and older as: a diagnosable mental, behavioral, or emotional disorder (excluding developmental and substance use disorders) that occurred within the past year. According to this definition:

- 1 in 5 adults (20 percent) experienced a mental illness, affecting 45.9 million adults.
    - Approximately 60 percent received no treatment for the condition.
    - The most common reason for not getting mental healthcare was not being able to afford it.
- 5 percent (11.4 million adults) suffered from *serious* mental illness.
- The rate of mental illness was more than twice as high among those age 18 to 25 (29.9 percent) than among those ages 50 and older (14.3 percent).
- Adult women were more likely than adult men to have experienced mental illness in the last year (23.0 percent versus 16.8 percent).
- Adults experiencing mental illness were more than three times as likely to have met the criteria for substance dependence or abuse in that period than those who had not experienced mental illness (20.0 percent versus 6.1 percent). In February 2013, another SAMHSA report found that 30.9 percent of all cigarettes consumed in the U.S. were smoked by the mentally ill. This is partly because the mentally ill population smokes more cigarettes per person than the rest of the population.
- 8.7 million Americans had seriously contemplated suicide over the past year.

People with mental disorders, including schizophrenia, depression, anxiety, personality disorders and substance abuse, have a significantly increased risk of dying from homicide. The likelihood of homicide was more than seven times greater among those with any mental disorder than in the general population, according to one recent analysis (Crump et al., 2013). For those with substance abuse disorders the risk was 16 times greater. People with mental illness are also four times more likely to be victimized in nonlethal violent incidents, than people in the general population. In fact, even mild psychological distress may almost double the likelihood of a subsequent diagnosis of somatic or psychiatric disability (Rai et al., 2012).

Given this situation, it is perhaps not surprising that overall use of psychiatric medications among adults also grew—by 22 percent from 2001 to 2010. Figures released in November 2011, are based on prescription-drug pharmacy claims of 2 million insured adults and children reported by Medco Health Solutions Inc., a pharmacy-benefit manager. The biggest increases were the growth of antipsychotic drug prescriptions for all ages, and the growth in adult use of drugs for ADHD.

Policy Developments

During this time, the economic recession has seen a dramatic decrease in spending across most sectors of state government, that is, support for mental health has dropped during a period of increasing demand. Between fiscal years 2009 and 2012, the National Association of State Mental Health Program Directors (NASMHPD) estimates that funding within the control of State Mental Health Authorities (SMHAs) in the 50 states was reduced by at least 3.49 billion dollars. In fiscal year 2011, 81 percent of states participating in the NASMHPD survey reported budget reductions during a time of increasing demand for mental health services.

This development is particularly unfortunate considering that between 2000 and 2009 public mental health systems saw important improvements. Positive changes began with the U.S. Surgeon General's report on mental illness in 1999, and gradually included recognition of evidence-based practices, new psychotropic medicines, and several federal initiatives. One example was the passage of insurance parity in 2008, which mandated that psychiatric disorders be covered in the same way as other illnesses. This was accompanied by increasing state mental health budgets. There was also an increase in integration of mental health and addiction with primary care among many of the states, to provide a comprehensive approach to multi-co-occurring conditions.

The result is that improvements begun in the previous decade have been followed by a retrenchment. One consequence is an increase in managed care strategies for mental health and addiction services. There is ongoing reassessment of which services can be outsourced, maintained in-house or eliminated without jeopardizing basic responsibilities.

The influence of health care expansion under the Affordable Care Act (ACA) remains to be seen. Although the ACA prohibits denial of coverage based on pre-existing mental or substance-use disorders, it did not require every insurance plan to offer benefits for those disorders, and it provided no way to monitor enforcement (Jeste, 2012). Some additional support was added in February 2010, but there were few details.

The shocking events of December 2012, in which 26 people, including 20 children, were killed in a single shooting incident in Newtown, Connecticut, renewed discussion about the role of mental illness in regard to gun-related violence. In January 2013 U.S. President Obama asked for $15 million to train teachers and others who interact with youth how to respond to and handle mental health issues. The proposal also calls for training 5,000 more social workers, counselors, and psychologists with a focus on serving students and young adults. Members of Congress also announced hearings from leading experts in regard to guns, violence and mental illness. Presumably, such ongoing discussions on mental health policy will include more provisions for support of mental health benefits, and implementation of parity with medical and surgical benefits.

Did You Know?

Treatment of Mental Illness Lowers Arrest Rates, Saves Money

It is well established that people with mental health problems, such as schizophrenia or bipolar disorder, make up a disproportionate percentage of defendants, inmates and others who come into contact with the criminal justice system. A total of 4,056 people who had been hospitalized for mental illness in 2004 or 2005 were tracked from 2005 to 2012. It was determined which individuals were receiving government-subsidized medication and which were receiving government-subsidized outpatient services, such as therapy, as well as who was arrested during the seven-year study period. People receiving medication were significantly less likely to be arrested. Outpatient services also decreased likelihood of arrest. Individuals who were arrested received less treatment and each cost the government approximately $95,000 during the study period. Individuals who were not arrested received more treatment and each cost the government approximately $68,000 during the study period. It cost about $10 less per day to provide treatment and prevent crime.

Clinical Developments: Diagnostic and Statistical Manual of Mental Disorders (DSM-5)

Publication of the fifth edition of the *Diagnostic and Statistical Manual of Mental Disorders* (DSM-5) in May 2013 marked one of the most anticipated events in the mental health field. Since the DSM-5 was opened for public comment, in early 2010, many changes have been suggested to improve the current volume, which was released in 1994. The chairman of the task force, David Kupfer, and the research director of the American Psychiatric Association (APA), Darrel Regier, led the initiative. Revisions were distributed across 13 workgroups, which were assigned to consider disorders in 20 categories. Revisions had to be approved by a scientific review committee, the task force leadership and the APA governing bodies. The final version had to be completed by December 2012, for publication and formal release at the annual APA convention in May 2013. Although detailed descriptions of the changes are beyond the scope of this text, a summary of the major revisions is warranted, because the DSM is crucial for designating the conditions for which psychotropic drugs are prescribed. Development and testing of new drugs must be directed toward the DSM diagnostic criteria.

In general, there was an overall effort to improve the relationship between behavioral/psychological disorders and other medical specialties, and toward a more global system. For example, some structural changes now incorporate influences of age, gender, and culture on diagnostic presentations. Another important change is that the new manual is more compatible with the *International Classification of Diseases (ICD) System*, which is used by the rest of the world, outside of North America. That is, the revisions of the DSM-5 are more aligned with the structure of the disorders in the upcoming ICD-11. As of October 1 2014, the ICD-10-CM will become the official health classification of the U.S. government. (This manual is available free at the National Center for Health Statistics Web site at www.cdc.gov/nchs/icd/icd10cm.htm; Clay et al., 2013.) A third difference is the use of a continuum of symptoms rather than discrete diagnostic boundaries. Fourth, the "multiaxial" system, which used five different axes (psychiatric diagnoses; co-morbid medical conditions; nonmedical factors; and other disabilities), is discontinued. In general, intellectual and personality disorders are given more equality with other diagnoses (Kupfer et al., 2013).

Here is a very brief overview of the major changes.

Organizational Changes

- Until now, the disorders in the DSM were organized into five main categories, or Axes. In the new edition this is replaced by 20 separate chapters of 'families of disorders.' Disorders will be arranged chronologically, starting with conditions usually seen in infants or childhood and moving to illnesses occurring in adults.

- A significant change is the addition of a measure of severity within the disorder categories. For example, symptoms of depression would be rated in regard to the *amount* of insomnia or the *frequency* of suicidal thoughts. Such ratings will be standardized to aid comparisons across therapists.

- Where available, objective test results will be part of the criteria, such as a polysomnogram for diagnosis of a sleep disorder.

Major Specific Changes

- Criteria from autistic disorder, Asperger disorder, childhood disintegrative disorder, and pervasive developmental disorder (not otherwise specified) have been combined into a single diagnosis of Autism Spectrum Disorder.

- Binge Eating Disorder is now in the Eating Disorder family.

- Disruptive Mood Dysregulation Disorder is a new designation for children who have persistent severe temper tantrums. This was done to address the increase in the diagnosis of pediatric bipolar disorder among children with severe emotional disturbance. Essentially, this diagnosis would be more likely for conditions of nonepisodic irritability, as opposed to episodic periods of mania, for which a bipolar diagnosis would be considered.

- Severe bereavement grief can be diagnosed as a type of major depression if the criteria are met. Previously, this diagnosis could not be applied if the death occurred within the preceding 2 months.

- Instead of separate diagnoses for substance "abuse" and "dependence," the diagnosis for these types of problems will be "Substance Use Disorders." A report of "craving" from the patient is now required. Postulated specific addictions to sex, food, caffeine, and the Internet were not included, although these decisions may be reconsidered depending on results of subsequent research. However, the specific word "addiction" is not included for any disorder. All such conditions are termed "use disorders."

- Posttraumatic Stress Disorder (PTSD) is in a chapter separate from anxiety disorders, with some revisions of symptoms.

- A variety of other syndromes are placed in a separate Section III, which is a category for conditions that may be reconsidered after more research.

The new manual will not only be available in print but also in electronic format so that it can be continuously updated.

Questioning the Efficacy of Psychotropic Medications

Public policy and diagnostic criteria are not the only aspects of mental health and substance abuse treatment that is undergoing upheaval. The therapeutic validity of psychotropic drugs and their clinical application have also been challenged and questions raised about the usefulness of even the newest drugs. One of the most powerful denunciations of the current state of psychopharmacology is found in the book, by Robert Whitaker, *Anatomy of an Epidemic: Magic Bullets, Psychiatric Drugs, and the Astonishing Rise in Mental Illness in America* (2009). This book criticizes pharmacotherapy on several levels, including the use of questionable diagnostic criteria, the reckless prescribing of psychotropic drugs for children, and the ethical corruption of pharmaceutical researchers, both in academia and industry. There is compelling support for all of these accusations. But Whitaker also argues that the psychiatric profession, in conjunction with the pharmaceutical industry, has even been responsible for causing more harm than good. Specifically, he charges that psychiatry has produced an iatrogenic epidemic, by promoting drugs that are either ineffective or inappropriate. He accuses the profession of being responsible for an unprecedented increase in unnecessary and coerced drug treatment, which has actually worsened the prevalence of mental illness. In brief, he argues that these drugs make "patients sicker than they would have been if they had never been medicated" (Horgan, 2012).

In regard to the consequences of antipsychotics, Whitaker's arguments have been refuted, most notably in an extensive article by E. Fuller Torrey (http://www.treatmentadvocacycenter.org/index.php?option=com_content&task=view&id=2085). In his rebuttal, Torrey discusses evidence *against* Whitaker's claim that outcomes for schizophrenia patients have worsened during the last few decades, and are now no better than they were a century ago. Torrey argues that the apparent increase in the number of people with mental illness, during a time when the use of drugs for depression and schizophrenia also increased dramatically, is a misreading or misinterpretation of the literature. In some cases the diagnoses are questionable, in other cases the stated results have not been replicated or even verified. Policy changes in medical coverage for mentally ill people who used to be on welfare or in hospitals, but who are now receiving social security disability or insurance benefits, give a false impression that the numbers have greatly increased. Torrey argues against Whitaker's conclusion that, for the most part, people with schizophrenia would do better without medications. In some of Whitaker's examples patients did not need long-term treatment because they had sufficiently recovered, in other situations the information about successful programs that did not use drugs was not published (so not evaluated by peers) or not confirmed. Torrey also criticizes the neurobiological process that Whitaker proposes to explain why antipsychotics worsen schizophrenia. In brief, Whitaker argues that because antipsychotic drugs block dopamine type 2 receptors, those receptors become supersensitive. If the drugs are stopped the symptoms then re-emerge, perhaps more intensely, leading to reinstatement of the antipsychotic, producing a vicious cycle. According to Torrey, a large number of stimuli, not just antipsychotics, can cause the same increase in dopamine receptors, and, furthermore, antipsychotics can also *decrease* these receptors if the receptors have previously been increased in number.

Aside from the controversy over the long-term efficacy of psychotropics in general, the specific benefit of antidepressant drugs for depression has also been questioned. Kirch and colleagues initiated this discussion in 1998, when they analyzed 38 published clinical trials involving more than 3,000 depressed patients. They found that 75 percent of the antidepressant effect was also produced by placebos. They pursued this unexpected result by using the Freedom of Information Act to get data that the drug companies had sent to the FDA in the process of getting their medications approved. They found that the difference between drug and placebo was even smaller in the data sent to the FDA than it was in the published literature. More than half of the clinical trials sponsored by the pharmaceutical companies showed no significant difference at all between drug and placebo. What they did find was a difference in side effects, like nausea and sexual dysfunction, produced by antidepressants. In fact, Kirsch argued that even the small statistical differences seen between placebo and drug might be due to the fact that patients can discern the physiological side effects produced by the active agents, which then potentiates the placebo influence. Kirsch concluded that antidepressants are not effective for mild or moderate depression, and that they only have a clinically meaningful benefit for severely depressed patients (Ioannidis, 2008; Kirsch, 2009).[1] This conclusion was supported by Fournier and colleagues (2010), who also reanalyzed archival datasets. Consistent with Kirsch, they found either no benefit or minimal improvement relative to placebo, in patients with mild or moderate symptoms, while the difference was substantial for patients with severe depression. A subsequent study by Barbui and colleagues (Barbui et al., 2011) confirmed the conclusion that for minor depression, antidepressants are unlikely to have an advantage over placebo.

The argument that antidepressants were largely ineffective was a dramatic challenge to their extraordinary success, especially of the newer antidepressants, ushered in by the first SSRI, Prozac. In his watershed book, *Listening to Prozac*, Peter Kramer even stated that Prozac made patients "better than well." Understandably, the reviews by Kirsch and Ioannidis elicited a reanalysis of the same evidence (Davis et al., 2011), which argued that antidepressants were indeed more effective than placebo for a substantial proportion of patients. Although a detailed analysis of the points made by these reviews is beyond the scope of this text, the current situation may be summarized as follows:

Antidepressants may not be very useful for mild depression because of the natural variability of this disorder. That is, the apparent substantial effect of placebo on the low baseline of a mild depression may be due to spontaneous changes in the course of the illness itself. However, as symptom intensity increases, to a "moderate" level, several studies have provided evidence of antidepressant benefit (Gueorguieva et al., 2011; Vöhringer and Ghaemi, 2011; Stewart et al., 2012). Some reasons for this difference are that the previous negative reviews used only a very few, select, perhaps unrepresentative, studies in their analyses, and that the studies used low doses or few drugs for comparison, and a variety of methods, rather than consistent treatment approaches. In this regard, Stewart et al. (2012) describe outcomes of six studies using data from the same outpatient clinic, which showed significant improvement even in patients with nonsevere depression, (HDRS ≤ 23) including remission (HDRS ≤7), regardless of the type of symptom or of illness duration. Outcomes of individual patients, rather than groups, may also show better prognoses (Gueorguieva et al., 2011), in that responders may be differentiated from nonresponders in the same sample, and independently compared with placebo-treated patients. Even Kirsch, in collaboration with other researchers, has shown that combining antidepressants and psychotherapy can offer some, albeit slight, advantage over either alone (Khan et al., 2012).

At this point, the literature supports short-term antidepressant efficacy for acute episodes of severe depression, and, at least in some individuals, for less severe, moderate symptoms as well. Yet, this evidence does not address the issue of long-term maintenance,

---

[1] Most of the data in these studies are obtained with the Hamilton Depression Rating Scale (HDRS). There are several versions of this scale; each of them consists of individual questions about symptom intensity, which are scored from 0 to either 2 or 4. For the 17-item version, scores can range from 0 to 54. A score of 0–7 on the HDRS is considered to be normal, scores of 20 or higher indicate moderately severe depression and are usually required for entry into a clinical trial. In these studies, a baseline score of 23 or less is considered not to be severe. In the Kirsch study, the baseline score had to exceed 28 for statistical improvement. Other rating scales and measures, such as the number or percent of patients who respond or recover may also be used.

that is, whether continued treatment, even when it is effective, prevents relapse. As discussed by Pies (2012), evidence supports a reduction of at least 6-month relapse rates from maintenance antidepressants compared with placebo. But it is not obvious if medications prevent relapse or recurrence beyond 6 to 12 months. In fact, the possibility that tolerance (Fava and Offidani, 2011) or a compensatory "tardive dysphoria" develops (El-Mallakh et al., 2011), to long-term antidepressant use has been proposed. At the very least, there is data that antidepressant discontinuation, especially if too sudden, greatly increases relapse risk.

Finally, it has been argued that the efficacy of psychiatric medications is comparable to that of other, nonpsychiatric medications. Leucht and colleagues (2012) noted that there is a lot of variability in the effect of drugs for many medical conditions, from a high rate of efficacy for drugs in gastric reflux treatment to a low rate of efficacy for statins for cardiovascular events. They concluded that, with respect to their effectiveness, psychiatric drugs fall in the middle compared to most drugs used in internal medicine.

But, notwithstanding this optimistic viewpoint, even when psychotropic drugs are effective it may take weeks before they show benefit and they have many side effects. They don't help enough people and, for some psychiatric disorders, there are still no medications available. Part of the problem is that we don't know the causes of mental illness, and current animal models are insufficient for addressing these needs. Yet these disorders take an enormous toll.

Pharmaceutical Developments

Given this situation, it is not surprising that the pharmaceutical pipeline for psychotropic drugs is shrinking. Until recently, nearly half the budget for research and development in brain disorders came from industry. However, the only new psychotropic medications approved by the FDA since the previous edition of this book were the antipsychotic drug, *lurasidone* (Latuda) and the antidepressant drug *vilazodone* (Viibryd). Currently, the pharmaceutical companies Novartis, Pfizer, GlaxoSmithKline, AstraZeneca, Merck and Sanofi, at the very least, have all cut back or terminated neuroscience research on brain diseases. Various suggestions have been made to break this impasse. In terms of financial support, perhaps insurance companies, or mental health research charity groups might provide new funding. Incentives, such as longer patent life, might be useful. Better collaboration among researchers and between researchers and clinicians might improve target identification and outcome measures. This includes more interaction between academia and industry. Early intervention and preemptive therapy might improve outcomes, if only by increasing adherence. And, one way of improving treatment effectiveness is by integrating medical and psychosocial approaches (Nutt and Goodwin, 2011; Insel and Sahakian, 2012; Schwab and Buchli, 2012).

Integrating Psychopharmacology and Psychological Therapies in Patient Care

About 10 years ago, in 2003, a U.S. Presidential Commission on Mental Health report noted that care for the mentally ill must go beyond prescribing medication and crisis management of symptoms (U.S. Department of Health and Human Services, 2003). The report called for counselors to help patients lead a fuller life, including (but moving beyond) administering drugs. The commission issued a vision statement as follows:

> We are committed to a future where recovery is the expected outcome and when mental illness can be prevented or cured. We envision a nation where everyone with mental illness will have access to early detection and the effective treatment and supports essential to live, work, learn, and participate fully in their community.

Following are the goals of the commission report:

- *Mental health is essential to health.* Every individual, family, and community will understand that mental health is an essential part of overall health.
- *Early mental health screening and treatment in multiple settings.* Every individual will have the opportunity for early and appropriate mental health screening, assessment, and referral to treatment.
- *Consumer/family-centered care.* Consumers and families will have the necessary information and the opportunity to exercise choice over the care decisions that affect them. Continuous healing relationships will be a key feature of care.
- *Best care science can offer.* Adults with serious mental illness and children with serious emotional disturbance will have ready access to the best treatments, services, and supports leading to recovery and cure. Research will be accelerated to enhance the prevention of, recovery from, and ultimate discovery of cures for mental illnesses.

The commission stated:

> These goals provide a set of ideals toward which to work. Symptom reduction via pharmacological means is only part of the plan: all mental health care should be delivered in an integrated fashion. All mental health personnel should understand their clients' medications well enough to allow them to interact meaningfully with other professionals.

With chronic physical diseases, such as hypertension, diabetes, and elevated cholesterol, medications will usually not work if life-style changes are not made. The same holds true for the treatment of psychological illnesses. This need to go beyond medication alone has been supported in numerous studies:

- In the STAR*D study (see Chapter 12), medication efficacy in treating depression in adults was only 30 percent with the first drug. With multiple medication switches or augmentation, the remission rate increased to about 60 percent. Thase and coworkers (2007) demonstrated that in depressed persons who failed to respond to citalopram therapy, an augmentation strategy adding cognitive therapy resulted in the same likelihood of remission and similar symptomatic improvement, as did switching from citalopram to either sustained-release bupropion or buspirone.

- In the TADS study (see Chapter 15), efficacy in treating depression in children and adolescents was only about 35 percent with medication alone. Adding cognitive-behavioral therapies markedly improved results.

- In the STEP-BD study (see Chapter 14), although remission of bipolar symptoms could be achieved in about 60 percent of people with the disorder, 50 percent of responders relapsed frequently.

- In the CATIE and CUtLASS studies (see Chapter 11), patients with schizophrenia were relatively noncompliant with medication prescription, regardless of which antipsychotic was prescribed

In all these cases, treatment with medication alone was less effective than anticipated by the prescriber, the client, the client's family, and even mental health practitioners. Therefore, it is important to recognize the limitations to pharmacological therapy.

Guidelines for this approach were offered in an editorial by Salzman et al. (2010), humorously presented as "The 7 Sins of Psychopharmacology," as follows:

1. The 3 "DS" - Diagnosis, Dose and Duration

   A comprehensive evaluation and accurate diagnosis is crucial. The diagnosis should be based on sound clinical criteria and the psychological context, background, family, ethnic and other considerations need to be part of the determination. Not all unhappiness is depression, not all excitement is mania, and not all nervousness is anxiety, requiring medication. Doses are derived from the analysis of pharmacokinetic and pharmacodynamic processes and an inadequate response or intolerable side effect may occur when these amounts are too low or too high. Ongoing assessment of the situation is necessary to determine the "best" dose for a particular patient. Likewise, the duration of drug treatment needs to be sufficient for the best response to be produced. Medication that is discontinued, altered, or augmented before an adequate assessment will not be in the best interest of the patient.

2. Try to avoid polypharmacy, unless there is a clear rationale, such as a co-occurring disorder. Adding drugs, even from a different therapeutic class, may only increase exposure to side effects without any benefit.

3. Drugs have limitations. Even the correct medication may not be the best solution.

4. Try to understand the psychological environment. Prescribing should be more than a 'mechanical' response to a list of symptoms. Some knowledge of the patient's circumstances can improve the therapeutic alliance and eventual outcome.

5. Obtain information about other diagnoses that might have been given to the patient and other treatments that the patient may also be taking.

6. Communicate with other practitioners and providers, as well as family members and significant others.

7. Keep up with the field, at least with the most important and relevant new findings. At the same time, be mindful of the source of the information and make an attempt to evaluate it appropriately.

Clinical Examples[2]

The following examples illustrate how clients can benefit from an integrated therapeutic system.

Client A is a 45-year-old male who was prescribed lithium for a diagnosis of bipolar II disorder. He presented with complaints of an 80-pound weight gain and an inability to remember names. Recognizing these problems as side effects of lithium therapy, the therapists noted a study on the efficacy of valproic acid for bipolar II and decided to make that medication switch. Thereafter, Client A lost about 40 pounds and his memory function improved, allowing him to continue working.

Five years later, Client A presented with complaints of listlessness, lack of energy, and sexual dysfunction. It was discovered that the client had been diagnosed with depression and had been prescribed *escitalopram* (Lexapro) in addition to the valproic acid. Escitalopram and valproate were discontinued and initiation of *aripiprazole* (Abilify) and/or *lamotrigine* (Lamictal) was recommended. Valproate and escitalopram were replaced with aripiprazole. About 2 weeks later, the client reported that the new drug was "intolerable" and complained of aches, myalgias, flulike symptoms, and electric shocks in his head. The psychologist determined that the client had serotonin discontinuation syndrome (rather than side effects of aripiprazole) and counseled the client about serotonin discontinuation syndrome. Three weeks later, the symptoms had ceased, the client was more energized, sexual function was improving, and no bipolar symptoms were reported. Continual progress was made over the next few months.

Client B was a man in his late twenties, referred by a physician for evaluation of cognitive difficulties. Neuropsychological testing was performed and diagnosis was made of notable cognitive dysfunction, with the greatest difficulty being with word finding. Medication review revealed that the client had recently been prescribed *topiramate* (Topamax). Replacement of the Topamax [prescribed for anxiety and posttraumatic stress disorder (PTSD)] with *pregabalin* (Lyrica) led to rapid resolution of the cognitive difficulties.

Client C was a 48-year-old woman diagnosed with depression and anxiety. She was prescribed *sertraline* (Zoloft) and showed some improvement. However, she gradually developed a panic disorder. Further history taking revealed that she had recently undergone surgery for breast lesions that were diagnosed as benign breast cysts. It turned out

---

[2] Although these vignettes are hypothetical, a real case was presented in the February 17th 2013 Sunday magazine issue of *The New York Times*. The patient was a 55 year old man, who suffered from depression and alcoholism, and who was admitted to the hospital after a fall down the stairs of his home. Because he hadn't been found for a few days, his condition was extremely serious and it took 5 weeks of medical treatment before he was able to transfer to a rehabilitation facility. After 2 weeks in rehabilitation, the patient began to have hallucinations and started talking to people who were not there, but whom he feared was going to hurt him. Even after his sleeping medication was changed (which was thought to be the source of the symptoms), the hallucinations continued. He also had a fever, racing heart rate, high blood pressure, and hyperreflexia. Fortunately, the attending physician noted that the patient had been prescribed a second antidepressant during the last two days of his rehabilitation treatment, as well as a heartburn medication, which all raised his serotonin level. Within 24 hours after being put on a drug that blocks serotonin, the patient was alert and talking, his hallucinations were gone, his heart rate and blood pressure were normal, and the tremors were resolving. This real-life incident illustrates the importance of communication as part of the collaboration among all medical personnel associated with patient care.

that Client C was a heavy coffee drinker. Sertraline interferes with the metabolism of caffeine, in essence doubling her blood level of caffeine. Caffeinism is associated with increasing anxiety (the panic disorder) and the development of benign breast cysts. Cessation of caffeine drinking (small amounts of caffeinated coffee and the remainder decaffeinated) led to resolution of the panic disorder.

Client D was a 28-year-old Gulf War veteran with severe PTSD presenting with night-time terror and threatening actions toward his wife. Moreover, he was amnestic for these episodes. Medication review revealed a prescription for *zolpidem* (Ambien) for sleep. It was determined that the Ambien might be causing the amnesia. Replacement of Ambien with gabapentin at bedtime improved PTSD symptoms, and the amnestic episodes were resolved.

Client E was an 88-year-old female care center resident whose family took her to therapy for increasing dementia. Medication review revealed that she had been receiving *imipramine* (Tofranil) for depression and *diazepam* (Valium) for anxiety and sleep difficulties. Because tricyclic antidepressants have anticholinergic difficulties, they can cause cognitive impairments. Benzodiazepines are widely known to worsen dementias. Cessation of these medicines and replacement with *quetiapine* (Seroquel) and *mirtazepine* (Remeron) at bedtime led to cognitive improvements, reductions in anxiety, better sleep patterns, and improvements in appetite.

Client F was a 5-year-old girl presenting with rages and aggressive behaviors made worse by psychostimulants and antidepressants. She was prescribed *valproic acid* (Depakote) and showed marked improvement in behavior. When she was referred to a psychologist, it was decided that with behavioral improvement, family therapy could be instituted to address problems underlying the client's behaviors. The possibility was also raised that, with effective family therapy, the valproic acid might eventually be stopped.

What do these cases have in common? First, all clients had been prescribed reasonable medications as therapy. Second, while efficacious, all the medications had significant side effects that limited optimal life functioning. Third, suggestions were made for reasonable modifications in therapy that often resulted in improved compliance, better life functioning, or amenability to the institution of psychological therapies.

To make specific suggestions for a client, it is important to be aware of three important factors that may affect patient compliance:

1. *Can the client afford the prescribed medication?* Patients and physicians alike are susceptible to ads for heavily promoted, expensive, brand-name medications. New medicines may have significant advantages over older medicines, but they also have their own constellation of side effects. Fortunately, in the last couple of years, numerous psychotherapeutic drugs have become available in less expensive generic forms.

2. *Can the client tolerate any degree of weight gain?* Some clients can tolerate a degree of weight gain, while undesirable weight gain might lead to noncompliance in others. In choosing an antidepressant, for example, *mirtazepine* (Remeron) might be appropriate for a client who can tolerate weight gain, while *duloxetine* (Cymbalta) or *bupropion* (Wellbutrin) might be appropriate for a client who wants to lose weight. The same considerations apply in the treatment of bipolar disorder and behavioral disorders associated with anger, agitation, and aggressive behaviors.

3. *Can the client tolerate any degree of cognitive dysfunction?* Many psychotherapeutic drugs are associated with drug-induced cognitive dysfunction; among them are benzodiazepines, tricyclic antidepressants, lithium, some anticonvulsant mood stabilizers, and some antipsychotic drugs. The young, the elderly, and people suffering from traumatic brain injury (for example) might not tolerate agents that can be detrimental to cognitive functioning. Others, however, might be able to tolerate some degree of cognitive slowing if the therapeutic benefit seems to outweigh the side effect. If these agents are prescribed, dysfunction may interfere not only with the efficacy of cognitive therapies but also with overall life functioning.

Considerations for Current Practice

Most relevant to this text, the convergence of economic, public health, academic, and professional developments has perhaps reinvigorated the discussion of collaborative interventions between psychology and primary medicine. For example, in patients with social anxiety disorder (SAD), the combination of the monoamine oxidase inhibitor (MAOI) antidepressant phenelzine, plus cognitive behavioral group therapy (CBGT) was found to be superior to either of the individual treatments alone. Surprisingly, neither the drug treatment alone nor the behavioral treatment alone differed in outcome from the placebo treatment. Because patients in the combination group had larger average improvements than the patients receiving the monotherapies, it was concluded that the combination produced an additive or synergistic effect (Blanco et al., 2010).

There is now also extensive evidence that psychological treatments have significant effects on depression (Cuijpers et al., 2008) and that combined treatments can be better than psychological therapy (Cuijpers et al., 2009a) or pharmacological treatment alone (Cuijpers et al., 2009b; Cuijpers et al., 2010). For chronic depression (lasting 2 years or longer) and especially for dysthymia, results of one meta-analysis show that psychotherapy may be less effective than it is in nonchronic depressive disorders and that pharmacotherapy is significantly more effective. However, a subsequent meta-analysis found equivalent short-term outcomes between psychotherapy and newer antidepressants, when only studies with appropriately trained therapists were included. In fact, psychotherapies had slightly better efficacy on depression rating scales at follow-up relative to Second Generation Antidepressants (Spielmans et al., 2011). Such results illustrate the complexity of treatment for psychiatric disorders and the importance of objective, scientific analyses in determining the respective benefits of psychological and pharmacological treatment.

In spite of the challenges to developing new, better psychotropic medications, the pharmaceutical industry has not abandoned the field. In a news release, the Pharmaceutical Research and Manufacturers of America stated "America's biopharmaceutical research companies are developing 187 innovative medicines to help the nearly 60 million patients in the United States who are suffering from some form of mental illness."

http://www.ifpma.org/fileadmin/content/Publication/2012/MNDs-Innovation.pdf

Hopefully, such commitment will be successful.

REFERENCES

Barbui, C., et al. (2011). "Efficacy of Antidepressants and Benzodiazepines in Minor Depression: Systematic Review and Meta-Analysis." *The British Journal of Psychiatry* 198:11–16.

Blanco, C., et al. (2010). "A Placebo-Controlled Trial of Phenelzine, Cognitive Behavioral Group Therapy, and Their Combination, for Social Anxiety Disorder." *Archives of General Psychiatry* 67: 286–295.

Carlat, D. (2010). "Psychologist Prescribing: The Best Thing That Can Happen to Psychiatry." The Carlat Psychiatry Blog. http://carlatpsychiatry.blogspot.com/2010/03/psychologists-prescribing-best-thing.html.

Clay, R. A. (2013). "The Next DSM." *Monitor on Psychology* April: 26–27.

Crump, C., et al. (2013)."Mental Disorders and Vulnerability to Homicidal Death: Swedish Nationwide Cohort Study." *British Medical Journal* doi: 10.1136/bmj.f557.

Cuijpers, P., et al. (2008). "Characteristics of Effective Psychological Treatments of Depression: A Meta-Regression Analysis." *Psychotherapy Research* 18: 225–236.

Cuijpers, P., et al. (2009a). "Psychological Treatment versus Combined Treatment of Depression: A Meta-Analysis." *Depression and Anxiety* 26: 279–288.

Cuijpers, P., et al. (2009b). "Adding Psychotherapy to Pharmacotherapy in the Treatment of Depressive Disorders in Adults: A Meta-Analysis." *Journal of Clinical Psychiatry* 70: 1219–1229.

Cuijpers, P., et al. (2010). "Psychotherapy for Chronic Major Depression and Dysthymia: A Meta-Analysis." *Clinical Psychology Review* 30: 51–62.

Davis, J., et al. (2011). "Should We Treat People With Drugs or With Psychological Interventions? A Reply to Ioannidis." *Philosophy, Ethics, and Humanities in Medicine* 6:8.

El-Mallakh, R. S., et al. (2011). "Tardive Dysphoria: The Role of Long Term Antidepressant Use in Inducing Chronic Depression." *Medical Hypotheses* 76: 769–773.

Fava, G. A., and Offidani, E. (2011). "The Mechanisms of Tolerance in Antidepressant Action." *Progress in Neuropsychopharmacology and Biological Psychiatry* 35: 1593–1602.

Fibiger, H. C. (2012). "Psychiatry, the Pharmaceutical Industry, and the Road to Better Therapeutics." *Schizophrenia Bulletin* 38: 649–650.

Fournier, J. C., et al. (2010). "Antidepressant Drug Effects and Depression Severity: A Patient-Level Meta-Analysis." *Journal of the American Medical Association* 6: 47–53.

Gueorguieva, R., et al. (2011). "Trajectories of Depression Severity in Clinical Trials of Duloxetine: Insights Into Antidepressant and Placebo Responses." *Archives of General Psychiatry* 68: 1227–1237.

Horgan, J. (2011). "Are Psychiatric Medications Making Us Sicker?" http://chronicle.com/article/Are-Psychiatric-Medications/128976/

Insel, T. R., and Sahakian, B. J. (2012). "A Plan for Mental Illness." *Nature* 483: 269.

Ioannidis, J. P. A. (2008). "Effectiveness of Antidepressants: An Evidence Myth Constructed From a Thousand Randomized Trials?" *Philosophy, Ethics, and Humanities in Medicine* 3: 14.

Jeste, D. V. (2012). "Mental Health and the 2012 US Election." *The Lancet* 380: 1206–1208.

Khan, A., et al. (2012). "A Systematic Review of Comparative Efficacy of Treatments and Controls for Depression." *PLoS One* 7: e41778.

Kirsch, I. (2009). *The Emperor's New Drugs: Exploding the Antidepressant Myth*. London: Bodley Head.

Kramer, P. (1993). *Listening to Prozac*. New York: Viking.

Kupfer, D. J., et al. (2013)."DSM-5 – The Future Arrived." *Journal of the American Medical Association* doi: 10.1001/jama.2013.2298.

Leucht, S., et al. (2012). "Putting the Efficacy of Psychiatric and General Medicine Medication Into Perspective: Review of Meta-Analyses." *British Journal of Psychiatry* 200: 97–106.

Nutt, D., and Goodwin, G. (2011). http://www.nature.com/news/2011/110614/full/news.2011.367.html

Pies, R. (2012). "Are Antidepressants Effective in the Acute and Long-Term Treatment of Depression? *Sic et Non*." *Innovations in Clinical Neuroscience* 9: 31–40.

Rai, D., et al. (2012). "Psychological Distress and Risk of Long-Term Disability: Population-Based Longitudinal Study." *Journal of Epidemiology and Community Health* 66: 586–592.

Salzman, C., et al. (2010). "The 7 Sins of Psychopharmacology." *Journal of Clinical Psychopharmacology* 30: 1–3.

SAMHSA "Results from the 2010 National Survey on Drug Use and Health: Mental Health Findings" HHS Publication 11-4667: 2012.

Schwab, M. E., and Buchli, A. D. (2012). "Plug the Real Brain Drain." *Nature* 483: 267–268.

Spielmans, G. I., et al. (2011). "Bona Fide Psychotherapy Appears as Effective as SGAs in the Short-Term Treatment of Depression, and Likely Somewhat More Effective Than SGAs in the Longer-Term Management of Depressive Symptoms." *Journal of Nervous and Mental Diseases* 199: 142–149.

Stewart, J. A., et al. (2012). "Can People With Nonsevere Major Depression Benefit from Antidepressant Medication?" *Journal of Clinical Psychiatry* 73: 518–525.

Torrey, E. F. (2011). http://www.treatmentadvocacycenter.org/index.php?option=com_content&task= view&id=2085.

U.S. Department of Health and Human Services. (2003). *President's New Freedom Commission on Mental Health, Final Report* (Publication SMA 03-3832). National Institute of Mental Health, Bethesda, MD. Available online at www.mentalhealthcommission.gov/.../FullReport.htm.

Vöhringer, P. A., and Ghaemi, S. N. (2011). "Solving the Antidepressant Efficacy Question: Effect Sizes in Major Depressive Disorder." *Clinical Therapeutics* 33: B49–B61.

Whitaker, R. (2010). *Anatomy of an Epidemic: Magic Bullets, Psychiatric Drugs, and the Astonishing Rise of Mental Illness in America*. New York: Crown Publishers.

CHAPTER 17 APPENDIX

Quick Reference to Psychotropic Medication

This appendix provides several quick-reference medication tables initially prepared by John Preston, Psy.D., ABPP, reproduced and modified by the authors of this textbook with his permission. The tables present a list of recommended doses and side effects for psychotherapeutic drugs. To our knowledge the information provided is accurate. However, the material is intended for general reference only, not as a guideline for prescribing for individual patients. It supplements the discussion of the pharmacology of these medicines presented in earlier chapters. The tables are designed to answer questions about the average doses of psychotherapeutic medicines encountered in clinical practice. They also detail the effects of therapeutic drugs on production of sedative side effects, potential for inducing weight gain, potential for producing cognitive impairments, and availability in generic (less expensive) formulations. Please check the manufacturer's product information sheet or the PDR for any changes in dosage schedule or contraindications. (Brand names are registered trademarks).

Antidepressants

| Names | | Usual daily dosage range | Sedation | Weight gain | Cognitive impairment | Generic available |
Generic	Brand					
imipramine	Tofranil	150–300 mg	mid	0–low	mid	yes
desipramine	Norpramin	150–300 mg	low	0–low	mid	yes
amitriptyline	Elavil	150–300 mg	high	0–low	mid	yes
nortriptyline	Aventyl, Pamelor	75–125 mg	mid	0–low	low	yes
protriptyline	Vivactil	15–40 mg	mid	0–low	mid	yes
trimipramine	Surmontil	100–300 mg	high	0–low	mid	yes
doxepin	Sinequan, Adapin	150–300 mg	high	0–low	mid	yes
clomipramine	Anafranil	150–250 mg	high	0–low	mid	yes
maprotiline	Ludiomil	150–225 mg	high	0–low	low	yes
amoxapine	Asendin	150–400 mg	mid	0–low	low	yes
trazodone	Desyrel, Oleptro (XR)	150–400 mg	mid	0–low	low–mid	yes
fluoxetine[1]	Prozac, Sarafem	20–80 mg	low	low	low	yes
bupropion-XL[1]	Wellbutrin-XL	150–400 mg	low	0	0	yes
sertraline	Zoloft	50–200 mg	low	low	low	yes
paroxetine	Paxil, Pexeva	20–50 mg	low	low	low	yes
venlafaxine-XR[1]	Effexor-XR	75–350 mg	low	low	0	yes
desvenlafaxine	Pristiq, Khedezla	50 mg	mid	low	0	yes
fluvoxamine	Luvox	50–300 mg	low	low	low	yes
mirtazapine	Remeron	15–45 mg	mid	low–mid	low	yes
citalopram	Celexa	10–60 mg	low	low	low	yes

Antidepressants (continued)

Names		Usual daily dosage range	Sedation	Weight gain	Cognitive impairment	Generic available
Generic	Brand					
escitalopram	Lexapro	5–20 mg	low	low	low	yes
duloxetine	Cymbalta	20–80 mg	low	low	0	no
atomoxetine	Strattera	60–120 mg	low	0	0	no
vilazodone	Viibryd	40 mg	low	low	low	no
vortioxetine	Brintellix	10–20 mg	low	low	0	no
MAO INHIBITORS						
phenelzine	Nardil	30–90 mg	low	0	0	yes
tranylcypromine	Parnate	20–60 mg	low	0	0	yes
selegiline	Emsam (patch)	6–12 mg	low	0	0	no

[1] Available in standard formulation and time release (XR or XL). Prozac available in 90-mg time-release/weekly formulation.

Bipolar Disorder Medications

Names		Serum level[1]	Weight gain	Cognitive impairment	Generic available
Generic	Brand				
lithium carbonate	Eskalith, Lithonate	0.6–1.5	high	high	yes
olanzapine/ fluoxetine	Symbyax	—[2]	high	high	yes
carbamazepine	Tegretol, Equetro	4–10+	low	low	yes
oxcarbazepine	Trileptal	—[2]	low	low	yes
valproic acid	Depakote	50–100	mid	mid	yes
gabapentin	Neurontin	—[2]	low	low	yes
lamotrigine	Lamictal	1–5	0	0	yes
topiramate	Topamax	—[3]	0	mid–high	yes
tiagabine	Gabitril	—[3]	0	low–mid	yes

[1]Lithium levels are expressed in mEq/l, carbamazepine, valproic acid, and lamotrigine levels in mcg/ml.
[2]Serum monitoring may not be necessary.
[3]Not yet established.

Psychostimulants

Names		Daily dosage range[1]
Generic	Brand	
methylphenidate[2]	Ritalin	5–50 mg
methylphenidate	Concerta[3]	18–54 mg
methylphenidate	Metadate	5–40 mg
methylphenidate[2]	Methylin	10–60 mg
methylphenidate	Daytrana (patch)	15–30 mg
dexmethylphenidate	Focalin	5–40 mg
dextroamphetamine[2]	Dexedrine	5–40 mg
pemoline	Cylert	37.5–112.5 mg
D- and L-amphetamine	Adderall	5–40 mg
modafinil	Provigil, Sparlon	100–400 mg
armodafinil	Nuvigil	150–250 mg
lisdexamfetamine	Vyvanse	30–70 mg

[1]Adult doses.
[2]Available in generic formulation.
[3]Sustained release.

Antiobsessional

Names		Daily dosage range[1]
Generic	Brand	
clomipramine	Anafranil	150–250 mg
fluoxetine	Prozac	20–80 mg
sertraline	Zoloft	50–200 mg
paroxetine	Paxil	20–60 mg
fluvoxamine	Luvox	50–300 mg
citalopram	Celexa	10–60 mg
escitalopram	Lexapro	5–20 mg

[1]Often higher doses are required to control obsessive-compulsive symptoms than the doses generally used to treat depression.

Antipsychotics

Names		Daily dosage range[1]	Weight gain	Cognitive impairment	Generic available
Generic	Brand				
LOW POTENCY					
chlorpromazine	Thorazine	50–800 mg	low	mid	yes
thioridazine	Mellaril	150–800 mg	low	mid	yes
clozapine	Clozaril	300–900 mg	high	low	yes
mesoridazine	Serentil	50–500 mg	low	mid	no
quetiapine	Seroquel (XR)	150–400 mg	low	0	yes
HIGH POTENCY					
molindone	Moban	20–225 mg	low	low	no
perphenazine	Trilafon	8–60 mg	low	low	yes
loxapine	Loxitane	50–250 mg	low	low	yes
trifluoperazine	Stelazine	2–40 mg	low	mid	yes
fluphenazine	Prolixin[2]	3–45 mg	low	low	yes
thiothixene	Navane	10–60 mg	low	low	yes
haloperidol	Haldol[2]	2–40 mg	low	low	yes
pimozide	Orap	1–10 mg	low	low	no
risperidone	Risperdal[3]	4–16 mg	mid	low	yes
paliperidone	Invega	3–12 mg	mid	low	no
olanzapine	Zyprexa	5–20 mg	high	low	yes
ziprasidone	Geodon	60–160 mg	0	0	yes
aripiprazole	Abilify	15–30 mg	0	0	no
iloperidone	Fanapt	12–24 mg	low	low	no
asenapine	Saphris	10–20 mg	low	low	no
lurasidone	Latuda	40–160 mg	low	low	no

[1]Usual daily oral dosage.
[2]Dose required to achieve efficacy of 100 mg chlorpromazine.
[3]Available in time-release IM format.

Hypnotics[1]

| Names | | Single-dose |
Generic	Brand	dosage range
flurazepam[2]	Dalmane	15–30 mg
temazepam[2]	Restoril	15–30 mg
triazolam[2]	Halcion	0.25–0.5 mg
estazolam[2]	ProSom	1.0–2.0 mg
quazepam[2]	Doral	7.5–15 mg
zolpidem	Ambien	5–10 mg
zaleplon	Sonata	5–10 mg
eszopiclone	Lunesta	1–3 mg
ramelteon	Rozerem	4–16 mg
diphenhydramine[2]	Benadryl	25–100 mg
doxepin[3]	Silenor	3–6 mg

[1]All hypnotics produce cognitive impairment.
[2]Available in generic formulation.
[3]Also marketed as Sinequan for the treatment of depression (Chapter 12).

Antianxiety (Anxiolytics)

Names		Single-dose dosage range
Generic	Brand	
BENZODIAZEPINES[1]		
diazepam	Valium	2–10 mg
chlordiazepoxide	Librium	10–50 mg
prazepam	Centrax	5–30 mg
clorazepate	Tranxene	3.75–15 mg
clonazepam	Klonopin	0.5–2.0 mg
lorazepam	Ativan	0.5–2.0 mg
alprazolam	Xanax, XR	0.25–2.0 mg
oxazepam	Serax	10–30 mg
OTHER ANTIANXIETY AGENTS[2]		
buspirone	BuSpar	5–20 mg
gabapentin	Neurontin	200–600 mg
hydroxyzine	Atarax, Vistaril	10–50 mg
propranolol[3]	Inderal	10–80 mg
atenolol[3]	Tenormin	25–100 mg
guanfacine[3]	Tenex	0.5–3 mg
clonidine[3]	Catapres	0.1–0.3 mg

[1]All benzodiazepines produce cognitive impairment and are available in generic formulation.
[2]All agents listed are available in generic formulation.
[3]Antihypertensive drugs.

Common Side Effects

ANTICHOLINERGIC EFFECTS
(block acetylcholine)

- Dry mouth
- Constipation
- Urinary retention
- Blurred vision
- Memory impairment
- Confusional states

EXTRAPYRAMIDAL EFFECTS
(dopamine blockade in basal ganglia)

- Parkinsonlike effects: rigidity, shuffling gait, tremor, flat affect, lethargy
- Dystonias: Spasms in neck and other muscle groups
- Akathisia: Intense, uncomfortable sense of inner restlessness
- Tardive dyskinesia: Often a persistent movement disorder (lip smacking, writhing movements, jerky movements)

Note: These are common side effects. All medications can produce specific or unique side effects.

Over-the-Counter

Name	Daily dose
St. John's wort[1,2]	600–1800 mg
SAMe[3]	400–1600 mg
Omega-3[4]	1–9 g

[1]Treats depression and anxiety.
[2]May cause significant drug-drug interactions.
[3]Treats depression.
[4]Treats depression, bipolar disorder, and perhaps psychosis.

GLOSSARY

Abstinence syndrome. State of altered behavior that follows cessation of drug administration. See also **Withdrawal syndrome**

Acamprosate. A structural analogue of glutamate, it is an anticraving drug used to maintain abstinence in alcohol-dependent patients.

Acetylcholine. Neurotransmitter in the central and peripheral nervous systems, which activates two types of receptors, muscarinic and nicotinic. See **Muscarine; Nicotine**

Additive effect. Effect that occurs when two drugs that have similar biological actions are administered. The net effect is the sum of the independent effects exerted by the drugs.

Adenosine. Chemical neuromodulator in the CNS, primarily at inhibitory synapses.

Adenylate cyclase. Intracellular enzyme that catalyzes the conversion of cyclic AMP to adenosine monophosphate.

Adrenaline (epinephrine). Hormone secreted by the adrenal gland that activates the sympathetic nervous system, as part of the "fight or flight" response.

Affective disorder. Type of mental disorder characterized by recurrent episodes of mania, depression, or both.

Affinity. Ability of a drug to bind to its receptor.

Agonist. Drug that attaches to a receptor and produces actions that mimic or potentiate those of an endogenous transmitter.

Akathisia. A movement disorder, characterized by a feeling of inner restlessness and an inability to sit still.

Aldehyde dehydrogenase. Enzyme that carries out a specific step in alcohol metabolism: the metabolism of acetaldehyde to acetate. This enzyme may be blocked by the drug disulfiram (Antabuse).

Allosteric. A substance that indirectly alters the effect of another molecule (such as an agonist or inverse agonist) at the receptor binding site.

Alzheimer's disease. Progressive neurological disease that occurs primarily in the elderly. It is characterized by a loss of short-term memory and intellectual functioning. It is associated with a loss of function of acetylcholine neurons.

Amyloid. A starch-like protein that is deposited in the liver, kidneys, spleen, or other tissues in certain diseases.

Amphetamine. Behavioral stimulant that acts by increasing the amount of biogenic amines in neuronal synapses.

Amygdala. A pair of almond-shaped neural structures in the cerebral hemispheres, which mediate emotional responses.

Anabolic steroid. Testosterone-like drug that acts to increase muscle mass and produces other masculinizing effects.

Anandamide. Endogenous chemical compound that attaches to cannabinoid receptors in the CNS and to specific components of the lymphatic system.

Anandamide receptor. Receptor to which anandamide and tetrahydrocannabinol bind.

Anesthetic. Sedative-hypnotic compound used primarily in doses capable of inducing a state of general anesthesia that involves both loss of sensation, amnesia, and loss of consciousness.

Antagonist. Drug that attaches to a receptor and blocks the action of either an endogenous transmitter or an agonistic drug.

Anticonvulsant. Drug that blocks or prevents epileptic convulsions. Some anticonvulsants (for example, carbamazepine and valproic acid) are also used to treat certain nonepileptic psychiatric disorders.

Antidepressant. Drug that is useful in treating mentally depressed patients but does not produce stimulant effects in nondepressed persons. Subdivided into several categories.

Antinociceptive. Decreasing sensitivity to painful (nociceptive) stimulation; analgesic.

Antipsychotic. Medication effective in the treatment of psychosis, particularly for reducing the positive symptoms of schizophrenia, such as hallucinations, delusions, and thought disorder.

Anxiolytic. Drug used to relieve the symptoms associated with defined states of anxiety. Classically, the term refers to the benzodiazepines and related drugs.

2-arachidonoyl glycerol (2-AG). One of the endogenous cannabis-like substances.

Arrythymia. A condition in which the heart beats with an irregular or abnormal rhythm.

Ataxia. A lack of muscle coordination that may affect speech, eye movements, the ability to swallow, walking, picking up objects and other voluntary movements.

Attention deficit/hyperactivity disorder (ADHD). Learning and behavioral disorder characterized by reduced attention span, impulsivity, and/or hyperactivity.

Atypical antipsychotic. Drug that alleviates the positive symptoms of schizophrenia (hallucinations, delusions, and thought disorder) without necessarily causing the neurological side effect of abnormal motor movements. Also used in the treatment of mania.

Autonomic nervous system. Portion of the peripheral nervous system that controls, or regulates, the visceral, automatic, usually involuntary functions of the body, such as heart rate and blood pressure.

Autoreceptor. A receptor located on the presynaptic neuronal membrane, which is activated by the neurotransmitter released by that neuron (or by substances that interact with that receptor).

Ayahuasca (also called hoasca). A hallucinogenic beverage made from the bark and stems of a tropical South American vine.

Barbiturates. Class of chemically related sedative-hypnotic compounds that share a characteristic six-membered ring structure.

Basal ganglia. An anatomical system in the brain consisting of three primary nuclei (the caudate nucleus, the putamen, and the globus pallidus) located at the base of the brain that are primarily responsible for coordinating and organizing smooth, voluntary motor functions. The basal ganglia are abnormal in a number of important neurological conditions including Parkinson's disease and Huntington's disease. This system may also be referred to as the *extrapyramidal system* to distinguish it from the pyramidal component of the motor system, which is responsible for controlling fine motor responses.

"Bath Salts." The term refers to a group of drugs containing one or more synthetic chemicals related to cathinone, an amphetamine-like stimulant.

Benzodiazepines. Class of chemically related sedative-hypnotic agents of which chlordiazepoxide (Librium) and diazepam (Valium) are examples. Primarily used in the treatment of anxiety and in alcohol withdrawal.

Bioavailability. The degree and rate at which a substance (such as a drug) is absorbed into a living system, and has access to the site of physiological activity.

Biomarker. A measurable substance in an organism whose presence is indicative of some phenomenon such as disease, infection, or environmental exposure.

Bipolar disorder. Affective disorder characterized by alternating bouts of mania and either depression or euthymia (normal affective state). Also called *manic-depressive illness.*

Blackout. Period of time during which a person may be awake but memory is not imprinted. It frequently occurs in people who have consumed excessive alcohol or to whom have been administered (or who have taken) large doses of sedative drugs.

Blood alcohol concentration (BAC). The weight of alcohol in a fixed volume of blood, used as a measure of the degree of intoxication in an individual. The BAC depends on body weight, the quantity and rate of alcohol ingestion, and the rates of alcohol absorption and metabolism.

Bradykinesia. Slowness and poverty of movement.

Brain syndrome, organic. Pattern of behavior induced when neurons are either reversibly depressed or irreversibly destroyed. Behavior is characterized by clouded sensorium, disorientation, shallow and labile affect, and impaired memory, intellectual function, insight, and judgment.

Brand name. Unique name licensed to one manufacturer of a drug. Contrasts with *generic name,* the name under which any manufacturer may sell a drug.

Bronchospasm. Abnormal contraction of the smooth muscle of the bronchi, resulting in an acute narrowing and obstruction of the respiratory airway.

Caffeine. Behavioral and general cellular stimulant found in coffee, tea, cola drinks, and chocolate. Acts by blocking an adenosine receptor.

Caffeinism. Habitual use of large amounts of caffeine.

Cannabis sativa. Hemp plant; contains marijuana.

Carbidopa. Drug that inhibits the enzyme dopa decarboxylase, allowing increased availability of dopa within the brain. Contained in the medication Sinemet.

Central nervous system (CNS). Brain and spinal cord.

Cerebellum. Structure located at the base of the brain, just above the brain stem, where the spinal cord meets the brain, whose function is to coordinate voluntary movements, posture, and balance.

Cerebral cortex. The outer layer of the cerebrum (cerebral hemispheres), composed of gray matter and responsible for mediating higher brain functions.

Cerebrum. The most dorsal, primary part of the brain, consisting of left and right hemispheres, separated by a fissure. It is responsible for the integration of complex sensory and neural functions and the initiation and coordination of voluntary activity in the body.

Chemoreceptor trigger zone. An area in the medulla oblongata that responds to blood-borne signals that cause nausea and vomiting.

Chromatin. Substance made up of DNA, RNA and proteins (histones), in the cell nucleus, which makes up chromosomes.

Chromosome. Composed of condensed chromatin fibers, it contains the genes.

Cirrhosis. Serious, usually irreversible liver disease. Usually associated with chronic excessive alcohol consumption.

Clonidine (Catapres). Antihypertensive drug useful in alleviating the symptoms of narcotic withdrawal.

Cocaine. Behavioral stimulant. Acts primarily by blocking reuptake of the transmitter dopamine into the neuron from which it was released.

Codeine. Sedative and pain-relieving agent found in opium. Structurally related to morphine but less potent; constitutes approximately 0.5 percent of the opium extract.

Comorbid disorder. Psychiatric disorder that coexists with another psychiatric disorder (for example, multisubstance abuse in a patient with major depressive disorder).

Compulsion. Repetitive or ritualistic behaviors or mental acts performed over and over in response to an obsessive thought, such as repeated hand washing.

Convulsant. Drug that produces convulsions (seizures) by blocking inhibitory neurotransmission.

Cotinine. The primary metabolite of nicotine.

COX inhibitors. Aspirin-like analgesic drugs that produce their actions by inhibiting the enzyme cyclooxygenase. Two variants of the enzyme occur: COX-1 and COX-2. Some drugs are specific for COX-2; others are nonspecific inhibitors.

Crack. Street name for a smokeable form of potent, concentrated cocaine.

Cross-dependence. Condition in which one drug can prevent the withdrawal symptoms associated with physical dependence on a different drug.

Cross-tolerance. Condition in which tolerance of one drug results in a lessened response to another drug.

Cytochrome P450 enzyme family. A large group of proteins, mostly (but not only) found in the liver, responsible for metabolizing a wide variety of endogenous and exogenous substances.

Delirium tremens (DTs). Syndrome of tremulousness with hallucinations, psychomotor agitation, confusion and disorientation, sleep disorders, and other associated discomforts, lasting several days after alcohol withdrawal.

Delta receptor. One of the 3 classes of opiate receptors (DOR), which is activated by the endogenous opiates, and synthetic opioids.

Dementia. Loss of mental ability severe enough to interfere with normal activities of daily living, lasting more than six months, not present since birth, and not associated with a loss or alteration of consciousness.

Detoxification. Process of allowing time for the body to metabolize and/or excrete accumulations of drug. Usually a first step in drug abuse evaluation and treatment.

Diagnostic and Statistical Manual of Mental Disorders (DSM-5). A classification system of mental disorders, published by the American Psychiatric Association, that proposes objective criteria to be used in diagnosis.

Diencephalon. The posterior part of the forebrain, whose major components are the thalamus and hypothalamus.

Differential diagnosis. Listing of all possible causes that might explain a given set of symptoms.

Dimethyltryptamine (DMT). Psychedelic drug found in many South American plants.

Disulfiram (Antabuse). An antioxidant used in the treatment of chronic alcoholism that interferes with the normal metabolic degradation of alcohol in the body, producing an unpleasant reaction when a small quantity of alcohol is consumed.

Dopamine. One of the monoaminergic (catecholamine) neurotransmitters in the central nervous system, considered to be the primary reward neurotransmitter in the brain, and important in mediating voluntary movement (loss of dopamine neurons produces Parkinson's disease). It is the precursor to norepinephrine.

Dopamine transporter. Presynaptic protein that binds synaptic dopamine and transports the neurotransmitter back into the presynaptic nerve terminal.

Dorsal root ganglia. A group of neurons on the dorsal roots of the spine that carry signals from sensory organs toward the appropriate part of the nervous system.

Dose-response relation. Relation between drug doses and the response elicited at each dose level.

Drug. Chemical substance used for its effects on bodily processes.

Drug absorption. Mechanism by which a drug reaches the bloodstream from the skin, lungs, stomach, intestinal tract, or muscle.

Drug administration. Procedures through which a drug enters the body (oral administration of tablets or liquids, inhalation of powders, injection of sterile liquids, and so on).

Drug dependence. State in which the use of a drug is necessary for either physical or psychological well-being.

Drug distribution. Movement of drug between the blood and various tissues of the body.

Drug interaction. Modification of the action of one drug by the concurrent or prior administration of another drug.

Drug misuse. Use of any drug (legal or illegal) for a medical or recreational purpose when other alternatives are available, practical, or warranted or when drug use endangers either the user or others with whom he or she may interact.

Drug receptor. Specific molecular substance in the body with which a given drug interacts to produce its effect.

Drug tolerance. State of progressively decreasing responsiveness to a drug.

DSM-IV, DSM-IV-TR. Abbreviation for *Diagnostic and Statistical Manual of Mental Disorders*, Fourth Edition, published by the American Psychiatric Association in 1994. A comprehensive classification of officially recognized psychiatric disorders. The Text Revision of the Fourth Edition was published in 2000.

Dual-action antidepressants. Antidepressant drugs that act by inhibiting the active presynaptic reuptake of more than one neurotransmitter, for example, norepinephrine and serotonin.

Dyskinesia. A movement disorder that consists of adverse effects including diminished voluntary movements and the presence of involuntary movements, similar to tics or chorea.

Dystonia. A state of abnormal muscle tone producing muscular spasm and abnormal posture, typically due to neurological disease or a side effect of drug therapy.

Efficacy. The ability of a drug to produce its intended effect.

Electroconvulsive therapy (ECT). A procedure in which an electric current is passed through the brain to produce controlled convulsions (seizures) to treat patients with depression, particularly for those who cannot take or are not responding to antidepressants, have severe depression, or are at high risk for suicide.

Electronic (e) cigarette (EC). A cigarette-shaped device containing a nicotine-based liquid that is vaporized and inhaled, used to simulate the experience of smoking tobacco.

Endorphin. Naturally occurring protein that causes endogenous morphinelike activity.

Enkephalin. Naturally occurring protein that causes morphinelike activity.

Entactogens. A class of psychoactive drugs that presumably produce distinctive empathic, emotional, and social effects.

Enteral route. Anything involving the gastrointestinal tract, from the mouth to the rectum.

Environmental tobacco smoke (ETS). Secondhand smoke; passive smoke. Exhaled smoke from cigarette smokers, which is inhaled by persons other than the smoker.

Enzyme. Large organic molecule that mediates a specific biochemical reaction in the body.

Enzyme induction. Increased production of drug-metabolizing enzymes in the liver, stimulated by certain drugs (inducers). As a result of induction, drugs that are metabolized by the induced enzyme will be degraded more rapidly. It is one mechanism by which pharmacological tolerance is produced.

Epigenetics. The study of heritable changes in gene expression caused by mechanisms other than changes in the underlying DNA sequence.

Epilepsy. Neurological disorder characterized by an occasional, sudden, and uncontrolled discharge of neurons.

Epinephrine. See **Adrenaline**

Exocytosis. Secretion of the substances in synaptic vesicles, out of the neuron terminal.

Extrapyramidal symptoms (EPS). Motor symptoms, such as tremors, slurred speech, dystonia, and anxiety that are side effects to neuroleptic drugs caused by effects on the basal ganglia and associated structures within the brain.

Fasciculation. A brief, spontaneous, contraction affecting a small number of muscle fibers, often causing a flicker of movement under the skin.

Fetal alcohol syndrome (FAS). A congenital syndrome caused by excessive consumption of alcohol by the mother during pregnancy, characterized by retardation of mental development and of physical growth, particularly of the skull and face of the infant.

Fibromyalgia. Fibromyalgia is a disorder of unknown etiology characterized by widespread pain, abnormal pain processing, sleep disturbance, fatigue and often, psychological distress.

First-order elimination. Elimination of a constant fraction of drug, per time unit, of the amount present in the organism. The elimination is proportional to the drug concentration.

First-pass metabolism (first-pass effect). The breakdown of drugs as they are transported through the liver, before they reach the rest of the body through the circulatory system.

Flashback. See **Hallucinogen persisting perception disorder (HPPD)**

Forebrain. The anterior part of the brain, made up of the telencephalon and diencephalon, which includes the cerebrum, parts of the basal ganglia and limbic system, and the thalamus and hypothalamus.

G protein. Specific intraneuronal protein that links transmitter-induced receptor alterations with intracellular second-messenger proteins or with adjacent ion channels.

Gamma aminobutyric acid (GABA). Inhibitory amino acid neurotransmitter in the brain.

Generic name. Name that identifies a specific chemical entity (without describing the chemical). Often marketed under different brand names by different manufacturers.

Genetic Opioid Metabolic Defects (GOMD). Genetic variants of the enzymes responsible for the breakdown of opioids in the body, which may cause either an abnormal decrease (fast metabolizers) or increase (slow metabolizers) in levels of opiate medications.

Glutamic acid. Excitatory amino acid neurotransmitter. It is the precursor to GABA, the inhibitory neurotransmitter.

Half-life. Time it takes for half of the amount of drug in the circulation to be eliminated.

Hallucinogen. Psychedelic drug that produces profound distortions in perception.

Hallucinogen persisting perception disorder (HPPD). An unexpected recurrence of the effects of a hallucinogenic drug long after its initial use. See **Flashback**

Harmine. Psychedelic agent obtained from the seeds of *Peganum harmala*.

Hashish. Extract of the hemp plant (*Cannabis sativa*) that has a higher concentration of THC than does marijuana.

Herbal Marijuana Alternatives (HMAs). Classes of synthetic cannabinoid drugs.

Heroin. Semisynthetic opiate produced by a chemical modification of morphine.

Hindbrain. The lower part of the brainstem, consisting of the cerebellum, pons, and medulla oblongata.

Hippocampus. Part of the brain (limbic system) involved in learning and memory formation

Histones. Proteins found in the cell nucleus, around which DNA is wound, so that it is condensed into a smaller space.

Hookah. An oriental tobacco pipe with a long, flexible tube that draws the smoke through water contained in a bowl.

Hyperalgesia. Abnormally heightened sensitivity to pain.

Hypercortisolemia. Elevated levels of cortisol in the blood.

Hyperkinetic. An abnormal amount of uncontrolled muscular action; like a spasm or tic.

Hypocretin. See **Orexin**

Hypomania. A condition similar to mania but less severe. The symptoms are similar with elevated mood, increased activity, decreased need for sleep, grandiosity, racing thoughts, and the like. However, hypomanic episodes differ in that they do not cause significant distress or impair one's work, family, or social life in an obvious way while manic episodes do.

Hypothalamus. Brain structure located below the thalamus and above the pituitary gland that regulates bodily temperature, certain metabolic processes, and other autonomic activities.

Hypoxia. State of relative lack of oxygen in the tissues of the body and the brain.

Ice. Street name for a smokeable, free-base form of potent, concentrated methamphetamine.

Intramuscular injection. An injection into a muscle.

Intravenous injection. An injection into a vein.

Ionotropic receptor. A receptor that works by directly opening or closing ion channels that alter ionic movement across cell membranes.

Isomers. Each of two or more compounds with the same formula but a different arrangement of atoms in the molecule and different properties.

Kappa receptor. One of several opiate receptor types.

Levodopa. Precursor substance to the transmitter dopamine; useful in alleviating the symptoms of Parkinson's disease.

Limbic system. Group of brain structures involved in emotional responses and emotional expression.

Lipid soluble. The ability of a chemical compound to dissolve in fats and oils.

Lithium. Alkali metal effective in the treatment of mania and depression.

Lysergic acid diethylamide (LSD). Semisynthetic psychedelic drug.

Major tranquilizer (archaic). See **Antipsychotic**

Mania. Mental disorder characterized by an expansive emotional state, elation, hyperirritability, excessive talkativeness, flights of ideas, and increased behavioral activity.

MAO. See **Monoamine oxidase**

Marijuana. Mixture of the crushed leaves, flowers, and small branches of both the male and female hemp plant (*Cannabis sativa*).

Medulla oblongata. The continuation of the spinal cord inside the skull, the lowest part of the brainstem, containing structures that control autonomic functions.

Mental Status Examination (MSE). An assessment of a patient's level of cognitive (knowledge-related) ability, appearance, emotional mood, and speech and thought patterns at the time of evaluation.

Mescaline. Psychedelic drug extracted from the peyote cactus.

Metabolic syndrome. The name for a group of risk factors that raises the risk for heart disease and other health problems, such as diabetes and stroke.

Metabotropic. A receptor type that is not linked directly to a membrane channel, but affects the channel indirectly through intermediate substances, such as second messengers.

Microtubule. Fibrous, hollow rods in the cells of body tissues, that function primarily to help support and shape the cell.

Midbrain. The short part of the brain, between the pons and the diencephalon.

Minor tranquilizer. Sedative-hypnotic drug promoted primarily for use in the treatment of anxiety.

Mixed agonist-antagonist. Drug that attaches to a receptor, producing weak agonistic effects but displacing more potent agonists, precipitating withdrawal in drug-dependent persons.

Monoamine oxidase (MAO). Enzyme capable of metabolizing norepinephrine, dopamine, and serotonin to inactive products.

Monoamine oxidase inhibitor (MAOI). Drug that inhibits the activity of the enzyme monoamine oxidase. Identifies one category of antidepressant medications.

Mood stabilizer. Drug used in the treatment of bipolar illness. Examples are lithium and any of the neuromodulator anticonvulsants.

Morphine. Major sedative and pain-relieving (analgesic) drug found in opium; makes up approximately 10 percent of the crude opium exudate.

Mu receptor. One of several types of opiate receptors, this type mediates the analgesic and rewarding effect of opiates.

Muscarine. Drug extracted from the mushroom *Amanita muscaria* that directly stimulates acetylcholine receptors.

Myelin sheath. A substance surrounding a nerve fiber which provides insulation and increases conduction speed.

Myristin. Psychedelic agent obtained from nutmeg and mace.

Neurodegenerative. Resulting in or characterized by degeneration of the nervous system, especially the neurons in the brain.

Neurofibrillary tangle. A pathological accumulation of paired helical filaments composed of abnormally formed tau protein that is found chiefly in the cytoplasm of nerve cells of the brain and especially the cerebral cortex and hippocampus and that occurs typically in Alzheimer's disease.

Neuroleptic malignant syndrome (NMS). The combination of hyperthermia, rigidity, and autonomic dysregulation that can occur as a serious complication of the use of antipsychotic drugs.

Neuromodulator. Antiepileptic drug used to treat bipolar illness, aggressive disorders, chronic pain, and a variety of other disorders.

Neuropathic pain. Pain caused by a primary lesion or dysfunction in the nervous system, that is, damage to nerves, to the brain, or the spinal cord.

Neurotransmitter. Endogenous chemical released by one neuron that alters the electrical activity of another neuron.

Neutrophil. Mature white blood cell.

Nicotine. Behavioral stimulant found in tobacco that directly stimulates acetylcholine receptors.

Nicotine replacement therapies (NRTS). Smoking cessation treatments that substitute another source of nicotine for the nicotine inhaled from smoking.

Nociceptive pain. Pain caused by damage to body tissue outside of the nervous system, and usually described as a sharp, aching, or throbbing sensation.

Nociceptor. The sensory receptor for painful stimuli

Norepinephrine (also called *noradrenaline*). One of the monoaminergic (biogenic) excitatory neurotransmitters, a catecholamine in chemical structure, involved in alertness, concentration, aggression and motivation, among other actions.

Norepinephrine-specific reuptake inhibitor. See **Selective norepinephrine reuptake inhibitor**

Nucleosome. Any of the repeating subunits of chromatin occurring at intervals along a strand of DNA, consisting of DNA coiled around histone.

Obsession. Intrusive thoughts that produce anxiety and that lead to repetitive behaviors (compulsions) aimed at reducing anxiety.

Off-label. Term applied to the clinical use of a drug for an indication other than that for which the drug was approved by the U.S. Food and Drug Administration. Use is usually justified by medical literature, even though formal USDA approval for the use was not sought by the manufacturer of the drug. The manufacturer is not permitted to promote a drug for an off-label use.

Ololiuqui. Psychedelic drug obtained from the seeds of the morning glory plant.

Opioid. Natural or synthetic drug that exerts actions on the body similar to those induced by morphine, the major pain-relieving agent obtained from the opium poppy (*Papaver somniferum*).

Opium. Crude resinous exudate from the opium poppy. Contains morphine and codeine as active opioids.

Orexin. An excitatory neuropeptide hormone that stimulates appetite, wakefulness and energy use. See **Hypocretin**

Orthostatic hypotension (also called Postural hypotension). A drop in blood pressure that occurs when standing up from a sitting or lying position.

Parenteral. Located outside the gastrointestinal tract.

Parkinson's disease. Disorder of the motor system characterized by involuntary movements, tremor, and weakness, resulting from the loss of dopamine-producing neurons.

Partial agonist. Drug that binds to a receptor, contributing only part of the action exerted by the endogenous neurotransmitter or producing a submaximal receptor response. Buprenorphine (in Suboxone) is an example.

Peptide. Chemical composed of a chain-link sequence of amino acids.

Periaqueductal gray. The neural tissue surrounding the cerebral aqueduct within the tegmentum of the midbrain. It plays a role in the descending modulation of pain and in defensive behaviour.

Peyote. Cactus that contains mescaline.

Pharmacodynamics. Study of the interactions of a drug and the receptors responsible for the action of the drug in the body.

Pharmacokinetics. Study of the factors that influence the absorption, distribution, metabolism, and excretion of a drug.

Pharmacology. Branch of science that deals with the study of drugs and their actions on living systems.

Phencyclidine (Sernyl, PCP). Psychedelic surgical anesthetic; acts by binding to and inhibiting ion transport through the NMDA-glutamate receptors.

Phenothiazine. Class of chemically related antipsychotic neuroleptic medications useful in the treatment of psychosis.

Physical dependence. State in which the use of a drug is required for a person to function normally. Physical dependence is revealed by withdrawing the drug and noting the occurrence of withdrawal symptoms (abstinence syndrome). Characteristically, withdrawal symptoms can be terminated by readministration of the drug.

Placebo. Pharmacologically inert substance that may elicit a significant reaction largely because of the mental set of the patient or the physical setting in which the drug is taken.

Plaque. A histopathologic lesion of brain tissue that is characteristic of Alzheimer's disease and consists of a dense proteinaceous core composed primarily of beta-amyloid that is often surrounded and infiltrated by a cluster of degenerating axons and dendrites.

Polypharmacy. The simultaneous use of multiple drugs to treat a single ailment or condition.

Pons. The part of the brainstem that links the medulla oblongata and the thalamus.

Postherpetic neuralgia. A painful condition that affects the nerve fibers and skin. Postherpetic neuralgia is a complication of shingles.

Potency. Measure of drug activity expressed in terms of the amount required to produce an effect of given intensity. Potency varies inversely with the amount of drug required to produce this effect—the more potent the drug, the lower the amount required to produce the effect.

Potentially reduced exposure products (PREPs). Cigarettes and smokeless tobacco products with purportedly lower levels of some toxins than conventional cigarettes and smokeless products.

Prodromal. Relating to or denoting the period between the appearance of initial symptoms and the full development of a disorder.

Prodrug. A biologically inactive compound that can be metabolized in the body to produce a drug.

Prolactin. A hormone released from the anterior pituitary gland that stimulates milk production after childbirth.

Psilocybin. Psychedelic drug obtained from the mushroom *Psilocybemexicana*.

Psoriasis. A skin disease marked by red, itchy, scaly patches.

Psychedelic. Drug that can alter sensory perception.

Psychoactive drug. Chemical substance that alters mood or behavior as a result of alterations in the functioning of the brain.

Psychological dependence. Compulsion to use a drug for its pleasurable effects. Dependence may lead to a compulsion to misuse a drug.

Psychopharmacology. Branch of pharmacology that deals with the effects of drugs on the nervous system and behavior.

Psychopharmacotherapy. Clinical treatment of psychiatric disorders with drugs.

Psychotherapy. Nonpharmacological treatment of psychiatric disorders utilizing a wide range of modalities from simple education and supportive counseling to insight-oriented, dynamically based therapy.

Racemate (racemic). Mixture of equal quantities of two enantiomers, substances whose molecular structures are mirror images of one another.

Rapid anesthesia-aided detoxification (RAAD). A procedure in which patients are placed under anesthesia while given treatment drugs, such as naltrexone, to avoid discomfort associated with drug detoxification.

Receptor. Location in the nervous system at which a neurotransmitter or drug binds to exert its characteristic effect. Most receptors are members of genetically encoded families of specialized proteins.

Receptor down-regulation (desensitization). Decrease in a cellular response to a drug or transmitter due to a decrease in the number of receptors on the cell surface.

Receptor upregulation (supersensitivity). Increase in a cellular response to a drug or transmitter due to an increase in the number of receptors on the cell surface.

Reward circuit. Nerve pathways of the central nervous system connecting the neuronal structures that mediate feelings of pleasure and satisfaction.

Reye's syndrome. Rare CNS disorder that occurs in children; associated with aspirin ingestion.

Risk-to-benefit ratio. Arbitrary assessment of the risks and benefits that may accrue from administration of a drug.

Schizophrenia. Debilitating neuropsychiatric illness associated with disturbances in thought, perception, emotion, cognition, relationships, and psychomotor behavior.

Scopolamine. Anticholinergic drug that crosses the blood-brain barrier to produce sedation and amnesia; antagonist at the muscarinic receptor.

Second messenger. Intraneuronal protein that, when activated by a G protein, mediates the response that is initiated when neurotransmitter molecules bind to an extracellular receptor.

Sedative-hypnotic. Chemical substance that exerts a nonselective general depressant action on the nervous system.

Selective norepinephrine reuptake inhibitor (SNRI). Drug that blocks the active presynaptic transporter for norepinephrine. Clinically used to treat ADHD, depression, and other disorders, including seasonal affective disorder.

Selective serotonin reuptake inhibitor (SSRI). Second-generation antidepressant drug that blocks the reuptake transporter for serotonin.

Serotonin (5-hydroxytryptamine, 5-HT). Indoleamine neurotransmitter in both the brain and the peripheral nervous system (gut) that is involved in depression, appetite, sleep, and sexual responsiveness, among other functions.

Serotonin syndrome. Clinical syndrome resulting from excessive amounts of serotonin in the brain. The syndrome can follow use of excessive doses of SSRIs, and it is characterized by extreme anxiety, confusion, and disorientation.

Serotonin withdrawal syndrome. Clinical syndrome that can follow withdrawal or cessation of SSRI therapy. The syndrome is characterized by mental status alterations, severe flulike symptoms, and feelings of tingling or electrical shock in the extremities.

Side effect. Drug-induced effect that accompanies the primary effect for which the drug is administered.

Signal transduction. A basic process in molecular cell biology involving the conversion of a signal from outside the cell to a functional change within the cell.

Speedball. A mixture of cocaine and heroin.

"Spice." Street name for synthetic cannabinoids.

Spinal cord. The large group of nerves that runs through the center of the spine and carries messages between the brain and the rest of the body.

Steady state concentration. The concentration of drug at which the rate of administration and the rate of elimination are equal.

Subcutaneous. Under the skin.

Substance P. Protein neurotransmitter that regulates affective behavior, increasing the perception of pain. Substance P antagonists exhibit analgesic and antidepressant actions.

Substantia nigra. A layer of large pigmented nerve cells in the midbrain that produce dopamine and whose destruction is associated with Parkinson's disease.

Sudden sniffing death syndrome. Death that occurs very quickly in response to inhaled fumes, most commonly from butane, propane, and aerosol abuse.

Supersensitivity. See **Receptor**

Synapse. The junction between two nerve cells, consisting of a presynaptic neuronal membrane (which releases neurotransmitter), a postsynaptic neuronal membrane (which receives the transmitter signal) and a minute space between the two.

Synaptic cleft. The gap between the pre- and postsynaptic membranes of a synapse, across which neurotransmitter molecules diffuse.

Synaptic plasticity. Ability of synapses to strengthen or weaken over time, as a result of increases or decreases in their activity.

Tardive dyskinesia. Movement disorder that appears after months or years of treatment with neuroleptic (antipsychotic) drugs. It usually worsens with drug discontinuation. Symptoms are often masked by the drugs that cause the disorder.

Tectum. The uppermost part ("roof") of the midbrain.

Tegmentum. The base, or floor, of the midbrain.

Teratogen. Chemical substance that induces abnormalities of fetal development.

Testosterone. Hormone secreted from the testes that is responsible for the distinguishing characteristics of the male.

Tetrahydrocannabinol (THC). Major psychoactive agent in marijuana, hashish, and other preparations of hemp (*Cannabis sativa*).

Therapeutic drug monitoring (TDM). Process of correlating the plasma level of a drug with therapeutic response.

Therapeutic index. The ratio of the toxic dose and the therapeutic dose of a drug, which provides a measure of drug safety.

Therapeutic window. The range of drug dose, or blood concentration, that maintains a safe therapeutic effect.

Tobacco harm reduction (THR). Procedures or substances taken to lower the health risks associated with using nicotine.

Tolerance. Clinical state of reduced responsiveness to a drug; can be produced by a variety of mechanisms, all of which require increased doses of drug to produce an effect once achieved by lower doses.

Torsades de pointes. Variant of ventricular tachycardia that can be the result of lengthening the QT interval.

Toxic effect. Drug-induced effect either temporarily or permanently deleterious to any organ or system of an animal or person. Drug toxicity includes both the relatively minor side effects that invariably accompany drug administration and the more serious and unexpected manifestations that occur in only a small percentage of patients who take a drug.

Tumor necrosis factor. A protein produced by macrophages in the presence of an endotoxin and shown experimentally to be capable of attacking and destroying cancerous tumors.

Unipolar depression (also called clinical depression, major depression, and unipolar disorder). Mental disorder characterized by an all-encompassing low mood accompanied by low self-esteem and loss of interest or pleasure in normally enjoyable activities.

Ventral tegmental area (VTA). Group of neurons, located on the floor of the midbrain (mesencephalon), that contain dopamine and serotonin; the VTA is a major component of the reward pathway in the brain.

Withdrawal syndrome. Onset of a predictable group of symptoms following the abrupt discontinuation or rapid decrease in dosage of a psychoactive substance on which the body has become dependent. May include anxiety, insomnia, delirium tremens, perspiration, hot flashes, nausea, dehydration, tremors, weakness, dizziness, convulsions, and psychotic behavior.

"Z drugs." Three drugs, whose names all start with the letter "z," that are structurally not benzo-diazepines, but which nevertheless bind to the same receptors to which benzodiazepines bind and exert the same agonist effects as the benzodiazepines.

Zero-order metabolism (kinetics). Condition in which the plasma concentration of a drug decreases (is metabolized) at a constant rate; the rate of metabolism does not depend on the amount (concentration) of the drug.

Index

Note: Page numbers followed by f indicate figures; those followed by t indicate tables; those followed by n indicate footnotes.